NEUROTRANSMITTERS, DRUGS AND DISEASE

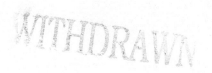

NEUROTRANSMITTERS DRUGS
AND DISEASE

Neurotransmitters, Drugs and Disease

EDITED BY

R. A. WEBSTER
BSc, PhD
Department of Pharmacology
University College
London

C. C. JORDAN
BSc, PhD
Glaxo Group Research Ltd
Ware

BLACKWELL SCIENTIFIC PUBLICATIONS

OXFORD LONDON EDINBURGH

BOSTON MELBOURNE

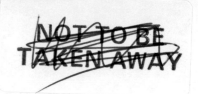
© 1989 by
Blackwell Scientific Publications
Editorial offices:
Osney Mead, Oxford OX2 0EL
  (*Orders:* Tel. 0865 240201)
8 John Street, London WC1N 2ES
23 Ainslie Place, Edinburgh EH3 6AJ
3 Cambridge Center, Suite 208
  Cambridge, Massachusetts 02142, USA
107 Barry Street, Carlton
  Victoria 3053, Australia

First published 1989

Set by Times Graphics, Singapore
Printed and bound in Great Britain
by Redwood Burn Ltd,
Trowbridge, Wilts

DISTRIBUTORS

USA
  Year Book Medical Publishers
  200 North LaSalle Street
  Chicago, Illinois 60601
  (*Orders:* Tel. (312) 726-9733)

Canada
  The C.V. Mosby Company
  5240 Finch Avenue East
  Scarborough, Ontario
  (*Orders:* Tel. (416) 298-1588)

Australia
  Blackwell Scientific Publications
  (Australia) Pty Ltd
  107 Barry Street
  Carlton, Victoria 3053
  (*Orders:* Tel. (03) 347-0300)

British Library
Cataloguing in Publication Data

Neurotransmitters, drugs and disease.
  1. Man. Nervous system. Synapses
  Neurotransmitters. Effect of drugs.
  I. Webster, R. A.   II. Jordan, C. C.
615′.8

  ISBN 0-632-00717-6

Contents

Section III: Applied neuropharmacology

List of contributors

N.J.M. Birdsall *Division of Molecular Pharmacology, National Institute for Medical Research, Mill Hill, London NW7 1AA*

N.G. Bowery *Department of Pharmacology, School of Pharmacy, 29/39 Brunswick Square, London WC1N 1AX*

J.H. Connick *Department of Physiology, St George's Hospital Medical School, Tooting, London SW17 0RE*

A.J. Cross *Astra Neuroscience Research Unit, 1 Wakefield Street, London WC1N 1PJ*

J. Davies *Department of Pharmacology, School of Pharmacy, 29/39 Brunswick Square, London WC1N 1AX*

A.H. Dickenson *Department of Pharmacology, University College London, Gower Street, London WC1E 6BT*

J.M. Elliott *Department of Pharmacology, St Mary's Hospital Medical School, Paddington, London W2 1PG*

R.J. Hardie *University Unit of Neurology, King's College Hospital, Denmark Hill, London SE5 9RS*

R.W. Horton *Department of Pharmacology, St George's Hospital Medical School, Tooting, London SW17 0RE*

C.C. Jordan *Glaxo Group Research Ltd, Ware, Herts SG12 0DJ*

B.S. Meldrum *Department of Neurology, Institute of Psychiatry, Denmark Hill, London SE5 8AF*

F. Owen *Division of Psychiatry, Clinical Research Centre, Harrow, Middlesex HA1 3UJ*

Christine M. Smith *Department of Pharmacology, London Hospital Medical School, Turner Street, London E1 2AD*

J.D. Stephenson *Department of Pharmacology, Institute of Psychiatry, Denmark Hill, London SE5 8AF*

T.W. Stone *Department of Physiology, St George's Hospital Medical School, Tooting, London SW17 0RE*

Sandra V. Vellucci *Department of Anatomy, University of Cambridge, Downing Street, Cambridge CB2 3DY*

R.A. Webster *Department of Pharmacology, University College London, Gower Street, London WC1E 6BT*

Preface

This book is based on a series of intercollegiate lectures in neuropharmacology organised annually for science and intercalated medical students in the University of London. Whilst many of the undergraduates were studying pharmacology the lectures proved useful for students in other disciplines, such as physiology, biochemistry and psychology. Postgraduates, research workers, lecturers and clinicians also attended and we hope this book will prove useful to anyone interested in the pharmacology of the central nervous system and in particular how various neurotransmitters may be implicated in the genesis of disorders of the central nervous system and in the modes of action of centrally acting drugs. Indeed it could be regarded as a textbook in basic and applied neuropharmacology. The contributors have lectured frequently on the topics about which they write. They are drawn from the numerous Colleges and Research Institutes in London and many of them are recognised experts in their own field.

Much emphasis is placed on neurotransmitters. We consider basic aspects of synaptic transmission and neurotransmitter function and outline and evaluate the methods used to study neurotransmitter systems, especially electrophysiological, biochemical and ligand binding techniques. Coverage of the general pharmacology of transmission at synapses utilising the main neurotransmitters (acetylcholine, noradrenaline, dopamine, 5-HT, the amino acids and peptides) includes their synthesis, release, postsynaptic action, destruction, neuronal organisation and possible physiological function. Particular attention is paid to the identification and classification of neurotransmitter receptors. Armed with such basic information we hope the reader will then be in a position to follow and evaluate the evidence presented by different contributors, in the second part of the book, for the involvement of the various neurotransmitters in disorders such as Parkinsonism, the epilepsies, schizophrenia, depression, anxiety and dementia as well as in the initiation and control of pain.

Generally references have been kept to a minimum, especially in the early chapters on basic neurotransmitter function, but in the applied section the reference lists tend to be longer and more detailed but they are selective rather than comprehensive.

R.A.W.

List of abbreviations

AIMS   abnormal involuntary movements
ACh   acetylcholine
AChE   acetylcholinesterase
AC   adenylate cyclase
Ad   adrenaline
αAA α-aminoadipic acid
α_1 alpha one (adrenoceptors)
α_2 alpha two (adrenoceptors)
AD   Alzheimer's disease
AA(s)   amino acid(s)
3-APS   3-aminopropane sulphonic acid
AADC   aromatic amino acid decarboxylase

β-CCE β-carboline-3-dicarboxylic acid ethyl ester
BBB   blood–brain barrier
BOL   2-bromo LSD (lysergic acid diethylamide)

CGRP   calcitonin gene-related peptides
CaM   calmodulin
COMT   catechol-O-methyl transferase
CNS   central nervous system
CSF   cerebrospinal fluid
CCK   cholecystokinin
ChAT   choline acetyltransferase
Cyclic AMP   adenosine 3',5',-monophosphate
Cyclic GMP   guanosine 3',5',-monophosphate

DADLE   D-ala, D-leu-enkephalin
δ delta (opioid receptor)
DAG   diacylglycerol
DABA   diaminobutyric acid
DOPAC   dihydroxy-phenol acetic acid
5,7-DHT   5,7-dihydroxytryptamine
DMT   N,N-dimethyltryptamine
DA   dopamine
DPDPE   D-penicillamine, D-penicillamine enkephalin

EEG	electroencephalogram
EOS	ethanolamine O-sulphate
EPSP	excitatory postsynaptic potential
E_xCCDI(s)	extracerebral dopa decarboxylase inhibitor(s)
GABA	gamma amino butyric acid
GABA-T	GABA-transaminase
GVC	γ Vinyl GABA
GAD	glutamic acid decarboxylase
GTP	guanosine triphosphate
GC	guanylate cyclase
HPLC	high pressure liquid chromatography
HA	histamine
HVA	homovanillic acid
HD	Huntington's disease
6-OHDA	6-hydroxydopamine
8-OH-DPAT	8-hydroxy-2-(n-dipropylamine) tetralin
5-HIAA	5-hydroxyindoleacetic acid
5-HT	5-hydroxytryptamine
5-HTP	5-hydroxytryptophan
IPSP	inhibitory postsynaptic potential
IP_3	inositol-1,4,5,-triphosphate
i.c.v.	intracerebroventricular
κ	kappa (opioid receptor)
LC	locus coeruleus
MFN	magnocellular forebrain nuclei
MOPEG	3-methoxy-4-hydroxyphenylglycol
MPTP	1-methyl-4-phenyl-1,2,3,6-tetrahydropyridine
MA(s)	monoamine(s)
MAO	monoamine oxidase
μ	mu (opioid receptor)
NT	neurotransmitter
NMDA	N-methyl-D-aspartate
NSAIDs	non-steroidal anti-inflammatory drugs
NA	noradrenaline
NRM	nucleus raphe magnus
NRPG	nucleus raphe paragigantocellularis
OMD	O-methyldopa (3-methoxytyrosine)

PCA	p-chloramphetamine
PCPA	p-chlorophenylalanine
PH	parathyroid hormone
PD	Parkinson's disease
PAG	periaqueductal grey matter
PNS	peripheral nervous system
PIP_2	phosphatidylinositol-4,5-biphosphate
PrBCh	propylbenzilyl choline
PG(s)	prostaglandin(s)
QNB	quinuclidinylbenzilate
REM	rapid eye movement
σ	sigma (opioid receptor)
SRIF	somatostatin (somatotrophin release inhibitory factor)
SPIP	spiroperidol (spiperone)
SP	substance P
SN	substantia nigra
SSADH	succinic semialdehyde dehydrogenase
TD	tardive dyskinesia
THIP	4,5,6,7, tetrahydroisoxazolo (5,4-c)pyridin-3, ol
TRH	thyrotrophin releasing hormone
TCA_s	tricyclic antidepressants
TH	tryptophan hydroxylase
VMA	vanillylmandelic acid
VIP	vasoactive intestinal peptide

I   Neurotransmitter systems and methodology

1   Basic aspects of neurotransmitter function

R.A. WEBSTER

Neuropharmacology may be described as the study of the actions of drugs and chemicals on the nervous system and in particular at the synapse. This book concentrates on the central nervous system (CNS) and will only deal with drugs that have a relatively specific effect, i.e. act on particular receptors rather than on some more general aspect of neuronal function, as with the general anaesthetics.

In order to understand how drugs produce relatively specific changes in CNS function it is necessary to know, not only how synaptic transmission is mediated by different neurotransmitters, but also how drugs alter synaptic transmission and which synapses and neurotransmitters they primarily affect. In essence we shall need to know a lot about neurotransmitters. Some questions that might be asked are:

1 What is a neurotransmitter?
2 How many neurotransmitters does the CNS need to function properly?
3 How do neurotransmitters work and what effects do they produce?
4 How may a substance be shown to be a neurotransmitter?

The first question is more difficult to answer than one might imagine. If a neurotransmitter (NT) is defined as a substance released from a nerve terminal to transmit an impulse to another neuron (or cell) then a NT must always be excitatory. If it is expected to produce a potential change postsynaptically that can be either a depolarisation (excitation) or hyperpolarisation (inhibition) then the NT could be either excitatory or inhibitory. Suppose, however, that it influences the function of an adjacent neuron indirectly by modifying a biochemical process or the release of another NT, without producing any detectable or marked potential change in the neuron. Is it still a NT? If not, what is it?

I will return to this later after considering the other questions.

How many neurotransmitters are needed in the central nervous system?

It is a principle of pharmacology that the effect of an agonist is not a direct function of the substance itself but of the receptor on which it acts and the cell function to which that receptor is linked. Thus acetylcholine (ACh) produces excitatory and inhibitory effects on smooth muscle through the same muscarinic receptor because in some tissues this is linked to excitation whilst in others it mediates inhibition, i.e. you cannot say that ACh itself is an excitatory or inhibitory substance. Could the CNS then function on one NT using different receptors?

Assume that neuron A in Fig 1.1 must excite neuron B and at the same time inhibit neuron C in order to optimise the excitation of B. It could achieve this with one NT able to activate receptors linked to different events on B and C. Of course neuron C would have other inputs, some of which would be excitatory (+) and if the same NT was used to produce this effect then it could not avoid activating the inhibitory mechanism on C as well (Fig. 1.1(a)). Also, this would mean that the NT released from A would be able to stimulate as well as inhibit neuron C. Even the provision of separate receptors linked to excitation and inhibition would not overcome these problems since both would be accessible to the NT. One possible solution is to separate physically the inputs and receptors linked to excitation from those linked to inhibition and, in fact, there is electrophysiological and morphological evidence that excitatory synapses are mainly on dendrites and inhibitory ones on the soma of large neurons. Unfortunately, although this might resolve the immediate problem the NT could still produce unwanted excitation at the adjacent dendrites of another neuron (D), (Fig. 1.1(b)).

Two NTs would be required to overcome this problem, one to activate receptors linked to excitation and another to evoke inhibition, i.e. place the determinant of function partly back on the NT. With this arrangement the inhibitory NT (I) could not stimulate neuron C (Fig. 1.1(c)) because it is released on to (−) receptors and could not activate any adjacent dendrites of another neuron since they would only have (+) receptors on them activated by the excitatory NT (E). This raises a fresh problem, which is receiving much consideration at present. Can a neuron release more than one NT?

It was generally assumed that it cannot and this became known as Dale's Law. During his studies on antidromic vasodilation he wrote (1935) 'When we are dealing with two different endings of the same sensory neuron, the one peripheral and concerned with vasodilation and the other at a central synapse, can we suppose that the discovery and identification of a chemical transmitter at axon reflex dilation would furnish a hint as to the nature of the transmission process at a central synapse. The possibility has at least some value as a stimulus to further experiments.'

This it certainly has been and in the last few years much evidence has been presented to show that more than one substance (but not necessarily more than one conventional NT) can co-exist in one nerve terminal. Fortunately this does not disprove Dale's Law (so called), as some claim (see Burnstock 1976) since he was referring to 'a' not 'the' NT and to different endings of one neuron. In fact he was simply saying that if a neuron uses a particular transmitter at one of its terminals it will use it at another irrespective of whether or not it uses more than one NT. This makes good sense especially since it is difficult to conceive how a neuron could differentially control the release of more than one NT from different

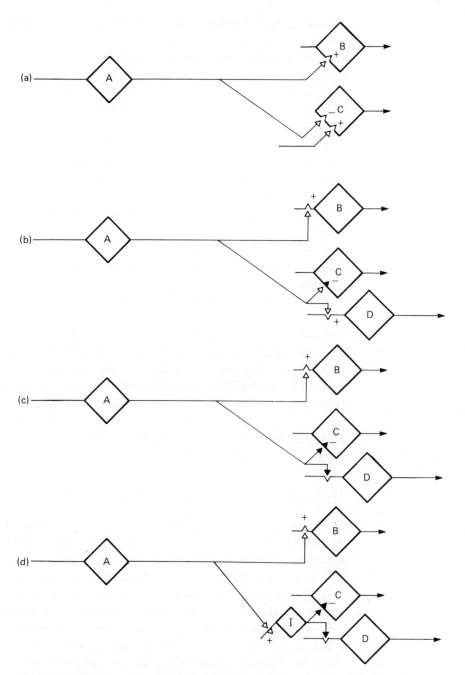

Fig. 1.1. Different synaptic arrangements whereby one neuron (A) can activate neuron (B) as well as inhibit neuron (C) without affecting other neurons (D). (a) Simplest arrangement. One NT activates one receptor linked to both (+) and (−), but these effects cannot be separated on (C). (b) Similar to (a) but (+) receptor is now on dendrite and separated from (−) receptor on soma. But A will still excite D. (c) A releases different (+ and −) NTs from different terminals. Unlikely to occur. (d) Neuron (A) releases same NT from all terminals but can inhibit (C) through an interneuron (I). For full details see text. ⟶ Excitatory (+) neurotransmitter (NT). ⟶ Inhibitory (−) neurotransmitter (NT). ⌄ Receptor for + NT (except in (a) where it is also linked to inhibition). ⌄ Receptor for − NT.

BASIC ASPECTS OF NEUROTRANSMITTER FUNCTION

terminals. On the other hand if the NTs were synthesised solely at the terminals and released by a propagated action potential then a neuron could release different substances from different terminals without, in essence, being aware of it or having to do anything special to achieve it. Thus neuron A (Fig. 1.1) could conceivably always release one NT at B and another at C but probably could not vary the proportion of each released.

Fortunately there is much evidence for another way in which one neuron can excite and inhibit different neurons using just one NT. Neuron A could excite B and inhibit C by the introduction of an inhibitory interneuron (I) the activation of which by A, using the same excitatory NT as at B, automatically inhibits C (Fig. 1.1(d)). This form of inhibition is quite common in the CNS and in fact much inhibition is mediated by these so-called short axon interneurons and a neuron may inhibit itself through feedback via a collateral onto an adjacent inhibitory short axon interneuron.

It might therefore be possible to set up a functional CNS with two NTs exerting excitatory and inhibitory effects through different receptors, situated on different parts of the neuron provided we were only interested in spreading activity of one kind and preferably at a constant rate. But this assumes that only two effects, i.e. fast excitation and inhibition, are wanted. In practice one neuron receives hundreds of inputs and some of these may need to exert a background conditioning effect. So we find there are many NTs working in a complex and integrated manner to control neuronal excitability and activity. Some of the ways in which they work will now be considered.

How do neurotransmitters work?

Before we can consider how NTs may work we must understand how the excitability of a neuron can be controlled and altered. The neuronal membrane is 20 times more permeable to K^+ than Na^+ ions and therefore K^+ moves out until the flow down the electrochemical gradient is balanced by the charge generated (Fig. 1.2). If this depended only on K^+ then it would occur when the inside is 80 mV more negative than the outside, which is the equilibrium potential for K^+, i.e. when K^+ influx $= K^+$ efflux. In fact the resting membrane potential at around -70 mV is less than this because of the contribution (inward flow) of Na^+. If Na^+ controlled the resting potential it would be $+50$ mV and if it was determined by chloride ions it would be -90 mV. On arrival of an excitatory input the Na^+ conductance channels open and there is an increased influx of Na^+ so that the potential starts to move towards the equilibrium potential for Na^+ but at 60–65 mV, the so called threshold potential, there is a sudden large increase in Na^+ influx (and in K^+ efflux). This depolarisation leads to the generation of an action (propagated) potential. The initial subthreshold change in membrane potential paral-

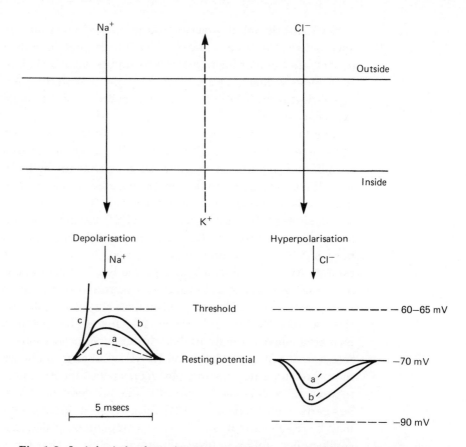

Fig. 1.2. Ionic basis for the excitatory post-synaptic potential (EPSP) and inhibitory post-synaptic potential (IPSP). Membrane potential (-70 mV) is maintained by Na^+ influx and K^+ efflux. Varying degrees of depolarisation, shown by different sized EPSPs (a and b), are caused by increasing influx of Na^+(c). Membrane potential moves towards threshold potential (60–65 mV) at which point an action potential is initiated (a′,b′). The IPSPs are produced by an influx of Cl^{-1}. Coincidence of an EPSP (b) and IPSP (a′) reduces the size of the EPSP (d).

lels the action of the excitatory transmitter and is known as the excitatory postsynaptic potential (EPSP). They last about 5 msec and are additive but not propagated. Such excitatory potentials are similar to the end plate potential (EPP) produced at the neuromuscular junction by activating the motor nerve. Unlike the neuromuscular junction, however, there are also inhibitory inputs to oppose and control the excitatory ones.

An inhibitory input increases the influx of Cl^- to make the inside of the neuron more negative. This hyperpolarisation, the inhibitory postsynaptic potential (IPSP), takes the membrane potential further away from threshold. It is the mirror-image of the EPSP and will reduce the chance of an EPSP reaching threshold voltage.

Such clear postsynaptic potentials are recorded intracellularly with microelectrodes in large quiescent neurons often after the synchronous activation of a number of presynaptic fibres and their production may be

BASIC ASPECTS OF NEUROTRANSMITTER FUNCTION

somewhat artificial. In practice, the activity of a neuron depends on a balance between a large number of excitatory and inhibitory inputs and, in fact, its bombardment by mixed inputs means that its potential is continuously changing and may only move towards the threshold for depolarisation if inhibition fails or is overcome by a sudden increase in excitatory input.

Not all influences on, or potentials recorded from, a neuron have the same time course as the EPSP and IPSP. If the preganglionic trunk to a peripheral sympathetic ganglion, such as that in the bullfrog, is stimulated then, in addition to the fast propagated potential (1 msec duration) that can be recorded from cells in the ganglion, there is a slow EPSP (5 sec), a slower IPSP and a very late EPSP lasting several minutes. Such potentials demonstrate the existence of different synaptic events that have some role not only in the control of the short and long term excitability of ganglion cells but probably of all neurons. Certainly slow potentials and prolonged changes in neuronal firing can be recorded in many parts of the CNS and neuronal activity is not merely controlled by the classical EPSPs and IPSPs. In ganglia the fast depolarisation is mediated conventionally by Na^+ influx after activation of the nicotinic receptors for ACh but the slower EPSP is linked to cholinergic muscarinic receptors and is accompanied by decreased conduction probably through reduced K^+ efflux (see Chapter 6). The mechanism of the slow IPSP is less certain but dopamine (DA) released from a ganglionic interneuron may be involved and, since it is accompanied by decreased membrane conductance and has a reversal potential close to that for Na^+, it may be due to a decreased Na^+ conductance.

Thus the fast EPSP and IPSP follow the rapid opening of Na^+ and Cl^- ion channels that are directly linked to NT receptors but this is not so for the slower potential changes, most of which appear to have a biochemical intermediary. It has been shown that preganglionic stimulation increases the levels of adenosine 3',5'-monophosphate (cyclic AMP) in the ganglion and this is believed to activate a protein kinase which in turn phosphorylates a protein constituent of the membrane to cause a change in ionic conductance (see Greengard 1976 and Chapter 5). The production of cyclic AMP at the start of this sequence is triggered by the NT activating a receptor linked to adenylate cyclase and many monoamines are believed to work through this mechanism. In some instances adenylate cyclase (AC) may be inhibited as it is linked to two distinct guanosine triphosphate (GTP) binding proteins in the cell membrane, (G_S and G_I). The former is stimulated by appropriate receptor activation (see Fig. 5.2) to a form that can stimulate AC whilst activation of G_I inhibits AC, possibly by reducing the effect of G_S. There are other protein kinases in the neuron apart from those linked to cyclic AMP and their activity appears to be controlled in a number of ways by the level of free cytosolic Ca^{2+}. This may enter the cell through distinct receptor controlled membrane channels or more probably it is displaced from intracellular stores. The latter depends on the stimulation of receptors controlling the hydrolysis of a membrane phospholipid, phosphatidylinositol-4,5-biphosphate (PIP_2) to both inositol-1,4,5-triphosphate (IP_3), which displaces Ca^{2+} and diacylglycerol (DAG). The elevated cytosolic Ca^{2+} facilitates the activation of a protein kinase C by DAG and can also affect other kinases and cell functions when it becomes bound to the intracellular (Ca^{2+} dependent) regulatory protein, calmodulin (CaM). It also seems that Ca^{2+} can activate guanylate cyclase (GC) to control the synthesis of guanosine 3',5'-monophosphate (cyclic GMP, cGMP) which is linked to another protein kinase. These procedures are summarised in Fig. 5.4 and dealt with in more detail in Chapter 5.

Such findings show that, although the activity of a neuron can be controlled in a number of ways by NTs activating appropriate receptors, two basic mechanisms are involved:

1 Those linked directly to Na^+ (ACh through nicotinic receptors, excitatory amino acids) or Cl^- (GABA) ion channels, involving fast events with increased membrane conductance and ion flux.

2 Those not directly linked to ion channels but initiating biochemical processes that mediate more long term effects and modify the responsiveness of the neuron. They are normally associated with reduced membrane conductance and ion flux (unless secondary to an increased Ca^{++} conductance) and may involve decreased Na^+ influx (inhibitory) or K^+ efflux (excitatory). Some amines (e.g. noradrenaline) may increase K^+ efflux (inhibitory).

These two mechanisms may also be distinguished by the fact that only the latter are voltage sensitive. Thus if current is passed through an intracellular electrode to modify membrane potential then the former are basically independent of the value of the resting potential whilst the latter are altered by it (see Chapter 3). This can mean that their effectiveness will vary with the state of the membrane potential. Thus different NTs produce different postsynaptic events, or is it that different NTs are needed to produce these different effects?

So far we have only considered how a NT may modify neuronal activity postsynaptically. Recently, interest has also turned to presynaptic events. It has been known for many years that stimulation of muscle or cutaneous afferents to the spinal cord produces a prolonged inhibition of motoneuron activity without any accompanying change in conductance of the motoneuron membrane, i.e. no IPSP. Such inhibition is not antagonised, like the conventional IPSP, by strychnine but it is associated with a depolarisation of afferent nerve terminals and is overcome by the GABA antagonist bicuculline. Since this inhibition does not directly modify the potential of the inhibited neuron but is accompanied by depolarisation of afferent fibres to the neuron it is presumably of presynaptic origin. If it is assumed that the amount of NT released from a nerve terminal depends on the amplitude of the potential change induced in it, then if that terminal is already partly depolarised when the impulse arrives it will release less transmitter (Fig. 1.3). There is no direct evidence for this concept from studies of NT release but electrophysiological experiments at the crustacean neuromuscular junction, which has separate excitatory and inhibitory inputs, show that stimulation of the inhibitory nerve, which releases GABA, reduces the EPSP evoked postsynaptically by an excitatory input without directly hyperpolarising (inhibiting) the muscle fibre.

Certainly when GABA is applied to various *in vivo* and *in vitro* preparations (spinal cord, cuneate nucleus, olfactory cortex) it will produce a depolarisation of nerve terminals that spreads sufficiently to be recorded in distal afferent axons. How GABA can produce this presynaptic depolarisation and conventional postsynaptic hyperpolarisation by the same receptor, since both effects are blocked by bicuculline, is uncertain, although an increased chloride flux appears to be involved in both cases. What is clear is that presynaptic inhibition can last much longer (50–100 msecs) than the postsynaptic form (5 msecs) and can be a very effective means of cutting off one particular excitatory input without directly reducing the overall response of the neuron. If some nerve terminals are depolarised rather than hyperpolarised by increased chloride flux then their resting membrane potential must be different from (greater than) that of the cell body so that when chloride enters and the potential moves towards its equilibrium potential there is a depolarisation instead of a hyperpolarisation. Alternatively, chloride efflux must be achieved in some way.

This form of presynaptic inhibition must be distinguished from another means of attenuating NT release, i.e. autoinhibition. At noradrenergic synapses the amount of noradrenaline (NA) released from the terminals is reduced by exogenous NA and increased by alpha adrenoceptor antagonists. The alpha$_2$ (α_2) adrenoreceptor mediating this effect can be distinguished from classical postsynaptic alpha$_1$ (α_1) adrenoreceptors by relatively specific agonists (clonidine and alpha-methylnoradrenaline for α_2, methoxamine and phenylephrine for α_1) and antagonists (yohimbine for α_2, and prazosin for α_1). This inhibition does not involve any change in membrane potential but the receptors are believed to be linked to and inhibit adenylate cyclase. To what extent autoinhibition occurs with other NTs is uncertain although there is evidence for it at GABA, dopamine and 5-HT terminals.

There is also the interesting possibility that presynaptic inhibition of this form, without potential changes, need not be restricted to the terminal from which the NT is released. Numerous studies in which brain slices have been loaded with a labelled NT and its release evoked by high K^+ or direct stimulation, show that such release can be inhibited by a variety of other NTs. A noradrenergic terminal has been shown to possess receptors for a wide range of substance (see Langer 1981) and although this may be useful for developing drugs to manipulate noradrenergic transmission it seems unlikely that many of the receptors could be linked to a physiological mechanism. One obvious difficulty is that a NT would

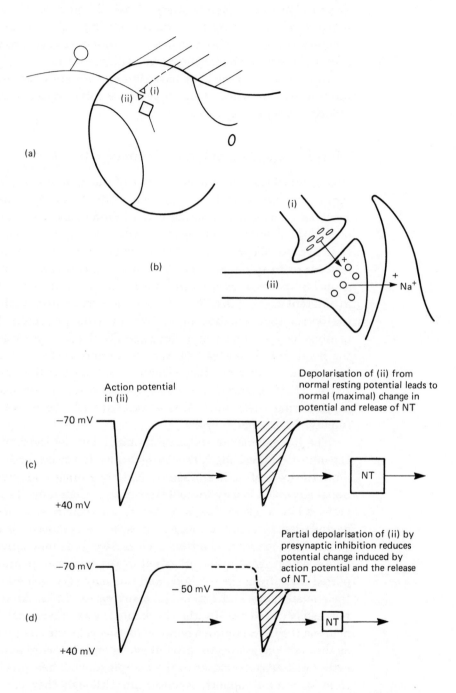

Fig. 1.3. Pre-synaptic inhibition of the form seen in the dorsal horn of the spinal cord (a). The axon terminal (i) of a local neuron makes an axo-axonal contact with a primary afferent excitatory input (ii), synapse shown enlarged in (b), to reduce the release of NT from it. This it does by partly depolarising terminal (ii) so that when an action potential arrives it produces less change in the potential of (ii) and a smaller release of NT (see (d)) than it could if (ii) had been at its resting potential (see (c)).

need to diffuse from the terminal at which it is released and avoid degradation long enough to affect release of a different NT at another terminal. Such an arrangement seems too imprecise for integrated CNS function although it could have a more long-term background effect and in fact there is some morphological evidence for it.

Obviously different NTs have different synaptic actions and it is of interest to see to what extent there are morphological correlates for these differing synaptic activities.

Morphological correlates of synaptic function

It is assumed that the reader is aware of the basic histological features of the neuron and synapse (see Shepherd 1979). Basically neurons consist of a cell body, the soma or perikaryon, with one major cytoplasmic process, termed the axon, which projects variable distances to other neurons, e.g. from pyramidal cortical cells to adjacent cortical interneurons, to striatal neurons or to spinal cord motoneurons. Thus by giving off a number of axonal branches a neuron can influence a large number of other neurons in different areas of the CNS. Primary sensory neurons with cell bodies in the dorsal root ganglion only have an axon projection but all other neurons have a number of other, generally shorter, projections which are the dendrites. These can be very numerous with projections running amongst a number of other neighbouring neurons like the branches of a tree. Their absence from sensory, i.e. initiating, neurons immediately suggests that their function is associated with the reception of signals (inputs) from other neurons.

The soma, dendrite and axon terminal, but not the axon itself, are all capable of synthesising NTs. Those formed in the cell body (soma) travel down the axon often in storage vesicles, for storage and release in the terminal alongside locally formed transmitter. Generally NTs are stored in vesicles but whether this is necessary for their release or to stop their degradation by metabolising enzymes in the cytoplasm is controversial. Whilst most neurotransmitters such as ACh, the monoamines (MAs) and amino acids (AAs) are synthesised in the terminal, peptides are transported there from the cell body and this may very well affect the level of their availability and action. In many cases (MAs, AAs) some of the released NT can be reabsorbed back into the axon terminal. In addition to neurons the CNS contains non-conducting cells the glia (neuroglia), such as the star-like astrocytes around axons and dendrites and oligodendrocytes (stellate cells) closer to the neuron soma. Their precise role, apart from structural support, is uncertain although they can take up and metabolise NTs, especially AAs.

An axon generally makes synaptic contact with the cell body of another neuron either on its dendrites, axo-dendritic synapses or soma, axo-somatic synapse. Gray (1959) has described subcellular features that distinguished two main types of synapse. Under the electron microscope his designated type I synaptic contact is broad (1–2 μm long) around a large cleft (300 Å) and shows assymetric thickening with an accumulation of dense material adjacent to the postsynaptic membrane. A type II junction is narrower (1 μm) with a smaller cleft (200 Å) and a more even but less marked membrane densification on both sides of the junction. Also the presynaptic vesicles are large (300–600 Å diameter), spherical and numerous at the type I synapse but smaller (100–300 Å), fewer in number and somewhat flattened or disc-like at type II. Although vesicles of varying shape can be found at both synapses, and some workers have claimed that the differences were due to fixation problems, the two types of synapse are widely seen and generally accepted. Type I synapses are predominantly axo-dendritic, i.e. excitatory and type II axo-somatic or inhibitory, although the distinction is not absolute and inhibitory type II contacts are found on the dendrites of some neurons (e.g. cerebellar Purkinje cells).

Unfortunately it is not yet possible to inspect a synapse under the electron microscope and identify the main NT involved although some terminals have characteristic vesicles. At cholinergic synapses the terminals have clear vesicles (200–400 Å) whilst monoamine terminals (especially NA) have distinct large (500–900 Å) dense vesicles. Even larger vesicles are found in the terminals of some neuro-secretory cells (e.g. the pituitary). One terminal can contain more than one type of vesicle and although all of them probably store transmitters it is by no means certain that all are involved in the release mechanism.

Recently dendro-dendritic synapses have been described which show characteristic synaptic connections and we need to abandon the belief that one neuron can only influence another through its axon terminals. In fact a release of DA from dendrites of dopaminergic neurons in the substantia nigra has been demonstrated. Dendro-dendritic synapses can also be reciprocal, i.e. one dendrite can make synaptic contact with another and be both pre- and postsynaptic to it.

Anatomical evidence can also be presented to support the concept of presynaptic inhibition and examples of one axon terminal in contact with another are well documented. These do not show the characteristics of either type I or II synapses but the shape of the presynaptic vesicle is of particular interest because even if the net result of activating this synapse is inhibition, the initial event is depolarisation (excitation) of the axonal membrane. This might suggest that the vesicles should be spherical but since the NT is GABA, normally an inhibitory transmitter, the vesicles could be flattened. Thus, does the type of synapse or the NT and its function determine the shape of the vesicle? Generally the vesicles at these axo-axonic synapses are flattened (or disc-like) but some have spherical vesicles and so whilst the situation is not resolved vesicle shape tends to be linked with the NT substance.

If NTs can also have distal nonsynaptic effects then nerve terminals that do not make definite synaptic connections should be apparent. In smooth muscle, noradrenergic fibres ramify along the muscle fibres and release NA from swellings or varicosities along their length. In certain parts of the brain, especially the cerebral cortex, some ultrastructural studies show that a high proportion of the varicosities of NA and 5-HT fibres do not appear to make specialised synaptic connections with other neurons. The implication is that the fibres meander through the cortex releasing amines that then diffuse to produce a general effect rather than a precise synaptic excitation or inhibition. Possibly they modulate the release of other NTs. One may wonder whether this is really feasible in view of the low level of NT released and the mechanisms available for NT degradation. However, very low concentrations (10^{-10} M) of NA are known to increase AA release from brain slices. Certainly the concept of non-synaptic NT release has recently been challenged by the demonstration, under appropriate histological conditions, of conventional synapses for the MAs (see references). Whichever view is correct it brings us back to the original question. Are the monoamines with the function just outlined really neurotransmitters or are they neuromodulators?

The synaptic arrangements referred to above are summarised in Fig. 1.4.

How may a substance be shown to be a neurotransmitter?

ACh is regarded as the prototype classical neurotransmitter at the neuromuscular junction. It transmits the excitatory impulse from nerve to muscle very quickly (synaptic delay 1 msec) and is then rapidly metabolised. The features of transmission at this synapse have in fact become a guide to synaptic neurotransmission generally and certain criteria have emerged which it is believed must be fulfilled before a substance can be regarded as NT. There are basically three criteria.

1 Presence. It perhaps goes without saying that the proposed transmitter must be shown to be present in the CNS and preferably in the area and at the synapses where it is thought to act.

2 Release. Simulation of the appropriate nerves should evoke a measurable release of NT.

3 Identity of action. The proposed NT must produce effects post-synaptically which are identical physiologically (appropriate membrane potential changes) and pharmacologically (sensitivity to antagonists) to that produced by neuronal stimulation and the released endogenous NT.

These criteria should be regarded as guidelines rather than rules. As guidelines they provide a reasonable scientific framework of the type of investigations that must be undertaken to establish the synaptic role of a substance. As rigid rules they could preclude the discovery of more than one type of neurotransmitter or one form of neurotransmission. Nevertheless the criteria have been widely employed and often expanded to include other features which will be considered as subdivisions of the main criteria.

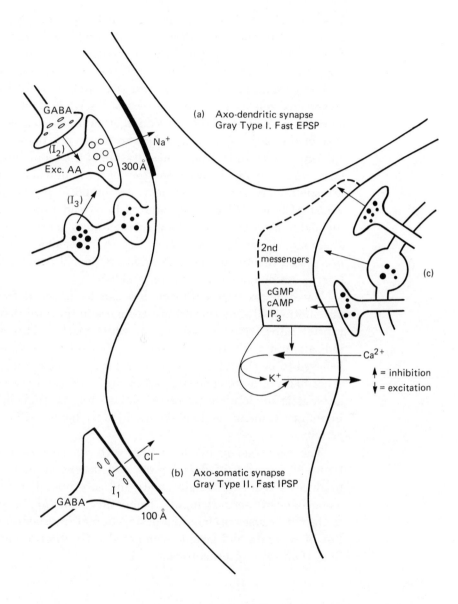

Fig. 1.4. Schematic diagram of different synaptic arrangements on a neuron. The hypothetical neuron has conventional axo-dendritic excitatory synapses (a) involving the fast and direct opening of Na^+ channels. Axo-somatic inhibition (b) involves the opening of chloride channels and hyperpolarisation (I_1). The microscopic organisation of these two synapses has been described by Gray (1959) and is outlined in the text. Slower changes in neuronal activity mediated through second messengers (see Fig. 5.4) and mainly altering K^+ flux are shown at (c) with the NT released at conventional synapses or from more distant varicosites. Pre-synaptic inhibition may be of the classical type (see Fig. 1.3) with depolarisation of the excitatory nerve terminal (I_2) or by an effect on NT release without a conventional synapse or potential change (I_3).

Presence

Distribution and concentration

It is generally felt that a substance is more likely to be a NT if it is unevenly distributed in the CNS although if it is widely used it will be widely distributed. Certainly the high concentration (5–10 μmol per g) of dopamine, compared with that of any other monoamine in the striatum or with dopamine in other brain areas, was indicative of its subsequently established role as a NT in that part of the CNS. This does not mean it cannot have an important function in other areas such as the mesolimbic system and parts of the cerebral cortex where it is present in much lower concentrations. In fact the concentration of the monoamines outside the striatum is very much lower than that of the amino acids or ACh. Thus in the spinal cord some amino acids are found at levels up to 10 μmol/g whilst ACh and NA are only present in 50 and 1 nmol/g amounts. This highlights a problem with some of the amino acids such as glycine and glutamate. Since they may have important biochemical functions that necessitate their widespread distribution, the NT component of any given level of amino acid is difficult to establish.

Nevertheless useful information can be deduced from patterns of distribution. Glycine is concentrated more in the cord than cortex and in ventral rather than dorsal grey or white matter. This alone would be indicative of a NT role for glycine in the ventral horn, where it is now believed to be the inhibitory transmitter at motoneurons. GABA on the other hand is more concentrated in the brain than the cord and in the latter it is predominantly in the dorsal grey so that although it is an inhibitory transmitter like glycine it must have a different pattern of activity.

The use of lesions in conjunction with concentration studies can also be useful. Section of dorsal roots and degeneration of afferent fibres produces a reduction in glutamate and substance P which can then be associated with sensory inputs. Temporary reduction of the blood supply to the cord causes preferential destruction of interneurons and a greater loss of asparate and glycine, compared with other amino acids, and so links them with interneurons.

Subcellular localisation

A NT should be concentrated in nerve terminals. When nervous tissue is homogenised the nerve endings break off from their axons and surrounding elements and then reseal. These elements are known as synaptosomes.

When crude homogenised tissue is centrifuged at a slow speed (1000 g for 10 minutes) the cell debris spins down (Fig. 1.5). If the supernatant is then spun at 20 000 g for 20 minutes the synaptosomes sediment with the mitochondria as a pellet leaving cytoplasmic (cell body) elements in the

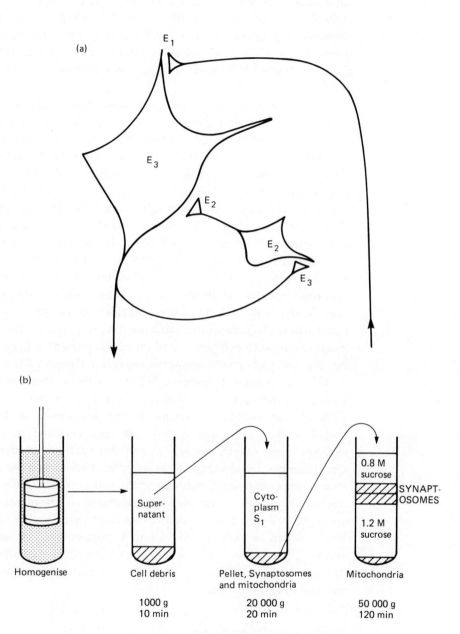

Fig. 1.5. Distribution of a neurotransmitter within different subcellular fractions.
(a) Within the hypothetical brain area shown, where it is assumed that this neuronal
arrangement is reproduced many times, the proportion of each NT found in the
synaptosome rather than the cell body (cytoplasmic) fraction will vary considerably. On
the assumption that although concentrated in nerve terminals the NT will also be found
in cell bodies and axons it is likely that E_1 will be almost entirely in synaptosomes, E_3
mostly in the cytoplasm whilst E_2 will be more evenly divided. (b) Procedure for
preparation and separation of synaptosomes. Tissue is homogenised and spun at 1000 g
for 10 min to remove cell debris. The supernatant is spun at 20 000 g for 10 min and the
pellet, containing synaptosomes and mitochondria is spun though two layers of sucrose
with the synaptosomes separating at the interface after 2 hours at 50 000 g.

supernatant. When the pellet is resuspended in 0.32 M sucrose and spun through layers of 0.8 and 1.2 M sucrose at 50 000 g for 2 hours most of the mitochondria will be recovered in the pellet whilst the synaptosomes are found at the 0.8–1.2 M sucrose interface (see Gray and Whittaker 1962 and de Robertis 1963). Such synaptosomes have been widely used to study NT release *in vitro*.

Of course it is important that some NT is always found in the synaptosome fraction (unless it is not preformed and stored before release) but it need not be restricted to it. A neuron consists basically of two parts: the soma (cell body) and the axon with its terminals. Even if the NT is concentrated in nerve endings there is always some in the soma from where it may be transported down the axon, and this element would appear in the early supernatant cytoplasmic fraction. If the area of CNS chosen for study (Fig. 1.5) contains only the cell bodies of neurons using a particular NT then that NT (E_3) will appear predominantly in the cytoplasmic fraction, but it could still be a NT at a distal site to which the neuron sends its axons or at local collaterals. Conversely if the area contains only the terminals of long axons from remote cell bodies then the NT (E_1) will be found almost exclusively in synaptosomes. Neuro-transmitters (E_2) associated with neurons intrinsic to the area, i.e. short interneurons with cell bodies and terminals present, will be found in both cytoplasmic and synaptosome fractions (see Chapter 6).

If it is reasonable to expect a NT to be present in nerve terminals how should it be preserved and stored so that it can be released on demand? This will obviously be determined by the mechanism of NT release. One theory is that NTs are stored and then released in predetermined amounts from special packets or vesicles that can be demonstrated in synaptosomes by electron microscopy and separated by centrifugation after disruption (osmotic shock) of the synaptosomes. Whether NTs are released from vesicles has been much debated (see References), but if they are to be released from vesicles they must certainly be found in them. Whilst it can be shown that 75% of synaptosomal NA (and ACh) is in vesicles there is less evidence that the amino acids are stored in this way. Of course, it is important to consider if it is necessary for all NTs to be released in the same way.

Synthesis and degradation

If a substance is to be a NT it should be possible to demonstrate the presence of appropriate enzymes for its synthesis from a precursor. There may be instances, as with peptides however, where the NT is transported to its site of location and action after synthesis in a distal neuronal cell body. Also re-uptake of released transmitter may conserve its concentration in the terminal without the need for very much new synthesis. The specificity of any enzyme system must also be established, especially if they are to be modified to manipulate the levels of a particular NT, or used as markers for it. Thus choline acetyltransferase may be taken as indicative of ACh and glutamic acid decarboxylase (GAD) of GABA but some of the synthesising enzymes for the monoamines (DA, NA and 5-HT) lack such specificity.

After release there must be some way of terminating the action of a NT but this is not always by chemical degradation as at the neuro-muscular junction. At peripheral noradrenergic synapses the NT is initially removed from the synaptic cleft by uptake into either the nerve (uptake one-U_1) or surrounding tissue (U_2) and it seems that the actions of many NTs in the CNS, especially the monoamines and amino acids are terminated by uptake into nerve terminals or the adjacent non-neuronal glial cells.

Such uptake processes can be quite specific chemically. Thus a high affinity uptake (activated by low concentrations) can be found for glycine in the cord where it is believed to be a NT, but not in the cortex where it has no such action. This specific uptake can be utilised to map terminals for a particular NT, especially if it can be labelled, and also for loading nerves with labelled NT for release studies.

Of course some transmitters may be released in small quantities or designed to have a prolonged action for which rapid destruction would be undesirable. Also since CNS function depends on changes in the rate of neuronal firing determined by a subtle balance between a number of different excitatory and inhibitory inputs it may be unnecessary to destroy the NT rapidly. Thus excessive firing of a neuron may be controlled by activating a feed-back inhibitory system to dampen down that neuron even in the presence of the excitatory NT, which could then diffuse away. Also the release of any additional excitatory NT could be avoided by reflex evoked presynaptic inhibition.

Pathways

If a substance (or its synthesising or degradative systems) can be demonstrated in particular neurons with a distinctive pattern of distri-bution or bunched together into well defined nerve tracts, then this is not only good evidence for its role as a NT but can tell us something of its function. Indeed the distinct patterns of distribution of ascending monoamine pathways from brain stem nuclei (Chapter 7) could probably be considered as adequate evidence for their neurotransmitter role. In practical terms we can only study the release (and actions) of an endogenous NT if it can be evoked by stimulating an appropriate nerve pathway. Also the neurological and behavioural consequences of lesion-ing such pathways can tell us much about the functions of the NT. It is therefore useful to know how NTs can be demonstrated histologically and their pathways mapped. These procedures are discussed in some detail later (Chapter 2).

Release

Before a substance can be considered to have a physiological role as a NT its release by nerve stimulation should be demonstrated. In reality of course it cannot be a NT unless it is released. Unfortunately it may be necessary to assume that this occurs in some instances for although it is possible to show the presence of a substance and some effect when it is applied directly to neurons its release may not be measurable for technical reasons. This is even more true if one strives for the ideal of demonstrating the release of an endogenous substance by physiological stimuli.

In the CNS access to the site of release is a major problem and attempts to achieve it have led to the development of a wide range of techniques of varying complexity and ingenuity or to short cuts of dubious value. These are considered in detail in Chapter 2. The feasibility of release studies in the CNS is to some extent dependent on the type of NT being studied. If we are dealing with a straightforward neural pathway with a number of axons going from A to B then by stimulating A and perfusing B we should be able to collect the NT. Unfortunately such arrangements are rare in the CNS and where they exist (e.g. corticospinal tract) it is not easy to perfuse the receiving (collecting) area. Sometimes the origin of a pathway is clear and easy to stimulate, e.g. NA fibres from their well defined nucleus in the locus coeruleus, but fibre distribution in the cortex is so widespread that collection of sufficient amounts for detection can be almost impossible by current methods.

These approaches are, in any case, only suitable for classical types of neurotransmitter. Those with slow background effects will not be released in measurable amounts over reasonable times. For such substances we require a measure of their utilisation, or turnover, over a much longer period of time. With NTs released from short axon interneurons there are no pathways to stimulate and it becomes necessary to activate the neurons intrinsically by field stimulation, which is of necessity not specific to the terminals of interneurons.

Apart from demonstrating release it is important to consider how NTs are released and whether they all need to be released in the same way, especially if they do different things. One concept of release is that on arrival of the action potential there is an influx of calcium ions: vesicles migrate to the membrane and then discharge their contents of stored NT into the synaptic cleft. It may be that some NTs must be released by this process, which is known as exocytosis, in order to produce their required effect but this may not be so for all NTs and so they may not all need to be stored. In this case their release may not depend on calcium. Also the different time courses of NT action referred to previously may require NTs to be released at different rates and in different ways, only some of which are achievable by vesicular mechanisms and exocytosis.

Identity of action

Many people (see Werman 1966) consider this to be the most important of all the criteria. Obviously a substance must have an effect of some kind if it is to be a NT but not all substances that have an effect on neurons need to be NTs. It may seem unnecessary to say this but the literature contains many accounts of the study of various substances on neuronal activity from which a NT role is predicted without any attempt to compare its effect with that of physiologically evoked (endogenous NT) effects. The importance of this safeguard is highlighted by the ease with which both smooth muscle and neurons will respond to a range of substances that cannot be released on to them as NTs. Thus the value of this criterion depends very much on the rigour with which it is applied and on its own is no more or less important than any other approach.

Ideally it should be shown that application of the proposed NT to a neuron, e.g. by iontopheresis (see Chapter 3), produces changes in membrane potential that are identical to and mediated by the same ionic mechanism as those produced by nerve stimulation and that the effects of both are equally overcome by an appropriate chemical antagonist. The basic system is outlined in Fig. 1.6. Clearly changes in membrane potential can only be recorded if the neuron is large enough to take an intracellular electrode and even if it can be shown that the applied and released NT produce similar changes in membrane potential and share a common reversal potential and ionic mechanism this would not be so surprising since the number of available ionic mechanisms is limited (i.e. both GABA and glycine produce hyperpolarisation by increasing chloride influx). Now that the properties of single ion channels can be recorded using modern patch clamp techniques it will be necessary to show that application of the presumed NT produces identical changes in the frequency (n) degree (γ, amount of current conducted) and duration (r) of channel opening to that achieved by synaptic activation. Unfortunately such a detailed analysis is presently only applicable to relatively simple systems with restricted innervations such as some neuromuscular junctions and cultured neurons.

The use of antagonists is absolutely vital but even they can give false positives. Thus GABA, β-alanine and glycine all produce hyperpolarisation of cord motoneurons by increasing chloride influx but only GABA is unaffected by strychnine. Since strychnine abolishes inhibition in the cord, GABA cannot be the inhibitory NT but either glycine or β-alanine could be and other features (distribution, release) had to be satisfied before glycine was preferred for that role. Perhaps the value of antagonists in elucidating synaptic physiology and pharmacology is most apparent from attempts to establish the identity of the major excitatory NT in the CNS. Although there is much indirect evidence which suggests that this should be glutamate it has not been possible to demonstrate that

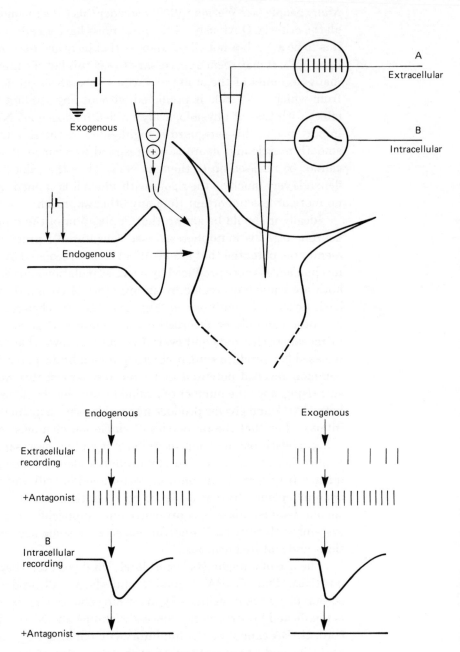

Fig. 1.6. Comparison of the effects of an endogenously released and exogenously applied neurotransmitter on neuronal activity (identity of action). Recordings are made either of neuronal firing (extracellularly A) or of membrane potential (intracellularly B). The proposed transmitter is applied by iontophoresis, although in a brain slice preparation it can be added to the bathing medium. In this instance the applied NT produces an inhibition like that of nerve stimulation, as monitored by both recordings, and both are affected similarly by the antagonist.

a particular synapse definitely uses it because of the lack of specific antagonists. Hopefully current progress in the classification of excitatory amino acid receptors and the development of specific antagonists effective at synapses *in vivo* (see Chapter 13) will soon rectify this situation.

It must also be remembered that a substance can only be shown to be identical in its action with that of a particular endogenous NT if the latter's precise mode of action is clearly established and easily studied. Thus it may be relatively easy to study those NTs mediating classical postsynaptic excitation and inhibition through distinct potential changes but more difficult for NTs which function over a much longer time course and possibly without producing recordable potential changes. Clearly this criterion should be fulfilled but the actions to be studied may not only vary but may not always be easily recorded or even known.

Neurotransmitter organisation

There can be no doubt that ACh is a NT at the mammalian neuromuscular junction where each muscle fibre is generally influenced by only one nerve terminal and where one NT acts on one type of receptor localised to a specific (end-plate) area of the muscle. Activation of the receptor leads to the opening of ion channels, depolarisation follows and the NT is rapidly destroyed by a highly localised concentration of metabolising enzyme. The system is fitted for the rapid release, action and destruction of the NT in a localised area, as required for induction of the rapid short postsynaptic event of skeletal muscle fibre contraction.

Whilst the study of this synapse has been of immense value in elucidating some basic concepts of neurochemical transmission it would be unwise to use it as a universal template of synaptic transmission since it is atypical in many respects.

Smooth muscle generally receives a dual opposing innervation from the autonomic nervous system. One sympathetic noradrenergic nerve fibre can influence a number of muscle fibres (or ganglion cells) by releasing NA from varicosities along its length without there being any defined 'end-plate' junctions. The result of receptor activation is a slow change in potential and inactivation of the NT is initially by uptake and then metabolism. In other words the NT function is geared to the slower phasic changes of muscle tone characteristic of smooth muscle. Even the cholinergic innervation is mediated through muscarinic receptors with a slower time course of action than achieved at the end plate of the neuromuscular junction.

In the CNS there are even more forms of neuronal organisation. One neuron can have many synaptic inputs and a multiplicity of NTs and NT effects are utilised within a complex inter-relationship of neurons. There are also positive and negative feedback circuits as well as presynaptic influences all designed to effect changes in excitability and frequency of neuronal firing, i.e. patterns of neuronal discharge. All of this is achieved with smaller intracellular spaces and synapses wrapped around with glia.

Whilst pharmacologists should try to exploit such differences between NT systems in developing drugs rather than adopting a blanket concept of neurotransmission it is still worthwhile trying to characterise different types of NT systems in the CNS in order to build up a functional framework and concept. The following patterns may be distinguished.

(Pa) Classical

These include not only pathways with very long axons, such as the cortico-spinal and spino-thalamic tracts but also numerous shorter interconnecting systems, e.g. thalamus to cortex etc. They may be regarded as the back-bone of the CNS. The axons, especially the very long ones, show little divergence and have a relatively precise localisation, i.e. activation of particular motoneurons by stimulating a precise part of the motor cortex. Their influences on neurons is phasic and generally rapid with conventional EPSPs. Distinct (type I) axo-dendritic synapses are common and these systems form the basic framework for the precise control of movement and monitoring of sensation. Such pathways are well researched and understood by neuroanatomists and physiologists, but their localised organisation makes them, perhaps fortunately, somewhat resistant to drug action. They are probably of less interest to pharmacologists than other systems and surprisingly little is known of the NTs they use, although amino acids such as glutamate are implicated.

(Pb) Short axon intrinsic systems

These are basically neurons whose cell body and axon terminals are both found in the same part of the CNS. They are not concerned with transmitting information from one part of the CNS to another but in controlling activity in their own area, although they may be influenced by inputs to them. They can be excitatory but are more often inhibitory. They may act postsynaptically through conventional IPSPs (or slower potential changes) or presynaptically by modifying NT release. The former systems are generally thought to use amino acids as NTs, e.g. GABA or glycine, whilst the latter systems may use GABA (presynaptic inhibition in cord) or peptides (enkephalin neurons). Excitatory interneurons may use ACh or an amino acid, like aspartate. Since they exert a background control of the level of excitability in a given area or system their manipulation by drugs is of great interest (e.g. attempts to increase GABA function in epilepsy), especially if this can be achieved without adversely affecting important primary (e.g. Pa) activity in the appropriate area. Although they can only have a localised action they may be influenced by long axon inputs to them and so incorporated into long pathway effects, such as the direct cortical inhibition of motoneurons or the reduction of afferent input to the cord by long descending spinal tracts.

(Pc) Controlling system

These are the amine (DA, NA and 5-HT) systems and employ some features of the two preceeding groups. They have long axons originating from neurons that are grouped together in nuclei of perhaps a few hundred cell bodies but spreading to vast areas of the brain and cord. The NTs are released at various sites along considerable lengths of the axon and distinct synaptic contacts may not always be seen. They may act either postsynaptically, or presynaptically to produce slow changes in activity or modify NT release. The tonic background influence of these systems and their role in behaviour have instigated the development and study of many drugs to manipulate their function. It also seems that the cholinergic input into the cortex from subcortical nuclei can be included in this category (see Chapter 6).

Of course whilst the identification of these distinct systems may be useful there are many neural pathways that would not fit easily into one of them. Thus some inhibitory pathways, such as that from the caudate nucleus to substantia nigra, utilising GABA, do not involve an inter-neuron. The dopamine pathway from the substantia nigra to striatum may start from a small nucleus but unlike other monoamine pathways it shows little ramification beyond its influence on the striatum. The object of the above classification is not to fit all neural pathways and mechanisms into a restricted number of functional categories but again to demonstrate that there are different forms of neurotransmission.

(Pd) Co-existence

Although it may be argued that this is not a pattern of NT organisation but merely a feature of some (or possibly all) neurotransmitter systems, it justifies separate consideration (Fig. 1.7). As mentioned previously it is now well established that more than one NT can coexist in the same nerve terminal. Since there is already good evidence for the existence of a fairly large number of different NTs, which it is assumed are released from their own specific neurons, and as they can produce a diversity of postsynaptic events one might consider the release of more than one NT from one terminal a somewhat unnecessary complication. Nevertheless since coexistence is established, its significance must be evaluated in respect of NT function and drug action. Some of the questions which require an answer are:

1 Which NTs co-exist and is there a definite pattern, i.e. does A always occur with B and never with C and is the ratio A:B always the same?

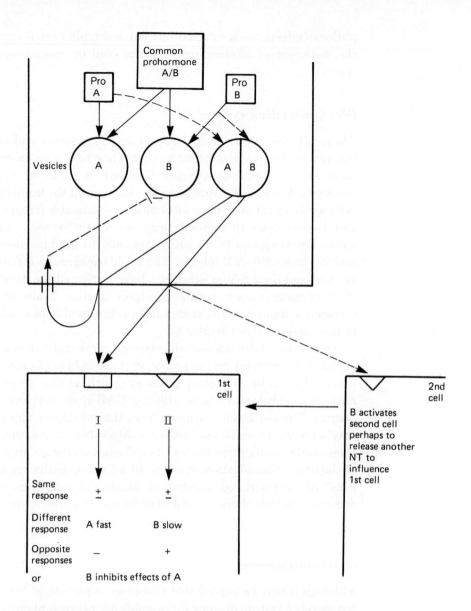

Fig. 1.7. Coexistence of neurotransmitters. The neurotransmitters (or modulators) A and B may be formed from the same or different prehormones and stored separately or together in vesicles. On release they can activate the same or different receptors on one cell, or one NT (B) can influence the function of the first cell indirectly by acting on a second cell. Their effects on the cell may be identical, the same but of different time course, or opposite. One NT could antagonise or augment some of the effects of the other or act presynaptically to affect its release.

2 Are NTs stored and released in a similar manner, i.e. do they come from different or the same vesicles or is one in vesicles and one in the cytoplasm?

3 What effects do NTs produce, how do they interact and are they both necessary for full synaptic transmission? The latter is a vital question for drug therapy based on NT replacement.

The answers, as far as they are available, imply that:

1 Although it is not certain that all nerves have more than one NT almost any NT can coexist with another so that localisation of one NT does not mean the nerve will necessarily always have the same second NT. Coexisting NTs may be;

(a) similar chemically and derived from a common precursor (or prehormone), e.g. leucine and methionine-enkephalin from pre-enkephalins or different chemically but derived from the same prehormone (or genes), e.g. ACTH and β-endorphin from pro-opiomelanocortin.

(b) two different peptides, e.g. substance P and CCK, which are formed from separate pre-hormones or genes (fibres found in dorsal roots)

(c) a peptide and a more conventional NT, e.g. substance P and 5-HT (spinal cord) CCK and DA (striatum and mesolimbic pathways)

(d) two non-peptide NTs, e.g. GABA and 5-HT (mid-brain).

Thus although there are some patterns of co-existence the permutations seem so numerous that one wonders if there is any limit to the possibilities without allowing for the fact that coexistence need not be limited to only two NTs.

2 Little is known about their release. Drugs like reserpine can, at certain dose levels, deplete adrenal chromaffin tissue of catecholamines but not enkephalins and the ratio of ACh to VIP (vasoactive intestinal polypeptide) released from nerves to the submandibular gland is known to vary with the frequency of nerve stimulation but little is known about what happens centrally under physiological conditions. Of course in any meaningful release study one would need to be certain that in any CNS area or neural pathway the two NTs coexist in all fibres in a similar ratio. Thus if there are some fibres with only one of the NTs then stimulation could appear to alter the ratio of released NTs by mainly affecting those fibres.

3 Once released the possibilities for action are almost endless. They would not need to act on the same postsynaptic receptors, although the enkephalins probably do, or even on the same cells (neurons). Thus in the periphery NA and VIP are both released from sympathetic nerves to salivary glands and cause vasoconstriction but only NA increases secretion (see below). They might react presynaptically with one reducing the release of the other or one NT may have no direct effect and simply increase (or decrease) in some way the postsynaptic response to the other (i.e. an endogenous benzodiazepine type compound released to increase the effectiveness of GABA). It is also possible that one NT may control the number of receptors for the other.

Co-operativity between NTs has been analysed most fully at peripheral sites such as the submandibular gland (see Lundberg & Hökfelt 1983) where secretion depends on organ blood flow and the two processes are closely interconnected. Here ACh and VIP are found in the same nerves probably in the small clear and large dense core vesicles respectively. Stimulating the parasympathetic nerves (Chorda lingual) at a low frequency (0.5 Hz) increases secretion and produces vasodilation, both of which are atropine sensitive. VIP does not increase secretion only blood flow and at higher stimulation frequencies (2 Hz) the vasodilation is not abolished by atropine suggesting that it is mediated in this instance partly by VIP, i.e. that VIP is necessary in addition to ACh to produce sufficient vasodilation and increase blood flow to enable the increased level of secretion to be achieved.

Thus it may be that a full understanding of how one NT works at a synapse will require knowledge of how that function depends on the actions of other NTs. It could unfold a whole new requirement and dimension to our understanding of synaptic physiology and pharmacology and the use of drugs. On the other hand it may be of little significance in some cases for although cholinergic mediated nicotinic and muscarinic responses as well as DA and peptide effects are observed in sympathetic ganglia, it is only nicotinic antagonists that actually reduce transmission; acutely anyway.

Having developed the above classification it is necessary to consider whether the tonic influences, e.g. Pc (Pb) are mediated by conventional NTs and if not what are they? Thus we return to the basic question.

What is a neurotransmitter?

Obviously a substance that meets all the criteria discussed above must be a NT but we have to consider if all NTs need to meet all the criteria especially since we have seen that NTs;

1 act at different types of synapses
2 occur in nerve fibres and pathways of differing organisation
3 are probably released and removed in different ways
4 produce a number of different postsynaptic effects with differing time courses of action.

Thus either NTs can differ considerably or not all the substances mediating synaptic events are NTs.

If a substance does not meet all the criteria for a NT it is rightly described as putative (i.e. presumed or possible). If it meets most of the criteria but perhaps has a very slow time course of action or does not directly affect the postsynaptic membrane potential then its status is questioned and it may be called a neuromodulator. It is important that the term neuromodulator is not also used, as is sometimes the case, to describe something which is not yet adequately established as a NT, i.e. a neuromodulator need not be a putative NT.

Apart from this one restriction I believe that generally it is more important to distinguish between the different effects that a substance can produce when released from a nerve, as detailed above, than to worry too much about what it is called. If, however, substances are to be given names like neurotransmitter and neuromodulator then we must be clear about what is meant by these terms and not use them vaguely or interchangeably. The main hindrance to the universal application of the term neurotransmitter to any substance released from a nerve is the fact that the criterion of identity of action, as defined by many workers, does not allow for postsynaptic events that are not recordable as a potential change or, at least, a fluctuation in neuronal firing. If a neurotransmitter can be regarded as a substance formed in and released from a neuron (axon, terminal or dendrite) to produce an effect on some parts (dendrite, soma or axon) of another (immediately adjacent or distal) neuron without passing into the blood, then the term is adequate to cover all the different effects I have considered and the term neuromodulator may be disgarded. If, on the other hand, realisation and acceptance of the fact that substances released from a neuron can produce a variety of effects on other neurons, is handicapped by the lack of appropriate terms to describe these actions, then acceptable terms must be introduced. This difficulty will become even more marked if some peptides or other substances are actually found to have trophic-like effects on neurons that take days or weeks to develop.

Acceptance of the fact that nerves can release substances that do more than just transmit impulses across a synapse, should encourage us to stop using neurotransmitter as a general term. Since substances mediate different effects they should, perhaps, be called neuromediators. Such a general term could include subclasses, i.e. neurotransmitter, neuromodulator, neurohormone, neurotrophic factor and there is no reason why one substance should not have more than one role. Whilst there can be slight differences in the actual mechanisms of their release, they will all originate from nerves and they are mainly distinguished by their subsequent actions. Whatever these actions it is assumed that it requires the participation of some active site or receptor and is therefore sensitive to chemical (drug) intervention and pharmacological manipulation. Although I may favour classification based on the term 'neuromediator' it will not be used in this book since it does not have universal acceptance. On the other hand since it has been established that a NT can produce a variety of different effects there is no merit in using the term neuromodulator to describe some substances. Thus all substances released from nerves will be referred to as neurotransmitters, irrespective of their subsequent action.

References and further reading

References

Burnstock G (1976) Do some nerve cells release more than one transmitter? *Neuroscience* **1**, 239–48.
Dale HH (1935) Pharmacology and nerve endings. *Proc. Roy. Soc. Med.* **28**, 319–32.
Gray EG (1959) Axo-somatic and axo-dendritic synapses of the cerebral cortex. An electronmicroscope study. *J. Anat.* **93** 420–33. See also Gray EG (1976) Problems of understanding the substructure of synapses. *Progr. Brain Res.* **45**, 208–34.

Gray EG & Whittaker VP (1962) The isolation of nerve endings from brain: An electron microscopic study of the cell fragments of homogenisation and centrifugation. *J. Anat.* **96**, 79–87.

Greengard P (1976) Possible role for cyclic nucleotides and phosphorylated membrane proteins in postsynaptic actions of neurotransmitters. *Nature* **260**, 101–8.

Langer SZ (1981) Presynaptic regulation of the release of catecholamines. *Pharmac. Rev.* **32**, 337–62.

Lundberg JM & Hökfelt T (1983) Coexistence of peptides and classical neurotransmitters. *Trends Neurosci.* **6** 325–32.

De Robertis E, de Iraldi AP, Rodriquez de Lores Arnaiz G & Gomez C (1961) On the isolation of nerve endings and synaptic vesicles. *J. Biophys. Biochem. Cytol.* **9**, 229–35.

Werman P (1966). Criteria for identification of a central nervous system transmitter. *Comp. Biochem. Physiol.* **18**, 745–64.

Mechanism of neurotransmitter release

Israel M, Dunnant Y & Manaranche R (1979) The present status of the vesicular hypothesis. *Prog. Neurobiol.* **13**, 237–75.

Tauc L (1982) Nonvesicular release of neurotransmitters. *Physiol. Rev.* **63**, 857–13.

Trends in *Neuroscience* (1979) and (1980) Papers, commentaries and comments by Marchbanks RM, Whittaker VP & Zimmerman H.

Synaptic and nonsynaptic release of monoamines

Beaudet A & Descarries L (1978) The monoamine innervation of rat cerebral cortex: synaptic and nonsynaptic axon terminals. *Neuroscience* **3**, 851–60.

Molliver ME, Grzanna R, Lidov HGW, Morrison JH & Olshowska JA (1982) Monoamine systems in the cerebral cortex. In: Chan-Palay V & Palay SL (ed.) *Cytochemical Methods in Neuroanatomy.* Alan R. Liss. New York. pp. 225–77.

Olshowska JA, Molliver ME, Grzanna R, Rice FL & Coyle JT (1981) Ultrastructural demonstration of noradrenergic synapses in the rat central nervous system by dopamine -hydroxylase immunocytochemistry. *J. Histochem. Cytochem.* **29**, 271–80.

Parnavelas JG, Moises HC & Speciale SG (1985) The monoaminergic innvervation of the rat visual cortex. *Proc. R. Soc. Lond. B.* **223**, 319–29.

Useful reference textbooks

Kuffler SW & Nicholls JG (1976) *From Neurone to Brain.* Sinauer Associates, New York.

Pycock CJ & Taberner PV (eds) (1981) *Central Neurotransmitter Turnover.* Croom Helm, London.

Shepherd GM (1979) *The Synaptic Organisation of the Brain.* 2nd Ed. Oxford University Press, New York.

Siegel GJ, Albos RW, Katzman R & Agranoff BW (1983) *Basic Neurochemistry.* 3rd Ed. Little, Brown and Company, Boston.

2 Neurotransmitter pathways and release

R.A. WEBSTER

Establishing the location and distribution of nerve fibres and pathways for a particular NT may not only give an indication of its possible function but is essential if its release is to be evoked through stimulating appropriate nerves.

Some useful data can be obtained about the utilisation of a NT by simply finding where it is concentrated through measuring its levels in different regions of the CNS or within different parts of a region. Unfortunately if the NT is formed predominantly in terminals, rather than cell bodies, this only tells us where that substance is likely to be released and not the origin of the axons that release it. Consequently it is necessary not only to detect and locate the NT but also trace the path of the fibres that contain and release it.

Location of neurotransmitters

Measurement

NTs can be measured in brain extracts by either chemical or biological procedures and their distribution roughly determined by performing such measures in a variety of brain areas. Special care is needed to ensure that the estimations are made as rapidly as possible after death and preferably from quick frozen tissue in which degradation is less likely to occur. Estimates of the levels of specific synthesising enzymes can also be useful, e.g. choline acetyltransferase (ChAT) for ACh and glutamic acid decarboxylase (GAD) for GABA.

Visualisation

Histological procedures

Stain for the NT or its synthesising or degrading enzymes by chemical, fluorescent or immunohistochemical procedures.

The monoamines can be detected by histo-fluorescent techniques in which freeze-dried tissue is exposed to formaldehyde vapour at 80°C for one hour. This gives condensation products which are not fluorescent in themselves but undergo dehydrogenation to yield isoquinoline derivatives that give a green or yellowish fluorescence when exposed to ultraviolet light. The emission peak for NA (green) can just be separated by chemical means from that for DA whilst 5-HT produces a yellow rather than a green fluorescence.

Immunohistochemical techniques have been used for the monoamines but are more easily used for larger antigenic molecules such as the peptides. In this case an antiserum is raised to the particular peptide and conjugated to a carrier protein such as bovine serum albumin. This is then applied to tissue sections and the antibody on the carrier reacts with and becomes fixed to the antigenic protein, which can then be visualised by fluorescent or other markers. The main problems are obtaining antibodies that will penetrate cells and which are specific to the peptide being studied.

In contrast to the monoamines and peptides other NTs such as GABA and acetylcholine have to be visualised indirectly; GABA by location of the enzyme glutamic acid decarboxylase, which synthesises it from glutamate and ACh by staining for its metabolising enzyme, acetylcholinesterase or its synthesising enzyme choline acetyltransferase, which is more specific to cholinergic fibres. There is now a procedure for the direct visualisation of GABA (Storm-Mathiesen *et al.* 1983).

Autoradiography

The existence of a neuronal uptake process for most NTs or their precursors means that tissues can be subjected to their [^{3}H]-labelled form, either *in vitro* (slice preparations) or *in vivo* (injection into brain or ventricles) and the NT then visualised, after appropriate preparation, by light or electron microscopy (Fig. 2.1). This procedure has been widely used to establish the neuronal localisation of the amino acids such as glycine and GABA as well as the monoamines but its value depends on the specificity of the uptake process, e.g. that GABA cannot enter neurons that do not release it, and in preventing uptake into non-neuronal tissue. The degree of binding of labelled substances to isolated membranes prepared from different brain areas can also be indicative of the likelihood of receptors for it occurring in those areas and for its function there.

Uptake

Although this is required for the localisation of labelled NT for autoradiography the mere demonstration of its existence in one brain area, compared to another, is also indicative of terminals in that area which normally take up and release the NT.

Response of neuron

Some idea of the site of release and therefore the location of a particular NT terminal can be obtained by determining the pattern of responsive-

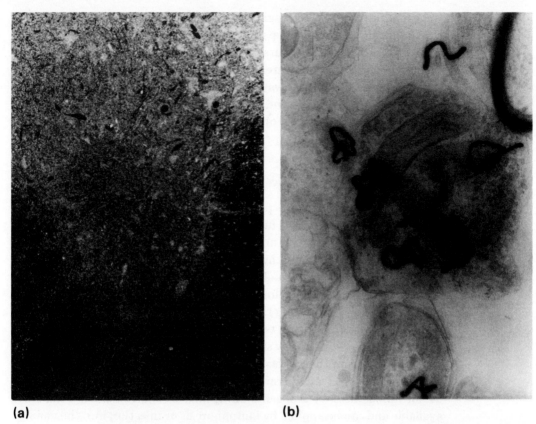

(a)   **(b)**

Fig. 2.1. Autoradiography of [^{3}H]-glycine in cat spinal cord after perfusion down the central canal of the anaesthetised animal. Cord fixed *in situ*. (a) Light microscopy. Note concentration of label (white area) in gray matter and cell bodies. Magnification: ×126. Development time: 6 months. (b) Electron microscope autoradiogram of glycine (black lines) over terminals (inhibitory?) with flat vesicles. Magnification: ×46 500. Development time: 2 months. (For details see Dennison *et al.* 1976.)

ness of neurons to its iontophoretic application. Whilst a neuron may well respond to a NT that is not normally released onto it and although all neurons seem to respond to most amino acids, there is some correlation between the degree of responsiveness of neurons to a NT and its physiological disposition. Unfortunately the effectiveness of a NT applied at a site where it is released from terminals and has an endogenous function can be reduced considerably in comparison with the activity of other substances simply by its uptake into the appropriate terminals.

Mapping neurotransmitter pathways

Not neurotransmitter specific

Pathways are normally traced by the use of horse-radish peroxidase. This is taken up by nerve terminals in the area to which it is applied and then travels antidromically (retrograde) up the axon to the cell body. Here it can be visualised and so the pathway, or at least its beginning and end, is traced. This does not, of course, tell you which NT is involved. Similarly lesioning (or ablating) an area which contains the neuronal cell bodies (origin) of a nervous pathway will be accompanied by degeneration of their axons and terminals and so by looking for such changes in different brain areas the distribution of neuronal pathways from the lesion can be mapped.

Neurotransmitter specific

If lesioning procedures are performed in conjunction with one of the measures of NT presence or function as outlined above, then it is possible to establish, by a reduction in the appropriate measure, which NT was used by the degenerating pathway (Fig. 2.2). This approach can be further refined if the NT can be visualised histochemically and some (or all) of it is formed in the cell body before being transported down the axon. In this case, after ligating or cutting the axon (axotomy), it will be possible to actually see a loss of NT distal to the lesion and its accumulation, especially at the lesion, on the cell body side. This is how monoamine pathways have been mapped from their subcortical nuclei (see Chapter 7).

One important way of confirming a particular NT pathway is by the use of antagonists. If a specific antagonist of the NT being studied is available and can be applied by iontophoresis or injection into the vicinity of the synapse being studied, then it should block the effects of any stimulated input to the area which uses that NT. Unfortunately it is not always easy to achieve the appropriate concentration of antagonist in relation to that of the NT released at the synapse to obtain a clear effect. Also it needs to be established that the input is a monosynaptic one and that the antagonist is not affecting an interneuron.

It may seem somewhat surprising that measures of NT uptake can be used to locate pathways but it has been shown that ablation of certain areas of the motor cortex leads to a loss of specific glutamate uptake in the striatum, which is indicative of a cortico-striatal pathway. The uptake mechanism has other uses. Certain neurotoxins such as 6-hydroxydopamine and 5,7-dihydroxytryptamine are taken up by catecholamine and 5-HT neurons respectively and cause degeneration of the whole neuron. Another less specific toxin is kainic acid which destroys cell bodies, possibly by overstimulated or increased Ca^{2+} influx and can therefore be used to remove intrinsic neurons in particular areas without affecting afferent terminals. Thus the loss of binding sites in a brain area after kainic acid is indicative of their post- rather than presynaptic location.

Brain imaging

There is one experimental approach to the study of neurotransmitter function that has probably advanced more in man than in animals and

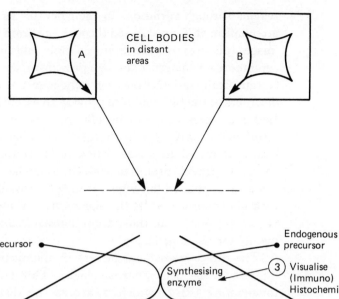

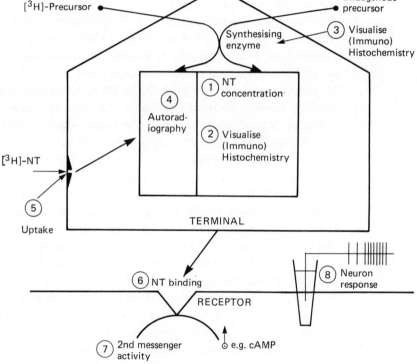

Fig. 2.2. Schematic representation of the methods (1–8) for localising and mapping the distribution of neurotransmitters and their pathways in the central nervous system. If measurements made by procedures 1–5 decrease following lesion of neurons in or axons from A but not B, then the terminals are likely to be those of axons that originate in A. Such lesions will not affect measures 6, 7 and 8, although they may tend to increase with time (denervation supersensitivity). If an antagonist blocks the response to stimulation of A but not B then the nerves probably originate in A.

that is the visualisation (imaging) of brain structures and chemicals *in situ*. Certainly the stimulus has come from clinical studies. Such neuro-imaging began just over a decade ago with the use of X-ray computer tomography (CT). This procedure distinguishes between different brain regions through variations in their density as measured by the varying attenuation of X-rays passed through the brain at different angles. A clear image (picture) of the brain is only obtained after very elaborate computerised analysis but it can provide precise details on the position of certain brain lesions that not only may be correlated with particular disorders of the CNS but also provide an essential guide for neurosurgery. Better pictures can now be obtained by the use of nuclear magnetic resonance (NMR) which utilises the signals given out from the many hydrogen nuclei in tissue, when it is irradiated with radiofrequency energy, to provide proton images. Other nuclei, such as $[^{31}P]$, $[^{28}Na]$, $[^{13}C]$, can also be studied but whilst it may be possible to measure brain ATP with phosphorous NMR the signals from these nuclei are much weaker (10^4 to 10^5 fold) than those from hydrogen, and NMR (like CT) is used mainly for anatomical studies.

The direct assessment of certain chemicals in the brain is of more interest to the neuropharmacologist. This relies on positron emission tomography (PET) which measures the distribution of a previously administered positron emitting isotope like $[^{15}O]$, $[^{13}N]$, $[^{11}C]$ and $[^{12}F]$ all of which have short half lives (2, 10, 20 and 110 min respectively). Each positive electron emitted from such relatively unstable isotopes collides within a few millimetres with a negative electron and their resulting mutual annihilation yields two gamma rays at 180° to each other which are picked up by gamma detectors arranged around the subject's head. Only rays arriving coincidentally at diametrically opposed detectors are counted and the level of detected emission reflects the concentration of ligand. Of course a low level of emission will be detected throughout the brain from the presence of the labelled substance and its metabolites in the blood and extracellular fluid, as well as that non-specifically located in all neuronal and glial tissue. Such background activity must be distinguished from more specific labelling. With due allowance for this fact PET has two basic uses in studying neurotransmitter function.

1 *Localising specific (NT) terminals.* After its injection a labelled precursor should be taken up and detected in appropriate nerve terminals (and possibly cell bodies) so that the intensity of emission reflects the density of innervation. Using this procedure it has been possible to show that very little $[^{18}F]$-fluorodopa is concentrated in the striatum of Parkinsonian patients compared with normals. Whether the label remains on dopa or is transferred to DA will not greatly affect the result since both will label DA neurons.

2 *Detecting NT receptors.* The injection and subsequent detection of an appropriately labelled ligand can give an indication of the density of the receptors to which it is bound. $[^{76}Br]$-bromospiperone has been used in this way to label and measure DA (D_2) receptors in schizophrenics (see Chapter 18). As with any binding study the validity of the approach depends on the specificity of the ligand for its receptor, i.e. it must show receptor selectivity and minimal non-specific binding. Of course there will

always be background activity as mentioned above but the extent of specific binding may be gauged by comparing the density of emission in any area where the NT is likely to function (e.g. striatum for DA) with that from one where it is not (e.g. cerebellum). The difference between these two levels should in fact increase as unbound drug is lost (excreted). To determine the precise number of receptors and see if that varies from brain to brain (e.g. between normal and schizophrenic) is somewhat more difficult. Normally the estimation of receptor number requires a measure of specific binding at two or more ligand concentrations under equilibrium conditions (see Chapter 4). This will clearly be difficult *in vivo*, not least because the effect of different doses may be unacceptable to the patient, but attempts have been made to achieve it and references are given to some reviews of this work (Frost 1986; Raichie 1986, Trimble 1986). It must also be remembered that unlike the membrane preparations used for *in vitro* binding studies much of the binding *in vivo* can be to presynaptic receptors and uptake sites.

Methods of studying the release of neurotransmitters

Although experiments may be performed *in vitro* or *in vivo* with a variety of preparations of varying degrees of complexity and physiological function, there are basically three components to any study of NT release. They are; **1** stimulation, **2** collection and **3** measurement. A further requirement may be the need to show that the release is calcium dependent.

Stimulation

Release may be evoked by:
1 chemicals, e.g. veratridine, which opens Na^{+2} channels
2 high levels (20–100 mM) of extracellular K^+ to produce general depolarisation of neurons
3 field stimulation between appropriately applied or implanted electrodes
4 electrical stimulation of defined neural pathways
5 physiological stimuli.
Procedures **1**, **2** and **3** can obviously only be used to show that a substance is releasable from neural tissue. They cannot be used to activate specific neurons or pathways.

Collection

This depends very much on the type of preparation being used but either some part of the CNS is taken out and maintained *in vitro*, just like an isolated organ, or the CNS is perfused *in situ* by introducing various cannulae into it. Commonly used preparation are outlined below.

Measurement

There are two approaches:

Exogenous neurotransmitters

In these studies the tissue is preloaded *in vitro* or *in vivo* with labelled NT (or its precursor), which is assumed to be taken up and released. This has been much used for studying the release of the amino acids and monoamines and depends very much on the specificity of the uptake process. The presumed NT may go into glia as well as nerve terminals and could go into and be released from nerves for which it is not the endogenous NT, especially if non-specific stimuli (**1–3** above) are being used. Also it assumes that the labelled NT exchanges and mixes with its endogenous counterpart and is released from the appropriate NT pool. Despite these problems this approach has the advantage of great simplicity and sensitivity since labelled NT can be detected by liquid scintillation counting at lower concentrations than achieved by most chemical methods. Unfortunately only one NT is usually studied at a time and so the data obtained are limited and interrelationships can be missed. A number of labelled amino acids can be produced from labelled glucose but since they will all contain the same label it is necessary to separate them by some form of chromotography before counting. This highlights another problem with labelled studies, namely that it is generally just the label [^{14}C] or [^{3}H] that is measured and in many cases no evidence is presented that the label has remained on the NT being studied, rather than on a metabolite or another NT. Thus without blocking its degradation, much of any labelled glutamate can end up as labelled GABA or glutamine.

A further problem centres on the fact that the proportion of labelled to endogenous NT released (specific activity) varies with time as the labelled NT mixes with more firmly bound NT or is depleted by use. This also makes it difficult to achieve repeated stimulations (releases) as the tissue runs out of labelled NT (Fig. 2.5).

Endogenous neurotransmitters

These measurements clearly require very sensitive assay procedures. They can be either biological, e.g. ACh on dorsal wall muscle of the leech (detection level 1 nM) or chemical, e.g. fluorescent detection of monoamines. The development of high pressure liquid chromatography (HPLC) and gas chromatography, as well as radioimmunoassays for the larger molecule peptides, has provided sensitive methods that will become more widely used. The value of HPLC is that it can be used to separate and detect a whole range of NTs, e.g. monoamines or amino acids and their metabolites (see Fig.2.3), so that their interrelationship can be studied. Of course this has to be avoided in radioimmunoassays when specificity of the antibody for the particular NT (peptide) being studied is

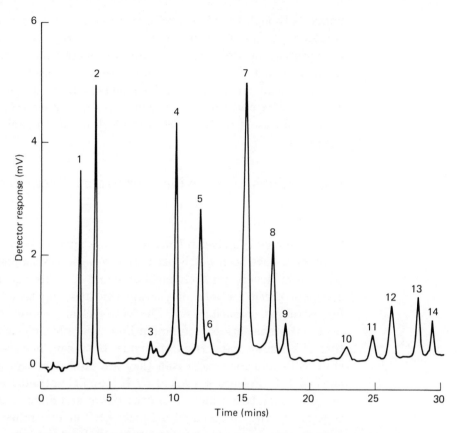

Fig. 2.3. Release of amino acids from cortical slices exposed to 50 mM K$^+$. Measurements by HPLC and fluorescence detection after reaction of amino acids with o-phthalaldehyde (see Farrrant *et al.* (1987). 1, aspartate. 2, glutamate. 3, asparagine. 4, serine. 5, glutamine. 6, histidine. 7, homoserine-internal standard. 8, glycine. 9, threonine. 10, arginine. 11, taurine. 12, alanine. 13, GABA. 14, tyrosine. Glutamate concentration is almost 1 pmol/μl which represents a release rate of 30 pmol/min/mg wet tissue.

of prime importance. One interesting technique combines both radio-labelled and endogenous forms of the same NT. In this the level of an endogenous NT in a sample (perfusate, CSF) is estimated by the ability of the NT to displace its labelled counterpart from a membrane preparation, as in a normal *in vitro* binding assay.

Preservation of the NT is of utmost importance in any release study. Generally, released NT is rapidly metabolised or taken up into nerve or glia and such processes may need to be blocked before sufficient NT escapes from the synapses to be detected. This introduces an important concept. All release studies (except perhaps voltammetry — see below) measure the overflow and not the amount of NT which is actually released. This overflow may not be detectable unless the NT can be preserved. Thus it is impossible to detect ACh, by biological procedures anyway, without stopping its hydrolysis by cholinesterase. Similarly the efflux of NA can be increased dramatically by blocking its neuronal uptake although in this instance the resulting increase in the synaptic concentration of NA can activate α_2-adrenoreceptors mediating auto-inhibition of release and so be counterproductive unless an α_2 antagonist is also included. Clearly the use of a variety of drugs to increase overflow can complicate any analysis and in some instances, as with DA release, it may be easier and safer to measure its metabolites (HVA or DOPAC) rather than use a range of drugs to block uptake, metabolism and auto receptors.

Preparations for studying neurotransmitter release

In vitro

Synaptosomes (pinched off nerve endings) prepared by centrifugation techniques have been widely used, as have various slice preparations. The latter may be very small chopped up cubes (0.1 mm square) of tissue or complete sliced sections of varying thickness up to 0.5 mm of cord, hippocampus, cerebellum etc. The 'cubes' clearly retain very little if any neuronal organisation or function and their physiological validity, like that of synaptosomes, is questionable. Both can, however, take up and store NTs and for this reason they are almost always preloaded with labelled NT. Release is evoked by K^+ or field stimulation in specially designed chambers which retain the tissue and allow it to be bathed or superfused with oxygenated artificial CSF at controlled temperatures. Despite the simplicity of these systems NT release can be shown to be Ca^{++} dependent and they have been much used to demonstrate the modification (generally inhibition) of the release of one NT by other NTs or drugs. The large 'proper' slices of CNS tissue are also used for electrophysiological studies (see Chapter 3); they retain some anatomical organisation as well as physiological function, and specific pathways may be stimulated. Again labelled NTs are often used but sensitive assay systems now make it possible to measure the release of endogenous NT (Fig. 2.3). Another *in vitro* system is the hemisected frog or young rat spinal cord which can be maintained *in vitro*, just like ganglia, for several hours. In all these cases there is a balance between the size (thickness) of the preparation for preserving structure and the difficulty of irrigating all the neurons adequately from the surface. Cultured cells may also be used in release studies.

In vivo

These systems have the advantage that functional synaptic activity is retained and may permit the use of physiological stimuli. Unfortunately the procedures that have to be used to obtain perfusates may cause considerable tissue damage and can sometimes merely create *in vitro* conditions *in situ*. There are basically two approaches (Fig. 2.4). Either

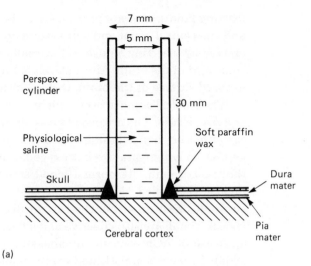

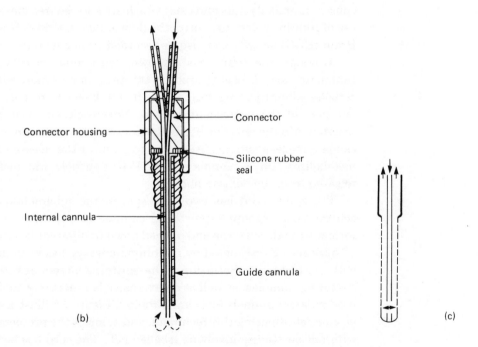

Fig. 2.4. Diagram of some cannulae used for the collection of perfusates *in vivo*.
(a) Cortical cup. The cup size obviously varies with the animal on which it is used. For
the rat the overall diameter is 6–7 mm and a common flow rate is 50 μl min^{-1} (b) Push-
pull cannula. The end of the guide cannula can be adjusted relative to that of the internal
cannula to obtain the correct fluid flow. Overall diameter of tip is about 0.75 mm and flow
rates of 10–20 μl min^{-1} are used. (c) The tip of a dialysis probe, which can otherwise
resemble a push-pull cannula, expanded to show dialysis tubing (broken line) around a
steel cannula through the base of which fluid can flow out and then up and over the
membrane. The length of membrane below the probe support can be altered (1–10 mm)
to suit the size of animal and the brain area being studied. Flow rates are normally below
5 μl min^{-1}.

existing fluid spaces are perfused, e.g. the ventricular spaces in the brain, and the central canal and sub-arachnoid space in the cord, or a space is created by inserting a push-pull cannula or length of dialysis tubing into some part of the brain. Alternatively a small cylinder can be placed on the exposed surface of the brain; the so-called cortical cup.

The cortical cup has been widely used, especially for the study of ACh and AA release. The arrangement is shown in Fig. 2.4. The artificial CSF can either be changed totally from time to time or superfused. It must be kept at body temperature but oxygenation should not be necessary since the tissue retains its normal blood supply. A release of endogenous or preloaded labelled NT can be evoked by K^+, current passed between electrodes near or within the cup, or distinct nerve stimulation. Physiological stimuli are also effective and a flashing light can be shown to evoke a release of ACh even in the anaesthetised animal (Collier & Mitchell 1966). In more sophisticated arrangements the cup can by fixed to the surface of the skull and the release of NTs monitored continuously in conscious animals (rats and cats) which are allowed free movement by the use of rotating valves to control the flow of fluid (Dodd & Bradford 1974). Brain (EEG) activity can also be recorded from electrodes in the cup.

Although the brain has its own ventricular spaces that can be cannulated for perfusion purposes, this procedure is more widely used for actually administrating drugs, since it is not easy to restrict fluid flow to one part of the ventricular system. Nevertheless a push-pull cannula inserted into the anterior horn of one lateral ventricle comes close to the caudate nucleus and has been used to monitor the release of DA and its metabolites and a cannula in the IVth ventricle will pick up GABA released from the dentate nucleus.

The spinal cord has two fluid spaces, the subarachnoid space and central canal. A simple polythene cannula can be introduced into the former from the cisterna and pushed down to different levels. The release of substance P, estimated by radioimmunoassay has been demonstrated with this technique. Perfusion of the central canal requires both input and collecting cannulae, as well as an extensive laminectomy, and can only be used in larger animals (cats and rabbits). Figure 2.5 illustrates a study of glycine release using this technique and some of the problems associated with release studies involving labelled NT. The cord has been preloaded with $[^{14}C]$-glycine and then perfused with artificial CSF whilst monitoring the efflux of label. When this had levelled off, both the sciatic and femoral nerves were stimulated to activate not only the orthodromic input but also the antidromic pathway to Renshaw cells, which are thought to release glycine. This failed to produce an increased efflux, probably due to re-uptake of released glycine, but when this was reduced by the non-specific amino acid uptake blocker para-hydroxymercuribenzoate (p-HMB), there was not only increased spontaneous efflux but the stimulus now evoked a measurable release. A second period of stimulation had very little effect, probably due to the depletion of labelled glycine.

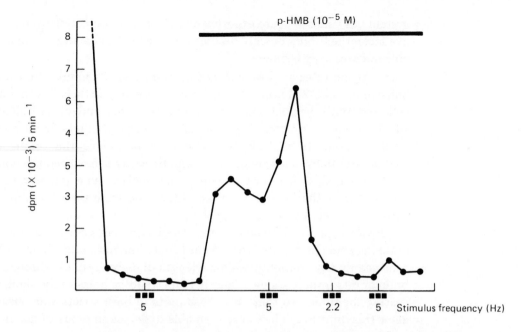

Fig. 2.5. Release of [^{14}C]-glycine into the perfused central canal of the halothane anaesthetised cat. The cord had been preloaded with [^{14}C]-glycine (1 μM). Each point represents the radioactivity (dpm) in a 5 min sample. Changing the perfusion medium to normal artificial CSF, with no labelled glycine in it, saw a rapid fall in the level of [^{14}C]-glycine in the perfusate as it was washed out of the extracellular spaces. Stimulation (■) (5 Hz for 3 × 2 min periods) of both femoral and sciatic nerves to activate orthodromic and antidromic inputs to the cord failed to alter efflux. Addition of $10^{-}-5$ M p-hydroxymercuribenzoate (pHMB), to block the uptake of glycine, caused an increased efflux and stimulation then produced a release. Subsequent stimuli were less effective probably due to the depletion of label. (See Jordan & Webster (1971).)

Release may be studied in a specific brain area by inserting a push-pull cannula into it with a micromanipulator using stereotaxic guidelines. This cannula simply consists of two tubes either adjacent to one another or more commonly one within the other, with fluid pumped down the central tube and collected under slight negative pressure from the outer (Fig. 2.4). They are of necessity somewhat large (1 mm o.d.) and may cause damage during insertion and become blocked. Despite their size they only perfuse a small area and they require backing from sensitive detection methods, or the use of preloaded labelled NT. Correctly positioned they can collect from a defined area receiving a particular NT input and may be implanted chronically.

A short loop of thin dialysis tubing can be fixed so as to link but protrude from adjacent tubes of a push-pull cannula, by which it is inserted into the brain. In this way fluid is simply passed through the tubing rather than into an artificial space, as with the push-pull cannula itself and, provided the NT can pass through the wall of the dialysis tubing, it can be collected without fear of blockage or contamination by blood. Unfortunately only a proportion of NT passes through the tubing and whilst the

NEUROTRANSMITTER PATHWAYS AND RELEASE

system has value in acute experiments, if sensitive detection systems are available, the tubing quickly becomes covered with glia and so impermeable in chronic experiments.

Perfusion rates are low with both systems, e.g. 20 μl min^{-1} for push-pull cannula and 2 μl min^{-1} for dialysis probes: very little NT is therefore collected. With the push-pull cannula (which is open ended) the pull must equal the push to prevent tissue damage and sensitive and reliable pumps must be used. In dialysis the fluid does not leave the tubing and so it is essentially a simple push system. Recently it has been possible to produce a dialysis cannula in which the dialysis tube (membrane) in essence forms the lower part of an outer concentric tube (or cannula). This reduces its overall size (Fig. 2.4).

Obviously more NT would be recovered with dialysis if a longer length of tubing could be exposed to nervous tissue. Imperato and Chiara (1984) achieved this by simply threading a length of dialysis tubing through the brain of rats from one side to another, via trephine holes in the skull, and coating the tubing so that only those parts in both striata were clear to allow free diffusion. They were then able to detect an efflux of dopamine and its metabolites from the striata.

Thus there are many methods available but few detailed studies of the release of any one NT at a particular site under varying physiological and pharmacological conditions, probably because the *in vivo* systems needed to achieve this are costly and difficult to establish. Also the methods used to study release vary from NT to NT. Early work on ACh release in the cortex could call on a large endogenous source plus proven methods of blocking degradation as well as a sensitive bioassay and so studies were performed *in vivo* using cortical cups and varied natural and other stimuli. Bioassays were not sensitive enough for monoamines and even with more sensitive chemical procedures the diverse nature of their pathways (except for DA in the striatum) meant that areas of concentrated release, in which a reasonable amount of NT could be detected, were difficult to find; even though an extensive innervation could be activated by electrodes placed in appropriate brainstem nuclei. For these and other reasons (see below) NA and 5-HT release has not been adequately studied directly in the CNS although there is much data on changes in their levels under various conditions. With the inhibitory amino acids like GABA and glycine, which are found predominantly in interneurons (although there are some GABA pathways, like that from the striatum to substantia nigra), their release requires somewhat crude field stimulation to activate the interneurons.

Turnover

Most of the above procedures permit the study of NT release in the short term. In many cases, especially when studying drug effects, one is not so much interested in which NT can be released from which neurons but how its release (perhaps in the brain as a whole) changes with time, i.e. on its utilisation or turnover (production, release, action and removal).

There are a number of ways to demonstrate and measure the turnover of a NT (see Pycock & Taberner 1981) The most obvious would be to determine the rate of production of its metabolites, on the assumption that the more NT there is released the more metabolites there will be formed. Obviously the metabolite must exist long enough to be measured. This is not the case with ACh since it is rapidly broken down to choline, which is then taken back into cholinergic nerves; whilst amino acids like glutamate and GABA are taken up and incorporated into biochemical pathways (see Chapter 11). Fortunately the metabolites of the monoamines have a long half-life and since they are not re-incorporated into further synthesis their measurement is much easier. If more than one metabolite is produced then in some studies, as when measuring the effect of a drug on NT turnover, it is really necessary to measure all the metabolites. This is because the drug might increase the production of one metabolite, not by increasing the turnover of the NT but by blocking the formation of other metabolites. Turnover studies are also most applicable to the monamines since, as discussed above, the wide distribution of their nerve endings does not provide a site of concentrated release to measure it directly and it is assumed to be of a slow nature. Consequently because many of the drugs used in behavioural disorders affect monoamine systems, their effects on the long term turnover of mono-amines are of equal interest to any effects on localised release. There are, in fact, many ways of manipulating the synthesis and metabolism of monoamines and these can be used to measure turnover (Fig. 2.6).

1 Block synthesis of the NT from its precursor. If the NT cannot be formed then the rate at which it is lost from the CNS gives a measure of turnover. The quicker it disappears the more it is being used. Blocking the synthesis of dopa from tyrosine will lead to depletion of DA and NA at a rate dependent on their utilisation. Loss of NA alone can be traced following block of its synthesis from DA.

2 Labelled precursor. Inject labelled precursor, e.g. $[^3H]$-tyrosine and measure rate of production of $[^3H]$-DA, $[^3H]$-NA and their metabolites. Measurements of the rate of loss of the labelled NT itself, after injection into the CNS, may not measure turnover since the NT can be lost without being incorporated into nerves and utilised.

3 Voltammetry. This might be more accurately described as *in vivo* electrochemistry. In it an appropriately coated carbon electrode serves as an oxidising agent to the hydroxy group(s) of a catechol (DA and NA) or indollamine (5-HT), which results in a transfer of electrons that is measured as current. The size of this current is proportional to the amount of amine oxidised. Since compounds vary in the ease with which they are oxidised and as the activity of the electrode as an oxidising agent depends on its energy state, i.e. the potential applied to it, the oxidation of compounds will vary with the potential of the electrode. Thus by applying

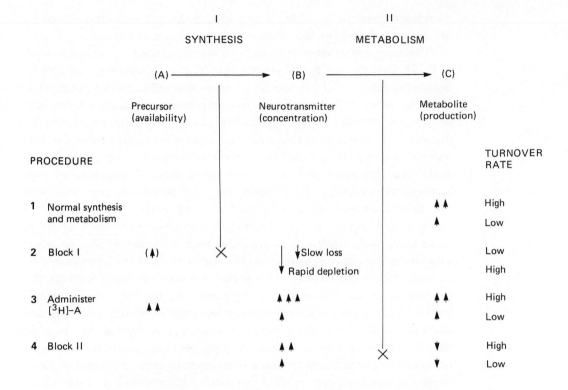

Fig. 2.6. Approaches to the study of neurotransmitter turnover. The NT (B) is formed from its precursor A and gives metabolites (C). Enzymes control its synthesis (I) and metabolism (II). Normally (I), with no drug modification of these stages, the turnover may be more rapid for one NT ↑↑ than another ↑. Blocking synthesis (2) may cause a rapid depletion of NT if turnover is high. Administration of labelled precursor (3) may lead to a rapid appearance of labelled NT if turnover is high. Also blocking NT metabolism (4) will lead to marked accumulation of NT if turnover (utilisation) is high.

an increasing voltage (up to 1 volt) to the electrode it is possible to record the oxidation of different compounds (as distinct current measurements) at different voltages. Unfortunately compounds of similar chemical structure oxidise with comparable ease and at a similar electrode potential so that NA, DA and 5-HT and their metabolites (as well as ascorbic acid) cannot be easily separated. Thus the method is best suited to studies in brain areas where one amine predominates (e.g. DA in the striatum) but the electrodes are relatively small (<10 μM) and can be inserted in discrete brain loci and combined with recording electrodes. When used in this way they record much higher extracellular concentrations of the NT than would be obtained by more conventional methods of monitoring NT release, possibly because of the proximity of the electrode to the site of concentrated release. Although the technique can be used to measure amines (if metabolism is stopped) and their metabolites, the electrode has a limited life (2–3 weeks) and so even though they may be implanted for chronic studies they really monitor release rather than long term turnover. For more detail see Marsden (1984) and Adams and Marsden (1982).

References and further reading

Adams RN & Marsden CA (1982) Electrochemical detection methods for monoamine measurements *in vitro* and *in vivo*. In: Iversen LL Iversen SD & Snyder SH (eds) *Handbook of Psychopharmacology*. Vol 15. Plenum Press, New York. pp. 1–74.

Bradley P (1975) *Methods in Brain Research*. John Wiley, Chichester.

Collier B & Mitchell JF (1966) The central release of acetlycholine during stimulation of the visual pathway. *J. Physiol.* **184**, 239–54.

Dennison ME, Jordan CC & Webster RA (1976) Distribution and localisation of tritiated amino acids by autoradiography in the cat spinal cord *in vivo*. *J. Physiol.* **258**, 55–6 P.

Dodd DR & Bradford HF (1974) Release of amino acids from the chronically superfused mammalian cerebral cortex. *J. Neurochem.* **23**, 284–92.

Farrant M, Zia-Gharib F & Webster RA (1987). Automated pre-column derivatization with o-phthaldehyde for the determination of neurotransmitter amino acids using reversed-phase liquid chromatography. *J. Chromatography* **417**, 385–90.

Frost JJ (1986) Imaging neuronal biochemistry by emission computed tomography. *Trends Pharmacol. Sci.* **7**, 490–6.

Hökfelt T & Ljungdahl A (1975) Uptake mechanisms as a basis for the histochemical identification and tracing of transmitter-specific neuron populations. In: Cowan WM & Cuenos M (eds) *The Use of Axonal Transport for Studies of Neuronal Connectivity*. Elsevier, Amsterdam. pp. 249–305.

Imperato A & Di Chiaro G (1984) Trans-striatal dialysis coupled to reverse phase high performance liquid chromotography with electrochemical detection: a new method for the study of the *in vivo* release of endogenous dopamine and metabolites. *J. Neurosci.* **4**, 966–77.

Iversen LL & Schon F (1973) The use of autoradiographic techniques for the identification and mapping of transmitter-specific neurons in CNS. *In*: Mangel A & Segal D (eds) *New Concepts in Transmitter Regulation*. Plenum Press, New York. 153–93.

Jones EG & Hartman BK (1978) Recent advances in neuroanatomical methodology. *Ann. Rev. Neurosci.* **1**, 215–96.

Jordan CC & Webster RA (1971) Release of acetylcholine and [^{14}C]-glycine from the cat spinal cord *in vivo*. *Br. J. Pharmac.* **43**, 411 P.

Marsden CA (1984) Measurements of neurotransmitter release *in vivo*. IBRO Handbook series, *Methods in Neuroscience*. John Wiley, Chichester.

Ottersen OP & Storm-Mathiesen J (1984) Neurons containing or accumulating transmitter amino acids. In: Björkland A, Hökfelt T & Kuhar MJ (eds) *Handbook of Chemical Neuroanatomy. Classical Transmitters and Transmitter Receptors in the CNS*. Vol. 3. Part 11. Elsevier, Amsterdam. pp. 141–246.

Pycock CJ & Taberner PV (1981) PP. 141–246. *Central Neurotransmitter Turnover*. Croom Helm, London.

Raichie ME (1986) Neuroimaging. *Trends Neurosci.* **9**, 525–9.

Storm-Mathiesen J, Leukes AK, Bor AT, Vaaland JL, Edminson P, Haug FMS & Ottersen OP (1983) First visualization of glutamate and GABA in neurones by immunohisto-chemistry. *Nature* **301**, 517–20.

Trimble MR (1986) *New Brain Imaging. Techniques in Phychopharmacology*. Oxford University Press, Oxford.

3 Electrophysiological methods in neuropharmacology

T.W. STONE

Electrophysiological methods for studying the nervous system are among the most useful techniques since they generally involve procedures which yield immediate answers to particular questions: the experimenter does not have to wait for hours for radioactive or biochemical analyses, or for weeks in anatomical studies of neuronal degeneration or autoradiography. Even more important, however, is the fact that electrophysiology usually involves the use of relatively intact tissues rather than disrupted tissue such as synaptosomes (nerve terminals), broken membrane preparations, or purified enzyme systems as in most biochemical studies. It is often impossible to know what relationship these severely abnormal preparations have to the normal nervous system.

Electrophysiological techniques range from those in which the activity of the entire brain is monitored in a conscious animal or human down to studies in which single ionic channels are studies in isolated patches of cell membrane.

Electroencephalography

For electroencephalographic (EEG) investigations, electrodes are fixed onto, or sometimes implanted through, the skull so that the electrical activity of the brain, and particularly the cortex, can be followed (Spehlmann 1985). In some cases the electrical activity of other brain regions is monitored by positioning the electrode tips stereotaxically (at coordinates determined from one of the several atlases available) within the target area of the brain. The records obtained are frequently difficult to interpret by the untrained eye but are useful for assessing the overall state of activity of an animal and the effects of drugs on the degree of arousal or sedation. The EEG of a resting animal for example consists usually of high amplitude (several hundred microvolts) slow wave activity whereas the alert and attentive brain tends to produce very low amplitude (microvolts) high frequency activity. The latter type of EEG is referred to as 'desynchronised' (Spehlmann 1985; Halliday et al. 1987).

EEG recordings are most often valuable in the study of the human brain since it can be a non-invasive technique and characteristic patterns can be recognised by experienced observers. Some of the most striking of these include very large amplitude, relatively high frequency 'spikes' which are detectable in electrodes placed close to the site of an epileptic focus. By examining the EEG taken from electrodes situated at different positions on the skull surface it is therefore often possible to localise the site of origin of epileptic abnormalities prior to surgery.

Another example of the use of the EEG is in the testing of anti-convulsant drugs which tend to depress the rhythmic waves produced in response to a sequence of flash stimuli.

The EEG is also particularly useful for monitoring the progress of sleep and therefore drug effects on sleep mechanisms. Normal sleep EEGs tend to be synchronised whereas dreaming sleep, which is associated with rapid eye movements (REM) is accompanied by a desynchronised rhythm. Since, as just noted, this is the pattern normally found in the waking state, REM sleep is often referred to as *paradoxical sleep.*

Evoked potentials

An extension of the EEG procedure is to deliver repeated stimuli to a subject and record the resulting electrical change in the brain. The usual type of response is a reasonably stereotyped, relatively low frequency waveform known as the evoked potential. This would be recorded of course in the appropriate area of brain, such as the occipital cortex following a visual stimulus, or the somatosensory cortex following a cutaneous stimulus etc. In animals, especially anaesthetised animals, the evoked potential may be clearly apparent in successive oscilloscope sweeps of an EEG record (triggered in synchrony with the stimulus). In man, however, the response is usually submerged beneath the complex activity of the waking brain's activity. For this reason evoked potential recordings are often connected to an electronic means of averaging the responses. Thus the summation, or averaging, of many evoked responses will emphasise the reproducible components of the evoked potential whilst flattening out the background EEG and random activity. Again these potentials are useful in animal studies for detecting sedation or other altered states of wakefulness and in man are frequently of diagnostic value since changes in the amplitude or latency of the evoked responses may indicate the onset of some neuronal disorders such as multiple sclerosis (Halliday *et al.* 1987).

Clearly both EEG and evoked potential recordings can be made on an acute basis in a conscious or anaesthetised animal or subject, or chronically over a period of many weeks or months following the implantation of suitable electrodes onto the brain. This confers many advantages for drug testing and analysis since the same animal can be used as its own control and different drugs can be used over a long period of time to compare directly their effects in the same preparation.

Single cell recordings

A more refined method for measuring the activity of the central nervous system is to use microelectrodes with a tip diameter of between 1 and 20 microns. Because of their high electrical resistance these electrodes record the activity of individual neurons or small groups of neurons around the conducting tip. Again, such recordings can be made in conscious animals following the chronic implantation of an electrode, or in anaesthetised animals. The effects of drugs injected peripherally in behaviourally effective doses can then be assessed by measuring and recording the firing rate and/or the pattern of firing of the cell(s) under study. It may be important, for example, to show that a suspected analgesic agent reduces the activation of dorsal horn neurons in the spinal cord in response to stimulation of C fibre afferent neurons, or potentially noxious cutaneous stimuli in anaesthetised animals (see Chapter 22).

Electrodes used for this purpose may be constructed from metals such as tungsten, which can be etched electrolytically or chemically to the tip size required or, alternatively, they can be made from glass capillaries pulled in a heating coil to produce very fine tips which may need to be broken slightly under microscopic control (Purves 1981). These latter pipette electrodes are then filled with a suitable conducting solution such as NaCl or KCl. All of these electrodes tend to have rather high resistances because of their small size, and so must be connected to an amplifier which itself has an input resistance several orders of magnitude greater.

Action potentials may be amplified and recorded directly either on an ultraviolet beam recorder, on photographic film or on magnetic tape. More usually the spikes are 'processed' in some way so that the potentials are counted and used to create records of spikes per second. It is also common to produce histograms of interspike intervals as an indication of firing patterns. If the neuronal responses to a particular pathway are of interest, an analysis of spike occurrences in small time 'bins' can be made by linking the analysis to the stimulation pulse. This yields a post-stimulus or peri-stimulus time histogram. It is akin to the averaging technique described earlier in that a number of sweeps are usually accumulated in order to emphasise small stimulus-linked excitatory or inhibitory responses which may not be clearly apparent within the background firing of a spontaneously active neuron (Fig. 3.1).

It is also frequently valuable to distinguish orthodromic and anti-dromic activation of cells in order to determine whether drug effects are being exerted primarily on the process of synaptic transmission (affecting transmitter release or its receptors) or directly upon the cell being monitored (producing depolarisation or hyperpolarisation). Synaptically evoked activity for example tends to yield spikes and postsynaptic potentials which vary slightly in latency whereas antidromic potentials have a fixed latency. Orthodromic activity tends not to follow stimulation rates of much more than about 20 Hz; antidromic spikes can follow stimulation at 200–300 Hz relatively easily. Finally, antidromic invasion can be identified most specifically by the 'collision test'. A spontaneously occurring spike is used to trigger the stimulating electrode. If the cell is be-

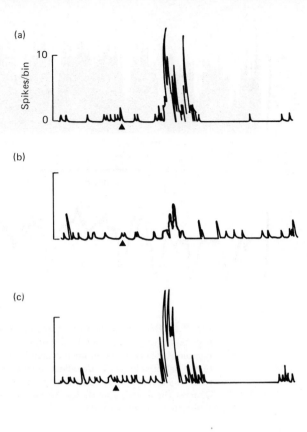

(a)

Spikes/bin

10

0

(b)

(c)

0   15 ms

Fig. 3.1. Peri-stimulus time histograms showing the type of the response seen after summating 128 sweeps of a slowly firing neuron excited by stimulation of an afferent pathway at the point indicated by the arrowhead (a). In (b) an amino acid antagonist, kynurenic acid, was applied by microiontophoresis and this clearly blocks activation of the cell. (c) shows recovery. Time calibration bar 15 ms. (MN Perkins & TW Stone, unpublished.)

ing activated antidromically, i.e. there are no synapses on the pathway, then the spontaneous and triggered spikes will collide and cancel each other out somewhere along the cell's axon. No response to the triggered stimulus would be seen.

Microiontophoresis

A further refinement of this technique is to combine the recording electrode with a micropipette consisting of one or more glass capillaries each of which has a tip diameter of around one micron and from which drugs can be applied into the immediate vicinity of the cell or cells being recorded. In most cases, substances which are soluble can then be ejected from the micropipette by passing the appropriate polarity of current through the solution: an outward going ('positive') current would eject cations such as acetylcholine whereas an inward ('negative') current causes the efflux of anions such as glutamate.

Drugs can of course be ejected in exactly the same way in order to examine their effects on the responses to locally applied neurotransmitters, and on the synaptically induced responses to stimulation of input

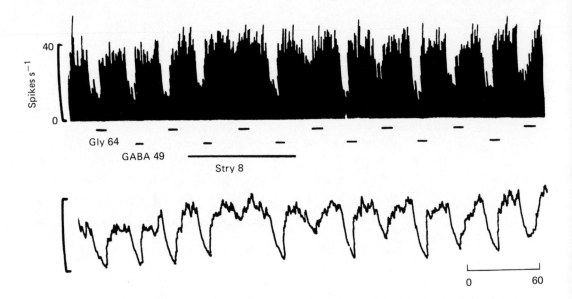

Fig. 3.2. Records of the firing rate of a spontaneously active neuron in response to the application of glycine (64 nA iontophoretic current) and GABA (49 nA) by microiontophoresis. Spontaneous activity is depressed by both agents but strychnine (8 nA) selectively blocks the effect of glycine. The two panels illustrate different means of recording cell firing rate. In the upper panel a spike integrator is reset every second, whereas the lower panel shows the responses seen via an instantaneous ratemeter. Time calibration bar: 60 seconds.

pathways. In this way the effects of drugs can be assessed for their pharmacological activities (Fig. 3.2) and, equally, compounds with a defined agonist or antagonist profile at transmitter receptors can be used to assess the identity of the transmitter released by a particular pathway of interest. One of the major criteria in transmitter identification has always been the ability to block the effects of synaptic activation and of the suspected transmitter in parallel.

The technique described above is known as *microiontophoresis* or *microelectrophoresis* (Stone 1985) although there are a number of variations upon the basic principle. For example, aqueous solutions in contact with a glass surface tend to have an overall positive charge and so passage of an outward current through the electrode to a distant ground reference will eject a very small volume of the total fluid. This is known as *electro-osmosis* and can be used to eject drugs which are only poorly soluble in solution, and therefore present only in small concentrations, or which are un-ionised and could not be ejected by the passage of current alone. Sometimes, use may also be made of the fact that some ions carry a hydration shell in which drugs molecules would be present. The ejection of sodium ions for example may be used in this way to increase the efflux of un-ionised molecules.

Finally, it is also possible to eject compounds from these micropipettes by applying a suitable pressure into the barrel (Stone 1985).

Clearly, microiontophoresis and its allied variants have a number of advantages in the study of neuropharmacology, since compounds are being applied directly to cells and therefore there is no uncertainty of access across the blood–brain barrier. Furthermore, it is possible to test a number of compounds over a short period of time without having to wait for the metabolism and removal of drugs from the animal. Indeed, in studies involving the peripheral administration of drugs, a different animal may be needed for each substance or dose to be tested. On the other hand by simply moving the iontophoretic electrode, it is possible to study many cells in the same animal.

Microiontophoresis also has disadvantages, however. For example, it is impossible to know accurately the amounts of substances ejected from the micropipettes and thus their local concentrations within the brain are uncertain. It is sometimes possible to calibrate electrodes by measuring their ability to release compounds at different currents *in vitro*, but this still leaves some uncertainty as to the distribution of the compounds when actually ejected within the brain. It is not possible therefore to perform conventional quantitative pharmacology constructing dose response curves, determining pA_2 values etc.; its use is largely confined to the qualitative examination of neuronal pharmacology (Fig. 3.2).

It is possible to combine these drug application techniques with intracellular recordings of neuronal or glial activity in order to further assess the effects of transmitters or drugs on membrane properties and ion channels. However, this technique is relatively difficult in the living animal because of movement artefacts introduced by cardiovascular and respiratory rhythms. For this reason such work is often carried out using isolated *in vitro* preparations of the central nervous system.

In vitro systems

As well as the greater mechanical stability of isolated brain tissue, *in vitro* techniques carry a number of other advantages (Kerkut & Wheal 1981). One is obviously the absence of any anaesthetic which often has unknown effects on the sensitivity of neurons to transmitters and drugs. Secondly, *in vitro* systems remove all problems of drug access such as the blood–brain barrier or the distribution of compounds into peripheral fat depots, and eliminate the complication of drug metabolism by peripheral tissues during the experiment.

Thirdly, it is possible to prepare slices of almost any portion of the brain for maintenance over periods of several hours in a small perfusion chamber. The effects of drugs can therefore be studied on any brain region with accurate localisation of the stimulating, iontophoretic and recording electrodes under visual guidance. This is a major advantage over the need for stereotaxis *in vivo* where the localisation of electrode tips may not be known until histology has been performed some time after the experiment.

In the same way specific pathways can often be stimulated electrically under visual control. The best examples of this are probably in hippocampal slices which are easily the most popular brain preparation for this type of work: the neurons are organised in discrete, clearly visible layers and orthodromic and antidromic activation of the cells can be performed at will by suitable placement of the stimulating electrodes.

Carrying this principle even further, it becomes possible *in vitro* to apply substances to different known parts of the cell surface, including the soma and portions of the dendritic tree, under visual control. This provides valuable information on the localisation of drug receptors which may be correlated with the presence of specific synaptic inputs in order to produce support for the identification of a particular transmitter being released by a neuronal pathway.

Next, it is possible in slice preparations to stabilise the incubation conditions or to manipulate these as desired. Thus, the oxygen tension, temperature, ionic concentrations in the medium etc. are now entirely under the experimenter's control. *In vivo*, parameters such as these may vary slightly during an experiment. Drug concentrations are also known accurately since they can be added to the bathing medium, and dose-response analyses become feasible. Of course, compounds can be applied iontophoretically also, if required for qualitative studies. A popular combination is to apply transmitter candidates iontophoretically whilst drugs of interest are perfused in the medium.

It is also possible to minimise indirect effects of compounds by suppressing synaptic transmission in low calcium, high magnesium solutions, or by adding tetrodotoxin, for example. This is obviously not feasible *in vivo* and it is frequently difficult to know whether drug effects are produced by direct actions on the cell being recorded or indirectly by affecting the uptake or release of other transmitters in the area.

Whenever possible, attempts are made to identify physiologically the cells being studied during the experiment. Some cells may respond only to certain types of sensory input or specific features of a sensory stimulus, for example. Others may give axons which form easily stimulated tracts such as the corticospinal tracts or thalamocortical radiations, and stimulation of these axons should permit identification of the cells of origin by the fact that they will be invaded antidromically.

As well as brain slice preparations, a popular system for studying CNS pharmacology is the isolated spinal cord since stimulation of the dorsal root will synaptically evoke ventral root activity which can be recorded with relatively coarse electrodes positioned on the roots, or microelectrodes can be used to record single units (Kudo 1978).

The effects of compounds on brain slices or spinal cord can also be assessed by measuring the standing potentials (DC potentials) between two parts of the preparation. A direct depolarisation or hyperpolarisation

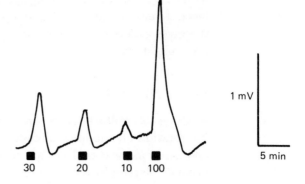

Fig. 3.3. Examples of DC recordings taken from a brain slice preparation to show the responses obtained to an excitatory amino acid applied as indicated by the black bars, and at concentrations of 10–100 μM. Calibration bars: 1 mV and 5 minutes (DAS Smith & NR Burton, unpublished.)

can then be detected simply by the direction of the DC shift. This is a relatively simple method, amenable to quantitative analyses, for screening large numbers of potentially useful drugs (Fig. 3.3).

Intracellular recordings

By making electrodes with submicron-sized tips, cells can be penetrated and records obtained of membrane potentials and synaptic potentials. If brief pulses of current are then passed through the recording electrode to ground, a transmembrane voltage change is seen which will vary with the membrane resistance (i.e. inversely with conductance). This provides a first indication of whether the net permeability of ions is increased or decreased. Some substances, such as GABA, may in some cells increase the membrane conductance for chloride without any change of membrane potential, since the chloride equilibrium potential is often close to resting potentials. Effects of GABA might be missed, therefore, if attention was paid only to voltage, not resistance changes. In an *in vitro* system, changes in the ionic concentration of the bathing medium and the use of substances blocking specific ionic channels may then yield more detailed clues as to the nature of the particular ions involved. It is by this means, for example, that we know that GABA often acts by increasing chloride permeability and that some excitatory amino acids increase sodium and calcium permeability.

The difficulty with such interpretations is that changes of membrane potential themselves may change some ionic permeabilities (voltage-sensitive channels). To circumvent this problem the technique of voltage-clamping was devised in which (ideally) two electrodes are inserted into a cell. The electronics are organised in such a way that any tendency for the membrane voltage to change is compensated instantly by a feedback system which passes current through the voltage clamp electrode. In other words, the membrane potential is held constant throughout the period of drug application. In this way the only change seen in the membrane is the change of current directly attributable to the drug. Again, in combination with suitable channel blocking agents (tetrodotoxin for sodium channels, tetraethylammonium or 4-aminopyridine for potassium channels, etc) this gives a more reliable indication of the involvement of ions in drug and transmitter action.

Single channel recording

Analysis of voltage noise in voltage clamp experiments can yield information on the ionic channels being opened but complex computer and mathematical analyses are required (McBurney 1983). Probably the ultimate electrophysiological technique is a method of observing activity in presumed individual ionic channels. This is often also known as 'patch-clamping' and involves applying relatively coarsely sized pipette tips very closely to the surface of a cell and then applying a negative pressure to the micropipette barrel. This causes, with experience, a very tight, very high resistance seal of the pipette tip to the cell surface. Agonist molecules within the solution in the pipette will then act on receptors in the membrane patch to open ionic channels, and if a low concentration of the agonist is used, these openings may be seen as discrete step jumps

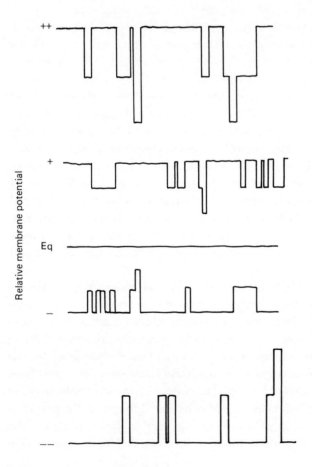

Fig. 3.4. Idealised records of single channel openings in a membrane patch containing two channels of differing conductances activated by the agonist. The step jumps of membrane current reflect the opening of one or both conductances. The conductance changes with membrane potential in the same way as other conductance events, for example it shows reversal at the equilibrium potential for the ion(s) involved. The duration of opening of many channels is around 1 ms.

of membrane current attributable to the opening of a single channel (Fig. 3.4). It is then possible to measure the mean open time and channel conductance due to the agonist action. Patch clamping is probably the most direct method we have of comparing the efficacy of different agonists in terms of their effects on ionic channels and has also led to many remarkable discoveries concerning drug action. Many drugs for example seem to act by interfering with the kinetics of channel opening or prolong the open time in response to an agonist.

Although many of these single cell techniques are carried out on brain slices, they may also be used to advantage in conjunction with cell cultures, where individual cells may be clearly distinguished and isolated from interfering influences of adjacent cells. Since such cells are normally used several days or weeks after isolation from the brain, however, the state of their development and differentiation, and their relationship to normal brain cells is often a matter of concern.

References

Halliday AM, Butler SR & Paul R (eds) (1987) *A Textbook of Clinical Neurophysiology.* John Wiley, Chichester.

Kerkut GA & Wheal (1981) *Electrophysiology of Isolated Mammalian CNS Preparations.* Academic Press, London.

Kudo Y (1978) The pharmacology of the amphibian spinal cord. *Progr. Neurobiol.* **11**, 1–76.

McBurney RN (1983) New approaches to the study of rapid events underlying neurotransmitter action. *Trends Neurosci.* **6**, 297–302.

Purves RD (1981) *Microelectrode Methods for Intracellular Recording and Ionophoresis.* Academic Press, London.

Spehlmann R (1985) *EEG Primer.* Elsevier, Holland.

Stone TW (1985). *Microiontophoresis and Pressure Ejection.* John Wiley, Chichester.

4 Receptor binding studies

N.J.M. BIRDSALL

Until the mid 1960s, the binding of a drug to its receptor had been inferred from analyses of the dose-response characteristics of specific whole tissue responses. With the development of receptor-specific ligands, radio-labelled to high specific activity, it became feasible to study *directly* the binding of drugs to their receptors. The pioneering investigation of Paton and Rang (1965) demonstrated that it was possible to observe the binding of [³H]-atropine to muscarinic receptor binding sites on longitudinal smooth muscle strips of the guinea-pig ileum. The usefulness of the technique was enhanced by the realisation that binding could also be observed in membrane preparations. This was demonstrated in 1971 in studies of the interaction of the snake toxin, α-bungarotoxin, with nicotinic acetylcholine receptors and of insulin with its receptor. There followed a 'lag period' of 2–3 years after which time a large number of papers on the characterisation of neurotransmitter receptors by binding studies appeared in the scientific literature. A testament to the current popularity of this approach can be judged from the number of papers (*c.* 150–200) that are published each month on this topic.

Most neurotransmitter receptors have now been characterised (with varying extents of rigour) by binding studies. In fact, some 'receptor' binding sites were delineated prior to the knowledge of the nature of the endogenous ligand. For example, the demonstration of the presence of opiate receptors in the CNS greatly aided the isolation and characteris-ation of the endogenous opioid peptides. To date, the endogenous ligand(s) for the benzodiazepine binding site are not unambiguously established.

It is not a trivial problem to establish that the binding of a radio-labelled drug to whole tissue, or to sub-cellular fractions derived from it, represents specific binding to the desired receptor and not to non-specific or other receptor sites. Several mistakes have been made, one example being the demonstration that the β-adrenoceptor, as originally defined by catecholamine binding was not the receptor but was probably catechol-O-methyl transferase.

It is the purpose of this section to discuss critically the principles, techniques and applications of binding studies to the study of drug-receptor interactions. Most of the examples will be taken from our studies on muscarinic acetylcholine receptors.

Principles

In order to demonstrate that the binding of a radiolabelled drug *in vitro* accurately reflects the binding to the receptors *in vivo*, it is necessary to satisfy certain basic criteria.

Specificity

A component of binding of the radiolabelled drug should be inhibited by pharmacologically effective concentrations of drugs which are known to act at the desired receptor, whereas pharmacologically effective concentrations of drugs which act primarily at other receptor sites should be ineffective. This is illustrated in a hypothetical case (Fig. 4.1) in which the binding of a radioactive drug is inhibited by increasing concentrations of two other non-radioactive drugs of the same pharmacological properties but not by another drug having a different pharmacological profile. This type of result allows the definition of *specific* and *non-specific* binding, the latter being the binding to sites other than the ones of interest. All drugs thought to interact with the receptor under consideration should (at sufficiently high concentrations) produce the same asymptotic level of inhibition of binding.

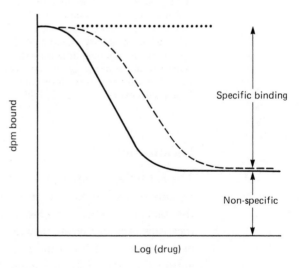

Fig. 4.1. Inhibition of binding of a radiolabelled drug as a function of increasing concentrations of three non-radioactive drugs. Binding is inhibited by two drugs (depicted by —— and ----) but not by a third drug (.....). The two active drugs exhibit different potencies in inhibiting the binding of the radiolabelled drugs but, at high concentrations, inhibit the same fraction of the total binding. This result allows definition of specific and non-specific binding of the radiolabelled drugs as illustrated.

Saturability

The specific component of binding, thus defined, should saturate with increasing concentrations of the radiolabelled drug (Fig. 4.2). In general, the non-specific binding is a linear function of increasing drug concentration.

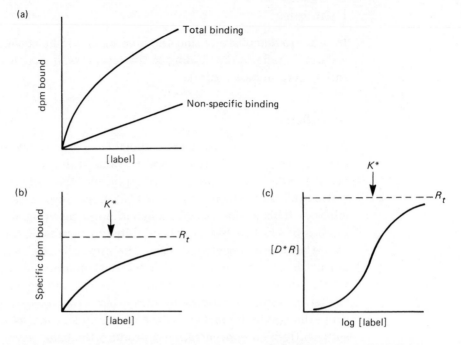

Fig. 4.2. Saturable binding. (a) Total and non-specific binding of a radiolabelled drug as a function of increasing concentration of the label. Non-specific binding is, in general, a linear function of increasing concentration of the radiolabelled drug. (b) Subtraction of the non-specific binding curve from the total binding gives the specific binding curve which asymptotes to a saturation level, R_t. The concentration of *free* radiolabelled drug at half saturation is the dissociation constant of the radiolabelled drug, the reciprocal of this value being the affinity constant K^*. (c) The binding curve becomes sigmoidal when the concentration of bound drug is plotted as a function of the logarithm of the concentration of free drug. In some ways this is a more convenient method of depicting a saturation isotherm as it allows data covering a wide range of concentrations of free ligand to be expressed in a single plot.

Localisation

The saturable component of binding should be detected in tissues and regions of tissues known from pharmacological experiments to contain the receptor. The converse does not necessarily hold; there may be receptor sites in tissues in which no pharmacological response has been detected because for some reason, the response is not expressed or the appropriate (possibly unknown) pharmacological response in that tissue has not been measured.

Quantitative correlations between binding and response

Ideally, any estimate of receptor occupancy, as a function of drug concentration, should agree with the estimates obtained by analysis of the whole tissue response. Whilst this correlation is relatively easy for antagonist binding where null methods (which assume that equal responses to an agonist in the presence and absence of an antagonist indicates equal occupancy of the receptors by the agonist) have provided a good quantitative approach in whole tissue pharmacology, the relationship between agonist binding and response is complicated by the non-linear nature of the intervening steps in the stimulus-response sequence. The determination of agonist *affinity constants* using classical pharmacological techniques has rarely been attempted, exceptions being those of the estimation of agonist affinity constants for muscarinic and β-adrenoceptors.

Choice of radioligand

One of the most important factors in binding studies is the choice of the radiolabelled ligand. It should be of high potency and have a 'clean' pharmacology in the sense that it should have a highly selective pharmacological profile for the receptor of interest. For most studies, it is advantageous to select an agonist and an antagonist because, as will be shown later, binding studies have revealed that the antagonist and, more often, the agonist binding properties of the receptor sites are complex and both ligands may be required to unravel the complexities.

The radioisotope most commonly used for binding studies is tritium, which can be relatively easily incorporated in high specific activity into most biological molecules. The other isotopes used are iodine[125] and iodine[131]. They are available at a higher specific activity than tritium but have shorter half-lives (60 days, 8 days versus 12.4 years for [^{125}I], [^{131}I] and [^{3}H] respectively) which necessitates more frequent resynthesis and greater expense. Sometimes there are problems with the purification of radioiodinated molecules, especially proteins and peptides and in some cases, the iodinated derivative(s) may not have the same binding characteristics as the unlabelled molecule.

Techniques

The basis of the binding technique is depicted by the equation below:

$$D^* + R \overset{K^*}{\rightleftharpoons} D^*R, \tag{1}$$
$$F \qquad\qquad B$$

in which a radiolabelled drug, D^*, binds with an affinity constant K^* (which is the reciprocal of the dissociation constant) to a receptor, R. The fraction of receptors, p, occupied by $[D^*]$, is given by:

$$p = \frac{K^*D^*}{1 + K^*D^*}. \tag{2}$$

The object of a binding experiment is to determine the concentration of D^*R, (B), at a *free* concentration of D^*, (F). The usefulness of this approach relies on the ability to measure the specific binding, B, in the presence of the non-specific binding of D^*, (NS). An acceptable minimum ratio of B/NS for accurate studies is $2 : 1$.

Typical conditions for a binding assay are:

1 0.1–1 mg membrane protein/ml.

2 A receptor concentration of $10^{-11} - 2 \times 10^{-9}$ M.

3 A radiolabelled ligand, specific activity 1–90 Ci/mmol, with an affinity for the receptor in the range $10^{11} - 10^7$ M^{-1}.

A radiolabelled ligand can also be used in a competition assay to determine the affinity constant for an unlabelled drug, L, (see [3] and Fig. 4.3).

$$
\begin{array}{c}
D^* + R \overset{K^*}{\rightleftharpoons} D^*.R. \\
+ \\
L \\
\kappa_L \updownarrow \\
L.R
\end{array}
\qquad [3]
$$

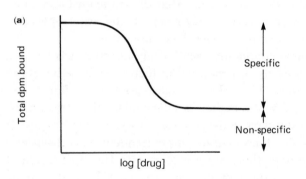

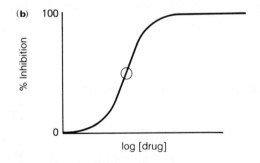

Fig. 4.3. Competition experiment. (a) The binding of a fixed concentration of a radiolabelled drug is inhibited by increasing concentrations of a non-radioactive drug. (b) Inhibition of *specific* binding of the radiolabelled drug as a function of concentration of non-radiolabelled drug. The mid-point on this curve, denoted by a circle represents the IC$_{50}$, the concentration of non-radioactive drug which inhibits 50% of the specific binding of the radiolabelled drug. Only under defined circumstances (see text) can the reciprocal of the IC$_{50}$ be equated with the affinity constant.

In such an experiment, it is usual to measure the inhibition of the specific binding of a fixed concentration of D^* as a function of varying concentrations of the unlabelled drug, L. The fractional inhibition of specific binding of D^*, I, is given by the equation:

$$
I = \frac{K_L[L]}{1 + K_L[L] + K^*[D^*]}.
\qquad [4]
$$

By a suitable choice of experimental conditions, $K^*[D^*] \ll 1$, and $K^*([R] + [RD^*] + [RL]) \ll 1$, equation [4] simplifies to

$$I = \frac{K_L[L]}{1 + K_L[L]} \qquad [5]$$

which is a simple binding function for L and is independent of D^*.

Whether the experiment be a direct binding [1] or a competition experiment [3], the concentration of RD^* is required to be measured at a given free ligand concentration. This is generally accomplished by one of three different assay procedures:

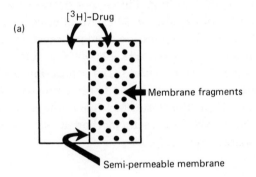

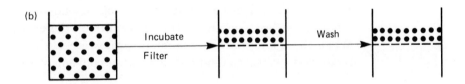

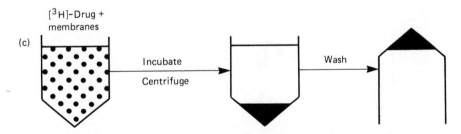

Fig. 4.4. Methods of measuring the binding of radiolabelled drugs to membrane bound receptors. (a) Equilibrium dialysis. Membrane fragments in one compartment are separated from buffer in a second compartment by a semi-permeable membrane. The binding of the radiolabelled drug to the membrane is estimated from the difference in concentrations of the [³H]-drug in the two compartments. (b) Filtration: membranes are incubated with the [³H]-drug. Unbound radioactivitiy is removed by rapid filtration and washing. (c) Centrifugation: membranes, incubated with the [³H]-drug are sedimented by centrifugation and the resulting pellet washed superficially.

RECEPTOR BINDING STUDIES

1 Equilibrium dialysis
2 Filtration assay
3 Centrifugation assay
which are depicted in Fig. 4.4.

Whilst method **1** is a rigorous method by which all the binding of D^* is determined, it is a relatively slow and inefficient procedure, and furthermore is rather insensitive because it relies on there being significant depletion of the total concentration of D^* caused by its binding to R. Method **2** is the procedure which is used overwhelmingly in binding studies. It is a rapid and sensitive procedure. However, its sensitivity relies on the assumption that the washing procedure only removes non-specific and not specific binding. This is not necessarily true, especially for ligands with affinities below 10^8 M^{-1}. An alternative procedure, **3**, is slowly gaining favour. The separation of membranes is accomplished by rapid centrifugation (30–120 seconds, 14 000 $\times$ g) and the pellet is only superficially washed. In this method, the separation and washing proceeds under equilibrium conditions and true estimates of 'non-specific' binding may be obtained. This latter fact inevitably results in a somewhat decreased ratio of B/NS relative to method **2** but for many purposes method **3** is probably preferable.

Data analysis

From a statistical viewpoint, it is preferable to analyse binding data using a non-linear least-squares fitting procedure on the untransformed data. When the appropriate computer programs are not available, or initial parameter estimates required, it is often convenient to use a linearised

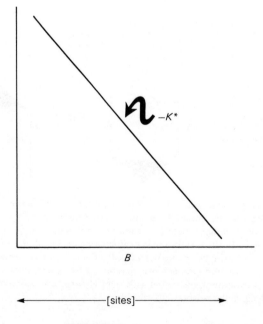

Fig. 4.5. Scatchard plot. B/F is plotted against B. For simple 1:1 mass action binding, the plot is a straight line, gradient $-K^*$, and intercept on the abscissa, the concentration of binding sites.

form of the binding equation and generate a Scatchard plot (Fig. 4.5) of the data for the binding of D^* to R. If there is one population of non-interacting receptor binding sites, a Scatchard plot (B/F vs B) of the data results in a straight line, the gradient being the affinity constant and the intercept on the abscissa being the total concentration of receptor binding sites in the experiment. Once this latter value has been estimated, it is possible to generate a Hill plot (Fig. 4.6) of the data, $\log[p/(1-p)]$ vs $\log D^*$, where p is the receptor occupancy. For simple 1:1 binding, the Hill plot is a straight line, gradient (H) 1.0. An example of these various forms

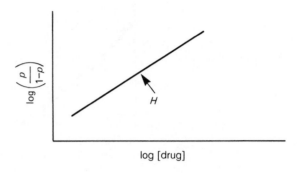

Fig. 4.6. Hill plot. Data from a direct binding curve (or a competition experiment) are plotted in the form $\log(p/1-p)$ versus $\log$ [drug] where p is the receptor occupancy. For simple 1:1 mass action binding, the Hill plot is a straight line, the gradient, H, being 1.0. For more complicated binding processes, the Hill plot may be non-linear (see e.g. Fig. 4.8(c)).

of data analysis is shown (Fig. 4.7) for an experiment in which the binding of the antagonist [³H]-propylbenzilylcholine to muscarinic receptors in the rat cerebral cortex was studied. The data are analysed in four ways: by non-linear least-squares analysis of total and non-specific binding, by non-linear least-squares analysis of the specific binding, by linear least-squares analyses of the Scatchard plot and Hill plot of the data. There is good agreement between the various parameter estimates and an absence of correlated deviations between the theoretical curves and experimental points. This evidence and the value of H being close to 1.0 suggests that [³H]-propylbenzilylcholine is binding to a uniform population of binding sites. As equations [2] and [5] are of the same form, it is possible to linearise [³H]-drug/unlabelled drug competition data and generate pseudo Scatchard plots (Hofstee plots) and Hill plots. Relatively often, Hill plots and Scatchard plots deviate from linearity. This will be discussed on pages 67 and 68.

Some problems associated with the interpretation of the results of binding studies

Whilst it is rather easy to perform binding studies, the analysis and, in particular, the interpretation of the data can be quite complex. Examples of some of the commonly occurring problems are given below.

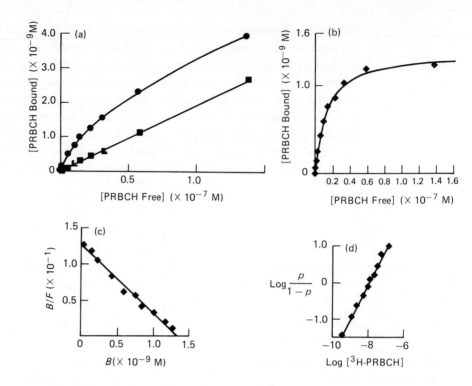

Fig. 4.7. Analysis of the binding of [^{3}H]-propylbenzilylcholine (PRBCH) to muscarinic acetylcholine receptors in a membrane preparation from rat cerebral cortex. (a) Total (●) and non-specific (■) binding as a function of concentration of free PRBCH. Non-linear least-squares analysis of the data indicates the presence of 1.43×10^{-9} M binding sites with an affinity constant for PRBCH of 7.6×10^7 M^{-1}. Non-specific binding is linear and under these experimental conditions is equivalent to 1.9% of the added [^{3}H]-PRBCH. (b) Specific [^{3}H]-PRBCH binding obtained by subtraction of the non-specific binding from total binding (see (a)). Non-linear least squares analysis indicates the presence of 1.38×10^{-9} M binding sites with an affinity for PRBCH of 8.3×10^7 M^{-1}. (c) Scatchard plot of the data in Fig. 4.7(b). Linear least squares analysis would suggest the presence of 1.33×10^{-9} M sites with an affinity for PRBCH of 9.4×10^7 M^{-1}. (d) Hill plot of the data in Fig. 4.7(b), the gradient being 0.98 ± 0.02 as determined by linear least squares analysis. The curves in Fig. 4.7(a)–4.7(d) are the least squares best fit curves.

Is the binding site a receptor?

Although the equation of the α-bungarotoxin binding site with the nicotinic acetylcholine receptor recognition site at the neuromuscular junction is not in doubt, the nature of a high affinity α-bungarotoxin binding site in the CNS and superior cervical ganglia has been in question for several years. This site shows elements of the properties of a nicotinic receptor in that nicotine and tubocurarine compete for binding to the site. However, in most species it has not been possible to show that α-bungarotoxin inhibits nicotinic electrophysiological responses in these tissues. Equally, the nature of the benzodiazepine 'receptor' binding site in the CNS was not clear when it was discovered. This binding site has the specificity for benzodiazepines which would be predicted for a benzodiazepine receptor from functional studies but subsequent work has shown that the 'receptor' is really an allosteric binding site on a class of GABA receptor (GABA$_A$ receptor — see Chapters 12 and 20).

Labelling of different neurotransmitter receptor sites

1 It has now been shown that certain radiolabelled drugs will label several different receptor sites. For example, [^{3}H]-dihydroergocryptine labels dopamine and α-adrenoceptors, [^{3}H]-spiperone labels dopamine and 5-HT receptors and [^{3}H]-LSD labels dopamine, α_1, α_2 and 5-HT receptors! By the ingenious use of combinations of non-radioactive receptor-specific drugs to define 'specific' binding it is now possible to use these radioligands for binding studies of particular receptor systems, but for some years there was confusion in the scientific literature caused by the use of these radiolabelled drugs which did not have a 'clean' pharmacology. Newer radiolabelled drugs, which have a greater receptor selectivity, are now available for α-adrenoceptor, dopamine and 5-HT receptor studies.

2 A more subtle pattern of binding is exhibited by most receptors in membrane preparations. Whereas the binding of antagonists indicates that there is a uniform population of binding sites, the binding of agonists to the same sites reveals heterogeneity. The ability of agonists to discriminate between the apparently homogenous population of antagonist sites is directly related to their efficacy.

The various forms of heterogeneity discussed above are clearly manifested in the binding curves. Consider a simple example in which two sites x and y have the same affinity for [^{3}H]-drug M but differ in their affinity for [^{3}H]-drug N (K_x, K_y) (Fig. 4.8(a)). In a binding experiment, [^{3}H]-drug M will bind equally to sites x and y whereas [^{3}H]-drug N will bind preferentially to site x, and only occupy site y to an appreciable extent at high concentrations. The Scatchard plot for the binding of M will be linear but that of N will be curved (Fig. 4.8(b)). It is possible to dissect the curved Scatchard plot into two components (dashed lines, Fig. 4.8(b)) and hence obtain the concentrations of sites x and y and their affinities for N. A Hill plot of the binding data for drug N will also deviate from linearity and have a gradient less than 1. Note that, in general, the Hill coefficient (H) is taken to be the average gradient in the middle region of the plot.

In many cases the affinity of N is so low that it cannot be observed in a direct binding experiment because of the poor specific/non-specific binding at the high concentrations of [^{3}H]-drug N necessary to occupy a significant fraction of y sites. In these circumstances, the binding data for drug N will appear to give a linear Scatchard plot, extrapolation of the data (Fig. 4.8(b)) giving a concentration of binding sites less than those labelled by drug M. The low affinity sites for drug N can be revealed in competition experiments using [^{3}H]-drug M. M monitors sites x

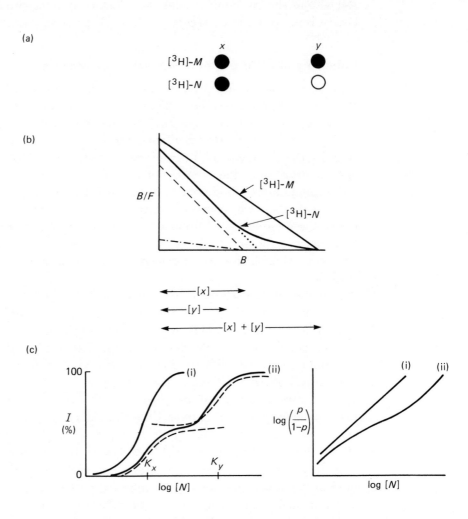

Fig. 4.8. Effects of receptor heterogeneity on binding curves: a simple two site model. (a) Two sites x and y have the same affinity for [³H]-drug M but [³H]-drug N has a higher affinity for x than y. Hence M binds equally to both x and y (closed circles) whereas N, at low concentrations, binds selectively to x (closed circle) and not y (open circle). (b) The Scatchard plot of specific [³H]-drug M binding is linear, the intercept on the abscissa being the sum of the concentrations of x and y sites. The Scatchard plot of specific [³H]-drug N binding is curved, and can be dissected into its two components (dashed lines) which yield the concentrations of x and y sites and the affinities of N for the two sites. If the binding of [³H]-N is not followed to high concentrations the Scatchard plot may then appear to be linear, extrapolation of the data (.....) suggesting (incorrectly) that [³H]-N labels fewer total sites than [³H]-M. (c) Low concentrations of [³H]-N and [³H]-N label different numbers of sites (see (a)) and hence the curves for inhibition of [³H]-N (i) and [³H]-M (ii) binding by N (or a drug with N-like specificity) are different. Inhibition of [³H]-N binding by N, gives a mass action curve ((i) left) and linear Hill plot ((i) right) with a gradient of unity. Inhibition of [³H]-M binding by N gives a biphasic curve ((ii) left), which is the sum of two mass action curves (dashed lines). The Hill plot is non-linear ((ii) right) and the gradient at the middle is less than one.

and y whereas N at low concentrations monitors x only, as shown by the filled circles in Fig. 4.8(a). Inhibition of binding of [^{3}H]-drug N by non-radioactive N (or another drug with N-like specificity) will give a mass action curve, affinity constant K_x and will not reflect the binding of N to site y. On the other hand, inhibition of binding of [^{3}H]-drug M by non-radioactive N (or another N-like drug) will reflect the binding of N to *both* sites x and y (Fig. 4.8(c)), the 'flat' inhibition curve being the sum of two (dashed) mass-action binding curves. It should be noted that in this latter inhibition curve, the IC_{50} value is not a measure of one affinity constant but is a function of both K_x and K_y. The Hill plots of the competition data are depicted in Fig. 4.8(c) (right).

'Functional' receptors

An enigmatic problem is that of how closely the binding properties of the site(s) measured *in vitro* correspond to those found *in vivo*. In membrane preparations, there is no membrane potential and the ionic environment is the same on both sides of the membrane which is certainly different from that found *in vivo*. In some instances it is possible to carry out binding studies on whole cells and, somewhat reassuringly, the results are often similar to those found from assays on broken cell preparations. This does not dispose of the problem of whether some or all of the binding sites seen in a binding study represent 'functional' receptors and in particular what is the significance of the various 'states' of the receptor found, for example, in muscarinic receptor binding studies. For some receptors it is now possible to look at the link between binding and a biochemical response in a broken cell preparation, and hence test the hypothesis.

Applications of binding studies

In this section it is only possible to give in most general terms and with a minimal number of examples, some of the uses of this powerful technique for studying neurotransmitter receptor systems.

Biochemical studies

These are usually addressed to the questions:
1 What is the structure of the receptor?
2 What are the differences between the binding of an agonist and an antagonist?
3 How is the binding of agonist to the receptor transduced into the physiological response?

Apart from the elucidation of the detailed quantitative equilibrium binding properties of the receptor, some of the other analytical biochemical approaches to the study of receptors are given in Fig. 4.9. The various 'states' of the receptor are enclosed in rectangles. Most receptors have now been solubilised but relatively few have been purified and reconstituted. Most of the advances have come from studies of the β-adrenoceptor

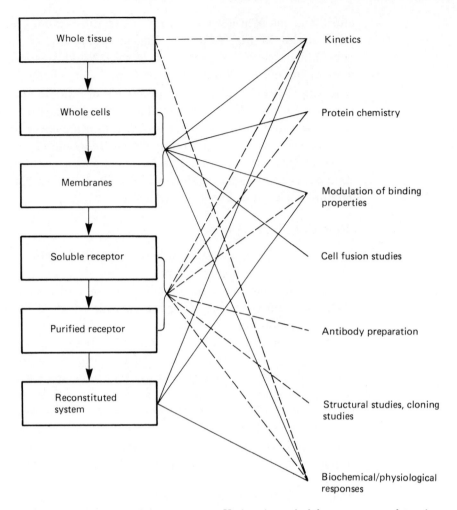

Fig. 4.9. Analytical studies on receptors. Various 'states' of the receptor are shown in the boxes and some of the analytical approaches which have been most commonly applied to these 'states' are linked by either full or dashed lines (for clarity).

and nicotinic receptor systems. One of the most informative facets of receptor binding studies has been the observation that various biologically relevant ligands (e.g. Mg^{2+}, monovalent ions, guanine nucleotides) can modulate the binding properties of certain receptors. In particular, it has been found that agonist binding to these receptors is enhanced by Mg^{2+} and inhibited by guanine nucleotides. There is now overwhelming evidence that this effect is caused by the binding of the nucleotides to heterotrimeric GTP-binding proteins (termed G- or N-proteins) which can act as a catalytic 'shuttle' between the agonist binding protein, R, and the effector component, E, of the system (see Chapter 5).

Initially it was assumed that the only effector system which could be modulated by G-proteins was adenylate cyclase but more recent work has shown that certain K^+ and Ca^{++} channels, cyclic GMP-phosphodiesterase, and probably phosphoinositide phospholipase C are all regulated by receptor activated G-proteins. Furthermore, at least eight different G-proteins have been characterised from biochemical or cloning studies, adding to the complexity of this transduction mechanism. In some instances it has been possible to clone genetic variants which are missing or have altered G and E components and to use these cells, or cells whose R, G or E components have been chemically altered, to reconstitute a functioning system. The initial breakthrough came from the work of Orly and Schramm (1976) when they fused two cell types with inactive β-adrenoceptors and adenylate cyclase respectively and created a functioning β-adrenoceptor adenylate cyclase system.

One of the pieces of information that only binding studies can give is the *number* of receptors. Admittedly, it is not possible to say that these receptors are all functional. Nevertheless, changes in receptor levels and binding properties in response to a variety of stimuli can be monitored. Some examples are given in Fig. 4.10 and below:

1 Ontogeny
2 Desensitisation, chronic drug administration
3 Physical lesions, e.g. denervation
4 Neurochemical lesions, e.g. 6-hydroxydopamine, kainate, ibotenate.
5 Neuropsychiatric disorders, e.g. Parkinsonism, Huntington's chorea, Alzheimers disease.

Receptor localisation

It is possible to pinpoint the precise anatomical location of the receptor binding sites using autoradiographic or immunohistochemical techniques at the light or electron microscope level in addition to detecting variations in the receptor distribution consequent upon *in vivo* 'perturbations' of the type listed above, which can result both in changes in the number of receptor binding sites and also in the binding properties of these sites. The basic technique involves the visualisation of ligands (agonists, antagonists or anti-receptor antibodies) bound to the receptor. An example is given in Fig. 4.10 of the use of the tritiated muscarinic antagonist, propylbenzilylcholine mustard, to label irreversibly muscarinic receptors in the hypoglossal nucleus of the rat brain and to investigate the effects of unilateral axotomy on receptor levels in the nucleus. It can be seen that the receptors are concentrated in the neuropil of the butterfly-shaped hypoglossal nuclei and that axotomy causes a decrease in number of sites on the operated but not contralateral nucleus.

Radioreceptor assays and drug screening

By analogy with the radioimmunoassay technique, it is possible to estimate drug or neurotransmitter concentrations by a radioreceptor assay. The principle of the technique is to estimate the ability of an unknown

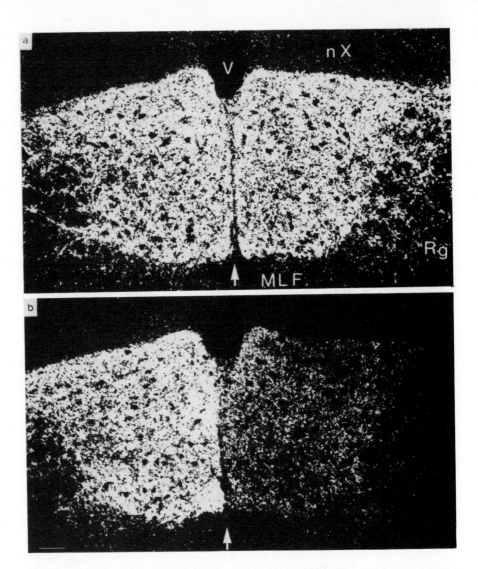

Fig. 4.10. Localisation of muscarinic receptors in the rat hypoglossal nucleus and the effect of unilateral axotomy on receptors levels. (a) Dark field photomicrograph of an autoradiograph of muscarinic receptors labelled with the tritiated irreversible antagonist propylbenzilylcholine mustard. There is heavy symmetrical labelling over both right and left hypoglossal nuclei in the normal rat. (b) There is a marked decrease in labelling of the hypoglossal nucleus on the side (right) ipsilateral to unilateral hypoglossal nerve section five days previously. Arrows, midline; MLF, medial longitudinal fasciculus; nX, dorsal motor nucleus of the vagus; Rg, gigantocellular reticular nucleus; V, caudal, closed part of the fourth ventricle. Scale bar, 100 μm. (Reprinted with permission from Rotter (1979) *Brain Res. Rev.* **1**, 207–24.)

concentration of a ligand, Z, in a sample to inhibit the binding of a radiolabelled ligand to its receptor. From the extent of inhibition, a knowledge of the structure of Z and a calibration competition curve for Z, it is possible to estimate the concentration of Z in the sample. The lower limit of the sensitivity depends on Z but is in the range 0.2–10 pmol. This technique has been used for example to estimate levels of adrenaline, noradrenaline, dopamine, acetylcholine, GABA, 5-HT, neurotensin, spiperone and diazepam. The limitation of this technique is its specificity: precautions should be taken to ensure that the only substance which inhibits binding of the radioligand in the assay is the compound itself. Any potent metabolite of a drug may interfere with the assay and give an incorrect estimate of drug concentration. The existence of this fact in itself is very useful information, especially for the pharmaceutical industry, and it leads to the final application of binding assays to be discussed in this section, that of the screening of drugs.

It is now possible to rapidly and accurately test newly synthesised drugs for their primary potency, that is, their affinity for the neurotransmitter receptor system with which they were designed to interact and, in some cases, to predict whether they will be agonists or antagonists. Furthermore, binding assays on other receptor systems can give information regarding the selectivity of the drug and hence the possible occurrence of side-effects. For example, some neuroleptics can bind with high affinity to α-adrenoceptors and muscarinic receptors as well as to dopamine receptors (as defined by [^{3}H]-spiperone binding).

The hypotensive side-effects of neuroleptics appear to be caused by high affinity binding to α-adrenoceptors whereas the Parkinsonian extrapyramidal side-effects result in part from the neuroleptics having a *low* affinity for muscarinic receptors. In some cases, therefore, the interaction of drugs with more than one receptor system may be beneficial rather than harmful.

Receptor binding assays are no substitute for *in vivo* or *in vitro* functional testing. Nevertheless, they provide a cheap and rapid primary screen for newly synthesised drugs as well as giving some insight into the mechanism of action of known drugs.

References and further reading

Birdsall NJM, Burgen ASV & Hulme EC (1978) The binding of agonists to brain muscarinic receptors. *Mol. Pharmac.* **14**, 723–36.

Cuatrecasas P & Hollenberg MD (1976) Membrane receptors and hormone action. *Adv. Protein Chem.* **30**, 251–451.

Hammer R, Berrie CP, Birdsall NJM, Burgen ASV & Hulme EC (1980) Pirenzepine distinguishes between muscarinic receptor subclasses. *Nature* **283**, 90–2.

Hulme EC, Birdsall NJM, Burgen ASV & Mehta P (1978) The binding of antagonists to brain muscarinic receptors. *Mol. Pharmac.* **14**, 737–50.

Orly J & Schramm M (1976) Coupling of catecholamine receptor from one cell with adenylate cyclase to another cell by fusion. *Proc. Nat. Acad. Sci., USA* **73**, 4410–14.

Paton WDM & Rang HP (1965) The uptake of atropine and related drugs by intestinal smooth muscle of the guinea pig in relation to acetylcholine receptors. *Proc. R. Soc.* **163B**, 1–44.

Yamamura HI, Enna SJ & Kuhar MJ (1987) *Neurotransmitter Receptor Binding*. Raven Press, New York.

5   Biochemical changes

J.H. CONNICK AND T.W. STONE

Whilst the electrochemical phenomena associated with the binding of a specific neurotransmitter (NT) to a membrane bound receptor have relinquished many of their secrets in response to the tenacity and ingenuity of experiments, the associated postsynaptic changes have proved more intractable.

A number of recent discoveries have, however, given new insight into the biochemical consequences of receptor activation. The first such event is the enzymatic production of a number of 'second messengers', the NT or hormone being the first messenger. The number of second messengers so far discovered is surprisingly small, and they appear to subserve similar roles in organisms at the extreme ends of the phylogenetic scale; from bacteria, to nerve cells in the mammalian central nervous system.

Cyclic AMP

One of the first of the second messengers to be recognised was cyclic adenosine $3',5'$ monophosphate (cyclic AMP) (Fig. 5.1).

During investigations into the mechanism by which adrenaline induced glycogenolysis in the liver in the late 1950s, Earl Sutherland and his colleagues (see Sutherland & Robison 1966), isolated a nucleotide from liver cells which they identified as cyclic AMP. Cyclic AMP was formed intracellularly by hydrolysis and cyclisation of adenosine triphosphate (ATP) by an enzyme complex now referred to as adenylate (or adenylyl) cyclase (Fig. 5.2). The significance of cyclic AMP was that it appeared to be the agent directly responsible for activating the intracellular biochemical machinery leading to glycogenolysis. Over the subsequent 20 years it has been recognised that cyclic AMP is a molecular mediator for the actions of a wide variety of hormones and NTs on cellular function.

In recent years Greengard (1976) and his colleagues have extended our knowledge of the mechanism of action of cyclic AMP with the discovery of protein kinases. These constitute a family of intracellular enzymes which form part of a cascade of reactions which are activated by cyclic AMP, and which then phosphorylate cellular proteins (Fig. 5.2). The phosphorylation of histones (associated with DNA) may, for example, mediate changes of gene transcription which underlie the effects of cyclic AMP on cell growth, division and differentiation. The phosphorylation of proteins lying within cell membranes may induce a change of confor-

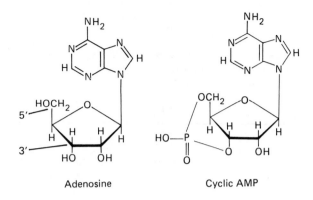

Adenosine   Cyclic AMP

Fig. 5.1. The structures of adenosine, cyclic adenosine 3'5'-monophosphate (cyclic AMP) and cyclic guanosine 3'5'-monophosphate (cyclic GMP). The purine bases, such as adenine or guanine linked to a ribose sugar molecule form the nucleosides adenosine and guanosine respectively. A nucleotide is a phosphorylated nucleoside. In referring to substituents, non-primed numbers refer to positions on the base, primed numbers to positions on the sugar molecule; 3' and 5' positions are indicated on the adenosine molecule.

Guanosine

mation which results in an alteration of the ionic permeability characteristics of the cell.

This latter concept, that cyclic AMP might mediate the effects of transmitters on membrane conductances, has attracted much research, although the problems of correlating the synaptic events involved in transmitter action with the underlying biochemistry represents a major challenge. The most complete analysis of this kind is still that performed by Bloom and his colleagues between 1969 and 1972 (see Bloom 1975). This study began with the demonstration that iontophoretic application of cyclic AMP to Purkinje cells in the cerebellum mimicked the effects of noradrenaline (norepinephrine), not only in depressing the firing rate, but also in producing a hyperpolarisation with an increased membrane resistance. In addition, compounds such as papaverine, which inhibit cyclic nucleotide phosphodiesterase, (the main catabolic enzyme destroying cyclic AMP, see Fig. 5.2) potentiated the effects of both noradrenaline (NA) and cyclic AMP. Substances which prevented activation of adenylate cyclase on the other hand, such as prostaglandin E_1 and nicotinate, blocked the noradrenaline responses, but not the effects of cyclic AMP. A particularly elegant contribution to this series of studies was the development of an immunocytochemical technique for cyclic AMP, by means of which it was shown that NA specifically enhanced cyclic AMP-

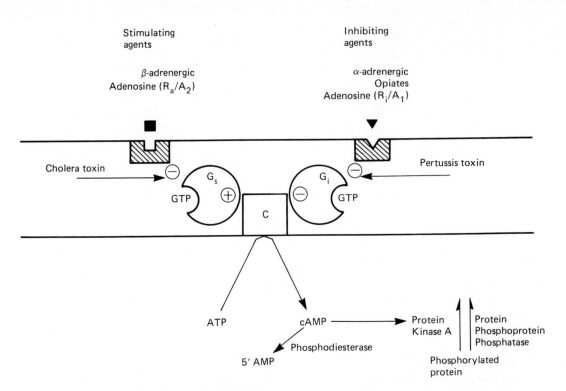

Fig. 5.2. A schematic diagram of the cyclic AMP system. Following the interaction of an agonist with its receptor in a cell membrane, the intracellularly directed catalytic subunit of adenylate cyclase [c] is activated, resulting in the catalysis of the hydrolysis of adenosine 5′-triphosphate (ATP) to cyclic adenosine 3′5′-monophosphate (cyclic AMP). Cyclic AMP may then be further hydrolysed to the 5′ monophosphate, but many of the actions of cyclic AMP probably result from the activation of protein kinases, which phosphorylate cellular proteins. The regulatory G-proteins possess sites on their α subunits at which cholera toxin or pertussis toxin can cause ADP-ribosylation (and thus inactivation) of the G_s and G_i protein respectively.

induced fluorescence in the Purkinje cell layer. Many aspects of this study also included correlation with the effects of locus coeruleus stimulation, as the site of origin of the cerebellar noradrenergic fibres. Subsequent studies have also been extended to the level of protein kinase involvement, with the finding that the effects on neuronal membrane properties of a series of cyclic AMP derivatives correlates well with their ability to activate protein kinases.

Similar, though not so extensive, studies in the cerebral cortex and hippocampus have supported the idea that cyclic AMP mediates amine effects on membrane properties.

An electrophysiological analysis by Greengard's group (Greengard 1976) of events at the superior cervical ganglion elicited a great deal of excitement by correlating the hyperpolarising effects of dopamine on the postsynaptic cells with the activation of a dopamine (DA) sensitive adenylate cyclase. However, these results have not proved to be readily reproducible in other laboratories.

Adenylate cyclase and transmitter receptors

The adenylate cyclase enzyme system is present throughout the central nervous system and can be activated by a number of putative NTs including NA, DA and histamine. The activity of the cyclase system is assessed by homogenising an area of brain, suspending that homogenate in a suitable incubating medium, and determining the amount of cyclic AMP formed, for example by radioimmunoassay, in the absence and presence of the substances being tested. However, the ability of transmitters to activate the cyclase from different regions does not always parallel the distribution either of the transmitter itself or of its receptors. In fact the current view is that some transmitters may act on two (or more) classes of receptors, only one of which is linked positively to adenylate cyclase. Some examples of this apparent receptor dualism are summarised in Table 5.1. In most cases the morphological localisation of the different receptor types is unknown, although the distribution of the dopamine D_1 receptor, which is linked to adenylate cyclase is well characterised in the striatum and substantia nigra (see Chapters 7 and 8).

Adenosine is included in Table 5.1 as it currently holds a unique role in CNS pharmacology. It is very unlikely that adenosine itself is a NT, but a number of depolarising agents, including glutamate and ouabain, cause the release of adenosine, and thus an indirect increase of cyclic AMP levels (probably via the P_1 receptors). The methylxanthines, such as theophylline, are quite potent antagonists of the activation of adenylate cyclase by adenosine. Indeed they are more potent in this respect than as inhibitors of phosphodiesterase, for which action they have often been used experimentally.

Table 5.1

Transmitter candidate	Receptor	Cyclase activation	Sample agonist	Sample antagonist
Noradrenaline	α	No	Phenylephrine	Phentolamine
	β	Yes	Isoprenaline	Propranolol
Dopamine	D_1	Yes	Dopamine	Ergot derivatives
	D_2	No	Ergot derivatives	Sulpiride
Histamine	H_1	No	2-methyl-histamine	Diphenhydramine
	H_2	Yes	Betazole	Metiamide
Adenosine	P_1	Yes	Adenosine	Theophylline
	P_2	No	ATP	Quinidine

The relationship between the externally directed neurotransmitter receptor (or receptor subunit) and the catalytic subunit of adenylate cyclase is unclear. The linkage may be an individual and permanent one (Fig. 5.3(a)) or several receptors may share one cyclase complex (Fig. 5.3(b)). The concept which has most support at present is a floating model

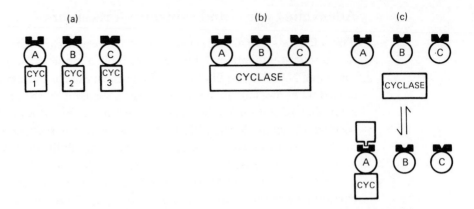

Fig. 5.3. Three possible ways in which transmitter and drug receptors might be related to adenylate cyclase. (a) Each receptor is permanently coupled to its own adenylate cyclase molecule. (b) Receptors for several different transmitters are permanently linked to a common cyclase. (c) The transmitter receptors and cyclase molecules lead independent existences except for a short period of time following the activation of a receptor by its agonist.

There is evidence favouring model (c) in the case of the β-adrenoceptor, whereas recent work suggests the adenosine receptor is permanently coupled to adenylate cyclase, as in models (a) or (b).

(Fig. 5.3(c)) in which receptors and cyclases lead essentially independent existences until a transmitter interacts with its receptor. Then the induced change in receptor conformation results in a functional link being established between the transmitter/receptor complex and cyclase. This model is supported by experiments in which turkey erythrocytes were treated with N-ethylmaleimide to inactivate adenylate cyclase but leave catecholamine receptors intact, and then fused with mouse leukaemia cells having the cyclase but no catecholamine receptor. After fusion, treatment with a catecholamine resulted in an increased level of cyclic AMP.

However, it has been found recently that the adenosine receptor appears to exist in permanent association with catalytic subunits of adenylate cyclase. Thus, progressive inactivation of adenosine receptors, or changes of membrane fluidity do not alter the kinetic parameters of cyclase activation. It therefore seems that different classes of agonist receptors may have different relationships with the cyclase enzyme.

The current molecular model for the linkage of a particular receptor with adenylate cyclase comprises at least three classes of component structured within the lipid membrane (Fig. 5.2).

Located at the outer membrane surface is the receptor component, containing a specific site for the binding of hormones or NTs. At the inner face of the membrane are the catalytic, cyclase component (C) and the nucleotide regulatory component (G). These nucleotide regulatory components contain sites for binding GTP and are responsible for mediating the effect of GTP and various transmitters on the activity of C.

Two functional classes of G have now been discovered; one mediates stimulation of the cyclase unit (G_s), the other inhibition (G_i). Each class appears to be linked to a separate class of receptor.

The current theory suggests that the receptor and G protein units normally exist as a complex, separate from the cyclase unit. The receptor inhibits the interaction of GTP with the G protein. When a transmitter binds to the receptor, this constraint is removed and the G protein forms a new complex with the cyclase. Depending on the type of G protein activated (G_s or G_i), the enzyme complex exhibits either increased or decreased production of cyclic AMP.

The study of these receptors is likely to assume considerable importance in view of the recent reports that desensitisation of adrenergic β-receptors involves uncoupling of the receptor from the cyclase catalytic subunit. As receptor desensitisation is of considerable pharmacological interest, methods of modulating the receptor–cyclase link may become of central importance.

A recent series of experiments has implicated cyclic AMP in the regulation of calcium influx into the nerve terminal; the cyclic AMP dependent phosphorylation of voltage sensitive sodium and potassium channels has also been demonstrated. Kaczmarek *et al.* (1978) working on bag cell neurons in the sea mollusc *Aplysia*, found that an afterdischarge following a brief synaptic activation could be mimicked by 5-HT or cyclic AMP. Recent voltage clamp studies have shown that the effects of cyclic AMP are due to inhibition of several different potassium channels, the effect of cyclic AMP being mediated by a cyclic AMP dependent protein kinase.

Guanylate cyclase

In general, the functional significance of this system is even less clear than that of adenylate cyclase, partly because the system operates at about one thousand fold smaller concentrations. Whereas the iontophoretic application of cyclic AMP generally depresses neuronal firing, however, Stone *et al.* (1975) reported that cyclic GMP often produces an excitation, and thus mimics, on some cells in the cerebral cortex at least, the increase of firing produced by acetylcholine. Opposing effects have also been seen by Swartz and Woody (1979) after the intracellular injection of the nucleotides so that penetration into the cells after extracellular iontophoresis is unlikely to have been a limiting factor. (Cyclic nucleotides can pass into and out of cells, but do so rather poorly. In many studies, derivatives such as dibutyryl cyclic AMP have been used which pass through cell membranes much more readily.)

Observations such as these, together with the voluminous literature on cyclic nucleotides in peripheral tissues, especially the heart, contributed to a concept of a dual control of cell function, activation of adenylate or guanylate cyclase mediating opposite effects on cell activity. However, it is unlikely that the situation will prove to be that simple. As would be expected for a possibly ubiquitous enzyme system responding to a number of NTs and hormones, the effects of various drugs on adenylate cyclase has been of great interest. In particular, while drug-receptor interactions are perhaps more immediately relevant to the acute effects of drugs, changes of adenylate cyclase activity appear to be of major importance in understanding the chronic effects of drug action. Morphine and related compounds, for example, are said to inhibit adenylate cyclase activity in acute experiments, but over a period of hours many of the test systems used adapt to the maintained application of the opiate so that cyclic AMP production in response to a control agonist reaches pre-opioid levels. A higher dose of morphine is then needed to suppress cyclic AMP production to a degree comparable with that of the first dose. Clearly this situation begs comparison with the phenomenon of opioid tolerance *in vivo*. The adaptation appears to be due to an increased synthesis of adenylate cyclase enzymes, and if the opiate is suddenly withdrawn, endogenous activators of the cyclase such as prostaglandin E are able to induce an exaggerated rise of cyclic AMP levels. Not a few authors have been tempted to relate this result with the opioid withdrawal syndrome *in vivo* (Collier 1980). (Note that prostaglandin E itself is an activator of adenylate cyclase in brain, but it inhibits cyclase activation by NA.)

Many other examples are known of drugs which, when administered chronically, result in an altered sensitivity of adenylate cyclase to appropriate agonists. Such drugs include neuroleptics and antidepressants, the latter being particularly interesting as all the classes of antidepressant drugs tested to date, including amine uptake inhibitors, monoamine oxidase inhibitors and miscellaneous compounds such as iprindole, are effective in producing a subsensitivity of the brain noradrenaline-sensitive adenylate cyclase system. Furthermore, electroconvulsive shock treatment, one of the most effective ways of treating endogenous depression, produces the same kind of change. As these modifications of the cyclase system only develop with chronic drug treatment, they correlate better with clinical signs of improvement than does, for example, inhibition of amine uptake, which is readily evident even after single doses of drugs. In some of these cases though, it is not absolutely clear whether the changed cyclase sensitivity is a direct result of the drug administration or a secondary consequence of a change in the number of receptors. In the case of the opiates, no change of receptor number or affinity accompanies the altered cyclase sensitivity.

Inositol phospholipids

The first suggestion that the metabolism of the inositol phospholipids, normal constituents of the plasma lipid membrane, might be of interest came in the early 1950s when Hokin and Hokin (1954) found that administration of acetylcholine to secretory cells in the pancreas caused

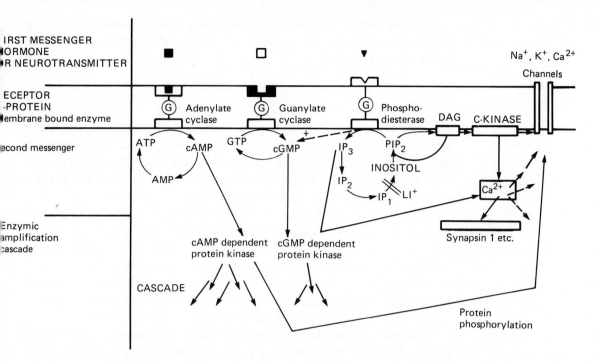

Fig. 5.4. A composite summary of some intracellular second messenger systems and interrelationships.

an increase in turnover of these compounds. It was not until the mid 1970s, however, that Michel (1975) proposed that the increased turnover of inositol phospholipids might be a general phenomenon, and showed that activation of the inositol phospholipid cascade (Fig. 5.4) led ultimately to the mobilisation of calcium within the cell.

Most of our knowledge of the inositol phospholipid cascade is very recent, and there is still much we do not know. It would appear that phosphatidylinositol is specifically phosphorylated at C4 and C5 of the six carbon ring, forming the compound PIP_2. In response to external stimuli, PIP_2 is hydrolysed to diacylglycerol (DAG) and inositol triphosphate (IP_3). It is at this point that the pathway bifurcates.

IP_3 is thought to mobilise calcium within the cell, releasing it from stores within the endoplasmic reticulum. The mechanism of this is unknown. The other branch, signalled by DAG remains localised in the membrane. DAG has been proposed to activate a membrane bound protein kinase-C-kinase.

Ultimately both IP_3 and DAG are reconstituted into PIP_2 via the inositol phospholipid cycle (Fig. 5.4).

The last stage of the lipid cycle, the conversion of inositol monophosphate (IP_1) to free inositol has been shown to be blocked by lithium ions. This has proved to be a very useful experimental tool and, in addition, has been proposed as a possible mechanism for the long established antimanic effect of lithium.

To date a large number of transmitter candidates including acetylcholine, amines and amino acids have been shown to modulate activity in the IP$_3$ system.

Calcium

The one common compound of all the secondary messenger systems discussed so far is calcium. The action of NA on heart muscle is mediated through the cyclic AMP cycle which modulates the intracellular level of calcium. The cyclic AMP dependent phosphorylation of voltage sensitive calcium channels has also been demonstrated.

As has already been mentioned guanylate cyclase is itself activated by an increase in intracellular calcium. The action of IP$_3$, as far as we can establish, is entirely due to its modulation of intracellular calcium whilst C-kinase is a calcium requiring enzyme, as are many protein kinases.

Calcium may, in fact, be regarded as the predominant second messenger. This is particularly so in nerve cells where depolarisation may directly open voltage sensitive calcium channels in the membrane.

Changes initiated by calcium are usually mediated by the protein kinases. Whilst it is outside the scope of this chapter to discuss these enzymes in any great detail at least one, synapsin I, is of direct importance since it is almost exclusively located in neurons.

Recent work suggests that synapsin I forms a net around small synaptic vesicles, and that the collagen tail of the protein is linked either directly or via the cytoskeletal network to the cell membrane. It is thought that phosphorylation of the collagen tail by calcium/calmodulin dependent processes allows synaptic vesicles to approach the membrane in order to release their contents.

References and further reading

Bloom FE (1975) The role of cyclic nucleotides in central synaptic function. *Rev. Physiol. Biochem. Pharmacol.* **74**, 1–103.

Collier HOJ (1980) Cellular site of opiate dependence. *Nature* **283**, 625–9.

Cramer H & Schulz J (eds) (1977) *Cyclic Nucleotides: Mechanisms of Action.* John Wiley, Chichester.

Greengard P (1976) Possible role for cyclic nucleotides and phosphorylated membrane proteins in postsynaptic actions of neurotransmitters. *Nature* **260**, 101–7.

Hokin MR & Hokin LE (1954) Effect of acetylcholine on phospholipids of the pancreas. *J. Biol. Chem.* **209**, 549–58.

Kaczmarek LK, Jennings K & Strumwasser F (1978) Neurotransmitter modulation, phosphodiesterase inhibitor effects and cyclic AMP correlates of afterdischarge in peptidergic neurites. *Proc. Nat. Acad. Sci. (USA)* **75**, 5200–4.

Michell RH (1975) Inositol phospholipids and cell surface receptor function. *Biochim. Biophys. Acta* **415**, 81–147.

Stone TW, Taylor DA & Bloom FE (1975) Cyclic AMP and cyclic GMP may mediate opposite responses in rat cerebral cortex. *Science* **187**, 845–7.

Sutherland EW & Robison GA (1966) The role of cyclic AMP in the responses to catecholamines and other hormones. *Pharmacol. Rev.* **18**, 145–61.

Swartz BE & Woody CD (1979) Correlated effects of acetylcholine and cyclic GMP on membrane properties of mammalian cortical neurones. *J. Neurobiol.* **10**, 465–88.

II **Synaptic pharmacology and neurotransmitter receptors**

6 Acetylcholine

R.A. WEBSTER

Acetylcholine (ACh) was the first neurotransmitter to be discovered when in 1921 Loewi demonstrated that stimulation of the vagus nerve released a chemical that slowed the beating of an isolated frog heart. Since then its mode of action at peripheral synapses and in particular at the neuro-muscular junction has been intensively studied but in many respects its central actions are still less well understood than those of some more recently discovered neurotransmitters like dopamine and GABA.

The cholinergic synapse

This is depicted in Fig. 6.1. Acetylcholine is synthesised in nerve terminals from its precursor choline which is not formed in the CNS but transported there in free form in the blood. Choline is taken up into the cytoplasm by a high affinity (K_m = 1-5 μM) saturable, uptake which is Na^+ and ATP dependent and whilst it does not appear to occur during the depolarisation produced by high concentrations of potassium it is increased by neuronal activity and is specific to cholinergic nerves. A separate low affinity uptake, or diffusion (K_m = 50 μM), which is linearly related to choline concentration and not saturable, is of less interest since it is not specific to cholinergic neurons. The reaction of choline with mitochondrial bound acetylcoenzyme A is catalysed by the cytoplasmic enzyme choline acetyltransferase (ChAT), although the precise location of the synthesis is uncertain and the ACh so formed is stored. As the rate of synthesis of ACh depends on the supply of choline it can be inhibited by drugs like hemicholinium or triethylcholine, which compete for choline uptake. The released ACh is broken down by membrane bound acetylcho-linesterase, often called the true or specific cholinesterase to distinguish it from a pseudo- or non-specific plasma cholinesterase, butyrylcholinester-ase. It seems that about 50% of the choline freed by the hydrolysis of ACh is taken back into the nerve. There is a wide range of anticholinesterases which can be used to prolong and potentiate the action of ACh. Some of these, such as physostigmine, which can cross the blood–brain barrier to produce central effects and neostigmine, which does not readily do so, combine reversibly with the enzyme. Others such as the pesticide, di-isopropylphosphofluorate (DYFLOS, DFP), form an irreversible complex requiring the synthesis of new enzyme before recovery.

Within the neuron, ACh is not distributed evenly. If brain tissue is homogenised in isotonic salt solution containing an anticholinesterase, about 20% of the total ACh is released into solution, presumably from cell bodies, and it is found in the supernatant fraction on centrifugation. The remaining 80% settles within the sedimenting pellet and if this is resuspended and spun through a sucrose gradient it is all found in the synaptosome (nerve ending) fraction. After lysis of the synaptosomes and further centrifugation about half of this ACh, i.e. 40% of the original total still remains in the spun down pellet. This is referred to as the firmly bound or stable 'pool' of ACh since it is not subject to hydrolysis by cholinesterase during the separation procedure. The other half (again 40% of the original) is found in the supernatant and undergoes hydrolysis unless protected by anticholinesterases. Whilst it is generally assumed that some of this latter ACh was always in the synaptosomal cytoplasm probably half of it (20% of the original) comes from disrupted vesicles. This mixture of vesicular and cytoplasmic (nerve ending) ACh is called the labile pool and is probably the most important source of releasable ACh, whether this is from vesicles or cytoplasm (see Chapter 1) and also where newly synthesised ACh is found. Thus in studies in which tissue has been incubated with labelled precursor choline not only is this pool (fraction) heavily labelled but most of the released ACh is also labelled. With the passage of time there is interchange of ACh between the labile and the so-called fixed pool and in the absence of adequate resynthesis, i.e. blockage of choline uptake, it is likely that ACh will be released from the latter source as well.

Whilst there is no uptake of ACh itself cholinergic nerve terminals do possess autoreceptors. Since these are activated by ACh rather than by the choline, to which ACh is normally rapidly broken down, it is unlikely that they would be operated unless the synaptic release of ACh was so great that it was not adequately hydrolysed by cholinesterase.

ACh is widely distributed throughout the brain and parts (ventral horn and dorsal columns) of the spinal cord. Whole brain concentrations of 10 nmol g^{-1} tissue have been reported with highest concentrations in the interpeduncular, caudate and dorsal raphe nuclei. Turnover figures of 0.15–2. 0 nmol g^{-1} min^{-1} vary with the area studied and the method of measurement, e.g. synthesis of labelled ACh from [^{14}C]-choline uptake or run down of ACh after inhibition of choline uptake by hemicholinium. They are all sufficiently high, however, to suggest that in the absence of synthesis depletion could occur within minutes.

Cholinergic receptors and postsynaptic effects

In the periphery ACh acts on two distinct receptors, (a) nicotinic, (b) muscarinic. The former mediate the fast excitatory effects of ACh at the first synapses outside the CNS involving the direct opening of Na^+ channels, membrane depolarisation and the initiation of impulses in

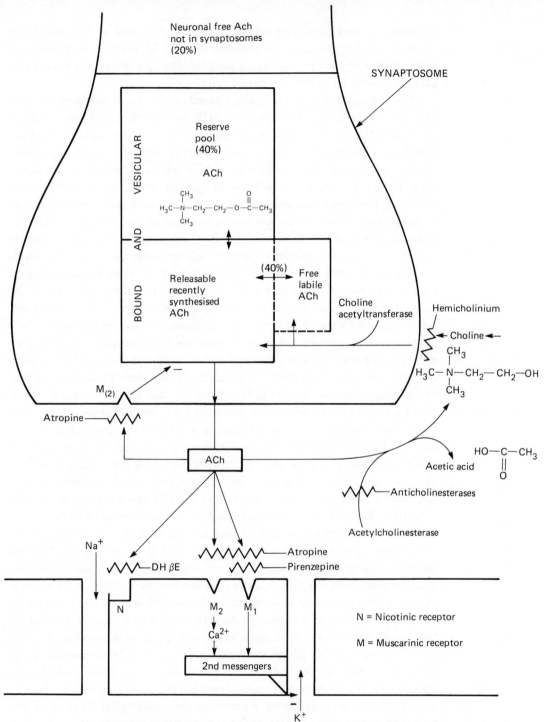

Fig. 6.1. Diagrammatic representation of a cholinergic synapse. Some 80% of neuronal acetylcholine (ACh) is found in the nerve terminal, or synaptosome and the remainder in the cell body or axon. Within the synaptosome it is almost equally divided between two pools, as shown. ACh is synthesised from choline, which has been taken up into the nerve terminal, and to which it is broken down again after release by acetylcholinesterase. Postsynaptically the nicotinic receptor is directly linked to the opening of Na^+ channels and can be blocked by compounds like dihydro-β-erythroidine (DHβE). Muscarinic receptors appear to inhibit K^+ efflux to increase cell activity. For full details see text.

sympathetic and parasympathetic ganglion cells and at the end plate (neuromuscular junction) of skeletal muscle. Muscarinic receptors are associated with slower excitatory and inhibitory effects on smooth and cardiac muscle as well as secretory cells.

This classification was originally based on the use of antagonists since atropine blocked the slow effects of ACh on smooth muscle etc, without modifying the faster events at ganglia and the neuromuscular junction, which were blocked by curare. Their naming derives from the fact that muscarine mimics the slow effects of ACh whilst nicotine first produces then blocks its faster responses at ganglia and the neuromuscular junction. The slower muscarinic effects of ACh on smooth muscle might be regarded as a feature of the tissue but it is in fact a characteristic of muscarinic receptor activation. This is clearly shown, perhaps somewhat surprisingly, in sympathetic ganglia where although transmission is nicotinic both receptors are found. The normal nicotinic response to pre-ganglionic nerve stimulation is the expected fast EPSP of some 20–30 msec duration from which the action potential arises. It is followed, however, by a further EPSP which takes several hundred milliseconds to develop and lasts several seconds. Unlike the fast response it is associated with an increase in membrane resistance, implying a reduction in ionic conductance and is blocked by atropine rather than curare, i.e. it is a muscarinic response. It also differs from the fast EPSP in that it is not capable of generating an action potential and therefore must have some background facilitatory effect. Whilst it must be admitted that antimus-carinic drugs have no detectable effect acutely on ganglionic transmission it is important to understand the basis of this slow muscarinic response since in the CNS there are far more (probably 100 times more), muscarinic than nicotinic receptors and the effects associated with their activation form the basis for many of the central actions of ACh.

The mechanism of the slow cholinergic EPSP has been much studied (see Adams and Brown 1982). Since the EPSP is accompanied by an increased membrane resistance and reduced conductance there must be some inhibition of ion flux and as there is a depolarisation, i.e. the inside of the neuron becoming less negative, this would necessitate a reduction either in the efflux of a positive ion or the influx of a negatively charged ion. It was found that if the ganglion cell was hyperpolarised then the slow EPSP became smaller whilst if it was depolarised the EPSP became larger suggesting that it depends on an ion conductance for which the equilibrium potential is more negative than the resting potential. In fact no EPSP was recorded at a membrane potential equal to that of the equilibrium potential for potassium. Thus it is assumed that the slow EPSP is produced by blocking the efflux of K^+. In practice since the K^+ equilibrium potential at 75 mV is some 10 mV greater than the resting potential, any reduction in K^+ efflux will make the inside of the neuron less negative and take the membrane potential towards that for Na^+, i.e. cause a small (slow) depolarisation. Recent experiments with the voltage clamp technique (Chapter 3) have shown that this involvement of K is not the result of any change in the passive K^+ flux but is associated with a particular type of voltage sensitive K^+ conductance termed the M (muscarinic) conductance (Gm or Im), which plays an important role in the control of neuronal activity. Since it is active even at resting membrane potential its inhibition will inevitably cause some depolarisation. More importantly it will be activated by any attempt to depolarise the neuron, when the opening of M channels and efflux of K^+ will tend to counter the depolarisation and act as a gate on firing. Thus during normal synaptic activity and despite the persistence of the excitatory neurotransmitter, the increased inward current will only generate a few spikes. Clearly if Gm is inhibited then the neuron will be more readily excited and more likely to discharge repetitively. The significance of this on the cortical function of ACh is discussed below.

Despite the wide variety of effects associated with the activation of muscarinic receptors on different organs it appeared that they were very similar and probably identical because all the many known muscarinic antagonists, like atropine, were equally effective (had the same affinity, K_D) against all muscarinic responses. More recently one drug, pirenzepine, was found to be about 100 fold more active against cholinergic (muscarinic) induced gastric acid secretion than against cholinergic activity in the heart of ileum. Although some of this difference may be explained on pharmacokinetic grounds it led to the subdivision of muscarinic receptors into M_1 (stomach) and M_2 (heart and most other smooth muscle). In respect of muscarinic control of neuronal function in the CNS it is probably of more significance that the muscarinic receptors on ganglionic neurons are of the M_1 type. It is also important to remember that whilst pirenzepine is more active at M_1 than M_2 receptors it is still weaker than atropine at both sites, the K_Ds for pirenzepine and atropine being 3.2 and 1.1 nM in ganglia but 620 and 1 nM in atria.

Binding studies show that muscarinic receptors are also not homogenous in the brain. Thus in the fore and hind brain, where the majority of muscarinic receptors are found, they show high affinity for pirenzepine and so are of the M_1 type whereas those in the mid-brain are M_2 and whilst pirenzepine can reduce ACh induced depolarisation of neurons in that area the Kd is high at 200 nM. Protection of either M_1 receptors with pirenzepine or M_2 receptors with carbachol, before measuring the binding of the tritiated non-specific muscarinic ligand quinuclidinyl benzilate ($[^3H](-)QNB$), show M_1 receptors predominantly in cerebral cortex, hippocampus, striatum and dorsal horn of the spinal cord and M_2 receptors in the cerebellum, nucleus tractus solitarius and vental horn of the spinal cord. Unfortunately pirenzepine does not easily cross the blood–brain barrier and so little is known of the function of the M_1 receptors in terms of general CNS activity although since they predominate and as atropine is a potent, albeit non-specific muscarinic antagonist, it is possible that an M_1 antagonist that enters the brain would not have effects vastly different from those of atropine even if M_1 and M_2 receptors are linked to opposing effects. Recent evidence obtained from binding studies on post-mortem tissue from Alzheimer's patients characterised by presynaptic cholinergic nerve terminal loss, show a reduction in M_2 but not M_1 binding. Thus if terminal autoreceptors are M_2 and postsynaptic ones at many synapses M_1, then M_2 antagonists would increase cholinergic activity by blocking the autoreceptors whilst M_1 antagonists would decrease cholinergic function. Clearly, specific manipulation of these different receptor mechanisms may have practical implications in the treatment of Parkinsonism, when there is increased cholinergic activity in the striatum and in Alzheimer's disease with reduced cortical ACh function. Possible second messengers for M_1 and M_2 receptors are discussed later.

Cholinergic pathways and function

Whilst the subcellular distribution of ACh, as described above, applies generally, the proportion of synaptosomal to cell body (cytoplasmic) ACh can vary from region to region depending on the neuronal organisation. Three distinct and basic CNS neuronal systems are illustrated in Fig. 1.6. In the hypothetical brain area shown the excitatory NT (E_1) would be found predominantly in synaptosomes since it is released from the nerve terminals of an afferent pathway whose origin (cell bodies) are far removed. E_2 is released from intrinsic neurons and will be distributed more evenly between synaptosomes and cytoplasm (cell bodies) whilst E_3 will be found mostly in the cytoplasmic rather than synaptosome fraction because despite its presence and concentration in the latter they form a relatively small proportion of the total mass when compared with the cell bodies of the large neurons. The ubiquitous nature of ACh as a NT is evidenced by it being employed in all three roles. Thus in the three regions of the CNS where it is most concentrated it behaves like E_3 in the ventral horn of the spinal cord as E_2 in the striatum and E_1 in the cortex (Fig. 6.2).

Since ACh is the transmitter at the skeletal neuromuscular junction one might also expect it to be released from any axon collaterals arising from the motor nerve. Such collaterals innervate (drive) an interneuron, the Renshaw cell, in the ventral horn which provides an inhibitory feedback on to the motoneuron. Not only is ACh (and ChAT) concentrated in this part of the cord but its release from antidromically stimulated ventral roots has been demonstrated both *in vitro* and *in vivo*. Also the excitation of Renshaw cells by such stimulation is not only potentiated by anticholinesterases but blocked by appropriate antagonists. In fact it illustrates both of the receptor characteristics of ACh since stimulation produces an initial rapid and brief excitation (burst of impulses), which is blocked by nicotinic antagonists, and this is followed, after a pause, by a more prolonged low frequency discharge that is blocked by muscarinic antagonists and mimicked by muscarinic agonists. Thus in this instance

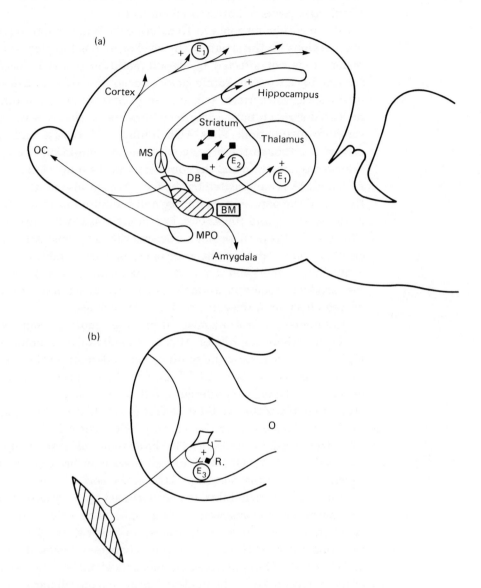

Fig. 6.2. (a) Acetylcholine is found in intrinsic neurons within the striatum (E_2 in text) but the main pathways are the cortical projections from the nucleus basalis magnocellularis (BM) which also sends axons to the thalamus and amygdala (E_1). There are other projections from the medial septum (MS) and nucleus of the diagonal band, or diagonalis broco (DB), to the hippocampus and from the magnocellular preoptic nucleus (MPO) and DB to the olfactory bulb. The DB and BM are sometimes referred to as the substantia inominata. Collectively these nuclei are known as the magnocellular forebrain nuclei (MFN). The effects of ACh mediated through these pathways are predominantly excitatory (slow) and involve muscarinic receptors. (b) In the ventral horn of the spinal cord ACh is released from collaterals of the motor nerves to skeletal muscle to stimulate (E_3) Renshaw cells (R) and activate inhibitory feedback on to the motoneuron. The initial activation of Renshaw cells is through nicotinic receptors.

although ACh is excitatory as in other areas of the CNS, it actually culminates in inhibition of motoneurons. Pharmacological manipulation of this synapse is not attempted clinically.

The nicotinic response at Renshaw cells is not found to any extent in other regions. In the striatum the level of ACh is the highest of any brain region. It is not affected by de-afferentation but is reduced by intra-striatal injections of kainic acid and so the ACh is associated with intrinsic neurons. Here ACh has an excitatory effect on other neurons mediated through muscarinic receptors and is closely involved with DA (inhibitory) function. Thus ACh inhibits DA release and atropine in-creases it although the precise anatomical connections by which this is achieved is uncertain and the complexity of the interrelationship between ACh and DA is emphasised by the fact that DA also inhibits ACh release. In view of the opposing excitatory and inhibitory effects of ACh and DA in the striatum and the known loss of striatal DA in Parkinsonism (see Chapter 16) it is perhaps not surprising that anti-muscarinic agents have been of some value in the treatment of that condition, especially in controlling tremor, and that certain muscarinic agonists, like oxotremor-ine, produce tremor in animals. Also anti-muscarinic drugs have long proved effective in the control of motion sickness.

Cholinergic neurotransmission has been most thoroughly studied in the cortex where the role of ACh as a mediator of afferent input (E_1 in Fig. 6.2) is indicated by the finding that undercutting the cortex leads to the virtual loss of ACh, ChAT and cholinesterase. That it is not the mediator of the primary afferent input has been shown by the inability of atropine to block the excitatory effect of stimulating those pathways and the fact that such stimulation causes a release of ACh over a wide area of the cortex and not just localised to the area of their cortical representation (see Collier & Mitchell 1967). Indeed there have been many experiments which show that the release of ACh in the cortex is proportional to the level of cortical excitability being increased by a variety of convulsants and decreased by anaesthesia (Fig. 6.3). The origins of this diffuse cholinergic input have been traced in the rat to the magnocellular forebrain nuclei (MFN) by mapping changes in cortical cholinesterase and ChAT after lesioning specific subcortical nuclei. The most important of them appears to be the nucleus basalis magnocellularis, similar to the nucleus of Maynert in man, which projects predominantly to the frontal and parietal cortex and is thought to be affected in Alzheimer's Dementia (Chapter 21). This nucleus together with the diagonal band form the substantia innominata and the dorsal neurons of this band also join with those in the medial septum to provide a distinct cholinergic input to the hippocampus, which is also atropine sensitive.

Despite the excitatory effect of ACh in the cortex and its increased release during convulsive activity, anti-muscarinic agents have only a slight sedative action (atropine may in fact cause stimulation) and no anticonvulsant activity except possibly in reducing some forms of

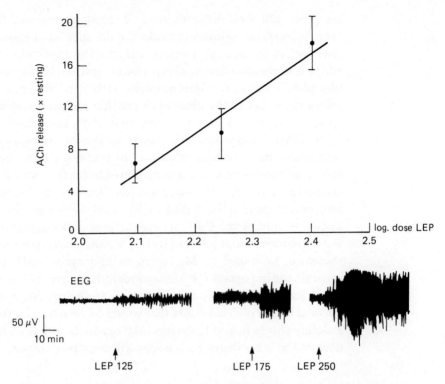

Fig. 6.3. Correlation between ACh release, EEG activity and injections of leptazol (LEP) (mg Kg^{-1} intravenously) in the urethane anaesthetised rat. ACh collected with a cortical cup incorporating EEG electrodes. Mean values $\pm$SE, n = 6. (Unpublished data, but see Gardner & Webster 1977.)

experimentally induced kindling. ACh appears to exert a background excitatory effect on cortical function and whilst it may not directly stimulate the firing of pyramidal cells it will sensitise them to other excitatory inputs through its muscarinic activity. Its role in the processing of memory and its possible malfunction in dementias has aroused considerable interest recently although drugs that modify cholinergic function in the CNS have little therapeutic use currently despite the recognised role of ACh as a neurotransmitter.

Thus ACh is an excitatory transmitter in the cerebral cortex. By its inhibitory effect on the voltage dependent K^{+} current (Gm or Im) it will lead to repetitive firing of neurons which appears to be important for memory fixation and could explain why a cholinergic malfunction may be involved in dementia. ACh may also induce repetitive firing in another way. Studies in the hippocampus have demonstrated a second K^{+} current which unlike Im is activated by (dependent on) Ca^{2+} and is involved in mediating the long hyperpolarisation of pyramidal cells after spiking. Again this is inhibited by ACh through a muscarinic mechanism and the reduction in post-spike hyperpolarisation will also lead to repetitive firing without producing the membrane depolarisation associated with the inhibition of Im. The precise link between activation of muscarinic receptors and their different ways of changing neuronal firing is uncertain. Muscarinic agonists increase the production of cyclic GMP, which itself activates cortical neurons, depress the synthesis of cyclic AMP, which is normally a neuronal depressant, and accelerate the breakdown of phosphatidylinositol-4,5-biphosphate (PIP_2) which could also have an excitatory effect as the phorbol esters that are produced will block post-spike hyperpolarisation. It seems that PIP_2 breakdown and probably cyclic GMP production, are linked to the M_1 (pirenzepine sensitive) muscarinic receptor and inhibition of cyclic AMP to the M_2 receptor. Which of these mechanisms is responsible for the various effects on K^+ conductance is currently uncertain (see Brown et al. 1986). Although M_1 receptors appear to be linked to PI breakdown and phorbol esters are known to inhibit the Ca^{2+} dependent post-spike hyperpolarisation, the latter response is not affected by the M_1 antagonist pirenzepine and may therefore, be linked to M_2 receptors and cyclic AMP production. In contrast the important Ca^{2+} independent K^+ current (Im), whilst blocked by pirenzepine and assumed to be controlled by M_1 receptors, is not affected by the phorbol esters that would be produced by their activation. Possibly this is linked to cyclic GMP production despite being independent of Ca^{2+}. No doubt such issues will soon be resolved.

References and further reading

Adams PR & Brown DA (1982) Pharmacology of the M (slow K^+) current. *J. Physiol.* **332**, 232–72 (2 papers).

Birdsall NJM & Hulme EC (1983) Muscarinic receptor subclasses. *Trends Pharmacol. Sci.* **4** 459–63.

Brown DA (1983) Slow cholinergic excitation — a mechanism for increasing neuronal excitability. *Trends Neurosci.* **6** 302–7.

Brown DA, Gahwiler BH, Marsh SJ & Selyanko AA (1986) Mechanisms of muscarinic excitatory synaptic transmission in ganglion and brains. *Trends Pharmacol. Sci. Suppl.* — Subtypes of muscarinic receptors II.

Collier B & Mitchell JF (1967) Release of ACh during consciousness and after brain lesions. *J. Physiol.* **188**, 83–98.

Fibiger HC (1982) The organisation of some projections of cholinergic neurons of the mammalian forebrain. *Brain Res. Rev.* **4**, 327–88.

Gardner CR & Webster RA (1977) Convulsant — anticonvulsant interactions on seizure activity and cortical acetylcholine release. *Eur. J. Pharmac.* **42**, 247–56.

Jordan CC & Webster RA (1977) Release of ACh in the perfused cat spinal cord in vivo. *Neuropharmacology* **17**, 321–7.

McIntosh FG & Collier B (1976) The neurochemistry of cholinergic terminals. In: Zaimis E & Maclagan J (eds) *Handbook of Experimental Pharmacology* **42** Springer-Verlag, Berlin.

Phillis JW (1976) Acetylcholine and synaptic transmission in the central nervous system. In: Hockman CH & Beiger D (eds) *Chemical Transmission in the Mammalian Central Nervous System.* University Park Press, Baltimore.

7 The catecholamines (noradrenaline and dopamine)

R.A. WEBSTER

The study of catecholamines (CAs) in the central nervous system (CNS) has been greatly facilitated by the wide range of methods available for their detection and estimation. For some 20 years it has been possible to detect CAs chemically by sensitive fluorescent procedures which involve oxidation of the amine to intermediary compounds that can be reacted either with ethylenediamine (condensation) or by the trihydroxyindole procedure (cyclisation) to give intensely fluorescent compounds. Fluorescent procedures have also been valuable in mapping CA pathways in the brain. Currently HPLC (or gas chromatography) are more commonly used for CA estimations because of their speed, sensitivity and ability to separate and measure a whole range of amines and metabolites in one sample. *In vivo* estimation of dopamine (DA) turnover by voltammetry is also now possible (see Chapter 2).

Analysis of the function and pharmacology of the CAs depends, like that of any other neurotransmitter (NT), on the availability of tools (drugs) to influence their activity specifically. Noradrenaline (NA) is well established as a peripheral NT but the development of drugs that affect its synthesis, storage, release and destruction, as well as the detailed classification of its receptors through the synthesis of specific agonists and antagonists, has been of less benefit than expected in attempting to understand its central action or manipulate its function to clinical advantage. One could argue in fact that it is the peripheral actions of NA which have retarded our understanding of its central function simply because no matter how specific may be the alpha (α) antagonists (like prazosin) or the beta (β) antagonists (like propranolol) their marked peripheral actions complicate the analysis of their central effects and also reduce their potential clinical use as centrally acting drugs. Clearly the value of a specific α_1 antagonist would be greatly reduced, even if activation of those receptors had a known and clinically undesirable central effect, if all the patients who received it suffered the consequences of a severe peripherally induced hypotension. The problem of specifically manipulating the CNS function of NA to advantage is compounded by the fact that the diffuse arrangement of its pathways precludes, or at least makes it difficult, to carry out a detailed analysis of its synaptic activity. It is for these reasons that we know more about the turnover and general function of NA and less about its release and precise synaptic activity than we do for the more conventional NTs, like ACh and GABA.

Dopamine (DA) has few peripheral actions, and its central pathways are more restricted than those of NA and better analysed. Thus a DA antagonist will not only have a central rather than a peripheral action but also tell us something about the central actions of DA.

So what is known of the central actions and function of NA and DA? Along with the indoleamine, 5-hydroxytryptamine (5-HT), they possess certain common features as central NTs which enable them to be grouped together. Monoamine (MA) neurons have three distinguishing characteristics:

1 Their axons arise from cell bodies in small distinct subcortical nuclei of perhaps only a few hundred neurons.

2 Despite these humble origins the axons ramify extensively to innervate most parts of the cortex as well as other brain areas and the spinal cord. In this respect the NA and 5-HT systems are more similar and although most of the cortex shows a high but variable fluorescence for both amines it should not be assumed that the arrangement of terminals is haphazard. Certainly NA and 5-HT fluorescence is seldom of equal intensity in one region. Whether or not the varicosities found along the axons make conventional synaptic contacts with adjacent neurons is considered below. The distribution of DA is more restricted than that of NA and 5-HT.

3 They produce a mixture of excitatory and inhibitory effects generally slow in onset and offset and involving second messengers.

In view of the radiating and diffuse projection of these pathways and their slow influence on neuronal activity it is perhaps not surprising that there has been much interest in their possible role in the control of behaviour.

Catecholamine pathways

The cell bodies of the catecholamine neurons are concentrated in nuclei originally labelled Al–A7 for NA and A8–A12 for DA by Dahlström and Fuxe (1964).

All of the NA nuclei are in the hind brain, i.e. pons, medulla region. By far the largest of these, but still only some 1500 cells in the rat, is the A6 locus coeruleus, which has smaller nuclei located ventral and caudal to it. The axons from these nuclei group into two main tracts, the dorsal medial bundle mainly running from the locus coeruleus (LC) to the cortex, thalamus, hypothalamus, geniculate bodies, colliculi and cerebellum and the ventral tegmental (or lateral) bundle from A1, 5 and 7 to the septal and pre-optic regions and the hypothalamus. Descending tracts to the spinal cord arise from A1, 2 and 6 but A2 neurons form the main NA innervation to the nucleus tractus solitarius which controls vagal innervation to the heart. In many cases the number of axons from NA neurons to certain brain area may not be sufficient to visualise directly but they become clearer after a lesion and the accumulation of the amine just rostral to it.

Most of the DA cell bodies (about 400 000) in human brain, are found in the A9 nucleus which forms the zona compacta (dorsal part) of the substantia nigra (SN), although a few cell bodies are found in the more ventral zona reticulata and in the zona lateralis as well. A8 is lateral, caudal and somewhat dorsal to A9 and A10 whereas A10 is ventral to A9 in the ventral tegmental mesencephalon. It is the axons from A9 (SN) which make the major contribution, together with some axons from A8, to the principal DA nigrostriatal pathway running to the striatum (caudate nucleus and putamen) and amygdala. This pathway is lateral to, but runs with, a more medial mesolimbic DA pathway, predominantly from A10, which innervates the nucleus accumbens and olfactory tubercle as well as parts of the cortex (mesocortical system) such as the prefrontal and perirhinal cortex. The DA innervation to the anterior cingulate cortex also comes from A10 but with some axons from A9. There is in fact no clear divide between A9 and A10 and some overlap of their pathways. A further totally separate DA pathway arises from A12 in the arcuate nucleus and forms the tuberoinfundibular tract in the median eminence to the pituitary gland for controlling prolactin release. The DA mesolimbic tract and the noradrenergic bundles come together in the medial forebrain bundle before entering the cortex.

Whilst the nigrostriatal pathways are ipsilateral some crossing occurs in fibres from the ventral tegmental A10 nucleus and also with some NA projections. These pathways are shown in Fig. 7.1. Further details can be obtained from Moore & Bloom (1978, 1979) and Lindvall & Bjorkland (1978). The nuclei provide distinct loci for activating the monoamine systems for electrophysiological, release and behavioural studies and for their destruction by electrolytic lesion or injection of the toxin 6-hydroxy-dopamine (6-OHDA).

The concentration of NA and DA in different brain areas of the rat is in keeping with the distribution of their pathways. Thus DA is concentrated in the striatum (10 μg/g), nucleus accumbens (5 μg/g) and olfactory tubercle (6 μg/g) but in the cortex there is much less (0.1 μg/g). By comparison NA reaches 0.25 μg/g in the cortex but even in the hypothalamus, where it is most concentrated, it only achieves 2.5 μg/g. 5-HT has a cortical concentration of about 0.5 μg/g. Generally whilst the cell body of a CA neuron may contain 10–100 μg/g CA, and its long, highly branched and mostly unmyelinated axon very little, the terminal varicosities boast some 1–3 mg/g.

It seems that the arrangement of CA neurons and pathways is similar in man although A10, which is the largest nucleus in the rat, is less well developed. In humans it has some 5000 cells compared with 50–80 times that number in A9 (SN). The SN cells in man and primates also differ from those in other species in containing granules of the lipoprotein pigment called neuromelanin. The melanin granules are free in the cytoplasm and give the SN a distinctive dark colour. Cells in this nucleus can also have hyaline inclusion bodies, the Lewy bodies, which are not

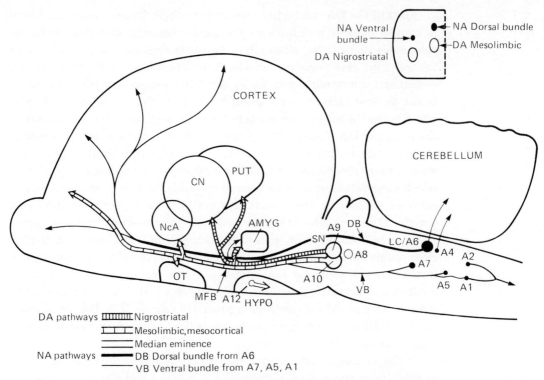

Fig. 7.1. Catecholamine pathways. AMYG, amygdala. CN, caudate nucleus. HYPO, hypothalamus. LC, locus coeruleus. MFB, medial forebrain bundle. NcA, nucleus accumbens. OT, olfactory tubercle. PUT, putamen. SN, substantia nigra.

common normally but appear to increase dramatically in patients with Parkinsonism. It has also been found that within the SN in man the neurons and blood vessels are very closely aligned. Capillaries and small vessels almost make direct contact with soma and dendrites without any glial intervention. This would obviously allow the neurons to be readily influenced by blood borne agents and might explain why they are more readily destroyed than other neurons. Certainly they will require considerable biochemical back-up to maintain function in all their terminals. Whilst similar detail is not available for the NA nuclei such as the LC the dependence of brain NA function on one such small concentrated nucleus must make it very susceptible to slight changes in blood and nutrient supply.

Catecholamine nerve terminals

It is not merely the concentration of cell bodies in discrete nuclei that characterises the CA system but the distribution and influence of their projections. In the striatum about 20% of all terminals are dopaminergic and most studies show that the nerve varicosities form classical synaptic contacts with the postsynaptic cells. This may not be so for all NA (and 5-HT) systems.

At one time it was thought that only a small percentage of noradrenergic terminals in the cortex showed conventional synaptic specialisations (membrane thickening) and the terminals appeared to resemble the varicosities seen in the peripheral sympathetic innervation of smooth muscle. This would have required NA to be released into the extracellular space and diffuse to its site of action. Whilst this 'non-synaptic' release may occur, more recent detailed EM studies have shown conventional synaptic contacts in the cortex (see references at end of Chapter 1). Nevertheless the distribution of NA fibres in the cortex is of considerable interest. They may be found in all layers of the neocortex but they are not arranged radially. They travel longitudinally through the grey matter and branch widely. Although the detailed cytoarchitecture varies from area to area, dense terminal fields are found in layers IV and V. Certainly the NA system has the organisation to modulate neuronal activity through a vast area of the neocortex.

Biochemistry of catecholamines

Synthesis

Since dopamine is the precursor of NA it is hardly surprising that its synthesis and metabolism are very similar to that of NA, even when it functions as a NT in its own right (see Fig. 7.2 and 7.3). Although both phenylalanine and tyrosine are found in the brain it is tyrosine which is the starting point for NA and DA synthesis. It appears to be transported into the brain after synthesis from phenylalanine (phenylalanine hydroxylase) in the liver rather than from phenylalanine found in the brain. Although the concentration of tyrosine in the brain is high (5×10^{-5} M) very little body tyrosine (1%) is used for the synthesis of DA and NA.

Tyrosine hydroxylase

Tyrosine is converted to dopa by the cytoplasmic enzyme tyrosine hydroxylase. This is the rate limiting step (K_m 5×10^{-6} M) in CA synthesis, it requires molecular O_2 and Fe^{2+} as well as tetrahydropteridine cofactor and is substrate specific. It can be inhibited by α-methyl-p-tyrosine, which depletes the brain of both DA and NA and it is particularly important for the maintenance of DA synthesis (see below).

Dopa decarboxylase

By contrast the cytoplasmic decarboxylation of dopa to dopamine by the enzyme dopa decarboxylase is about 100 times more rapid (K_m 4×10^{-4} M) and indeed it is difficult to detect endogenous dopa in the CNS. This enzyme, which requires pyridoxal phosphate (vitamin B6) as cofactor, can decarboxylate other amino acids (e.g. tryptophan and tyrosine) and in view of its low substrate specificity is known as a general L-aromatic amino acid decarboxylase.

Whilst a number of drugs, e.g. α-methyl dopa, inhibit the enzyme they have little effect on the levels of brain DA and NA compared with α-methyl-p-tyrosine and they also affect the decarboxylation of other amino acids. Some compounds, e.g. α-methyl dopa hydrazine (carbidopa) and benserazide, which do not easily enter the CNS have a useful role when given in conjunction with levodopa in the treatment of Parkinsonism (see Chapter 16). Of course in those neurons in which DA is the NT, synthesis stops at this stage and it becomes stored in vesicles.

Dopamine β-hydroxylase

In noradrenergic nerves the vesicles contain a synthesising enzyme, dopamine β-hydroxylase, which rapidly (K_m 5×10^{-3} M) converts DA to NA. Whilst it will act on other phenylethylamines, e.g. converting tyramine to octopamine, its restricted localisation to vesicles in noradrenergic terminals gives it functional specificity *in vivo*. Being a Cu^{2+} containing protein it can be inhibited by copper chelating agents like diethyldithiocarbamate or disulfiram. Such drugs can be used experimentally to deplete the brain of NA without affecting DA levels for although the latter might be expected to increase it is probable that excess DA is deaminated by monoamine oxidase (MAO).

In a few central neurons NA becomes the substrate for phenylethanolamine-N-methyl transferase, as in the adrenal medulla, and is converted into adrenaline.

Summary

Thus it is possible to deplete the brain of both DA and NA by inhibiting tyrosine hydroxylase but whilst NA may be reduced independently (by inhibiting dopamine β-hydroxylase) there is no way of specifically losing DA other than by destruction of its neurons. In contrast it is easier to augment DA than NA by giving the precursor dopa due to its rapid conversion to DA and the limit imposed on further synthesis by the restriction of dopamine β-hydroxylase to the vesicles in NA terminals.

Metabolism

Just as the synthesis of DA and NA is similar so is their metabolism. They are both substrates for monoamine oxidase (MAO) and catechol-O-methyl transferase (COMT). In the brain MAO is found in, or attached to, the membrane of the intraneuronal mitochondria. Thus it is only able to deaminate CAs after their uptake into nerve endings and blockade of uptake leads to a marked reduction in the level of deaminated metabolites. Nevertheless the final metabolite of both amines is one that has been both deaminated and O-methylated so it must be assumed that most of any released amine is taken up intraneuronally, deaminated and then O-methylated (Figs 7.2 and 7.3). Certainly the brain contains much more DOPAC (the deaminated metabolite of DA) than the corresponding 0-methylated derivative, 3-methoxy tyramine. The final metabolite of DA in both brain and urine is homovanillic acid (HVA). It is possible, however, that the high levels of DOPAC in the brain partly reflect intraneuronal metabolism of unreleased DA and it is by no means certain the metabolism of DA by MAO and COMT is always sequential.

Noradrenaline basically follows the same degradative pathway as DA except that after intraneuronal deamination to the aldehyde in the CNS it is not necessarily dehydrogenated to the acidic compound 3,4-dihydroxy-mandelic acid (DOMA) to the same extent as in the periphery. Instead it is reduced to the corresponding glycol (dihydroxyphenylglycol). Both these intermediaries are then further broken down by COMT with DOMA giving vanillylmandelic acid (VMA) and the glycol forming 3-methoxy-4-hydroxyphenylglycol (MOPEG). Certainly the intracerebral injection of [^{3}H]-NA gives rise to a preponderance of MOPEG rather than VMA, as does stimulation of the LC and its NA pathways. Thus MOPEG is considered to be the main metabolite of brain NA and estimates of its concentration in CSF and urine are taken as a guide to NA function in the CNS.

It is generally accepted that COMT is an extracellular enzyme in the CNS that catalyses the transfer of methyl groups from S-adenylmethion-ine to the meta-hydroxy group of the catechol of both amines. Whilst it may be inhibited by pyrogallol and catechol this does not seem to potentiate noradrenergic activity and neither of these toxic compounds has any clinical use. In contrast a whole range of drugs inhibit MAO and have been used clinically in the treatment of depression (Chapter 19) even though they are of dubious effectiveness. Recently much interest has centred on the finding that MAO exists in two forms, MAO_A and MAO_B, but although one (A) may be more active against NA and 5-HT than DA, which is a substrate for both and whilst (B) is more effective against β-phenylethylamine and DA, they do not show absolute substrate specificity. It seems likely that MAO_B is the dominant enzyme in human brain. This classification is substantiated to some extent by antagonists (inhibitors) with clorgyline being a specific inhibitor of the A form and selegiline (deprenyl) of the B. Unfortunately many of the inhibitors used clinically in the past, e.g. iproniazid, tranylcypromine and pargyline affect both forms of the enzyme. These mixed inhibitors may not only reduce the deamination of both DA and NA (as well as 5-HT) centrally but will almost certainly potentiate the effects of the amines peripherally. It is for this reason that patients given a MAO_A, or mixed, inhibitor develop severe hypertensive reactions to foods like cheese. This contains tyramine and since neither this amine, which is normally deaminated in the gastrointestinal tract, nor the NA which it releases systemically, will be

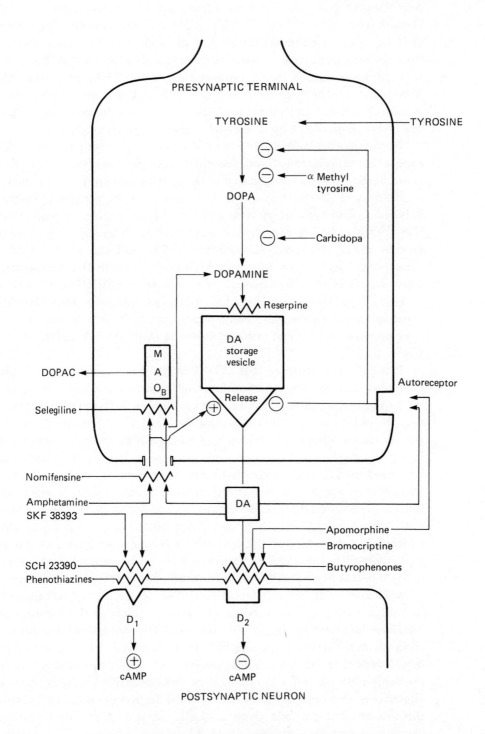

Fig. 7.2. A diagrammatic representation of a dopaminergic synapse. The biochemical pathway for the synthesis and degradation of DA is shown opposite together with the structures of amphetamine and apomorphine.

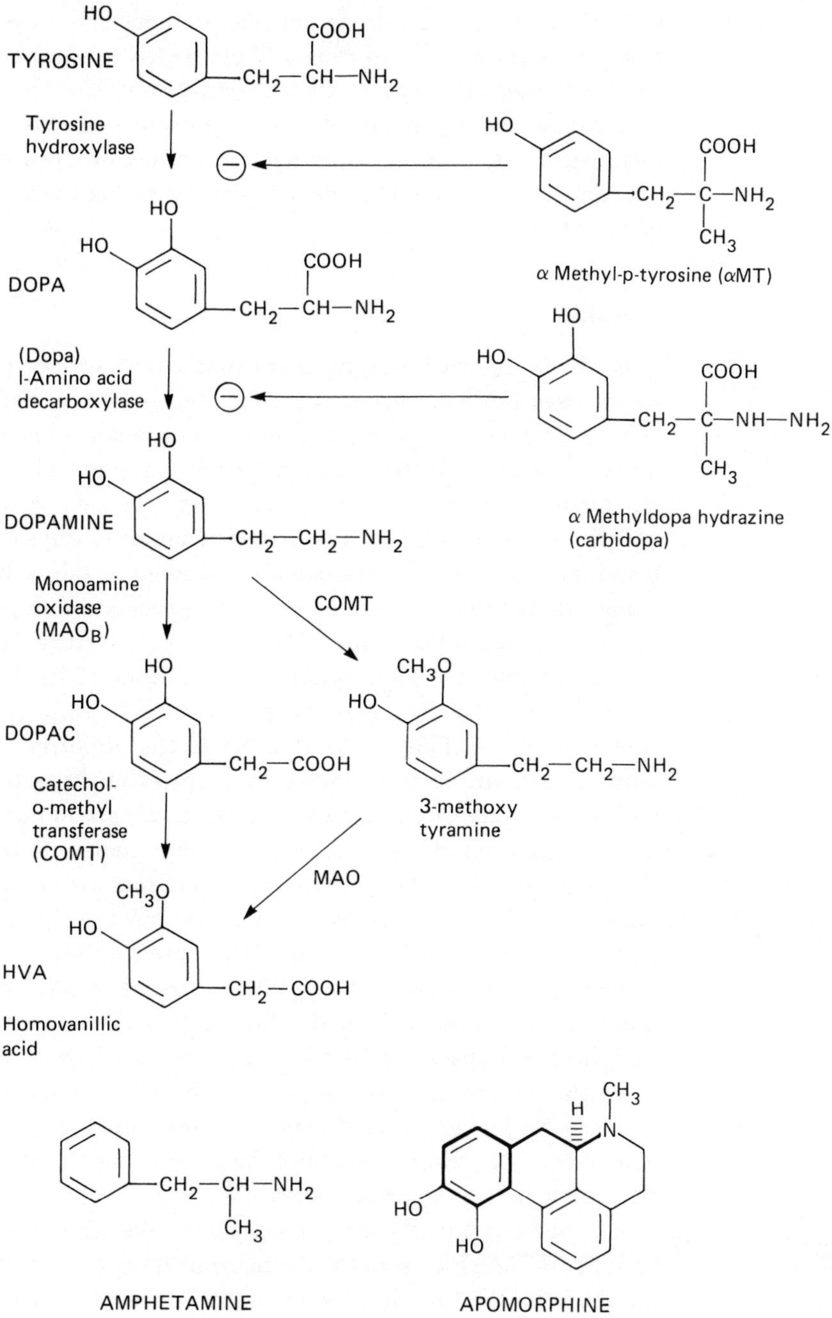

TYROSINE

Tyrosine hydroxylase

α Methyl-p-tyrosine (αMT)

DOPA

(Dopa) l-Amino acid decarboxylase

α Methyldopa hydrazine (carbidopa)

DOPAMINE

Monoamine oxidase (MAO$_B$)

COMT

DOPAC

Catechol-o-methyl transferase (COMT)

3-methoxy tyramine

MAO

HVA

Homovanillic acid

AMPHETAMINE

APOMORPHINE

Fig. 7.2. *Cont.*

THE CATECHOLAMINES (NORADRENALINE AND DOPAMINE)

deaminated, not only will more NA be released but it may be more effective as a pressor agent. Much interest has been shown recently in the use of the more specific B inhibitors since if this enzyme is mainly in the CNS they should have little peripheral effect. Of course if the B rather than the A form is found centrally and yet NA is a substrate for MAO_A, then NA may be deaminated differently centrally from peripherally. It also raises the question of the importance of MAO if it is found intraneuronally and can only act on amines in the nerve terminal. Its function may be to control the cytoplasmic rather than the synaptic levels of the MAs.

Uptake

It has been known for many years that after its intravenous injection in large doses NA will become concentrated in sympathetically innervated tissues, such as the spleen, and that this capacity is lost after denervation and degeneration of the sympathetic nerve supply. The advent of labelled NA made it possible to show that this 'uptake' also occurred with the low concentration of NA that might be encountered physiologically at nerve terminal synapses. Uptake was first studied in detail by Iversen (1967) using isolated rat hearts. It is an active process which proceeds against a concentration gradient (up to 1000:1), is temperature, energy and sodium dependent and can be blocked by inhibitors of its Na^+/K^+ activated ATPase, as well as by a wide range of substrate inhibitors. Whilst uptake shows some specificity, in that L-NA is the preferred substrate (100:1), many drugs can be transported by it into the nerve terminal (amphetamine, tyramine, guanethidine, 6-hydroxydopamine) and it is blocked by a wide range of drugs, e.g. cocaine, and many of the tricyclic antidepressants such as desmethylimipramine and nortryptiline. The importance of uptake in the control of synaptic NA levels is established by the fact that even when MAO and COMT are inhibited any stimulation of sympathetic nerves causes very little increase in NA overflow unless the uptake process is also blocked. Thus neuronal uptake (referred to as U_1 at peripheral synapses) is the first stage in the destruction of NA. Peripherally there is also uptake into smooth muscle (U_2) but it is less important and it is not known to what extent non-neuronal (glial) uptake of NA occurs in the CNS. Blockade of uptake potentiates the effect of iontophoretic NA on central neurons, at least acutely.

DA nerve terminals also possess an uptake system. This appears to be specific for DA since striatal DA neurons do not concentrate NA and DA uptake is blocked by drugs such as nomifensine which do not affect NA uptake. Despite this selectivity some compounds, e.g. amphetamine and 6-OHDA, can be taken up by both types of neuron.

Studies with labelled NA (and DA) show that freshly taken up amine is released preferentially. This suggests that recaptured NA could be an important source of supply for release although there is no evidence that blocking uptake, even over the long term, normally impairs release.

Storage and release

Most (up to 75%) of the DA and NA in nerve terminal is stored in vesicles (sometimes called granules or particles) and so protected from MAO. Studies of their composition and function, mainly in peripheral nerves and chromaffin cells, show that they contain NA in a 4:1 ratio with ATP in chromaffin cells but possibly 8:1 in nerves. In addition there is the enzyme dopamine β-hydroxylase and a soluble protein, chromogranin, as well as a Mg^{2+}- and Ca^{2+}-dependent ATPase. The quantity of NA in vesicles is such that if it was in free solution this would be sufficiently hypertonic to cause lysis of the vesicle. Apart from providing a site for synthesising NA and protecting it from MAO it seems likely that vesicles also provide the source of NA released by nerve stimulation. Vesicles come in two sizes and are usually referred to as dense cored because of their appearance after fixation for electron microscopy. The larger (75 nm diameter) are found in the cell body and transported to the terminal by axoplasmic flow (5 mm/hour in rat, 10 mm/hour in cat) during which time NA is synthesised within them. Smaller vesicles are mainly formed in the nerve terminal from endoplasmic reticulum (although some are transported from the cell body). They contain dopamine β-hydroxylase and can synthesise NA which is again complexed with ATP but in a much higher ratio of 20:1 (NA:ATP). It is generally considered unlikely that vesicles are reused but since some released NA is taken back into the nerve terminal and freshly taken up [^{3}H]-NA is preferentially released, presumably from vesicles, it seems that not all vesicles synthesise their NA or at least not all of it. Release is considered to be by exocytosis and Ca^{2+} dependent (see Fillenz 1984).

Storage can be disrupted by the Rauwolfia alkaloid, reserpine and by drugs like tetrabenazine. The latter seems to be more active in CA neurons but reserpine depletes all amines (NA, DA and 5-HT) from both neurons and chromaffin cells and storage does not return until new vesicles are synthesised. It should be emphasised that these drugs deplete the neurons of amines by stopping amine being incorporated into vesicles so that it leaks out and is deaminated. They do not cause a release of amines to induce synaptic activity.

It is likely that up to 30% of terminal NA is free in the cytoplasm rather than retained in vesicles.

Turnover

Autoreceptors: short term control

It was emphasised above that in order to obtain maximum overflow of released NA it is necessary to block its metabolising enzymes and neuronal uptake. It is now known that the resultant increase in synaptic NA inhibits its own further release by activating receptors on the nerve terminal. Thus the synapse has a local mechanism for controlling NT

　THE CATECHOLAMINES (NORADRENALINE AND DOPAMINE)

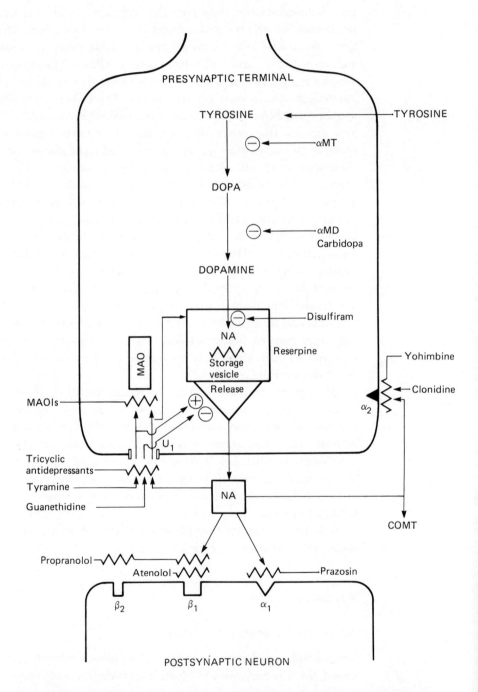

Fig. 7.3. A diagrammatic representation of a noradrenergic synapse. The biochemical pathway for the synthesis and degradation of NA is shown opposite.

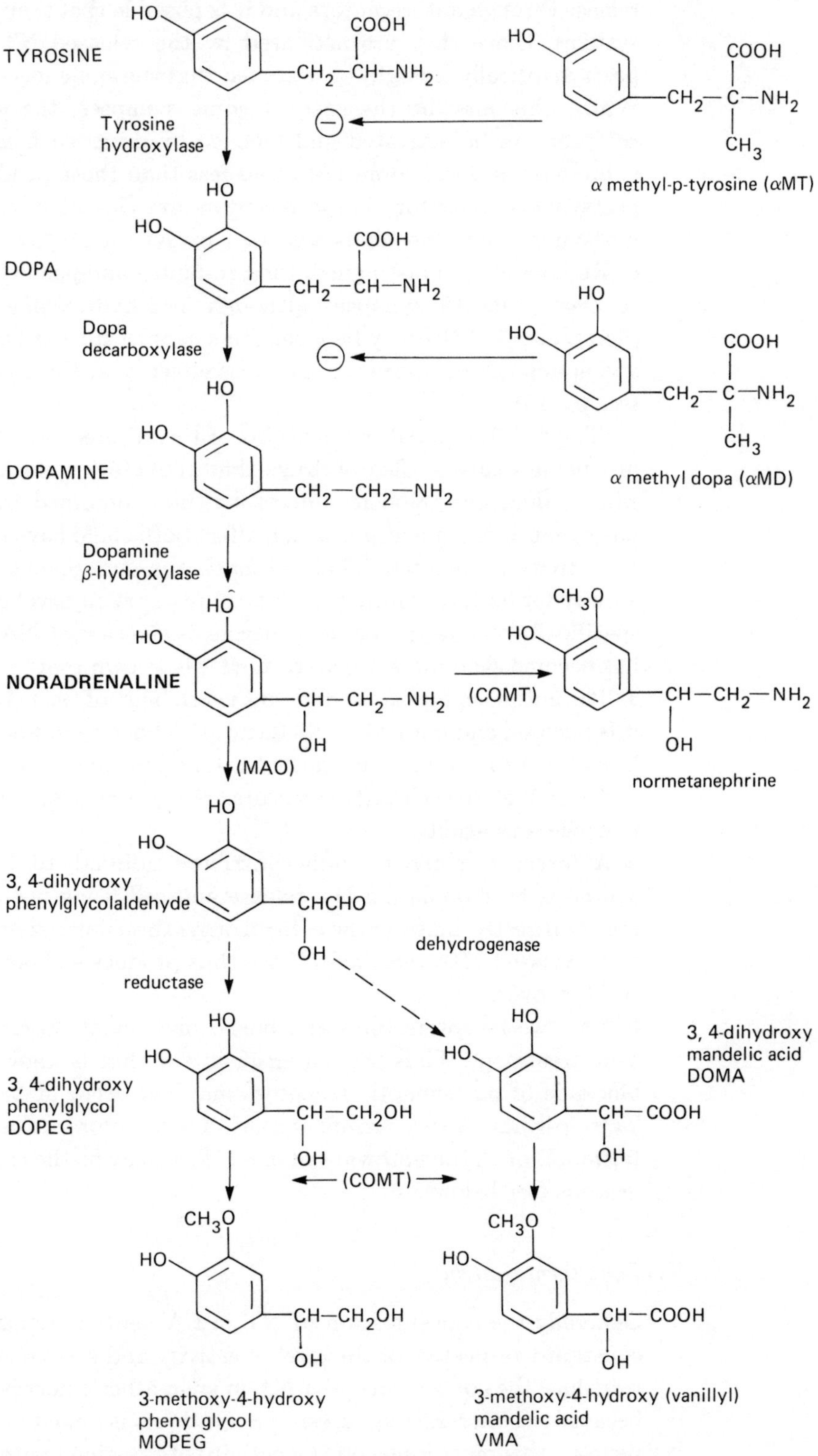
TYROSINE
Tyrosine
hydroxylase
α methyl-p-tyrosine (αMT)
DOPA
Dopa
decarboxylase
α methyl dopa (αMD)
DOPAMINE
Dopamine
β-hydroxylase
NORADRENALINE
(COMT)
normetanephrine
(MAO)
3, 4-dihydroxy
phenylglycolaldehyde
dehydrogenase
reductase
3, 4-dihydroxy
phenylglycol
DOPEG
3, 4-dihydroxy
mandelic acid
DOMA
(COMT)
3-methoxy-4-hydroxy
phenyl glycol
MOPEG
3-methoxy-4-hydroxy (vanillyl)
mandelic acid
VMA

Fig. 7.3. *Cont.*

release through autoreceptors and it is possible that they exist for all NT systems. Since they are activated by the released NT that also acts postsynaptically it might be assumed that the same receptor is involved. Whilst this may be the case at some synapses, the presynaptic NA receptor can be activated and blocked by drugs such as clonidine and yohimbine in doses some 100 times less than those needed to affect the postsynaptic receptor. These receptors are classified as alpha one (α_1) postsynaptically and alpha two (α_2) presynaptically. So far it has not proved possible to distinguish the pre-(auto) and postsynaptic receptors so clearly at DA synapses although 3-(3-hydroxyphenyl)-N-n-propyl piperidine (3-PPP) may be a selective agonist for the DA autoreceptors and apomorphine appears to be more effective at these presynaptic sites (see p. 115).

The full functional implications of the autoreceptor system are only just being realised. Clearly drugs that activate (or block) autoreceptors will produce the opposite effects to those obtained by acting at the postsynaptic site and drugs which affect both could have their postsynaptic activity attenuated. Thus although the endogenous NT must have affinity for both receptors it is important to try to develop drugs that act specifically on one site or the other, as is the case at NA synapses. This has become even more apparent now it is known that:

1 The autoreceptors are found on the cell body of the neuron from which it is released and not just on its terminals. Thus clonidine (α_2 agonist) inhibits the firing of neurons in the LC (and DA that of neurons in the SN) and even if all the cell body receptors are not innervated they will respond to exogenous agents.

2 Autoreceptors may not only contribute indirectly to the control of NT synthesis by modulating NT release and cell firing but their activation may be directly linked to the control of synthesising enzymes, e.g. tyrosine hydroxylase in DA terminals. They thus produce a short term control of NT turnover.

3 The two receptors (pre- and post-) may adapt differently to chronic drug treatment. Thus the supersensitivity that is known to follow the blockade of postsynaptic receptors may not occur at presynaptic sites. This will have extra significance if autoreceptors do not exist on the terminals of all the pathways of one NT, as may be the case with DA projections (see below).

Long term control

Generally the concentration of NT in CA neurons remains remarkably constant irrespective of the level of activity and it is virtually impossible to reduce the concentration of NA in sympathetic nerves by stimulation because this increases synthesis, i.e. synthesis is linked to demand. In CA neurons this must hinge on the activity of tyrosine hydroxylase which is increased by nerve stimulation. *In vitro* studies show it is controlled by end product feedback inhibition and possibly therefore *in vivo* by the level of free intraneuronal NA and DA. Recent evidence suggests that whilst this may play some part it seems that nerve stimulation increases the activity of tyrosine hydroxylase more directly, probably by a change in the affinity of the hydroxylase enzyme for its pteridine cofactor rather than for tyrosine with which it is normally saturated. This is perhaps not too surprising since only free cytoplasmic CA could influence hydroxylation and this should be kept constant by MAO even though MAO only prevents the elevation of CA and it is its reduction that would stimulate synthesis. The precise role of cytoplasmic CA is uncertain for although there is no evidence of NA being released from the cytoplasm by nerve stimulation it is recaptured into the cytoplasm by uptake. Possibly there is a special pool of NA directly linked to hydroxylation and reflecting release requirements without there being an overall change in cytoplasmic amine. Kunczenski (1973) describes two forms of striatal tyrosine hydroxylase — soluble and particulate. For more detailed analysis of synthesis control see Walker (1986) and Cooper *et al.* (1982).

Values for tyrosine hydroxylase activity, CA levels and turnover, as determined by Bacopoulos and Bhatnager (1977), are shown in Table 7.1.

Table 7.1.

	Tyrosine hydroxylase activity (nmol dopa synthesised/mg protein/ hour)	Concentration $\mu g/g$	Turnover $\mu g/g$/hour
DA			
Substantia nigra	17.5	1.73	1.7
Caudate nucleus	12.0	2.12	7.4
Nucleus accumbens	11.1	0.62	2.6
Amygdala	4.3	0.25	0.9
NA			
Locus coeruleus	4.6	0.22	0.99
Cortex	0.27	0.10	0.33
Pons-medulla	0.23	0.13	0.99

These values emphasise the greater synthesis of dopa and turnover of amine in DA neurons and the higher activity of tyrosine hydroxylase in areas containing CA cell bodies (SN and LC) rather than terminals.

Neurotoxins

These may show specificity by utilising the appropriate uptake mechanisms. Thus guanethidine, an adrenergic neuron blocking agent, may reduce the release of NA from peripheral nerves without affecting ACh terminals not because of a particular mechanism of action in NA terminals but because it is transported into and concentrated within them. In fact large and repeated doses of this compound produce a chemical sympathectomy but its effect can be reduced by drugs that block the uptake process. Although this compound has not been used centrally other toxins have been. The most widely used is the 6-hydroxylated form of DA, 6-hydroxydopamine (6-OHDA) which is taken up into both DA and NA nerve terminals where it is readily oxidised to compounds that cause degeneration of the terminals over a period of days. To produce a central effect it must be administered directly into the brain by intracerebroventricular (i.c.v.) injection. NA terminals can be protected by prior injection of the uptake inhibitor desmethylimipramine and DA terminals by nomifensine. Alternatively small amounts may be injected directly by stereotaxic techniques into particular DA and NA nuclei where uptake takes place even if terminals are not present.

Recently much interest has centred on a very specific toxin for DA neurons. This is 1-methyl-4-phenyl-1,2,3,6-tetrahydropyridine (MPTP). It was discovered when a student, who was addicted to pethidine, tried to manufacture 1-methyl-4-phenyl-4-propionoxypiperidine (MPPP) but took a short cut in synthesis and produced MPTP. When he administered this to himself he developed Parkinsonism. MPTP destroys DA neurons. Again this process depends on the uptake mechanism since MPTP itself is not the active material. It needs to be deaminated to MPP^+ which is then taken up by DA nerve terminals (see Chapter 16).

Receptors and neuronal responses

Adrenoceptors: classification

Four distinct adrenoceptors have been characterised peripherally and classified as α_1 and α_2 as well as β_1 and β_2. The actions associated with these receptors and specific agonists and antagonists for them are shown in Table 7.2.

With so many tools with which to study adrenoceptors one might have expected their central location and functions to have been fully analysed. Unfortunately this is not so. As mentioned at the start of this chapter many of these drugs do not cross the blood-brain barrier and all have peripheral effects, which can complicate the analysis of their central actions. Thus our understanding of the central distribution and function of adrenoceptors depends almost entirely on the results of electrophysiological, binding and biochemical studies which cannot be easily extrapolated to physiological changes.

Despite these problems there is evidence for all four adrenoceptors in the CNS although since NA is not an agonist at β_2 receptors it does not mean that they are all innervated. Their distribution has been mapped by three different ligand binding studies:

1 Autoradiographic localisation of specific tritiated ligands.
2 Calculation of the number of specific binding sites in different brain regions.

Table 7.2. Adrenoceptor classification. Agonists and antagonists

Receptor	a_1	a_2	β_1	β_2
Peripheral actions	Smooth muscle Generally contraction $\uparrow IP_3$ Ca^{2+}	Presynaptic Reduces NA release $\downarrow cAMP$	Heart Stimulation $\uparrow cAMP$	Smooth muscle Relaxation $\uparrow cAMP$
Agonist				
Specific	Methoxamine Phenylephrine	Clonidine Methyl noradrenaline	— —	Salbutamol —
Mixed	Noradrenaline —	Noradrenaline —	Noradrenaline Isoprenaline	— Isoprenaline
Antagonists				
Specific	Prazosin	Yohimbine Piperoxane	Atenolol Practolol	— —
Mixed	Phentolamine	Phentolamine	Propranolol	Propranolol

Specificity is seldom absolute. Thus clonidine will activate α_1 as well as α_2 receptors, and salbutamol β_1 as well as β_2 when the concentrations are increased (100 fold).

3 The effect of 6-OHDA lesions and degeneration of NA pathways on receptor number. Increases (with supersensitivity to agonists) indicate a postsynaptic location and decreases a presynaptic one.

Visualisation of [³H]-prazosin (α_1) binding sites shows their presence in layer IV and parts of V in most of the neocortex, where NA terminals are known to be concentrated, also in the thalamus and dorsal raphe nucleus. In contrast α_2 receptors ([³H]-clonidine binding) were found mostly in the locus coeruleus on NA cell bodies and in the nucleus tractus solitarius. Detailed autoradiography of the separate β receptors is not available but conventional binding studies show that the cerebral cortex contains predominantly β_1 and the cerebellum β_2 receptors (displacement of the mixed β antagonist [³H]-dihydroalprenolol by more specific β_1 and β_2 agonists and antagonists). Lesion of the noradrenergic dorsal bundle produces a loss of cortical NA but an increase in β_1 receptors in all forebrain areas except the hypothalamus and in α_1 receptors in the frontal cortex, thalamus and septum. Surprisingly such lesions also increase α_2 binding in frontal cortex, but not in other areas and the more widespread destruction of NA pathways by 6-OHDA given into the ventricles does not produce the expected loss of α_2 binding in the brain. β_2 receptor number increases in the cerebellum after 6-OHDA (see Uprichard *et al.* 1980 and Palacios 1984).

Thus it seems that α_1 and β_1 receptors are found in various parts of the cortex, the main fields of influence of NA pathways, but the pathways to the cerebellum seem to innervate β_2 receptors, despite the fact that NA is not an agonist for these receptors. It is probable that α_2 receptors are not restricted to and may not even be primarily associated with, NA nerve terminals.

Adrenoceptors: functional aspects

NA does not behave like a classical NT, by producing rapid depolarisation or hyperpolarisation of neurons. Instead it produces a mixture of slowly developing and more maintained excitatory and inhibitory effects. Most studies have involved iontophoretic application *in vivo*, when the anaesthetic may modify the response (barbiturates reduce excitatory effects), but recently brain slices have been used. In only a few instances has it been possible to compare directly the effect of endogenous (nerve released) and exogenous NA, despite the ease with which NA cell bodies in the LC can be stimulated, and there are few reports on the intracellular monitoring of membrane potential. Most neurons, irrespective of whether they are innervated by NA pathways, will respond to NA but in analysing its physiological function it is important to consider primarily the results from innervated areas such as parts of the cortex, hippocampus and cerebellum, as well as the LC itself.

Exogenous and endogenous NA have been compared in the cerebellum (Hoffer *et al.* 1973). Iontopheresis of NA to rat Purkinje cells produces a depression of spontaneous discharge mimicked by the β agonist isoprenaline and blocked by mixed β antagonists. Intracellular recording shows an hyperpolarisation with no change, or an increase, in membrane resistance, i.e. reduced ion conductance. Stimulation of the LC projection to cerebellum produces a similar depression and hyperpolarisation. Both LC stimulation and applied NA also have a similar depressant effect on pyramidal cells in the hippocampus. However, in both instances despite the inhibition of spontaneous firing NA can apparently increase the response to other inputs. In hippocampal slices, NA augments the effect of both applied glutamate and depolarising currents and intracellular recording indicates that it blocks a Ca^{2+} activated K^+ conductance, which attenuates spiking in pyramidal cells. Thus the accommodation (dampening) which normally follows a depolarising stimulus is reduced and the number of spikes it generates is increased (Madison and Nicoll 1982). This appears to be a beta effect since not only is it blocked by propranolol but isoprenaline and cyclic AMP also reduce the Ca^{2+}/K^+ conductance like NA. These effects have a long latency (50 msec) but prolonged duration (400 msec). The depression of spontaneous background firing by NA, coupled with the increased response to other imputs, has lead to the suggestion that it improves the signal to noise ratio.

In the neocortex generally NA produces some β_1 mediated inhibition but mainly α_1 excitatory effects (mimicked by methoxamine, blocked by prazosin). In other regions, e.g. dorsal raphe nucleus and dorsal lateral geniculate nucleus, which have a strong innervation from LC, both iontophoretic NA and LC stimulation facilitate the response of neurons to other inputs through an α_1 (prazosin sensitive) mechanism. Again the response to LC stimulation lasts for hundreds of milliseconds and although NA does not generate firing it produces enough depolarisation (a few millivolts), probably by decreasing K^+ conductance, to make the neuron more readily fired by other inputs. The decreased conductance could also enhance the voltage changes produced by excitatory inputs and again improve the signal to noise ratio. Thus irrespective of whether NA increases (α_1) or decreases (β) background firing it can still enhance input signals and these could be inhibitory or excitatory.

Iontophoretic application of both NA or clonidine to neurons in the LC produces an inhibition that is blocked by yohimbine. Since these are NA neurons the response can be ascribed to activation of autoreceptors even though they are on the cell bodies rather than terminals. It might seem that such receptors would not be innervated but antidromic stimulation of the dorsal noradrenergic bundle, which arises from LC, does suppress LC neuron firing for up to one second through an α_2 (piperoxane blocked) mechanism. Intracellular recordings show that the α_2 agonist clonidine hyperpolarises LC neurons probably by increasing K^+ efflux through a Ca^{2+} activated mechanism. Little is known of the role of the apparently large number of other postsynaptic α_2 binding sites in the CNS.

It seems from these experimental findings that all the neuronal effects of NA involve changes in K^+ conductance coupled with facilitation of the response to other NTs. The slow onset and long duration of its activity are also in keeping with the concept of a background effect widely distributed in the brain areas. (See Aghajanian 1984 and Szabadi 1979.)

Dopamine receptors: classification

When discussing adrenoceptors in the CNS it was possible to assume a classification based on experimental evidence obtained from peripheral studies and concentrate on their central actions. With DA any classification of its receptors must depend on more recent central studies and these are therefore considered separately in Chapter 8. It appears that there are at least two well defined DA receptors, D_1 linked to adenylate cyclase and stimulation of cyclic AMP production and D_2 that might reduce the enzyme's activity, although this is probably not their main mode of action. It is the D_2 receptors to which most of the effective neuroleptic drugs bind, which are activated by DA agonists like bromocriptine and are thought to be the important postsynaptic receptors mediating behavioural and extrapyramidal activity.

Dopamine receptors: functional aspects

Because DA is more localised to one brain area (striatum) than is the case with NA and since there is such a pronounced DA pathway from SN to the striatum it would be reasonable to assume that the effect of this pathway on striatal neurons would be well established. Unfortunately this is not the case.

Over the years a large number of studies using extracellular recording in the striatum have shown that iontophoretic DA depresses 75–100% of all neurons responding to it, irrespective of whether spontaneous, excitatory amino acid induced, or synaptic evoked activity, was being monitored. Most striatal neurons are in fact quiescent in anaesthetised animals and therefore need to be activated by an amino acid or the studies are biased by selecting only the few spontaneously active neurons. As with NA this inhibitory response is slow in onset (up to 15 seconds) and long in duration (possibly minutes). Stimulation of SN can produce inhibition, excitation or mixed effects but it is unlikely, despite the high proportion of DA neurons in this nucleus that all the effects are elicited by DA. By the same line of argument it would be surprising, considering the density of the DA innervation to striatum compared with that of NA in the cortex, if the role of DA was just a modulatory one. All neuroleptics block the inhibitory effects of applied DA but some, e.g. haloperidol, are less active against SN evoked inhibition.

DA induced inhibition is mimicked by cyclic AMP and this has been implicated as the second messenger. Although both DA and cyclic AMP induced inhibitions are potentiated by phosphodiesterase inhibitors it should be remembered that it is the D_1 receptor which is linked to stimulation of cyclic AMP and the D_2 receptor which is implicated in most DA function (e.g. in Parkinsonism) and probably being studied electrophysiologically in the striatum. Although the new D_1 agonist SKF 38–393, is a potent stimulant of adenylate cyclase in rat striatum, it has not been evaluated on neuronal firing. It does not, however, reduce electrically evoked ACh release in striatal slices which could be considered the outcome of the electrophysiological changes and which is inhibited by the D_2 agonist bromocriptine.

The picture is complicated rather than clarified by intracellular recordings from striatal neurons since they show that SN stimulation invariably produces a monosynaptic depolarisation, which is blocked by haloperidol. This may proceed to a hyperpolarisation if the stimulus is strong enough, but DA iontophoresed on to the same neuron also causes depolarisation (Kitai *et al.* 1976), although this may be accompanied by the reduced discharge usually seen with extracellular recording. DA infused in increasing concentrations into the striatum through a push-pull cannula also generally depresses extracellularly recorded cell firing but low concentrations can produce excitation or bimodal excitation-inhibition (Schoemer & Elkins 1984). Thus it seems that whether applied iontophoretically or released by low levels of afferent nerve stimulation DA may depolarise of striatal neurons and can be regarded as an excitatory NT even though the overall effect of both applied and released DA (with higher stimulus strengths) is a reduction in cell firing (see Siggins 1978 and Ryall & Kelly 1978). One may assume that it is this latter effect that is more likely to be achieved when augmenting DA function with large doses of levodopa or bromocriptine. The question of how an excitatory NT can depress cell firing remains to be elucidated but it may involve interneurons. DA increases the release of GABA in the striatum and this would involve an initial excitation of GABA neurons even if the released GABA inhibited the firing of other neurons such as the excitatory cholinergic neurons that are also present in the striatum. Alternatively there is evidence that DA inhibits the effects of the excitatory corticostriatal pathway which is believed to release glutamate. Since appropriate cortical lesions cause degeneration of this pathway and loss of DA binding sites, it is possible that the inhibition of glutamate release by DA, that can be demonstrated in striatal slices, is due to a presynaptic action of DA on glutamate nerve terminals. Conceivably then, the initial direct postsynaptic effect of DA may be excitatory but the resultant overall response is inhibitory through some of the mechanisms discussed above. Of course since intracellular recordings are only made from relatively large neurons the depolarisation they show may not be representative of striatal neurons generally. The implications of these effects in the use of DA agonists is considered later.

In other brain areas receiving a DA input, i.e. nucleus accumbens and amygdala (mesolimbic) or prefrontal cortex (mesocortical) the iontophoretic application of DA to neurons invariably causes an inhibition of firing (spontaneous or evoked). These effects are blocked by neuroleptics but they have not been compared with those of DA released by A10 stimulation.

Dopamine receptors: autoreceptors

It is most probable that the DA effects on neuronal activity just discussed are mediated through the same receptor (D_2). There are claims that these postsynaptic receptors may differ from DA autoreceptors although the distinction is nowhere near as clear as for the α_2 and α_1 receptors of NA neurons. It is based on the finding that low doses of apomorphine decrease striatal DA turnover and locomotor activity in rats. This would have to be a presynaptic affect for a DA agonist, which normally increases locomotor activity by a postsynaptic action. It is achieved with a dose of apomorphine 100 fold less than that which induces locomotor activity. This does not necessarily mean that the receptors are different although some neuroleptics, e.g. metoclopramide are more effective than others in blocking these low dose (presumed presynaptic) effects of apomorphine than in affecting postsynaptic sites. There are no antagonists with a clear presynaptic as opposed to postsynaptic effect. In fact studies with a whole range of agonists and antagonists on DA release (reduced through autoreceptor activity) and ACh release (decreased by postsynaptic receptor activity) in striatal slices, show no difference between the two responses and in the receptors involved. Even 3PPP, which is claimed to be a specific autoreceptor agonist, because it inhibits tyrosine hydroxylase activity in striatal homogenates, had no effect on DA release. It thus seems that the autoreceptor is the same or very similar to the postsynaptic D_2 receptors. It is not a D_1 receptor as D_1 agonists like SKF 38393 and the D_1 antagonist SCH23390 do not modify DA release or the apomorphine decrease in locomotor activity (Cuomo *et al.* 1986). If autoreceptors are activated by high synaptic concentrations of neurotransmitter they could possibly be more important at DA than NA synapses, especially in regions like the striatum where the synaptic concentration of DA must exceed that of NA in any brain region. Indeed voltammetry measurements imply that it can reach 10^{-4} M after SN stimulation, when activation of autoreceptors would presumably be unavoidable. They may also be important in the SN itself, where they are known to occur on the neuronal cell bodies, since it has been shown that DA can be released from the dendrites of these DA neurons and this would then inhibit their firing. Autoreceptors may not be so vital in other regions with a DA innervation and the possible consequences of their absence on the mesocortical pathway is discussed later.

Functional significance of catecholamine pathways

With such distinct pathways and a whole range of drugs to manipulate their activity one might be forgiven for thinking that it would be easy to establish the function of the CAs in the CNS. In reality it has proved most difficult. Drugs which reduce the concentration or activity of DA or NA generally decrease CNS function (α-methyltyrosine, reserpine) whilst drugs which increase CA activity (amphetamine, cocaine) are stimulators. One conclusion from such observations is that NA is needed to maintain normal behaviour whilst DA activates more abnormal behaviour.

Noradrenaline

Stimulation of locus coeruleus (LC) does not produce any clearly defined effects although there is some evidence that it supports self stimulation in animals. In cats it produces electroencephalographic (EEG) arousal and a rise in blood pressure (Koella 1977). There are claims that LC controls the sleep-waking pattern because the discharge of neurons within it increases during waking (Chu & Bloom 1973). Others claim that the increase occurs in non-adrenergic neurons although considering the preponderance of NA neurons in the LC it would be surprising if some were not involved. Lesions of LC reduce paradoxical REM sleep and also lead to EEG synchrony and whilst they do not reduce simple locomotive activity more complex response activity is impaired.

Since LC neurons are inhibited by α_2 agonists this provides another means of reducing central NA function. Unfortunately when clonidine or NA are infused into the LC region, the rat's spontaneous motor activity is increased whilst it is reduced by yohimbine (Weiss *et al.* 1986). Also the depressed state induced in rats by strong uncontrolled shock is overcome by clonidine infusion to LC. Thus these observations imply that since inhibition of LC (and NA function) increases activity then NA must be behaviourally depressant although of course since neuronal firing of the LC was not monitored in these experiments such conclusions may not be justified. Also when clonidine is administered i.v. or i.c.v. it has the opposite effect, i.e. it is depressant and sedative, as are α_1 and β_1 agonists like phenylephrine and isoprenaline after injection into the lateral ventricle. Clearly although direct application of NA and related agonists to the CNS has interesting possibilities it is only of real value if it can be restricted to particular areas where its effect on neuronal firing, as well as behaviour, can be monitored.

Alpha and β antagonists are used clinically. Prazosin is a specific α_1 antagonist employed to treat hypertension but no consistent central effects have been reported. By contrast β blockers have often been used to treat anxiety although it is not known whether their efficacy in this condition is due to a β-blocking action in the CNS or in the periphery (e.g. reducing cardiac function), or even to some other effect. Despite the availability of isomers with or without β-blocking activity and some that do not readily penetrate the CNS the situation is not resolved. The D isomer of propranolol does appear, however, to retain its calming effect on animals despite the loss of β antagonism and it is anxiolytic in man, like practolol, which does not easily cross the blood-brain barrier. The peripheral effects may therefore predominate (see Kielholz 1977).

Thus it is difficult to define a central functional role for NA. It must be involved in some way in the control of behaviour not only because so many drugs that modify its function have a behavioural effect in animals but many of the drugs used to treat behavioural disorders in man alter NA function. Possibly in no instance is NA the primary NT involved. This would be true of benzodiazepine induced sedation which is accompanied by reduced NA turnover (see Chapter 20) even though the benzodiazepines have no direct effect on NA synapses. Also it seems that the antidepressants must work, at least in part, by modifying NA function but even here controversy rages over whether this has to be increased or decreased to obtain a beneficial effect (see Chapter 19). Possibly the electrophysiological finding that NA increases signal to noise ratio, like a high frequency filter, is really its function, i.e. it facilitates (is required for) normal behaviour and the activity of other NTs rather than initiating function itself. In the evolutionary development of nervous system complexity it in fact appears after DA and 5-HT.

Dopamine

It is easier to allocate a central function to DA not only because it has few peripheral effects but its central distribution is more restricted than that of NA.

Of course the assessment of DA also starts with the knowledge that many people unfortunately suffer from a reasonably specific degeneration of its main neuronal pathway (nigrostriatal) and the akinesia that develops is such a clear symptom of Parkinsonism that DA must be linked to the control of motor function. It is also known that an imbalance of DA function on the two sides of the rat brain, either by stimulation or lesion of one SN, causes off-line or rotational movement (Ungerstedt & Arbuthnott 1970). This is best shown some days after 6-OHDA lesion of one SN and its nigrostriatal (NS) pathway when systemic apomorphine (DA agonist) causes animals to turn away from the lesioned side (contraversive), presumably because the denervated striatum has become supersensitive and therefore more responsive than the control side to DA agonists. Conversely amphetamine promotes movement towards the lesioned side (ipsiversive) because it can only release DA in the intact striatum. Thus animals move away from the side with the most responsive and active striatum. These drugs also produce other motor activity including increased locomotion and a so called 'stereotype' behaviour in which rats sniff avidly around the cage and spend much time licking and rearing. It appears that stereotypy is due to activation of the NS pathway as it is absent after lesion of the substantia nigra and follows apomorphine and amphetamine injection into the striatum whereas locomotor responses to amphetamine are reduced by lesions to A10 and can be induced by its injection into the nucleus accumbens. Another indication of the importance of DA in motor control is the observation that in man its precursor levodopa, and DA agonists like bromocriptine, not only overcome the akinesia of Parkinsonism but in excess will actually cause involuntary movements, or dyskinesia. Also it is well known that all the DA antagonists like chlorpromazine and haloperidol, produce Parkinsonian-like symptoms in man (and catalepsy in animals). In fact such drugs may be used to block DA activity and reduce the dyskinesia of Huntington's Chorea. Thus DA seems to sit on a knife edge in the control of motor function.

The main use clinically of DA antagonists, however, is in the treatment of schizophrenia and the control of mania. Since psychotic symptoms are also a side-effect of levodopa therapy in Parkinsonism and as amphetamine causes hallucinations and schizophrenic like symptoms in man, presumably by releasing DA, it appears that DA also has an important part to play in the control and induction of psychotic symptoms. It is possible that the role of DA in psychotic behaviour is mediated primarily through the mesolimbic and mesocortical pathways and its control of motor function through the striatum. The differential effect of amphetamine and apomorphine on the striatum and mesolimbic areas, as discussed above, also points to the possibility that these DA pathways subserve different functions. There is also evidence that the neurons from which they arise may have different characteristics. Although there is some overlap in the location of the cell bodies of the different DA pathways between the various DA nuclei they can be identified by antidromic activation of their terminal axons in the appropriate projection areas. Recordings from neurons so identified show that they have differing firing patterns. Thus cells innervating the prefrontal cortex have a much higher firing rate (9.7 Hz) than those to the cingulate and piriform cortex (5.9 or 4.3) and the striatum (3.1). Unlike the NA neurons they are also remarkably little affected by the state of the animal, i.e. its wake-sleep cycle. The cells in A10 which form the mesocortical pathway are also less easily inhibited by DA agonists suggesting that they probably have fewer autoreceptors.

Unfortunately it seems that the DA postsynaptic receptor is identical at both sites so that even if they control different functions it has been difficult to divorce the antischizophrenic from the extrapyramidal inducing activity of DA antagonists (see section on DA antagonists). Evidence for a malfunction (hyperactivity) of DA in schizophrenia is considered in Chapter 18. Those interested in a detailed and critical analysis of CA function in the control of behaviour, especially in animals, should consult Mason (1986).

DA has two other well established central actions. It appears to be the mediator of activity in the chemoreceptor trigger zone and responsible for the induction of all vomiting other than that of vestibular origin. Such vomiting is an unfortunate side-effect of levodopa therapy, it is induced by apomorphine and controlled by the DA antagonists. The separate DA pathways in the hypothalamic median eminence control (inhibit) the release of prolactin.

Levodopa and DA agonists

Levodopa is used in the treatment of Parkinsonism (see Chapter 16). It is converted to DA and therefore may produce all the effects expected of this NT. On the credit side it overcomes the akinesia but it may cause nausea and vomiting, psychotic symptoms and dyskinesias. In addition it will reduce prolactin secretion.

Where the conversion of levodopa to DA takes place is uncertain since it is estimated that Parkinsonian patients have lost over 80% of their DA innervation to the striatum. It is perhaps fortunate that dopa decarboxylase is not only a very fast acting enzyme with spare substrate capacity but it is also widely distributed. Thus some decarboxylation probably occurs in the capillary walls as the drug enters the CNS. On the debit side these properties of the enzyme also mean that only 30% of any orally administered levodopa actually enters the circulation and only 10% of that (i.e. 3% of the original dose) gets into the CNS. This proportion can be increased by combining levodopa with a drug that inhibits dopa decarboxylase but does not itself cross the blood-brain barrier (BBB) so that decarboxylation still occurs in the CNS. They are known as extracerebral dopa decarboxylase inhibitors (ExCDDIs). Such drugs, e.g. α-methyl dopa hydrazine (carbidopa) and benserazide are now routinely combined with levodopa. This means that less levodopa is needed and vomiting is avoided, presumably because the chemoreceptor trigger zone, although in the CNS, is not protected from the circulation by the BBB. If levodopa cannot be decarboxylated peripherally something has to happen to it and it is mainly o-methylated by COMT to give 3-methoxy tyrosine. This has a much longer half-life (24 hours) than levodopa (2 hours) and competes with dopa for entry into the CNS. How it may affect levodopa therapy, especially in the long term, is uncertain.

Although DA will not cross the BBB it has been possible to develop D_2 agonists that do. These include bromocriptine, lisuride, pergolide and apomorphine. Of these bromocriptine has been most widely used and although longer acting than levodopa it suffers from the same side-effects. Since it acts directly, the only way of avoiding vomiting is to combine it

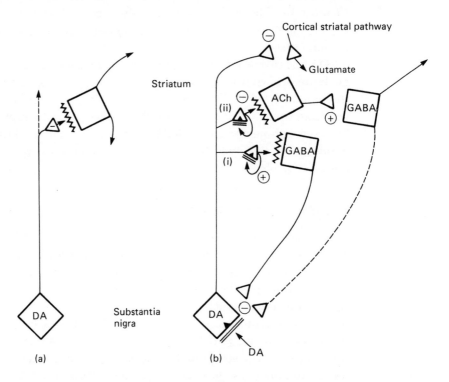

Fig. 7.4. Influence of autoreceptors and different DA receptors on dopaminergic neuron function between substantia nigra and striatum. (a) No autoreceptors (▲) on DA neuron cell body or nerve terminals. There is less inhibitory control and a higher turnover of DA and neuronal discharge rate. Antagonists only act postsynaptically and therefore cannot influence these parameters. (b) In this arrangement there is inhibitory control of DA activity by autoreceptors on the terminals and cell bodies (therefore less turnover and lower discharge rate). Antagonists acting only postsynaptically (∿) would just allow inhibitory neuronal feed-back to substantia nigra to increase with (i) or without (ii) ACh interneurons. Blocking autoreceptors (=) would further increase synthesis and release of DA and firing of DA neurons. There is evidence that the DA inhibitory effect on glutamate release and ACh neurons is mediated by D_2 receptors whereas effects of DA on GABA neurons in the striatum and on GABA nerve terminals in the substantia nigra follow D_1 activation. ⊖ inhibition; ⊕ excitation.

with a DA antagonist that does not cross the BBB, like domperidone, and which will therefore not attenuate its required central effect. It has also been widely used to treat disorders like amenorrhoea and galactorrhoea which are caused by high plasma prolactin levels through insufficient DA inhibition. There is an indication that bromocriptine is more effective in the presence of some residual DA function. Certainly it would not produce the D_1 effects of DA. Although the function of D_1 receptors remains uncertain they are in fact more numerous than D_2 receptors in the CNS and recent studies with the D_1 agonist SKF38393 and the antagonist SCH23390 suggest that they may be involved in the control of grooming in rats (Starr & Starr 1986). It also seems that although the D_1 agonist itself does not induce stereotypy it will potentiate the effects of D_2 agonists in producing this response. A possible basis for this effect is becoming apparent. As mentioned above the inhibition of striatal activity by DA may involve three processes.

1 Direct inhibition of glutamate release from terminals of the cortico-striatal pathway. Blocked by D_2 antagonists.

2 Inhibition of ACh release (D_2 receptors).

3 Increase in GABA release from striatal neurons. This is mimicked by the D_1 agonist SKF38393 and blocked by the D_1 antagonist SCH23390 (Girault *et al.* 1986). Since D_1 receptors are also found on striato-nigral nerve terminals in the SN (they are lost by lesion of GABA neurons in striatum), they could also control SN activity (see Dubois *et al.* 1986).

These findings are summarised in Fig. 7.4. Clinically it could mean that the D_2 agonists will lack the full effect of levodopa as they would not increase GABA release in the striatum.

The clinical potential of the different approaches to augmenting DA function in Parkinsonism are considered in Chapter 16.

DA antagonists

These drugs produce catalepsy, reduced motor function and sedation in animals and counteract the sterotype activity induced by amphetamine (DA release) and apomorphine (DA agonists). In man they are anti-emetic, cause akinesia (Parkinsonism), control mania and reduce the symptoms of schizophrenia. Additionally, they facilitate the release of prolactin and so produce the effects associated with its raised plasma levels. It is assumed, that these effects are achieved by blocking postsynaptic DA (D_2) receptors. By acting presynaptically they block autoreceptors and experimental studies show that they increase the synthesis, release and turnover of DA, and raise HVA. This they do more effectively in the striatum than in other DA innervated regions (Fig. 7.4).

Because they induce a tranquil state in major psychotic disorders, affect motor function and are used in the treatment of schizophrenia, the DA antagonists are known variously as major tranquillizers, neuroleptics or anti-psychotics. Neuroleptic seems to be the currently preferred term.

Chemically they include a number of phenothiazine derivatives (e.g. chlorpromazine, Fig 19.1), butyrophenones (e.g. spiroperidol, Fig. 18.9), thioxanthenes (e.g. flupenthixol, Fig 18.1) and benzamides (e.g. sulpiride, Fig 18.6).

There is a very strong correlation, certainly amongst the phenothiazines and butyrophenones, between DA antagonism (at least as measured by $[^3H]$-haloperidol displacement) and the clinical dose for treating schizophrenia (Fig 8.2). All neuroleptics also produce Parkinsonism to some extent, as would be expected of a DA antagonist, and with few exceptions their potency in treating schizophrenia is unfortunately paralleled by their ability to induce Parkinsonism. Also after long-term use in schizophrenia most of these derivatives eventually produce a dyskinesia (tardive) even though the anti-psychotic activity persists. These observations pose two clear questions:

1 If all neuroleptics are D_2 receptor antagonists and if this receptor is involved in both their anti-schizophrenic and Parkinsonian inducing properties, could a compound really be developed that was effective in schizophrenia without readily causing Parkinsonism?

2 How can a dyskinesia develop (requiring increased DA activity) if anti-psychotic activity (necessitating decreased DA activity) is retained?

There are some compounds, e.g. thioridazine, clozapine and sulpiride, often called 'atypical' neuroleptics, which do appear to control schizophrenia without producing extrapyramidal side-effects as clearly as the other neuroleptics, and one DA antagonist (metoclopramide) which produces extrapyramidal effects with little antipsychotic activity. Not surprisingly, therefore, there have been many attempts to demonstrate differences between the DA pathways to the striatum (presumed involvement in Parkinsonism) and its mesolimbic and mesocortical projections (presumed importance in schizophrenia). As the functional postsynaptic receptors appear identical (D_2) in all regions and since they also cannot be distinguished by current antagonists from those found presynaptically, there is much interest in the possibility that the main difference between the pathways might be in the actual presence or absence of autoreceptors. There is in fact some evidence that the mesocortical projections lack autoreceptors (Bannon & Roth 1983). DA agonists do not reduce DA synthesis in the cortex to the extent they should do if autoreceptors controlling synthesis were present, nor do DA antagonists increase it. As autoreceptors are also found on cell bodies it is interesting to note that if DA agonists are applied to neurons identified in A9 and A10 by antidromic stimulation as sending axons to the cortex they are less easily inhibited than those feeding the striatum. This again indicates fewer autoreceptors on the neurons with cortical projections and presumably also on their terminals as does the higher basal firing rate of A10 neurons to cortical areas than of SN neurons (see above) to the striatum. Even if mesocortical projections do not posses autoreceptors can this really explain why some neuroleptics produce fewer extrapyramidal side-effects?

There is certainly no firm evidence linking anti-psychotic activity to non-striatal areas and the increased DA receptor number found in postmortem schizophrenic brain is most marked in the striatum (see Chapter 18). Also those antagonists which appear to block autoreceptors preferentially as measured by DOPA production rather than DA release or cell firing, produce more extrapyramidal side-effects (see Anden *et al.* 1984). This is perhaps somewhat surprising in view of the fact that these compounds would presumably increase DA synthesis and release preferentially in the striatum, where the autoreceptors are thought to occur and so reduce the danger of extrapyramidal effects. In fact *in vivo* voltammetry shows that clozapine, thioridazine and metoclopromide all increase DA release (Stamford *et al.* 1988) much more in the striatum than the nucleus accumbens despite the fact that only the latter is noted for its extrapyramidal side-effects, whilst the others are typical neuroleptics.

Of course the striatum has been described as the chemical factory of the CNS and the degree of extrapyramidal activity induced by the neuroleptics could also depend on how they affect other NTs. ACh is an excitatory NT in the striatum and antimuscarinic drugs (atropine-like) not only have some value in treating Parkinsonism but also reduce neuroleptic induced akinesia. Not surprisingly, therefore, those neuroleptics with strong antimuscarinic as well as DA antagonistic activity, such as clozapine and thioridazine produce less signs of Parkinsonism than those like fluphenazine or haloperidol that have no such activity and even potentiate ACh peripherally. Such drugs also have varying degrees of α_1, histamine and 5-HT blocking activity, which may affect their ability to produce extrapyramidal symptoms. Nevertheless, clozapine blocks the hyperactivity induced by DA injected into the nucleus accumbens but not the striatum whilst metoclopramide has the opposite effect. This still needs to be explained.

The question of how these drugs can actually induce dyskinesia (increased DA function) and yet also retain their antipsychotic activity might be related to the different properties of the various DA projections. Experimental evidence shows that tolerance develops to the DA blocking action of the neuroleptics after chronic treatment over a few weeks in rats so that not only does the increase in DA turnover and reduction in apomorphine induced stereotypy, which they produce acutely, gradually subside but on drug withdrawal apomorphine induced stereotypy and DA receptor number are enhanced. After months of treatment such supersensitivity can be shown even without stopping the drugs (Clow *et al.* 1980). This increase in DA function could explain how some neuroleptics produce tardive dyskinesias in man, although this may not be the only explanation (see Waddington *et al.* 1986) and there is no firm evidence of increased endogenous DA activity. Also it requires that such supersensitivity does not develop in other brain areas, like the mesocortical DA pathway, which might be more important in mediating the symptoms of schizophrenia. An absence of autoreceptors and feedback facilities in the latter might explain why DA supersensitivity does not develop there and why antipsychotic activity is retained. Of course it is also possible that there are different cotransmitters for DA in different brain areas and they affect its activity differently. In fact CCK binding sites increase in mesolimbic areas and frontal cortex but not in the striatum, after chronic neuroleptic treatment (Wong *et al.* 1984).

References and further reading

Aghajanian GK (1984) The physiology of central α and β adrenoceptors In: Usdin E, Catlsson A, Dahlström A & Engel J (eds) *Catecholamines. Part B Nevropharmacology and the Central Nervous System.* Alan R. Liss, New York. pp. 85–92.

Anden NE, Lander TA, Anden MG, Liljenberg B, Lindgren S & Thornström U (1984) The pharmacology of pre- and postsynaptic dopamine receptors: differential effects of dopamine receptor agonists and antagonists. In: Usdin E, Carlsson A, Dahlström A & Engel J (eds) *Catecholamines. Part B Neuropharmacology and the Central Nervous Systems.* Alan R. Liss, New York. pp. 19–22.

Bacopoulus NG & Bhatnagar RK (1977) Correlation between tyrosine hydroxylase activity and catecholamine concentration or turnover in brain regions. *J Neurochem* **29**, 631–43.

Bannon MJ & Roth RH (1983) Pharmacology of mesocortical dopamine neurons. *Pharmacol. Rev.* **35**, 53–668.

Chu NS & Bloom FE (1973). Norepinephrine containing neurones: changes in spontaneous discharge patterns during sleep and waking. *Science* **179**, 908–10.

Clow A, Theoporou A, Jenner P & Marsden CD (1980) Changes in rat striatal dopamine turnover and receptor activity during one year's neuroleptic administration. *Eur. J. Pharmacol.* **63** 135–44.

Cooper JR, Bloom FE & Roth RH (1983) *The Biochemical Basis of Neuropharmacology* 4th edition. Oxford University Press, New York.

Cuomo V, Cagiano R, Colonna M, Renna G & Racagni G (1986) Influence of SCH 23390, a D_1 receptor antagonist on the behavioural response to small and large doses of apomorphine in rats. *Neuropharmacology* **25**, 1297–300.

Dahlström A & Fuxe K (1964) Evidence for the existence of monoamine-containing neurons in the central nervous systems. I. Demonstration of monoamines in the cell bodies of brain stem neurons. *Acta. Physiol. Scand.* **62** (suppl 232), 1–55.

Dubois A, Savosta M, Curet O & Scatton B (1986) Autoradiographic distribution of the D_1 agonist ^3H SKF 38393 in the rat brain and spinal cord. Comparison with the distribution of D_2 dopamine receptors. *Neuroscience* **19** 125–37.

Fillenz M (1984) Norepinephrine. In: Lajtha A (ed) *Handbook of Neurochemistry*, Vol 6. Plenum, New York. pp. 51–69.

Girault JA, Spampinator U, Glowinski J & Beson MJ (1986) In vivo release of $[^3H]\gamma$-aminobutyric acid in the rat neostriatium- II. Opposing effects of D_1 and D_2 dopamine receptor stimulation in the dorsal caudate putamen. *Neuroscience* **19**, 1109–18.

Hoffer BJ, Siggins GR, Oliver AP & Bloom FE (1973) Activation of the pathway from locus coeruleus to rat cerebellum Purkinje neurons: Pharmacological evidence of noradrenergic central inhibition. *J. Pharmac. Exp. Ther.* **184**, 553–69.

Iversen LL (1967) *The Uptake and Storage of Noradrenaline in Sympathetic Nerves.* Cambridge University Press, London.

Kielholz P (1977) *Beta-Blockers and the Central Nervous System.* Hans Huber, Berne.

Kitai ST, Sugimori M & Kocsis JC (1976) Excitatory nature of dopamine in the nigro-caudate pathway. *Exp. Brain. Res.* **24**, 351–63.

Koella WP (1977) Anatomical, physiological and pharamacological findings relevant to the central nervous effects of the beta-blockers. In: Kielholz P (ed) *Beta-Blockers and the Central Nervous System.* Hans Huber, Berne. pp 21–34.

Kuczenski R (1973) Striatal tyrosine hydroxylase with high and low affinity for tyrosine:

implications for the multiple-pool concept of catecholamines. *Life Science***13**, 247-55.

Lindvall O & Björland A (1978) Organisation of catecholamines neurons in the rat central nervous system. In: Iversen LL, Iversen SD & Snyder SH *Handbook of Psychopharmacology Vol. 9* Plenum, New York. pp. 139-231.

Madison DV & Nicholl RA (1982) Noradrenaline blocks accommodation of pyramidal cell discharge in the hippocampus. *Nature* **299**, 636-8.

Mason ST (1984) *Catecholamines and Behaviour.* Cambridge University Press, Cambridge.

Moore RY & Bloom FE (1978) Central catecholamine neuron systems, anatomy and physiology of the dopamine system. *Ann. Rev. Neurosci.* **1**, 129-69.

Moore RY & Bloom FE (1979) Central catecholamine neuron systems, anatomy and physiology of the norepinephrine and epinephrine systems. *Ann. Rev. Neurosci.* **2**, 113-48.

Palacios JM (1984) Light microscopic autoradiographic localization of catecholamine receptor binding sites in brain. Problems of ligand specificity and use of new ligands. In: Usdin E, Carlsson A, Dahlström A & Engel J (eds) *Catecholamines. Part B. Neuropharmacology and the Central Nervous System.* Alan R. Liss, New York. pp. 73-84.

Ryall RW & Kelly JS (1978). Iontophoresis and transmitter mechanisms in the mammalian central nervous system. North Holland, Biomedical Press. Amsterdam. Various papers, pp. 11-77.

Schoener EP & Elkins DP (1984) Neuronal response to dopamine in rat neostriatum. A push-pull perfusion study. *Neuropharmacology* **25**, 611-16.

Siggins GV (1978) Electrophysiological role of dopamine in striatum: excitatory or inhibitory? In: Lipton MA, Di Mascio A & Killam KF (eds) *Psychopharmacology: A Generation of Progress.* Raven Press, New York. pp. 143-57.

Stamford JA, Kruk ZL & Millar J (1988) Actions of dopamine antagonists on stimulated striatal and limbic dopamine release; an *in vivo* voltammetric study. *Br. J. Pharmac.* **94**, 924-32.

Starr BS & Starr MS (1986) Differential effects of dopamine D_1 and D_2 agonists and antagonists on velocity of movement, rearing and grooming in the mouse. Implication for the role of D_1 and D_2 receptor. *Neuropharmacology* **25**, 455-64.

Szabadi E (1979) Adrenoceptors on central neurons: microelectrophoretic studies. *Neuropharmacology* **18**, 831-43.

Ungerstedt U & Arbuthnott GW (1970) Quantitative recording of rotational behaviour in rats after 6-hydroxydopamine lesions of the nigrostriatal dopamine system. *Brain Research* **24**, 485-93.

U'Prichard DC, Yamamura HI & Reisine TD (1980) Characterization and differential in vivo regulation of brain adrenergic receptor subtypes. In: Pepeu G, Kuhar MJ & Enna SJ (eds) *Hormones.* Raven Press, New York. pp. 213-21.

Usdin E, Carlsson A, Dahlström A & Engel, J (1984) *Catecholamines Part B. Neurophamacology and the Central Nervous System.* Also *Part A. Basic and Peripheral Mechanisms* and *Part C. Theroretical Aspects.* Alan. R. Liss, New York.

Waddington JL, Youssef HA, O'Boyle KM & Molloy AG (1986) A reappraisal of abnormal involuntary movement (tardive dyskinesia) in schizophrenia and other disorders: animal models and alternative hypothesis. In: Winslow W & Markstein P (eds) *The Neurobiology of Dopamine Systems.* Manchester University Press. pp. 266-86.

Walker RJ (1986) Biosynthesis, storage and release of dopamine. In: Winslow W & Markstain P (eds) *The Neurobiology of Dopamine Systems.* Manchester University Press. pp. 3-24.

Wang RY, White FJ & Voigt MM (1984) *Cholecystokinin, Dopamine and Schizophrenia.* *Trends Pharmacol. Sci.* **6**, 436-8.

Weiss JM, Simson PG, Hoffman LJ, Ambrose MJ, Cooper S & Webster A (1986) Infusion of adrenergic receptor agonists and antagonists into the locus coeruleus and ventricular system of the brain. Effects on swim motivated and spontaneous motor activity. *Neuropharmacology* **25**, 367-84, also 385-91.

8   Dopamine receptors

A.J. CROSS AND F. OWEN

There is now a great deal of evidence to suggest that dopamine (DA) acts as a neurotransmitter both in the brain and in some sympathetic ganglia. In addition, DA has potent effects in some vascular systems and in the parathyroid gland, and may also act as a hormone involved in the hypothalamic control of pituitary function. In parallel with the realisation that DA acts as a neurotransmitter in its own right (as distinct from being a precursor of noradrenaline (NA)) it has become clear that DA interacts with receptors which are also quite distinct from those for other catecholamines. The interaction of many psychoactive drugs with DA receptors has added impetus to the study of the pharmacology of these receptors. The combination of these pharmacological studies with physiological and biochemical experiments has demonstrated that DA can interact with a heterogeneous population of receptors, and that stimulation of these receptors may be coupled to a variety of intracellular events.

Although DA is considered primarily as a neurotransmitter in the brain, study of its actions in peripheral systems has provided information relevant to the classification of DA receptors. The study of such model systems has also enhanced our understanding of DA receptor — effector systems, and their relationship to cellular function. The availability of these established model systems combined with the well-defined anatomical and functional organisation of DA neurons in the brain are probably the major reasons why the mechanisms of DA-mediated neurotransmission are so well understood.

The study of DA receptors expanded greatly with the introduction of ligand binding techniques. The application of these techniques produced many reports of multiple DA receptor subtypes or states. Pharmacological experiments and biochemical studies of receptor-effector coupling have clarified the situation and provided a simplified framework for DA receptor classification. The classification of DA receptors will be discussed in terms of these ligand binding studies along with other pharmacological and biochemical studies. Electrophysiological and behavioural studies of DA receptors have been extensively reviewed elsewhere (e.g. Waddington 1986, Costall & Naylor 1981) and will not be included in the present discussion.

The chapter is organised in more or less chronological order to show how concepts of DA receptor classification have evolved and led to the present widely accepted scheme.

Approaches to the classification of two dopamine receptors

Dopamine stimulation of adenylate cyclase

The first biochemical demonstration of a DA receptor mechanism distinct from those for other catecholamines came from the studies of Greengard, Kebabian and colleagues in 1971 (see Kebabian 1978 and Iversen 1977 for review) on bovine superior cervical ganglia (SCG). Stimulation of the SCG induces an increase in cyclic AMP content which is mediated via an interneuron within the ganglia. DA was known to be contained in SCG interneurons, and it was subsequently shown that exogenously applied DA could increase cyclic AMP production in the SCG tissue. Noradrenaline is considerably less potent than DA, and the DA mediated stimulation is not blocked by propranolol or by NA synthesis inhibitors. Thus, the effect of DA is direct, is not mediated by the release of NA, and does not involve stimulation of the β-adrenoceptor.

This finding was followed by observations that DA can stimulate cyclic AMP production in the retina and the corpus striatum of mammalian brain, (Fig. 8.1) and that this was due to activation of the

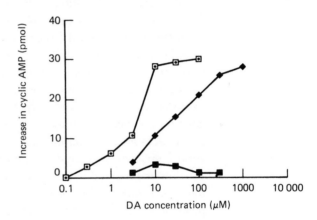

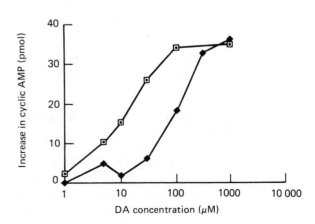

Fig. 8.1. Dopamine-stimulated adenylate cyclase in rat striatum. *Upper*: stimulation of cyclic AMP production by dopamine (□), noradrenaline (◆) and apomorphine (■). *Lower*: Dose response curves for dopamine in the absence (□) and presence (◆) of fluphenazine (0.1 μM). Data taken from Kebabian (1978).

enzyme adenylate cyclase. A number of DA agonists were able to mimic the effects of DA in rat striatum, most notably some naphthalene derivatives such as ADTN, and other catecholamines such as epinine and NA. The 'classical' DA agonist apomorphine, although of high affinity, acted as a partial agonist in this system.

It was also shown at this time that a number of antipsychotic drugs (the neuroleptics) were potent competitive antagonists of DA stimulation of adenylate cyclase in rat striatum (Fig. 8.1). The ability to antagonise DA was shown by neuroleptics of many chemical classes. Thus flupenthixol (a thioxanthene) has high affinity for inhibition of DA stimulated adenylate cyclase and is a highly potent neuroleptic, whereas chlorpromazine (a phenothiazine) is less potent in both systems and diethazine and promazine, phenothiazines devoid of antipsychotic activity are also virtually inactive *in vitro*. Whilst the correlation between antipsychotic potency and inhibition of DA stimulated adenylate cyclase holds true for phenothiazines and thioxanthenes, several other chemical classes of neuroleptics display clinical potencies which are not predicted by their activity *in vitro*. This is particularly the case for the butyrophenones such as haloperidol, which is of high potency clinically but is at best only weakly active in the adenylate cyclase system of rat striatum.

Further anomalies are observed with a series of DA agonists derived from the ergot alkaloids. Many of these compounds, such as bromocriptine, lisuride and lergotrile act as DA agonists in behavioural models of postsynaptic DA receptor function (Goldstein *et al.* 1978). Indeed, several of these compounds have been used successfully in the treatment of Parkinson's disease and hyperprolactinaemia. When studied in the adenylate cyclase system in rat striatum, bromocriptine, like apomorphine, acts as a partial agonist. Moreover, lergotrile displays no agonist action, but acts as a weak non-competitive antagonist.

The unexpected actions of many dopaminergic drugs in rat striatum have been mirrored in other tissues in which DA stimulates cyclic AMP production. Thus in the teleost retina, apomorphine acts as a DA antagonist and the butyrophenone, domperidone, is inactive as a antagonist. The bovine parathyroid gland has provided a particularly useful model system to study the effects of dopaminergic drugs on both cyclic AMP production and a physiological response (pp. 135–136). In this tissue, apomorphine and lisuride both act as antagonists and the butyrophenone spiperone is of low potency.

Ligand binding to dopamine receptors

Initial studies of DA receptors with ligand binding techniques used either [^{3}H]-dopamine or [^{3}H]-haloperidol as ligands and membrane preparations of mammalian corpus striatum as a source of receptors. Neither of these ligands proved to be entirely suitable for binding studies and they were replaced by [^{3}H]-spiperone, a butryophenone neuroleptic of extremely high clinical potency. It was immediately apparent in studies using either [3H]-haloperidol or [3H]-spiperone that the rank order of potencies of neuroleptics was quite different to that of inhibition of DA-stimulated adenylate cyclase (for reviews of ligand binding studies see Seeman 1980 and Creese et al. 1983). In particular, the butryophenones were considerably more potent in the ligand binding assay. The order of potencies of neuroleptics for inhibition of [3H]-spiperone binding did however correlate with their clinical potencies as antipsychotic agents (Fig. 8.2). It had been shown previously that the order of potencies of neuroleptics clinically correlated well with their potencies in many behavioural tests of DA receptor function.

The anomalous behaviour of some DA agonists and the novel antagonists was not observed in [3H]-spiperone binding. Thus neuroleptics of the butyrophenone structure had potencies well correlated with their potencies in vitro. Other atypical neuroleptics, such as the substituted benzamides sulpiride and metoclopramide, also inhibit [3H]-spiperone binding, interestingly neither compound inhibits DA-stimulated adenylate cyclase in rat striatum (Schimdt & Hill 1977). The correlation between in vitro and in vivo potencies also extends to DA agonists, correspondingly the ergot alkaloids are potent inhibitors of [3H]-spiperone binding, although of course this does not allow an assessment to be made of their efficacy as agonists.

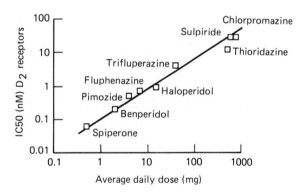

Fig. 8.2. Relationship between the clinical potency of neuroleptic drugs (average daily dose) and their affinity at the D_2 receptor. Data taken from Seeman (1980).

Dopamine receptors in the bovine anterior pituitary

It is well established that DA acts as a release inhibiting hormone controlling prolactin secretion from the anterior pituitary. The source of DA in the portal vein appears to be the cells of the median eminence. In man, the administration of neuroleptics results in a rapid rise in circulating prolactin levels and, conversely, apomorphine induces a fall in basal serum prolactin concentrations. The preparation of isolated mammotrophs from the bovine anterior pituitary has provided an extremely useful model system in which to study DA receptor function (Caron et al.

1978). In this system many DA agonists, including the ergot alkaloids and apomorphine, are capable of inhibiting prolactin release. Moreover, apomorphine acts as a full agonist in this preparation. The neuroleptic drugs inhibit the effects of DA agonists, and their order of potency is similar to that observed in [^{3}H]-spiperone binding either in the rat striatum or in anterior pituitary membranes. A number of studies have shown that DA agonists do not induce a rise in intracellular cyclic AMP content in mammotrophs, suggesting that the DA receptors in this tissue do not stimulate adenylate cyclase activity.

Two pharmacologically distinct DA receptors

The clear pharmacological distinction between DA stimulation of cyclic AMP production in bovine parathyroid, teleost retina or rat brain and the inhibition of prolactin release from bovine anterior pituitary led to the classification of DA receptors into two distinct forms, which were termed D_1 and D_2 by Kebabian and Calne (1979). A summary of this classification scheme is given in Table 8.1 (see also Stoof & Kebabian 1984).

Table 8.1. Classification of dopamine receptors

Receptor	D_1	D_2
Cyclase linkage	Yes	No
Location	Bovine parathyroid	Anterior pituitary
Apomorphine	Partial agonist	Full agonist
Dopaminergic ergots	Antagonists	Potent agonists
Selective antagonist	None	Sulpiride
Radiolabelled ligand	[^{3}H]-Flupenthixol	[^{3}H]-Spiperone [^{3}H]-Dihydroergocriptine

At this time the D_1 receptor was seen as being invariably associated with stimulation of adenylate cyclase, whereas the D_2 receptor was independent of adenylate cyclase, at least in the anterior pituitary. It has, however, become clear that D_2 receptors may be linked to adenylate cyclase in an inhibitory fashion (see below). In anterior pituitary, D_2 receptors can be labelled with the ergot [^{3}H]-dihydroergocriptine or with the butyrophenone [^{3}H]-spiperone. The pharmacological profile of [^{3}H]-spiperone binding in the rat striatum was also consistent with the D_2 receptor; thus the rat striatum contains both D_1 and D_2 receptors. The behavioural effects of the neuroleptics and DA agonists in experimental animals all appear to be mediated via the D_2 receptor, and the behavioural consequences of D_1 receptor stimulation are not clear.

The pharmacology of D_1 and D_2 receptors

Studies of the D_1 receptor

The initial classification scheme for DA receptors suffered from the lack
of drugs with a high degree of selectivity for the D_1 receptor. The
development of several 1–phenylbenzazepine derivatives has provided
a series of compounds which act as selective D_1 receptor agonists and
antagonists (Fig. 8.3). It is this development which has provided one of
the cornerstones of DA receptor classification.

AGONISTS   ANTAGONIST

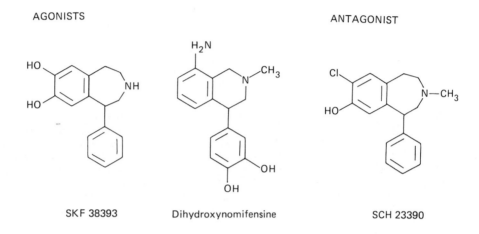

SKF 38393   Dihydroxynomifensine   SCH 23390

Fig. 8.3. Structures of compounds with selective actions at the D_1 receptor.

The first compound of this series to become widely available was SKF
38393, and it is at present the most selective D_1 receptor agonist
identified. Thus SKF 38393 is capable of stimulating cyclic AMP production in the rat striatum, the effect being competitively inhibited by D_1
receptor antagonists such as fluphenazine. SKF 38393 is more potent
than dopamine but acts as a partial agonist. Interestingly none of the
benzazepine derivatives so far available is devoid of at least some
antagonist action. In the [³H]-spiperone binding model of D_2 receptors,
SKF 38393 is at least 100 times less active, and the compound does not
inhibit prolactin release. It thus has a high degree of selectivity for the D_1
receptor compared to the D_2 receptor. The action at the D_1 receptor is
stereoselective, only the R-isomer being active. More recently developed
D_1 agonists include SKF 82526 (fenoldopam) and dihydroxynomifensine.
Slight modifications of the SKF 38393 structure have led to a series of
compounds which act as selective D_1 receptor antagonists (Fig. 8.3). Most
prominent amongst these is SCH 23390, which acts as a highly potent D_1
receptor antagonist in the adenylate cyclase system, and is 2–3 orders
of magnitude less potent in [³H]-spiperone binding to the D_2 receptor.

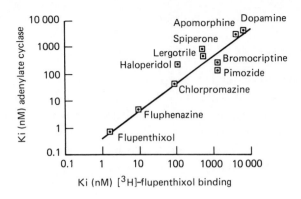

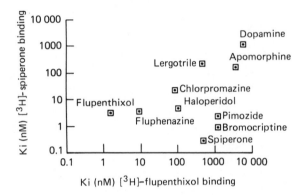

Fig. 8.4. [³H]-flupenthixol binding to the D₁ receptor. *Upper*: relationship between potency at DA-stimulated adenylate cyclase and potency in [³H]-flupenthixol binding. *Lower*: relationship between potency at D₂ receptors ([³H]-spiperone binding) and [³H]-flupenthixol binding.

Replacement of the chlorine in position 7 by other halogens or a methyl group maintains the antagonist activity and selectivity. These compounds are also stereoselective, the R-isomer being considerably more active than the S-isomer. SCH 23390 is a potent antagonist of cyclic AMP production in the bovine parathyroid and teleost retina, whereas it is inactive against prolactin release in the anterior pituitary.

The high potency and selectivity of SCH 23390 for the D₁ receptor has led to its use in the tritiated form as a ligand for D₁ receptors in binding assays. Previous ligand binding studies had used [³H]-flupenthixol (or the closely related [³H]-piflutixol) as ligand (Fig. 8.4). However, these ligands are equipotent at D₁ and D₂ receptors and in order to study binding to the D₁ receptor, selective D₂ antagonists have to be included in the binding assay. Ligand binding studies using [³H]-SCH 23390 show a pharmacological profile similar to DA stimulation of adenylate cyclase. Of particular importance, these studies have demonstrated the presence of high and low affinity agonist binding states of the D₁ receptor. Thus in the rat striatum, agonists inhibit ligand binding to the D₁ receptor with shallow displacement curves consistent with binding to high and low affinity states. In the presence of GTP (or stable analogues) the displacement curves are converted to those consistent with binding to a single low affinity site (Fig. 8.5). Previous studies using [³H]-agonists such as [³H]-dopamine had demonstrated the presence of a binding site with

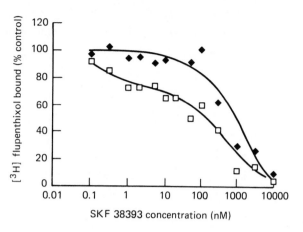

Fig. 8.5. Effects of guanine nucleotides on D_1 receptors. The graph shows the inhibition of [^{3}H]-flupenthixol binding by SKF 38393 in the absence (□) and presence (◆) of GppNHp, a stable analogue of GTP. Data from Sibley *et al.* (1982). In the absence of GppNHp, SKF 38393 interacts with two apparent sites with affinities of 0.2 and 270 nM. In the presence of GppNHp, the binding is consistent with a single class of sites affinity = 380 nM.

properties distinct from D_1 and D_2 receptors. These binding sites were termed D_3 sites. The D_3 binding sites are sensitive to modulation by guanine nucleotides and it is now clear that they represent agonist binding to the high affinity state of the D_1 receptor. The modulation of agonist binding to the D_1 receptor by guanine nucleotides is consistent with the involvement of a GTP-binding protein in receptor-effector coupling.

The activities of the selective D_1 receptor agonists and antagonists, which were initially identified using rat striatal preparations are also maintained in model systems in which D_1 receptors can be studied in the absence of D_2 receptors. Thus in the bovine parathyroid gland, SKF 38393 stimulates cyclic AMP production, although it is only a partial agonist. In teleost retina SKF 38393 again acts as a partial agonist and SCH 23390 is a potent antagonist of DA-stimulated adenylate cyclase.

Studies of the D_2 receptor

Along with the development of a selective D_1 receptor agonist and antagonist, a variety of compounds from different chemical classes have been identified as having selective actions on the D_2 receptor (Fig. 8.6). The ergot alkaloids have long been recognised for their dopaminergic activity, and one such derivative the partial ergoline LY 141865 acts as a selective D_2 agonist. Other compounds of quite distinct structure also act as selective D_2 agonists. Included in this group are the substituted phenylethylamines such as N 0434 and some of the tetralin derivatives such as RU 24926.

Substituted benzamides and butyrophenes were classified as selective D_2 antagonists, and indeed the benzamides such as ($-$)sulpiride and the butyrophenones such as domperidone or spiperone are devoid of activity at DA-stimulated adenylate cyclase. Further modifications of the benzamide structure have produced the so-called 'second generation' neuroleptics which retain the selectivity for the D_2 receptor but are considerably

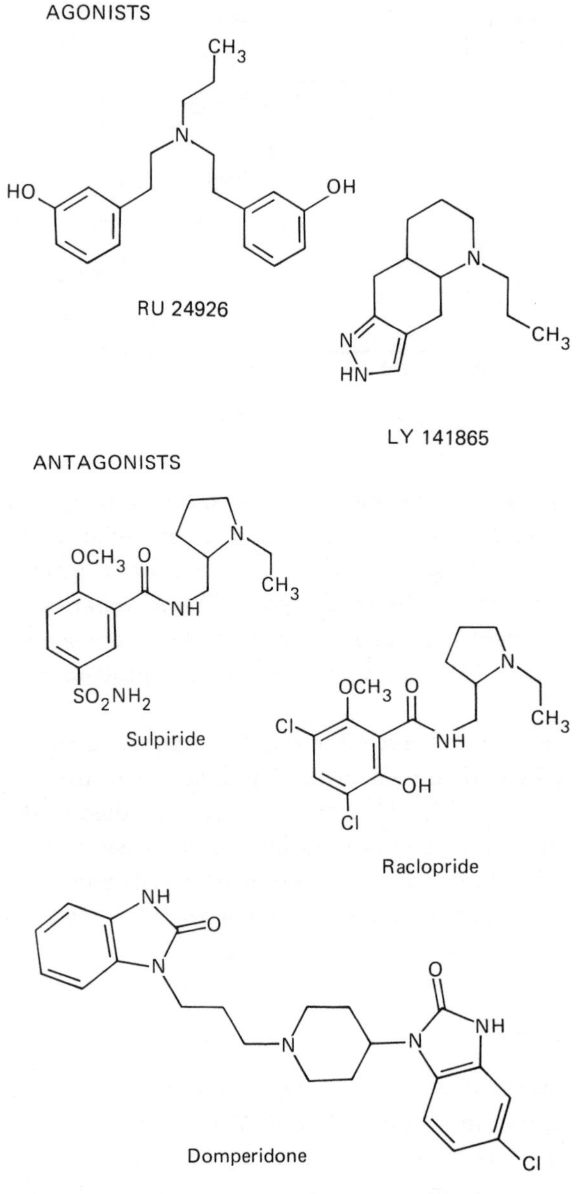

Fig. 8.6. Structures of compounds with selective actions at D₂ receptors.

more potent. Included in this group of compounds are YM 09151-2 and raclopride. Both of these compounds have been produced in tritium-labelled form as ligands for the D_2 receptor, and have proved in binding assays to have the expected pharmacological profile.

Considerable attention has been paid to ligand binding studies on D_2 receptors in both the rat striatum and anterior pituitary. In these tissues the displacement of [³H]-spiperone binding by agonists is consistent with binding to high and low affinity states of the receptor (Sibley *et al.* 1982a, Grigoriades & Seeman 1984). As in many other systems, the addition of guanine nucleotides to receptor preparations results in the conversion of the agonist state from one of high affinity to one of low affinity. It remains controversial whether the conversion is complete in the striatum, although this seems to be the case in the pituitary (Sibley et al. 1982b). This ligand binding data is further complicated by the actions of certain benzamides, which may also show heterogeneity of binding in rat striatum, but not in pituitary (Martres et al. 1984). These binding sites (termed D_4 sites) appear to have high affinity for certain benzamide drugs and dopamine agonists such as apomorphine, and do not convert to a low affinity agonist state in the presence of guanine nucleotides. Recent evidence suggests that in the globus pallidus DA receptors labelled with $[^3H]$-spiperone do not convert to the low affinity state and may thus also be consistent with the D_4 site. Whether this binding site represents a third DA receptor remains unresolved at the present time.

Dopamine receptors in the periphery

In the periphery, DA acts at low concentrations to induce relaxation of vascular smooth muscle in the renal blood vessels and also to inhibit NA release from certain sympathetic nerve terminals (Hilditch & Drew 1985). The pharmacological characteristics of these systems suggests that DA is acting at receptors distinct from both α- and β-adrenoceptors. Moreover, the DA induced vasodilatation differs pharmacologically from the action of DA on sympathetic fibres and these so called 'peripheral DA receptors' have been classified as DA_1 and DA_2 respectively. The development of selective dopaminergic agents has enabled this classification of peripheral DA receptors to be incorporated into a broader scheme. Observations that DA_1 receptors are potently inhibited by SCH 23390, and that fenoldopam acts as a potent agonist suggests that this receptor is analogous to the D_1 receptor. This conclusion is strengthened by the finding that $(-)$ sulpiride is only weakly active in this system. The presynaptic DA_2 receptor is particularly sensitive to antagonism by $(-)$ sulpiride and is insensitive to SCH 23390. The DA_2 receptor is also stimulated by LY 141865, suggesting that it is similar to the D_2 receptor.

Dopamine receptors and intracellular signalling

D_1 receptors and stimulation of adenylate cyclase

The bovine parathyroid gland has provided a particularly useful model system for studying the physiological consequences of D_1 receptor stimulation (Brown et al. 1977, 1980) (Fig. 8.7). In isolated parathyroid cells, DA agonists induce a rise in intracellular cyclic AMP content (via an increase in the activity of adenylate cyclase), and hence activate cyclic AMP dependent protein kinase. The selective D_1 agonist SKF 38393 is a potent dopaminemetic in this system, whereas D_2 selective drugs are inactive and ergot alkaloids such as lisuride are antagonists. DA agonists

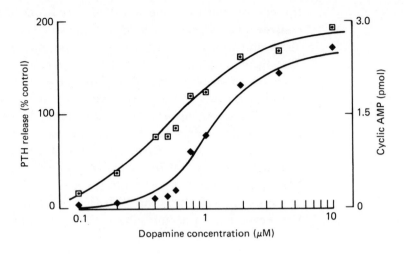

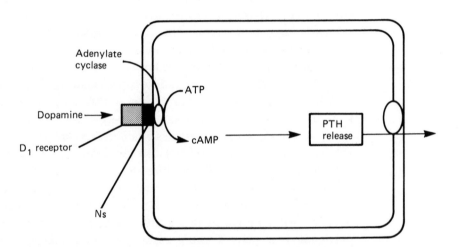

Fig. 8.7. D_1 receptors in the bovine parathyroid gland. *Upper*: the effect of dopamine on cyclic AMP production (▣) and parathyroid hormone release (◆). Data from Brown *et al.* (1977). *Lower*: schematic representation of the organisation of D_1 receptor effector mechanism. Dopamine binding to the receptor activates adenylate cyclase, presumably via the regulatory protein N_S. The resulting increase in intracellular cyclic AMP is related to an increase in PTH release.

also stimulate the release of parathyroid hormone (PTH), and there is an excellent correlation between the rise in intracellular cyclic AMP concentrations and the release of PTH. There would thus seem to be little doubt that, within the parathyroid gland, increased cyclic AMP production acts as the intracellular signal resulting from D_1 receptor stimulation.

In the teleost retina, DA is present in a population of amacrine cells which synapse onto horizontal cells. DA stimulates cyclic AMP production in the horizontal cells with the pharmacological profile expected of D_1 receptor stimulation (Watling & Dowling 1981). DA also induces a marked potentiation of specific hyperpolarising potentials in these cells, which may be involved in controlling the light sensitivity of responses. These effects of DA can be mirrored either by treatment with dibutyryl cyclic AMP or a phosphodiesterase inhibitor, and again this suggests that cyclic AMP acts as the 'second messenger' in D_1 receptor stimulation in the teleost retina. In other tissues which contain D_1 receptors, such as mammalian striatum or the vascular system, receptor stimulation induces an increase in cyclic AMP content, although the physiological consequences of such an increase are not clear (see Kelly & Nahorski 1986 for discussion). This process has been studied indirectly using cholera-toxin, which contains an enzymatic activity which ADP-ribosylates the guanine nucleotide binding protein N_S, resulting in a permanent activation of adenylate cyclase. When injected bilaterally into nucleus accumbens of the rat, cholera toxin induces an increase in the locomotor behaviour of the animals. Although bilateral injections of DA into the nucleus accumbens induces a similar locomotor activity, the presence of other adenylate cyclase activating receptors (e.g. VIP and β-adrenergic) in the basal ganglia does not permit any definite conclusions to be drawn. The biochemical consequences of D_1 receptor stimulation are better understood. It has recently been demonstrated that a specific phosphoprotein (DARPP 32-DA and adenosine $3'5'$-monophosphate regulated phosphoprotein) is phosphorylated in rat striatum in the presence of either DA, 8-bromo cyclic AMP or cyclic AMP-dependent protein kinase (Browning *et al.* 1985). The distribution of DARPP-32 closely parallels the distribution of D_1 receptors in the brain. Although it has been shown that phosphorylated DARPP-32 acts as a potent phosphoprotein phosphatase inhibitor, and as such could modulate many intracellular processes, the functional consequences of these changes remain to be determined.

D_2 receptors and the inhibition of adenylate cyclase

A number of studies using isolated cell preparations have provided evidence for D_2 receptor mediated inhibition of adenylate cyclase. In the melanotrophs of the intermediate lobe of the pituitary, NA stimulates adenylate cyclase activity via activation of a β-adrenoceptor. The resulting increase in intracellular cyclic AMP content is paralleled by increased α-MSH release (Munemura *et al.* 1980). In this preparation, DA is able to inhibit the adenylate cyclase activity induced either by β-adrenoceptor stimulation or by treatment with cholera toxin. The DA-induced inhibition of adenylate cyclase activity and α-MSH secretion is antagonised by $(-)$sulpiride and mimicked by LY 141865, consistent with a D_2 mediated effect (Cote *et al.* 1981). Treatment of the intermediate lobe with pertussis toxin, which ADP-ribosylates and so inactivates N_i, blocks the effect of DA. As the inhibitory action of DA requires the presence of GTP it seems likely that the inhibitory GTP-binding protein

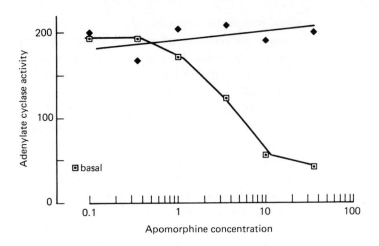

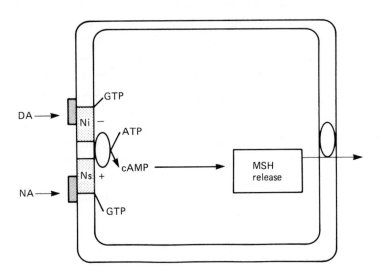

Fig. 8.8. D_2 receptors in the intermediate lobe of the rat pituitary. *Upper*: The effects of dopaminergic agents on adenylate cyclase activity in rat intermediate lobe. Basal activity (45 pmol) is stimulated (to 200 pmol) by isoproterenol (via β-adrenoceptor activation). Addition of apomorphine (□) inhibits the isoproterenol-stimulated adenylate cyclase activity. The effect of apomorphine is blocked by 10 μM fluphenazine (◆). *Lower*: Schematic representation of the organisation of the D_2 receptor and β-adrenoceptor in the melanotroph. Noradrenaline stimulates adenylate cyclase via a β-adrenoceptor linked to N_S. Dopamine inhibits the noradrenaline-stimulated adenylate cyclase via a D_2 receptor linked to N_i. Cellular cyclic AMP concentrations are closely related to MSH release from the melanotroph. Data from Cote *et al.* (1981)

N_i is involved in linking the D_2 receptor to adenylate cyclase (Fig. 8.8). A similar situation appears to occur in the anterior pituitary, where DA inhibits prolactin release from the mammotrophs via a D_2 receptor (see above). In the anterior pituitary DA inhibits both basal and VIP-stimulated adenylate cyclase via a D_2 receptor (Onali *et al.* 1981). Moreover, the inhibition of prolactin release from the anterior pituitary is sensitive to pertussis toxin, suggesting an involvement of N_i. These findings are consistent with the results of ligand binding experiments in the anterior pituitary (see above) demonstrating the involvement of a GTP binding protein in receptor action.

Within the rat striatum, selective D_2 receptor agonists such as LY 141865 have been found to inhibit the D_1 receptor stimulated accumulation and efflux of cyclic AMP from intact cells, and to inhibit basal adenylate cyclase activity. In such preparations the stimulation of cyclic AMP accumulation by DA can be enhanced by selective D_2 antagonists such as $(-)$ sulpiride. In addition, treatment of rat striatal slices with amphetamine induces a slight increase in cyclic AMP accumulation which can be markedly enhanced in the presence of $(-)$ sulpiride. Taken together these observations suggest that D_2 receptors are capable of inhibiting adenylate cyclase in rat striatum. Interestingly, D_2 receptor agonists do not inhibit cyclic AMP accumulation induced by isoprenaline, VIP or cholera toxin, suggesting that the inhibitory D_2 receptors are closely associated with at least some of the striatal D_1 receptors. The inhibition of adenylate cyclase activity by D_2 receptor agonists requires the presence of GTP and is inhibited by prior treatment with pertussis toxin suggesting that N_1 protein is involved. These findings are in agreement with ligand binding studies in rat striatal membranes in which agonist binding to D_2 receptors is GTP-modulated and sensitive to pertussis toxin treatment. However, as noted previously it is at present unclear whether all striatal D_2 receptors are associated with N_1.

Dopamine receptors in the CNS

The basal ganglia

The distribution and properties of DA receptors within the basal ganglia have been studied using experimental lesions, ligand binding techniques and a variety of biochemical approaches.

In the rat, lesions of intrinsic striatal cell bodies with excitotoxins such as kainic acid induce a marked loss of striatal D_1 receptors, with a less pronounced loss of D_2 receptors. It has thus been suggested that the majority of D_1 receptors are located on striatal cell bodies whereas D_2 receptors may be distributed approximately equally between intrinsic striatal cells and striatal efferents. The bulk of the D_2 receptors associated with the terminals of neurons projecting to the striatum are thought to reside on the cortico-striatal tract, as lesions of this tract may eliminate up to half the striatal population of D_2 receptors. The functional role of striatal D_2 receptors has been elucidated to some extent, thus selective D_2 agonists inhibit striatal ACh turnover and release, presumably by a direct action on striatal cholinergic neurons. In addition, D_2 selective drugs also modulate the release of glutamate and cholecystokinin (CCK). As striatal glutamate release is predominantly from the terminals of the cortico-striatal tract, and CCK release is from terminals of a pathway originating in the temporal lobe, both these effects may be mediated by D_2 receptors located on nerve terminals (i.e. presynaptic heteroreceptors). It has been shown that the D_2 receptors located on cortical-striatal terminals may not be modulated by GTP (Creese et al. 1979) (the so-called D-4 site). This may merely reflect differences in receptor effector coupling or different affinity states of the D_2 receptor and remains an area of controversy.

Whilst it is clear that D_1 receptors are present on intrinsic striatal cells, the effects of D_1 receptor stimulation on other striatal transmitters are not clear. Interestingly, D_1 agonists such as SKF 38393 do not modulate striatal ACh release, suggesting that D_1 receptors are not present on cholinergic cells (which may well contain D_2 receptors). The inhibition of DA-stimulated adenylate cyclase by D_2 agonists suggests that some cells do possess both D_1 and D_2 receptors. However, these cells are clearly not cholinergic.

Within the substantia nigra a clear anatomical distinction between D_1 and D_2 receptors can be made. Thus neurotoxin-induced degeneration of dopaminergic cells induces a marked reduction in D_2 receptor binding sites with no effect on DA-stimulated adenylate cyclase activity. In contrast, destruction of the striato-nigral pathway results in a large loss of D_1 receptors in the substantia nigra with no effect on D_2 receptors.

Other brain regions

Ligand binding techniques have identified D_1 and D_2 receptors in areas of cerebral cortex, amygdala, hippocampus, hypothalamus and carotid body. Within the hypothalamus D_2 receptors modulate the release of β-endorphin. D_2 receptors are also present in the septum, and modulate the activity of the septal cholinergic neurons which project to the hippo-campus.

Presynaptic DA receptors

There is much evidence to suggest that within the rat striatum DA can inhibit its own release by acting on receptors present on dopaminergic terminals (presynaptic autoreceptors) (Roth 1984). Although a great deal of difficulty has been encountered in studying the pharmacology of this system, there are now indications that these presynaptic receptors may be of the D_2 type. Thus, under the appropriate conditions DA release is inhibited by LY 141865 and this effect is blocked by sulpiride. The D_1 agonist SKF 38393 is inactive in this system, thus suggesting a D_2 mediated effect in the absence of D_1 receptors. These findings are of course in agreement with studies showing that D_2 receptor antagonists increase striatal DA turnover whereas D_1 antagonists have no effect, although the D_2 receptors mediating this action may equally be located on the dopaminergic cells of the substantia nigra as on the terminals in the striatum.

The effector system involved in the D_2 inhibition of DA release is not known. Both DA release and the activity of tyrosine hydroxylase are enhanced by cyclic AMP derivatives. Thus it is possible that D_2 mediated inhibition of cyclic AMP formation may be involved, although there is no direct evidence to support this.

Conclusions

It is now clear that DA receptors can be classified into two subtypes, the D_1 and D_2 receptors, which are summarised in Table. 8.2. The evolution of this concept, which we have attempted to outline, was dependent upon the development of selective and specific drugs suitable for ligand binding and pharmacological experiments. Perhaps of more importance was the identification of model systems in which the receptor subtypes could be studied in isolation. The application of the information gained in these peripheral systems to the study of DA receptors in the central nervous system has led to a much greater understanding of the role of DA receptor subtypes in brain function. It is the importance of DA as a neurotransmitter in the brain, and its involvement in many neuropsychiatric disorders, which stimulates this interest and will hopefully lead to the development of therapeutic agents with improved efficacy and safety.

Table 8.2. Dopamine receptor classification

Receptor	D_1	D_2
Adenylate cyclase linkage	Stimulatory (N_S)	Inhibitory (N_i)
Peripheral localisation	Bovine parathyroid	Anterior pituitary Intermediate lobe pituitary
	Renal blood vessels (DA_1)	Sympathetic terminals (DA_2)
Central localisation	Striatal cell bodies	Striatal cell bodies Striatal afferent terminals *S. Nigra* dopaminergic cell bodies
Selective agonists	SKF 38393 Dihydroxynomifensine	LY 141865 RU 24926
Selective antagonists	SCH 23390	Sulpiride Domperidone
Radiolabelled ligand	[³H]-SCH 23390 [³H]-Flupenthixol	[³H]-Spiperone [³H]-Raclopride

References and further reading

Brown EM, Carroll, RJ & Aurbach GD (1977) Dopaminergic stimulation of cyclic AMP accumulation and parathyroid hormone release from dispersed bovine parathyroid cells. *Proc. Natl. Acad. Sci.* **74**, 4210–13.

Brown EM, Attie MF, Reens S, Gardner DG, Kebabian J & Aurbach GD (1980) Characterisation of dopaminergic receptors in dispersed bovine parathyroid cells. *Mol. Pharmacol.* **18**, 335–40.

Browning MD, Huganier R & Greengard P (1985) Protein phosphorylation and neuronal function. *J. Neurochem.* **45**, 11–23.

Caron MC, Bealieu M, Raymond V, Gagne B, Drouin J, Lefkowitz R J & Labrie F (1978) Dopaminergic receptors in the anterior pituitary gland. Correlation of [^{3}H] dihydro-ergocriptine binding with dopaminergic control of prolactin release. *J. Biol. Chem.* **253**, 2244–53.

Costall B & Naylor RJ (1981) The hypothesis of different dopamine receptor mechanisms. *Life Sci.* **28**, 215–29.

Cote TE, Crewe CW & Kebabian JW (1981) Stimulation of a D_2 receptor in the intermediate lobe of the rat pituitary gland decreases the responsiveness of the β-adrenoceptor: biochemical mechanisms. *Endocrinology* **108**, 420–6.

Creese I, Usdin T & Snyder SM (1979) Guanine nucleotides distinguish between two dopamine receptors. *Nature* **278**, 577–8.

Creese I, Sibley DR, Hamblin HW & Leff SE (1983) The classification of dopamine receptors: relationship to radioligand binding. *Ann. Rev. Neurosci.* **6**, 43–71.

Goldstein M, Lew JY, Nakamura S, Battista AF, Lieberman A & Fuxe K (1978) Dopaminephilic properties of ergot alkaloids. *Fed. Proc.* **37**, 2202–6.

Grigonades D & Seeman P (1984) The dopamine/neuroleptic receptor. *Can. J. Neurol. Sci.* **11**, 108–13.

Hilditch A & Drew GM (1985) Peripheral dopamine receptor subtypes — a closer look. *Trends Pharm. Sci.* **6**, 396–400.

Iversen LL (1977) Catecholamine — sensitive adenylate cyclases in neuronal tissues. *J. Neurochem.* **29**, 5–12.

Kebabian JW (1978) Dopamine — sensitive adenylate cyclase: a receptor mechanism or dopamine. *Adv. Biochem. Psychopharm.* **19**, 131–54.

Kebabian JW & Calne DB (1979) Multiple receptors for dopamine. *Nature* **277**, 93–6.

Kelly E & Nahorski SR (1986) Dopamine receptor — effector mechanisms. *Rev. Neurosci.* **1**, 35–54.

Martres MP, Sokoloff P, Delandre M, Schwartz JP, Protais P & Costentin J (1984) Selection of dopamine antagonists discriminating various behavioural responses and radioligand binding sites. *Arch. Pharmacol.* **325**, 102–15.

Munemura M, Eskay RL & Kebabian JW (1980) Release of β-melanocyte-stimulating hormone from dispersed cells of the intermediate lobe of the rat pituitary gland: involvement of catecholamines and adenosine 3'5'-monphosphate. *Endocrinology* **106**, 1795–807.

Onali P, Schwartz JP & Costa E (1981) Dopaminergic modulation of adenylate cyclic stimulation by vasoactive intestinal peptide in anterior pituitary. *Proc. Natl. Acad. Sci.* **78**, 6531–34.

Roth RM (1984) CNS dopamine autoreceptors: distribution, pharmacology and function. *Ann. N.Y. Acad. Sci.* **430**, 27–53.

Schmidt MJ & Hill LE (1977) Effects of ergots on adenylate cyclase activity in the corpus striatum and pituitary. *Life Sci.* **20**, 789–98.

Seeman P (1980) Brain dopamine receptors. *Pharmacol. Rev.* **32**, 229–313.

Sibley DR, Leff SE & Creese I (1982a) Interactions of novel dopaminergic ligands with D-1 and D-2 dopamine receptors. *Life Sci.* **31**, 677–45.

Sibley DR, Delean A & Creese I (1982b) Anterior pituitary dopamine receptors. Demonstration of interconvertible high and low affinity states of the D-2 dopamine receptor. *J. Biol. Chem.* **257**, 6351–61.

Stoof JC & Kebabian JW (1984) Two dopamine receptors: biochemistry, physiology and pharmacology. *Life Sci.* **35**, 2281–96.

Waddington JL (in press) Behavioural correlates of the action of selective D-1 dopamine receptor antagonists. *Biochem. Pharmacol.*

Watling KJ & Dowling JE (1981) Dopaminergic mechanisms in the teleost retina. 1. Dopamine-sensitive adenylate cyclase in homogenates of carp retina: effects of agonists, antagonists and ergots. *J. Neurochem.* **36**, 559–69.

9 5-Hydroxytryptamine

A.H. DICKENSON

5-hydroxytryptamine (5-HT) or serotonin has had a somewhat chequered career as a central transmitter. Early histofluorescence techniques indicating the widespread nature of 5-HT projections in the central nervous system (CNS) led to much interest in the possible roles of this monoamine which subsequently fell from grace due mainly to a large degree of confusion regarding subdivision of 5-HT receptor types. However, a recent consensus on the receptor classification and many 5-HT agents should give impetus to elucidation of the central effects of serotoninergic systems.

Anatomy of CNS 5-HT pathways (Fig. 9.1)

Almost all CNS 5-HT originates from groups of cell bodies situated on or close to the midline of the caudal brainstem through to the midbrain. These cell groups comprise the raphe nuclei complex and have also been labelled B1 to B9 on the basis of fluorescence studies corresponding to the

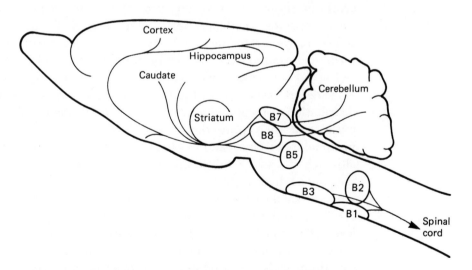

Fig. 9.1. Major 5-HT pathways in a longitudinal of the rat brain. The cell groups B1–B8 correspond to the 5-HT containing raphe nuclei with the exception of the minor groups B4 and B6. B1, nucleus raphe pallidus; B2, nucleus raphe obscurus; B3, nucleus raphe magnus; B5, nucleus raphe pontis; B7, nucleus raphe dorsalis; B8, nucleus raphe medianus.

A groups of catecholamine nuclei. The most prominent groups are B1 (nucleus raphe pallidus), B2 (nucleus raphe obscurus), B3 (nucleus raphe magnus), B7 (nucleus raphe dorsalis) and B8 (nucleus raphe medianus). In simplified terms B1–B3 give rise to descending projections to the spinal cord whereas the bulk of ascending projections and hence forebrain 5-HT derives from B7–B8.

The mapping of 5-HT pathways has used fluorescence, immunohisto-chemical and receptor autoradiography techniques coupled with the use of neurotoxins and degeneration studies. Nuclei raphe dorsalis and medianus project in the medial forebrain bundle to widespread areas of the forebrain, principally the hypothalamus, olfactory complex, colliculus, caudate nucleus, geniculate, hippocampus and cortex and also the cerebellum. The caudal group of nuclei project to the lower brainstem, trigeminal complex and both dorsal and ventral horns of the spinal cord. Some ascending projections to thalamus, hypothalamus and midbrain arise from nucleus raphe magnus.

Studies on inputs to the raphe nuclei are sparse but cerebellar, cortical and spinal cord projections have been described, although few studies of this nature have identified the transmitter in the pathways.

Although classical synaptic connections of 5-HT neurons have been observed, non-synaptic release from varicosites on axons may also occur in certain areas of the CNS.

Pharmacology of 5-HT neurons (Fig. 9.2)

5-HT is synthesised from L-tryptophan, present in the diet, and increased synthesis results from loading with this amino acid for which active transport across the blood–brain barrier occurs. There is also an active transport system for neuronal uptake of the precursor. Synthesis proceeds via formation of L-5 hydroxytryptophan (5-HTP) and the enzymes concerned are cytoplasmic located tryptophan hydroxylase (TH) and 5-HTP decarboxylase, with the former being the rate limiting step. The distribution of tryptophan hydroxylase reflects the location of the raphe nuclei and their projection zones. 5-HTP can be used to augment neuronal 5-HT levels and has been a useful research tool in this respect although it can be taken up by other neuronal types. Inhibition of tryptophan hydroxylase by para-chlorophenylalamine (PCPA) causes, after several days treatment, a marked and almost complete depletion of 5-HT although the usefulness of PCPA is reduced by a lesser drop in NA levels. Alpha methyl 5-HTP is an inhibitor of 5-HTP decarboxylase but since this enzyme is not rate limiting and is also found in non-serotonin containing cells this inhibitor is not of great practical use. Tryptophan hydroxylase is not fully saturated under normal conditions so loading with tryptophan can usefully increase 5-HT synthesis, although due to complex interrelations between plasma tryptophan levels and 5-HT synthesis, mainly due to plasma protein binding and active uptake mechanisms, the final effects are not clearly predictable.

Once released from the terminal much 5-HT seems subject to reuptake into the terminal where breakdown to 5-hydroxyindole acetic acid (5-HIAA) is produced by monoamine oxidase. Thus MAOI such as iproniazid cause a build up of neuronal stores of 5-HT and it then seems that more is released per impulse. Uptake of 5-HT can be reduced by many of the tertiary tricyclic antidepressants reasonably specifically *in vitro* but in practice the formation of secondary derivatives that reduce NA uptake precludes this selectivity *in vivo*. However, fluoxetine, citalopram and zimelidine seem quite selective 5-HT uptake blockers and fenfluramine and para-chloroamphetamine (PCA) both inhibit the uptake pump but unlike the drugs above also release 5-HT from the intraneuronal stores so leading ultimately to a reduced synaptic concentration of 5-HT due to rundown of the stores. This is probably the major action of these agents. Release of 5-HT can be provoked by amphetamines and some tricyclic antidepressants such as chlorimipramine. It is worth noting that chloroamphetamines are more potent in this regard than the non-halogenated derivatives.

Reserpine and tetrabenazine deplete 5-HT by interference with the vesicular storage of the monoamine and the resultant leakage leads to catabolism by monoamine oxidase.

Two neurotoxins, 5,6 and 5,7-dihydroxytrypramine (5,6-DHT and 5,7-DHT) gain access to the neuron via the uptake process and thence cause an irreversible destruction of the neuron and so a marked depletion of 5-HT. Recovery of the 5-HT levels is slow (months) and sprouting of the regrowing axons, at least near the cell bodies in the raphe nuclei has been described so that some terminal zones may subsequently receive a greater innervation.

A variety of studies *in vivo* and *in vitro* have used electrophysiological techniques to record the firing of 5-HT containing raphe neurons (identified by fluorescence, etc. following electrode impalement) which is typically slow (around 0.5 Hz) and highly regular. This is reduced by a variety of agents that increase synaptic 5-HT levels such as uptake blockers and MAOI and also by 5-HT itself, LSD and 8-OH-DPAT. This lead to the idea of a receptor (autoreceptor) on the soma of the neuron, activated by 5-HT released from recurrent collaterals or other raphe neurons nearby to reduce impulse production in the cell. There is also evidence that synthesis of 5-HT is dependent on impulse flow in 5-HT neurons, possibly through 5-HT restricting TH conformation to an inactive form. This slowing of 5-HT neuronal activity through 5-HT receptor activation may explain some of the effects of LSD on man, particularly the sensory hallucinations and perceptual changes, since the widespread projections of the raphe nuclei to sensory relay areas of the brain such as the geniculate, colliculus and spinal cord implies a role for

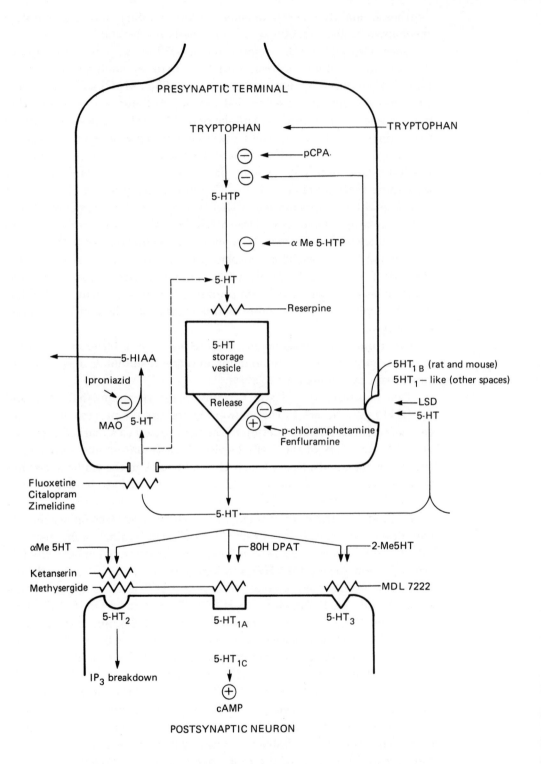

Fig. 9.2. A diagrammatic representation of a 5-HT synapse. The biochemical pathways for the synthesis and degradation of 5-HT are shown opposite.

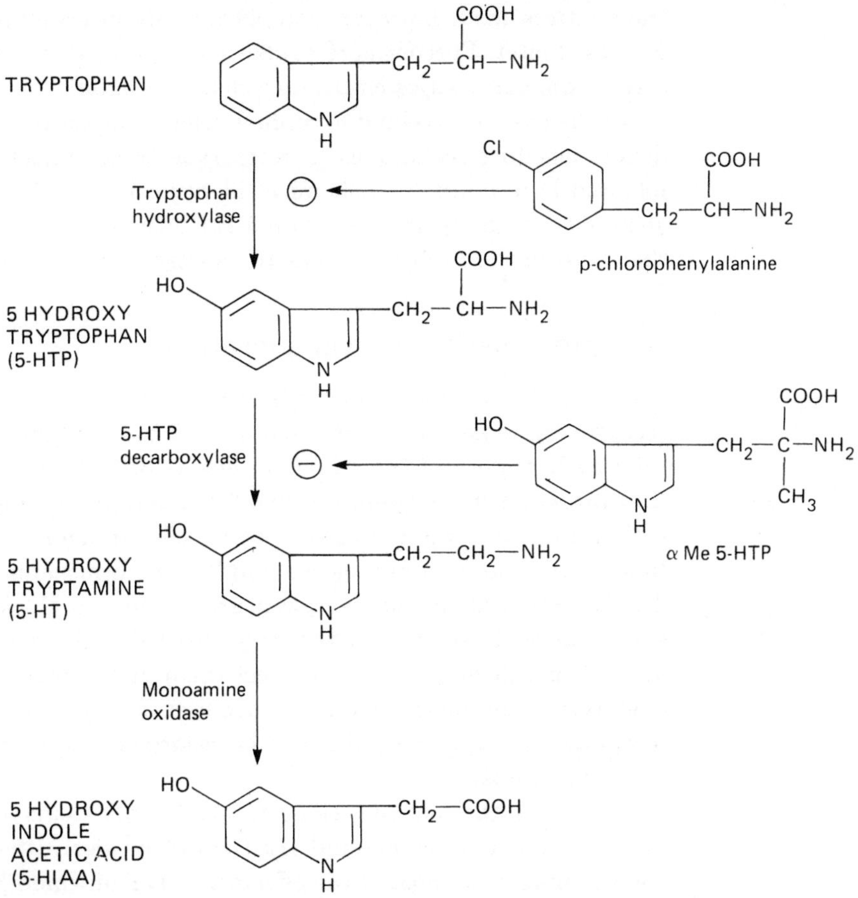

TRYPTOPHAN

COOH
|
—CH$_2$—CH—NH$_2$
N
H

Tryptophan hydroxylase ⊖ ←

Cl— ... —CH$_2$—CH—NH$_2$, COOH

p-chlorophenylalanine

5 HYDROXY TRYPTOPHAN (5-HTP)

HO— ... —CH$_2$—CH—NH$_2$, COOH
N
H

5-HTP decarboxylase ⊖ ←

HO— ... —CH$_2$—C—NH$_2$, COOH, CH$_3$
N
H

α Me 5-HTP

5 HYDROXY TRYPTAMINE (5-HT)

HO— ... —CH$_2$—CH$_2$—NH$_2$
N
H

Monoamine oxidase

5 HYDROXY INDOLE ACETIC ACID (5-HIAA)

HO— ... —CH$_2$—COOH
N
H

Fig. 9.2. *Cont.*

5-HT in somatosensory integration. The ability of a variety of hallucinogenic agents such as dimethyltryptamine, psiloytin and mescaline to reduce raphe unit activity correlates quite well with their hallucinogenic effects. In many raphe nuclei projection areas the effect of 5-HT is to elicit a slow hyperpolarisation (although depolarisation seems the rule in the facial nucleus) so there would be resultant disinhibition of these postsynaptic elements which may partly be the basis for visual, tactile and auditory hallucinations elicited by these agents. Unfortunately, unit recordings in chronically prepared animals indicate that the depression of raphe nuclei activity by LSD is of shorter duration than the behavioural effects. Tolerance occurs to the effects of LSD on behaviour but not to the depression of neuronal activity suggesting that direct postsynaptic effects may also be involved.

The raphe serotonergic axons are unmyelinated and so conduct slowly. This may, to some extent, account for the delay in postsynaptic hyperpolarisation elicited following raphe stimulation, especially in the long ascending and descending systems. Co-existence of 5-HT with other transmitters may, however, complicate this interpretation and will be discussed later. Furthermore evidence exists for non-synaptic release of 5-HT from varicosities *en passage* along the axon.

In the case of descending raphe nuclei projections to the spinal cord, double labelling techniques (a retrograde tracer injected into the cord followed by immunohistochemical identification of 5-HT) suggest that about 80% of the neurons contain 5-HT although early studies indicated that most of the raphe-spinal neurons were non-serotoninergic.

Receptor classification and location

There has been a recent upsurge of interest in a classification of 5-HT receptors to replace that proposed in 1957 by Gaddum & Picarelli. From their early studies of the stimulant effects of 5-HT on guinea-pig ileum they proposed the existence of two 5-HT receptors. One was associated with a direct contraction of smooth muscle, antagonised by dibenzyline (phenoxybenzamine) and designated 'D', the other appeared to mediate depolarisation of the cholinergic neurons and was blocked by morphine and so termed 'M'. Whilst the drugs used did distinguish between the direct (smooth muscle) and indirect (neuronal) effects of 5-HT neither phenoxybenzamine (an alkylating agent at adrenoceptors and histamine receptors, etc.) nor morphine can be regarded as specific or even useful 5-HT antagonists.

Interest in the central actions of 5-HT partly stems from the fact that the hallucinogenic compound (LSD) and its derivative 2-bromo LSD (BOL) antagonise most of the effects of 5-HT on smooth muscle as does the related ergot derivative methysergide. The finding that ketanserin (as well as mianserin) blocked some of those actions, e.g. vasoconstriction, contraction of trachea and uterus but not contraction of the guinea-pig ileum and rat fundus meant that there were at least two peripheral 5-HT receptors on smooth muscle, those blocked by ketanserin (designated 5-HT_2) and those unaffected by it but blocked by methsergide, i.e. 5-HT_1. Thus, in the periphery there appear to be at least three 5-HT receptors. The 5-HT_1 and 5-HT_2 sub-types (originally covered by D) on smooth muscle and the 5-HT_3 (M) receptors on nerves for which more selective antagonists such as MDL72222, ICS 205–930 and GR38032 have since been developed (see Fig. 9.3). There also appears to be evidence for a number of receptors for 5-HT in the CNS, although their classification may not be directly comparable to that adopted for the periphery. Much depends on binding studies with the neuroleptic [^{3}H]-spiperone. Like haloperidol this is primarily a dopamine (DA) antagonist but comparisons of the regional distribution of their binding showed that whilst [^{3}H]-haloperidol binding was confined to areas of high DA concentrations, e.g. striatum, nucleus accumbens and olfactory tubercle and could be displaced by the DA ligand (+)butaclomol, [^{3}H]-spiperone binding was more widespread in the cortex, especially in occipital and frontal areas

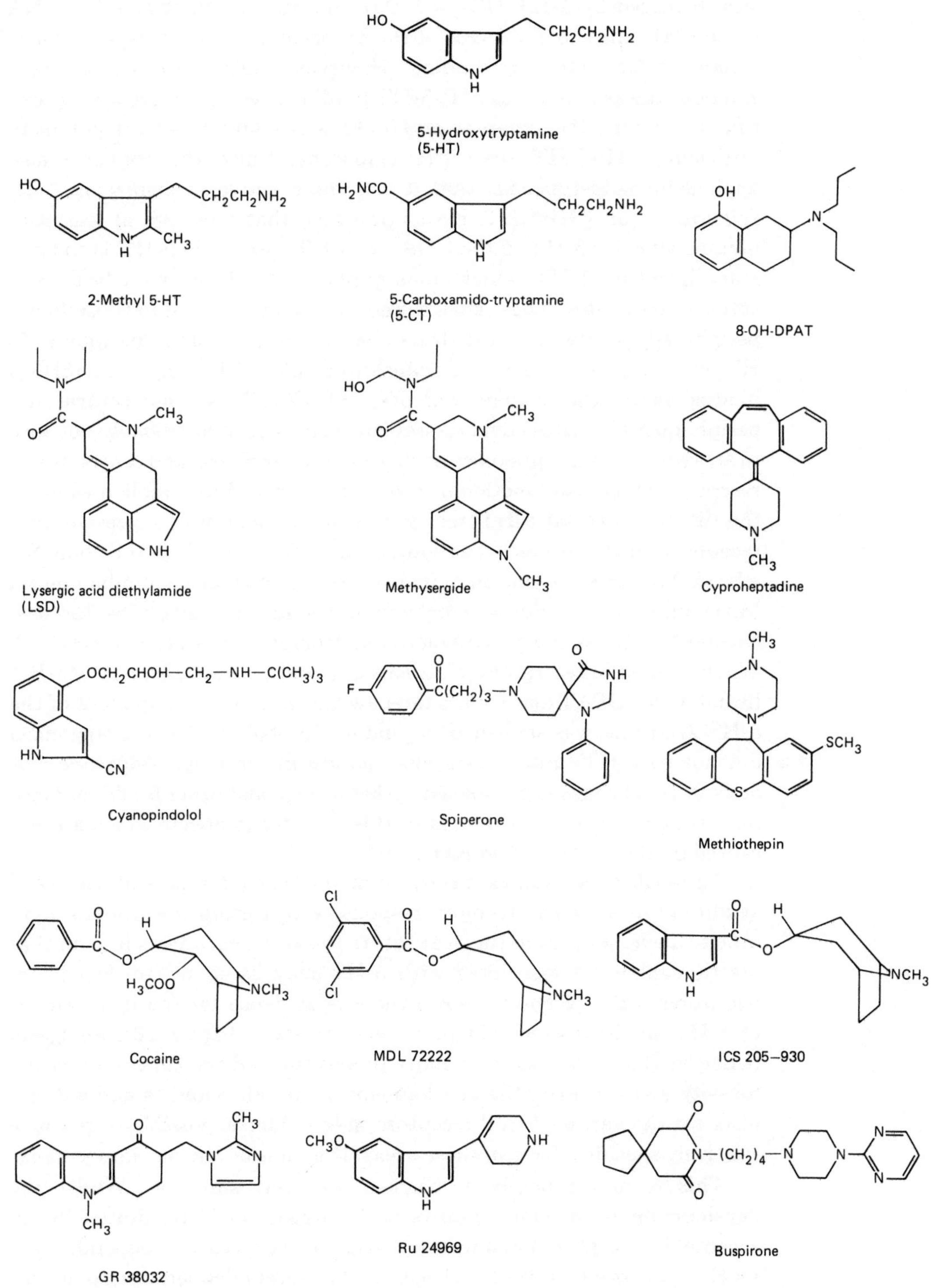

Fig. 9.3. Some agonists and antagonists used in the classification of 5-HT receptors.

where no DA is found. Also, in these cortical areas [³H]-spiperone binding was displaced by 5-HT (IC_{50} 4.4 μM) and not by DA (240 μM) or NA (1000 μM). The same was true of the hippocampus where spiperone also competed for [³H]-LSD binding. However, when these studies were extended it was found that [³H]-5-HT binding sites were more widespread than those for [³H]-spiperone and 5-HT was 1000 times more potent in displacing [³H]-5-HT than [³H]-spiperone. Since the converse also applied for spiperone, i.e. that it was more active in displacing [³H]-spiperone than [³H]-5-HT, it was proposed that there are at least two binding sites for 5-HT in the CNS, i.e. 5-HT_1 for which 5-HT is the primary ligand and 5-HT_2 which binds spiperone; LSD appears to be equally active at both sites. These sites cannot be directly related to those found peripherally. Certainly those drugs that are antagonists at peripheral 5-HT_2 sites, e.g. ketanserin and mianserin displace [³H]-spiperone ($5HT_2$) binding more readily than that of 5-HT (5-HT_1) so that central and peripheral 5-HT_2 sites could be similar. At present it is probably not wise to attempt to use a common classification for peripheral and central 5-HT receptors. Of course functional studies are required to establish whether the different central 5-HT recognition or binding sites represent true receptors. In this respect it is somewhat easier to study 5-HT than NA effects. Thus administration of its precursor 5-HTP or tryptophan plus a MAO inhibitor, produces a behavioural syndrome involving forepaw treading, head weaving, hyperactivity, tremor and Straub (erect) tail. When studied in reserpinised animals to avoid indirect effects, the 5-HT ligand 8-OH-DPAT also causes forepaw treading. This component of the 5-HT syndrome was abolished by pindolol (probably a 5-HT_1 antagonist) but not by 5-HT_2 antagonists like ketanserin (although spiperone was active). Head shakes are blocked by ketanserin and other 5-HT_2 antagonists supporting an involvement of this receptor in effects which are not caused by the 5-HT_1 ligand 8-OH-DPAT.

Although these studies merely show that some features of the 5-HT syndrome in animals are more responsive to certain antagonists than others one hopes that in the near future those central effects in man that are thought to be associated with 5-HT may be shown to depend on particular 5-HT receptors. Since there is evidence for the involvement of 5-HT in depression (Chapter 19), anxiety (Chapter 20), analgesia (Chapter 22), as well as in memory processing and the control of eating (obesity and anorexia) the development of specific agonists and antagonists for the various 5-HT receptors may render it possible to produce relatively specific effects in these areas. It is thus of obvious importance.

This is unfortunately a 'chicken and egg' situation. Whilst the development of specific agonists and antagonists is facilitated by an acceptable receptor classification, such a classification depends very much on the availability of such agents. The recent deliberations of an appropriate working party (see Bradley *et al.* 1986) reached a consensus on a proposed classification and the subsequent part of this section will be

Table 9.1. The classification of 5-HT receptors based on Bradley *et al.* (1986)

	5-HT$_1$-like	5-HT$_2$	5-HT$_3$
Selective agonist	5-Carboxyamidotryptamine (5-CT)	—	2Me5-HT
Antagonist	No selective antagonist Methysergide*	Ketanserin Methysergide	MDL 72222 ICS 205-930
Not antagonised by	Ketanserin MDL 72222	MDL 72222	Ketanserin Methysergide
Corresponds to	D?	D	M
Subdivisions	5-HT$_{1A}$ 5-HT$_{1B}$ 5-HT$_{1C}$	—	—

*Weak antagonist or partial agonist

based on that. Table 9.1 lists the three subclasses of receptor: 5-HT$_1$-like, 5-HT$_2$ and 5-HT$_3$ together with the selective agonists and/or antagonists for the three types. Attention is drawn to the lack of a selective antagonist for the '5-HT$_1$-like' and a selective agonist for the 5-HT$_2$ receptor. Responses due to the three subtypes may be differentiated by the antagonists methsergide, ketanserin and MDL 72222. The 5-HT$_2$ type seems to correspond to the earlier D type (so too may the '5-HT$_1$-like') whereas the M type seems closest to the 5-HT$_3$ type of receptor. The second messenger for the '5-HT$_1$-like' subtype seems to be adenylate cyclase whereas the 5-HT$_2$ subtype seems linked to the IP$_3$ cycle: stimulation of adenylate cyclase and IP$_3$ breakdown are believed to occur, respectively.

On the basis of radioligand binding studies the '5-HT$_1$-like' receptor has been further subdivided into three types, 5-HT$_{1A, 1B}$ and $_{1C}$ which under appropriate conditions can be labelled using 8-OH-DPAT, cyano-pindolol and mesulergine respectively although the selectivity of these agents is less than perfect. Therefore, the distinction between these binding sites hinges on use of ligands which have affinity for other sites (receptors). Thus β-blockers such as cyanopindolol bind to 5-HT$_{1A}$ and 5-HT$_{1B}$ sites.

Two major problems are posed by these sub-classes of binding site:

1 How do they relate (if at all) to receptor sub-types defined by measurements of functional activities?

2 Are the apparent affinities measured in binding studies a reflection of agonist or antagonist activity?

The roles of the functionally-defined receptor types can be gleaned by use of the agonists and/or antagonists listed in the table and likewise the use of labelled versions of these agents can be a powerful tool for probing the location of the binding sites in the CNS tissue using autoradiographic techniques.

'5-HT₁-like' receptor

A major effect of activation of this receptor seems to be inhibition of neurotransmitter release and neuronal inhibition. A reduction in neurotransmitter release has been shown for ACh and NA (the latter may be relevant to the interconnections between raphe and noradrenergic cell bodies in the brain) and also for 5-HT itself, which is indicative that the autoreceptor on the 5-HT neuronal soma is of this subtype. Likewise LSD and 8-OH-DPAT label this receptor and as discussed previously slow raphe unit activity. The resultant disinhibition of visual and sensory relay nuclei (colliculi, spinal cord, etc.) may underlie the visual and tactile changes caused by LSD. The neuronal inhibition produced by 5-HT has been observed in cortical hippocampal and spinal cord areas where 5-HT₁-like sites are labelled. Interestingly, in the rat spinal cord the dorsal horn has a high density of 5-HT$_{1A}$ sites whilst 5-HT$_{1B}$ receptors are found in the ventral horn. An exception to the inhibitory effects of 5-HT is the depolarisation of facial nucleus motoneurons, although this seems to be mediated by 5-HT₂ receptors.

The '5-HT behavioural syndrome' has long been used as a model for activation of 5-HT-dependent systems in the CNS and consists of a variety of motor and behavioural changes induced by increasing 5-HT levels (usually 5-HTP and a MAOI or an uptake blocker are used). As described above certain aspects of this syndrome can be attributed to 5-HT₁ receptors, namely forepaw treading and Straub tail (an elevation of the tail). It may be that the high levels of '5-HT₁-like' receptors in some motor areas (ventral cord, basal ganglia and motor cortex) are implicated.

The '5-HT₁-like' receptor also is likely to mediate some cardiovascular effects (hypotension, tachycardia, relaxation and contraction of vascular smooth muscle) and these effects may have some central components since high numbers of '5-HT₁-like' receptors are found in the solitary tract.

Finally the '5-HT₁-like' receptor also seems involved in stimulation of sexual behaviour: the receptor binding sites in hypothalamic areas may underlie these effects, and also the well documented role of 5-HT in thermoregulation.

The effects on temperature of 5-HT, usually microinjected or given i.c.v, depend on the species tested, the ambient temperatures and the site of injection in the hypothalmus. The effects of 5-HT in these studies are usually countered by NA, verifying the original monoamine hypothesis of thermoregulation of Feldberg and Myers whereby these two transmitters balanced thermoregulatory drive (see Hellon 1975). Supporting this premise are studies showing that 5-HT turnover depends on ambient temperature, that raphe serotoninergic neurons respond to body and skin temperature changes and that electrical stimulation of the raphe and locus coeruleus have opposing effects on thermoregulation. Very recent evidence is that hypothermia is mediated by 5-HT_1 and hyperthermia by 5-HT_2 receptors. 5-HT_{1A} receptors may also play a role in the action of some anxiolytics (see Chapter 20).

5-HT_2 receptors

Some of the functional effects of 5-HT_2 receptor activation have already been mentioned (depolarisation of motoneurons and thermoregulatory influences). In addition to the 5-HT_1-like components of the 5-HT behavioural syndrome the headtwitch and shaking produced by 5-HT stimulation seem to be mediated via the 5-HT_2 receptor, as do the clonic seizures elicited by tryptamine. In keeping with the motor effects 5-HT_2 receptors are found in the motor cortex.

Hypertension and vascular contraction can be broadly assumed to result from this receptor type and bearing on the $D\text{-}5\text{-HT}_2$ correspondence, contraction of smooth muscle in gut, bronchi and bladder can be attributed to the 5-HT_2 receptors, although the results may depend on species.

There are reports that both 5-HT_2 sites in cortex and 5-HT_{1A} type sites in hippocampus are reduced in Alzheimer's disease (see Chapter 21).

5-HT_3 sites

These sites have only very recently been identified in the CNS but in peripheral systems seem involved in depolarisation of autonomic ganglia and the stimulation of release of ACh and NA seen in peripheral tissue. Pain induced in blister base preparations in man by 5-HT seems to occur via this receptor type as does flare which may relate to an involvement in migraine. This site corresponds well to the original M class of 5-HT receptor. The previous failures to demonstrate the presence of 5-HT_3 sites in the CNS seem due to technical problems with the binding studies and high levels in human cortex have now been reported. A recently described 5-HT_3 antagonist (GR38032) is reported to have anxiolytic (see Chapter 20) and possibly antipsychotic potential, as gauged by behavioural studies in animals, as well as antiemetic effects.

Other functions of 5-HT

The roles of 5-HT in sensory modulation in the spinal cord are discussed in the chapter on Pain and Analgesia (Chapter 22) and serotonin in anxiety in Chapter 20. Several aspects of 5-HT function attributable to receptor subtypes have been mentioned; finally we shall discuss sleep and punishment.

Sleep

Again, similar to the situation with regard to temperature regulation a close interrelationship exists between NA and 5-HT in the generation and maintenance of sleep patterns. There are, however, several discrepancies in the literature and this account is thus only a summary of certain aspects of 5-HT and sleep (see also Chapter 20).

The role of 5-HT in sleep has been extensively studied by Jouvet and co-workers (see Jouvet 1974). The main lines of evidence are that pCPA which blocks 5-HT synthesis causes insomnia which can be reversed, leading to normal sleep by injection of 5-HTP which restores the 5-HT levels. Raphe lesions produce an insomnia which is proportional both to the extent of the lesion and the decrease in 5-HT turnover in projection areas. The catecholamine systems are also intimately involved and the general scheme suggested is that the serotonergic raphe neurons are responsible for slow wave sleep and for triggering paradoxical sleep whilst catecholamine and cholinergic systems in the brainstem maintain paradoxical sleep and behavioural and EEG arousal. With reference to the postulated roles of the raphe system in both sleep and temperature regulation, it is interesting to note that hypothalamic temperature regulation alters over the sleep cycle.

It is likely, however, that 5-HT and NA are not the only transmitters involved in sleep and recently emphasis is tending to shift away from the monoamines.

Punishment

Many behavioural studies indicate that 5-HT is involved in punishment behaviour such as 'freezing' in the presence of inescapable electric shock, the 'conditioned emotional response', since reducing 5-HT function blocks this response. Likewise signalled avoidance studies provide additional evidence for this rôle, and in general the effects of reducing 5-HT function are comparable to those of the benzodiazepines (see Stein *et al* 1977).

Co-existence of 5-HT with other neurotransmitters

The increasingly frequent co-existence of peptides with other non-peptides, neurotransmitters or peptides in CNS neurons also holds for 5-HT neurons. Particular emphasis should be made of the descending 5-HT projections to the spinal cord from the caudal brainstem raphe nuclei since, in addition to 5-HT, the cells in these nuclei contain thyrotrophin releasing hormone (TRH), substance P (SP) or enkephalins. It is interesting to note that electrical stimulation of the raphe magnus inhibits most dorsal horn nociceptive neurons in normal animals yet in animals with a full depletion of cord 5-HT, by pCPA pretreatment, the same stimulation inhibits very few neurons but excites in a powerful and prolonged fashion, a large proportion of cells. It is tempting to speculate that this results from excitatory effects of TRH or SP which are normally masked by serotoninergic inhibitions (see Rivot *et al.* 1980).

Tryptamine

Tryptamine is found in 5-HT neurons, including those in man, and also in catecholamine cells. Its role as a transmitter is controversial however, since its release by nerve stimulation has not been demonstrated. Tryptamine levels are elevated by various drugs such as pCPA, MAOI as well as by tryptophan loading. It is formed from tryptophan by decarboxylation whilst the additional action of a methyltransferase, requiring a methyl group donor (such as methionine) produces N,N-dimethyltryptamine (DMT). Methoxy-DMT can also be formed from 5-HT itself. Neither of these pathways is likely to be important in normal states but may be involved in some pathologies in man since DMT is able to produce hallucinations, spatial perception changes, euphoria and speech impairment. Some of these effects are also seen with LSD and interestingly, the actions of DMT in animals resemble those of LSD. There seems little tolerance to the effects of DMT but this may result from its short half-life. An involvement of tryptamine in disorders such as schizophrenia has been hypothesized but remains unproven. (For further details on tryptamine see Chapter 10.)

References and further reading

Bradley PB, Engel G, Feniuk W, Fozard JR, Humphrey PPA, Middlemiss DN, Mylecharane EJ, Richardson BP & Saxena PR (1986) Proposals for the classification and nomenclature of functional receptors for 5-hydroxytryptamine. *Neuropharmacology* **25**, 563–76.

Dahlstrom A & Fuxe K (1964) Evidence for the existence of monoamine-containing neurones in the central nervous system. *Acta. Physiol. Scand.* **62**, suppl 232, 1–55.

Fuller RW (1980) Pharmacology of central serotonin neurons. *Ann. Rev. Pharmacol.* **20**, 111–27.

Hellon RF (1975) Monoamines, pyrogens and cations. *Pharm. Rev.* **27**, 289–321.

Jacobs BL (1976) An animal behaviour model for studying central serotonergic synapses. *Life Sci.* **19**, 777–86.

Jacobs BL & Gelperin A (eds) (1981). *Serotonin Neurotransmission and Behaviour.* MIT Press, Cambridge MA, USA.

Jouvet M (1974) The role of monoaminergic neurons in the regulation and function of sleep. In: PetreQuadens O & Schlag JD (eds) *Basic Sleep Mechanisms* Academic Press, New York. pp. 207–36.

Pazos A & Palacios J (1985) Quantitative autoradiographic mapping of serotonin receptors in the rat brain. I and II. *Brain. Res.* **346**, 205–49.

Peroutka SJ (1984) 5HT receptor sites and functional correlates. *Neuropharmacology* **23**, 1487–92.

Rivot JP, Chaouch A & Besson JM *et al.* (1980) Nucleus raphe magnus modulation of response of rat dorsal horn neurons to unmyelinated fiber inputs: partial involvement of serotonergic pathways. *J. Neurophysiol.* **44**, 1039–57.

Stein L, Wise D & Balluzi J (1977) Neuropharmacology of reward and punishment. In: Iversen LL, Iversen S & Snyder SH (eds) *Handbook of Psychopharmacology 8.* Plenum Press, New York. pp. 25–54.

Steinbusch HW (1981) Distribution of serotonin immunoreactivity in the central nervous system of the rat — cell bodies and terminals. *Neuroscience* **6**, 557–618.

10 Trace amines and other possible mediators in the central nervous system

R.A. WEBSTER

Acetylcholine and noradrenaline serve as neurotransmitters in both the central and peripheral nervous systems but a number of other established central neurotransmitters like dopamine, GABA and 5-HT, do not appear to have that role in the periphery. Nevertheless 5-HT is known to be released from enterochromaffin cells and functions as a chemical mediator of various effects on smooth muscle. It is perhaps pertinent to ask whether other substances, not normally found in neurons but classified as chemical mediators in the periphery, also exist in the CNS and have a functional role there. These include adrenaline, histamine, adenosine and the prostaglandins as well as the so called trace amines such as tryptamine, phenylethylamine, tyramine and octopamine. Their central pharmacology will be briefly reviewed.

Adrenaline

The enzyme β-phenylethanolamine-N-methyl transferase, which is required to convert noradrenaline (NA) to adrenaline (Ad) is present in the CNS and there is histofluorometric evidence (positive staining with antibodies not only to this enzyme but to tyrosine hydroxylase and dopamine β-hydroxylase as well) for adrenergic cell bodies in two groups (nuclei) alongside NA neurons of the locus coeruleus (LC) but ventral and lateral (C_1) and dorsal and medial (C_2) to it. Projections go to the hypothalamus and in particular to the dorsal motor nucleus of the vagus as well as to the LC itself. Little is known of the normal function of these relatively minor pathways although stimulation of C_1 causes a release of adrenaline in the hypothalamus and a rise in blood pressure which is blocked by mixed β-antagonists but not by β_1 antagonists administered i.c.v. (Marsden 1987). Such a β_2 mediated response would be better mediated by Ad rather than NA, which has little activity at such receptors (see Chapter 7).

Histamine

In the periphery histamine (HA) is found mainly in mast cells and is known to act on two receptors. Basically H_1 receptors are linked to contraction of most smooth muscle (gut and bronchi) and increased capillary permeability, whereas H_2 receptors control gastric acid secretion. Histamine is found in the CNS at a whole brain concentration of 50–70 ng/g and there is evidence for the presence of both receptors. Its concentration is highest in the hypothalamus and although some of this may be in mast cells, undercutting the cortex leads to a marked reduction in content of both histamine and histidine decarboxylase, the enzyme required for histamine synthesis from the amino acid precursor histidine. This has been taken as evidence for histamine being present in neuronal pathways rather than mast cells but it has not been possible to

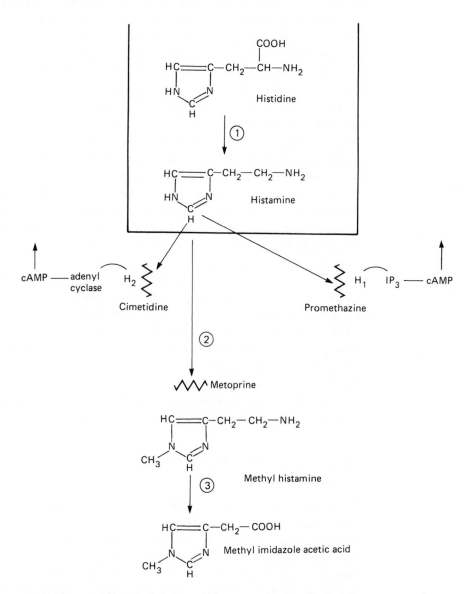

Fig. 10.1. Synthesis, actions and metabolism of histamine. 1, Histidine decarboxylase. 2, Histamine-n-methyl transferase. 3, Monoamine oxidase (MAO_B). Cimetidine and promethazine are H_2 and H_1 receptor antagonists and metoprine inhibits the methylation of histamine. IP_3, inositol triphosphate

demonstrate the low levels of its condensation products by the conventional histofluorometric techniques used for catecholamines. Fortunately histidine decarboxylase is a specific enzyme distinct from the more general amino acid decarboxylase found in monoamine neurons and so it provides a marker for HA neurons. Recently an antibody has been raised to this enzyme (Pollard & Schwartz 1987) which has allowed HA neurons and pathways to be definitely established by immunohistochemistry. A group of about 1000 cells is found in the magnocellular nucleus very close to the ventral lateral surface of the brain and a smaller nucleus near the tip of the third ventricle, i.e. all the neurons are close to the internal and external brain CSF spaces. Their projections are divergent like those of NA and 5-HT with many going to limbic structures and the hippocampus, although other fibres in the median eminence of the hypothalamus may control hormone release from the pituitary.

Histamine is metabolised by histamine-n-methyl transferase to methylhistamine which is then deaminated into methylimidazole acetic acid by monoamine oxidase (MAOB) (Fig. 10.1). Like NA it depresses neuronal firing, when applied by iontophoresis in most brain areas but potentiates excitatory signals in the hippocampus. Here it blocks the long lasting hyperpolarisation (accommodation) that normally follows firing through a Ca^{2+} activated K^+ conductance; again like NA (Haas 1985). It has been implicated in arousal since not only does intraventricular HA produce EEG arousal but most H_1 antagonists are sedative in man. In contrast, raising brain HA with metoprine, an inhibitor of histamine-N-methyltransferase, protects animals from maximal electroconvulsive shock (Tuomisto & Tecke 1986). High levels of histamine and H_2 receptors in the hypothalamus have implicated HA in food and water intake and thermoregulation (see Hough & Green 1983). Both H_1 and H_2 receptors are linked to an elevation of cyclic AMP in the CNS either through adenylate cyclase (H_2) or the inositol triphosphate system (H_1) but their respective functions are not known. No clear central effects have been noted during the widespread use of H_2 antagonists and HA has not been implicated in any disorders of the CNS (see Green et al. 1978).

Trace amines (tryptamine, phenylethylamine, tyramine and octopamine)

Decarboxylation, instead of hydroxylation, of the amino acid precursors of DA and 5-HT results in the formation of amines that are only found in trace amounts in the CNS but have distinct effects when administered into the brain. Since such decarboxylation can be achieved by the non-specific L-aromatic amino acid decarboxylase there is considerable potential for its occurrence, especially if there is a rise in the concentration of the appropriate precursor or some malfunction in their normal hydroxylation through rate limiting processes. This could shunt tyrosine, tryptophan and phenylalanine though to tyramine, tryptamine and

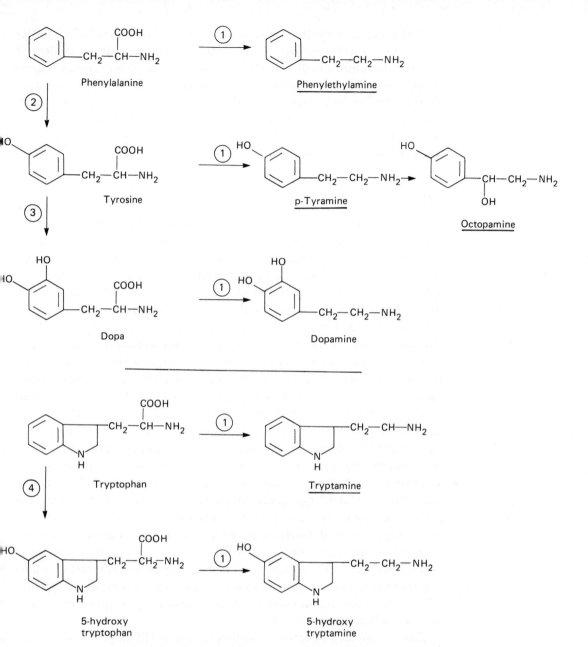

Fig. 10.2. Synthesis of the trace amines (underlined). 1, Decarboxylation by aromatic L-amino acid decarboxylase. 2, Phenylalanine hydroxylase. 3, Tyrosine hydroxylase. 4, Tryptophan hydroxylase.

phenylethylamine rather than to the more normally formed dopa, 5-HT and tyrosine (see Fig. 10.2). It is this potential for synthesis together with the known central effects of these amines when injected, that preserves an interest in them despite their very low concentrations in whole brain, i.e. phenylethylamine 1.8, p-tyramine 2.0, m-tyramine 0.3 and tryptamine 0.5 ng/g. Generally concentrations are highest in the striatum (4, 11,

0.3 and 1.5 ng/g respectively) but still very much lower than DA (10 μg/g). Unlike the catecholamines their concentration rises dramatically (50 times) after inhibition of MAO. Turnover can also be increased easily by the provision of extra substrate since decarboxylation is not rate limiting. Distinct anatomical pathways have not been identified since there is no specific enzyme involved in their synthesis that can be used for immunohistochemistry, and they are not sufficiently concentrated for ordinary histofluorescence.

Tryptamine

Although tryptamine can be detected in brain there has been much debate over whether it exists separately from 5-HT or merely coexists with it. Specific high affinity binding sites have been demonstrated for tryptamine in rat cortex. These appear to be different from 5-HT sites but until appropriate antagonists are found it remains possible that they form a subset of the ever increasing number of 5-HT receptors (see Chapter 9). The behavioural response in rats to tryptophan plus a MAO inhibitor (Grahame-Smith 1971) is accompanied by an elevation of brain tryptamine as well as 5-HT and is less marked if the synthesis of tryptamine is reduced by a decarboxylase inhibitor, even when it does not have a significant effect on 5-HT levels. In fact after a MAOI, tryptamine produces a behavioural response in rats similar to that of tryptophan apart from the absence of certain features like tremor and wet-dog shake. The complexity of the situation is illustrated by studies of the effect of intra-hypothalamic injections of 5-HT and tryptamine on rat body temperature (Cox *et al.* 1981). In these it was shown that 5-HT decreased temperature whilst tryptamine actually increased it but it was not possible to block one effect preferentially with a whole range of antagonists, despite some differences in effectiveness. Also although it was the tryptamine, and not the 5-HT response, which was abolished after destruction of 5-HT neurons with 5,7-dihydroxytryptamine, which implies that tryptamine was releasing 5-HT, it was found that raphe (5-HT) neuron stimulation produces hyperthermia, like tryptamine, rather than hypothermia, like 5-HT.

These opposing effects of tryptamine and 5-HT are also seen when they are applied directly to cortical neurons by iontopheresis. Tryptamine is predominantly depressant whilst 5-HT is mainly excitatory. Surprisingly the 5-HT antagonist metergoline is more effective against tryptamine and the depressant effects. When the medial raphe nucleus is stimulated this produces inhibition of cortical neurons followed by excitation but it is the inhibition (tryptamine-like) that is blocked by metergoline. In keeping with this finding is the observation that depletion of 5-HT with pCPA reduced only the excitatory (5-HT) response whilst 5,7-dihydroxytryptamine which destroys the neurons, abolished both effects (see Jones 1982). The inference from these studies and those on temperature is that some neurons in the raphe nucleus release something other than 5-HT. This might be tryptamine but if it is not, then its effects are presumably modified by tryptamine.

The above findings suggest that there is a subclass of 5-HT receptors preferentially activated by tryptamine and blocked by metergoline. Unfortunately it seems likely that at appropriate concentrations they will also be stimulated by 5-HT whilst high concentrations of tryptamine can affect other 5-HT receptors. Possibly the term tryptamine receptor, as first used by Gaddum to describe the effects of indole amines, may be one to which we should return.

Phenylethylamine

The relationship of phenylethylamine to dopamine is not unlike that of tryptamine to 5-HT. Present in low concentrations in the brain there is some evidence for distinct binding sites but not for specific neurons. When injected i.c.v. it causes stereotyped behaviour similar to, but more marked than, that seen with amphetamine. These effects are blocked by neuroleptics (DA antagonists) and since phenylethylamine does not bind directly to DA receptors it is assumed to release DA, like amphetamine. This is substantiated by the fact that in rats with unilateral 6-OHDA lesions of the SN its systemic administration causes ipsilateral rotation like amphetamine. Phenylethylamine certainly increases the overflow of [³H]-DA from striatal synaptosomes and slices and of endogenous DA *in vivo*, but part of this may be due to block of DA uptake (see Phillips & Robson 1983). In any case such effects only occur with concentrations of 5×10^{-5} M, which are not likely to be encountered *in vivo* and it is not Ca^{2+} dependent. Peripherally phenylethylamine causes contractions of the rat fundus, like amphetamine, tryptamine and 5-HT which are reduced by some 5-HT antagonists, like methysergide, but not by DA antagonists. Thus some of its central effects may be mediated through a tryptamine receptor. Needless to say the DA and amphetamine like activity and structure of phenylethylamine, together with the facility for its synthesis in the CNS, has lead to suggestions of its involvement in schizophrenia.

In fact there is some evidence for increased excretion of its metabolite (phenyl acetic acid) in the subgroup of paranoid schizophrenics.

Tyramine

p-Tyramine is decarboxylated from tyrosine and is present in the CNS in higher (threefold) concentrations than m-tyramine, the hydroxylated derivative of phenylethylamine. In the periphery p-tyramine is easily hydroxylated to octopamine, which has some direct effects on α_1 adrenoceptors, unlike tyramine which functions by releasing NA. When tested on central neurons tyramine always produces the same effects as NA but they are slower and less marked, implying an indirect action. By contrast octopamine often produces the opposite effect to NA and it is probable that octopamine may have a functional role in the invertebrate CNS where it is found in higher concentrations (5 μg/g) than in the mammalian brain (0.5 ng/g). Neither tyramine nor octopamine have distinct behavioural effects, unlike phenylethylamine and little is known of their central effects, although depressed patients have been shown to excrete less conjugated tyramine than normal subjects after challenge with tyrosine (Bonham-Carter *et al.* 1978).

For further details of the trace amines see Usdin & Sandler (1976), Jones (1983) and Boulton *et al.* (1984).

Prostaglandins

The main problem with any study of prostaglandins (PGs) is that although brain concentrations can exceed 0.1 μg/g, they appear to be formed on demand, rather than preformed and stored. Also specific effective antagonists remain to be developed. PGs are widely and evenly distributed, unlike most NTs. Thus any analysis of their central effects rests heavily on either studying PG release, or their effects when applied directly (i.c.v. injection). Certainly the brain has the enzymatic ability to synthesise both prostaglandins (cycloxygenase) and leukotrienes (lypoxygenase) from arachidonic acid (Fig. 10.3).

When injected into the brain (often in rather large concentrations) PGEs but not PGF_2 are depressant and cause sedation and catatonia. PGEs can be found in superfusates of cat cortex and their concentration is increased by direct electrical stimulation as well as by afferent nerve activation. In fact, when given intraventricularly PGE_1 and PGE_2 antagonise convulsions induced by leptazol and electroshock but whether they

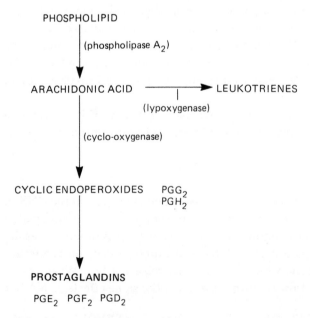

Fig. 10.3. Metabolic products of arachidonic acid. Cyclo-oxygenase is inhibited by aspirin and related drugs.

have any role in initiating or controlling convulsive activity is uncertain. The levels of a number of PGs, especially PGD_2 and PGE_2 are reported to be significantly lowered in spontaneously convulsing gerbils and in these animals the levels of brain lypoxygenase derivatives have also been found to increase after the onset of seizures (Simmet *et al.* 1987), although such changes can result from, rather than cause, the convulsions.

One area of particular interest, in view of the anti-pyretic effects of cyclo-oxygenase inhibitors like aspirin, is the possible role of PGs in the control of body temperature. Thus i.c.v. injections of PGE_1 and PGE_2 elevate body temperature and PGE levels increase in CSF following pyrogen induced fever. Unfortunately this release does not occur near the anterior hypothalamus, which is considered to control body temperature, and iontophoretically applied PGE_2 does not affect the firing of hypothalamic neurons. Also lesions of the anterior hypothalamus abolish PGE-but not pyrogen-induced fever. The situation remains to be resolved (see Wolfe 1983).

Adenosine

Studies of the so called non-adrenergic, non-cholinergic (NANC) nerve induced inhibition of certain smooth muscle preparations has lead to the discovery of distinct adenosine receptors in such tissues and to the neural evoked release of adenosine. Adenosine works through at least two receptors (A_1 and A_2) distinguished by the order of activity and effects of a range of agonists on cyclic AMP production. Activation of A_1 receptors depresses adenylate cyclase activity and reduces cyclic AMP whilst A_2 receptors have a stimulant effect. Although adenosine is found in the CNS it has not been possible to establish a clear presence of adenosine binding sites in the brain probably because of competition from the high levels of the endogenous ligand (100 ng/g) and other nucleotides (0.5 μg/g). The fact that theophylline is an antagonist at both adenosine receptors and a CNS stimulant has implicated adenosine in CNS function.

When applied to central neurons adenosine has a strong inhibitory effect. In addition it can reduce NT release and is known to be released during intense neuronal activity. It is this observation that has lead to the proposal that adenosine is an endogenous limiter of neuronal function which is formed, as a result of neuronal activity, to produce inhibition. Thus it has been postulated to play an important role in controlling convulsant activity (Dragunow 1986). Certainly adenosine and its analogues are anti-convulsant and this effect is reversed by theophylline, which is proconvulsant. Also the brain concentration of adenosine rapidly increases during the development of seizures and this response does not appear to be secondary to changes in blood flow or oxygen supply. Adenosine is another compound that enhances the after-hyperpolarisation of pyramidal cell, by a Ca^{2+} dependent change in K^+ conductance. If adenosine release after excessive neuronal activity really can arrest seizures it is interesting that the most effective drugs in the treatment of continuous epileptic attacks, i.e. status epileptics, are the benzodiazepines (e.g. clonazepam and diazepam). These have been shown to increase the efflux of [^{3}H]-adenosine from rat cortex, presumably by blocking its uptake (Phillis *et al.* 1980) and to potentiate its depressant effects on cortical neurons. Since the depressant effects of flurazepam on cortical neurons is reduced by theophylline and as adenosine competes with benzodiazepines for their binding sites, some interrelationship may exist, even if the primary action of the benzodiazepines remain dependent on GABA. For a full analysis of the central actions of adenosine and its possible involvement in the effect of other centrally acting drugs refer to Phillis and Wu (1981). (See also Chapters 5, 17 and 20.)

References and further reading

Bonham-Carter SM, Sandler M, Goodwin BL, Sepping P & Bridges PK (1978). Decreased urinary output of tyramine and its metabolites in depression. *Br. J. Psychiat.* **132**, 125–32.

Boulton AA, Baker GB, Dewhurst WG & Sandler M (eds) (1984) *Neurobiology of the Trace Amines*. The Humana Press Inc.

Cox B, Lee TF & Martin D (1981) Different hypothalamic receptors mediate 5-hydroxytryptamine and tryptamine induced core temperature changes in the rat. *Br. J. Pharmac.* **72** 472–82.

Dragunow M (1986) Adenosine, the brain's natural anticonvulsant? *Trends Pharmacol. Sci.*, 128–9.

Grahame-Smith DG (1971) Studies *in vivo* on the relationship between brain tryptophan, brain 5-HT synthesis and hyperactivity in rats treated with a monoamine oxidase inhibitor and l-tryptophan. *J. Neurochem* **18**, 1053–66.

Green JP, Johnson CL & Weinstein H (1978) Histamine as a neurotransmitter. In: Lipton MA, Dimascio A & Killam KF (eds) *Psychopharmacology. A Generation of Progress.* Raven Press, New York. pp. 319–32.

Haas HC (1985) Histamine actions in the mammalian central nervous system. *Adv. Biosci* **51**, 215–24.

Hough LS & Green JP (1983) Histamine and its receptors in the nervous system. In: Lajtha A (ed.) *Handbook of Neurochemistry*, Vol. 6. Plenum Press, New York. pp. 187–211.

Jones RSG (1982) Response of cortical neurones to stimulation of the nucleus raphé medianus: a pharmacological analysis of the role of indoleamines. *Neuropharmacology* **21**, 511–20. (also pp. 209–14, and pp. 1273–7)

Jones RSG (1983) Trace biogenic amines: a possible functional role in the CNS. *Trends Pharmacol. Sci.*, **4**, 426–9.

Marsden CA (1987) Measurement of hypothalamic adrenaline release *in vivo* — effects of drugs and electrical stimulation. *Neuropharmacology* **26**, 823–30.

Phillips SR & Robson AM (1983) *In vivo* release of endogenous dopamine from rat caudate nucleus by phenylethylamine. *Neuropharmacology* **22**, 1297–303.

Phillis JW, Siemens RK & Wu PH (1980) Effect of diazepam on adenosine and acetylcholine release from rat cerebral cortex: further evidence for a purinergic mechanism in action of diazepam. *Br. J. Pharmac.* **70**, 341–9.

Phillis JW & Wu PH (1981) The role of adenosine and its nucleotides in central synaptic transmission. *Progress in Neurobiology* **16**, 187–239.

Pollard H & Schwartz JC (1987) Histamine neuronal pathways and their functions. *Trends Neurosci.* **10**, 86–9.

Simet Th, Seregia A & Hertting G (1987) Formation of sulphidopeptide-leukotrienes in brain tissue of spontaneously convulsing gerbils. *Neuropharmacology* **26**, 107–10.

Tuomisto L & Tecke U (1986) Is histamine an anticonvulsive inhibitory transmitter? *Neuropharmacology* **25**, 955–8.

Usdin E & Sandler M (eds) (1976) *Trace Amines and the Brain*. Dekker, New York.

Wolfe CS (1982) Eicosanoids: Prostaglandins, thromboxanes, leukotrienes, and other derivatives of carbon-20 unsaturated fatty acids. *J. Neurochem.* **38**, 1-9.

11 Amino acid neurotransmitters

R.W. HORTON

By the mid 1960s, the ability of certain amino acids to reversibly increase or decrease neuronal firing when applied directly to the exposed cerebral cortex or microiontophoretically to single spinal or cortical neurons had been demonstrated in several laboratories. The potent actions of amino acids known to be present within the brain were of particular interest. Gamma Aminobutyric Acid (GABA) and glycine inhibited neuronal firing, while L-glutamate and L-aspartate were excitatory. The idea was advocated that these amino acids might play a physiological role as neurotransmitters in synaptic transmission in the mammalian CNS.

This hypothesis was slow to reach acceptance, partly because of the widespread nature of their distribution and action in the brain. The concentrations of the main putative amino acid transmitters in the rat brain (glutamate, 12; aspartate, 4; GABA, 2; glycine, 1 μmol/g wet weight) were three orders of magnitude greater than acetylcholine and the monoamines, the other major putative transmitter candidates of the era. Their transmitter function seemed, in most cases, to be of secondary importance to their established metabolic role within the brain. Further, their electrophysiological effects were considered non-specific since all or almost all neurons were excited by glutamate or aspartate and inhibited by GABA. These factors were considered by many to be inappropriate to transmitter candidates by comparison with the 'classical' neurotransmitters.

During the last twenty years, many of the accepted requirements for neurotransmitters have been satisfied with respect to GABA, glutamate/aspartate and glycine at synapses within the mammalian CNS. Specific release by stimulating certain pathways, mechanisms for synaptic inactivation, the pharmacological and molecular characterisation of specific receptors, associated ion channels and other mediators of their postsynaptic actions, and an identity of action between synaptically mediated events and those induced by local application of neurotransmitter have been demonstrated. It has been estimated that 30–40% of synaptic connections in the CNS utilise GABA as their transmitter and 15-20% utilise glutamate/aspartate as their transmitter. This chapter will describe the metabolic events, release and inactivation mechanisms associated with amino acid neurotransmission and how these events are influenced by drugs. Some specific pathways which utilise amino acid neurotransmitters are detailed. The receptors which mediate the effects of amino acid neurotransmission are considered in detail in Chapters 12 and 13.

General properties

Amino acid neurotransmitters are the only neurotransmitters that have a major metabolic function in addition to their transmitter role.

Glutamate, aspartate and glycine (but not GABA) are incorporated into proteins within the brain, are precursors of intermediates of glucose metabolism — a vital pathway for the maintenance of CNS function and are precursors and intermediates in pathways unrelated to neurotransmission. Glutamate, by conversion to glutamine, plays a vital role in ammonia detoxification within the brain. Glutamate holds a key position since it is a potent excitatory substance and the immediate precursor of a potent inhibitory substance, GABA.

The separate regulation of metabolic and transmitter function is possible because glutamate exists in several 'pools' within the brain, which only slowly equilibrate with each other, rather than one homogeneous pool. Glutamate is said to be compartmented. For example, glutamine is actively formed from a pool of glutamate not in equilibrium with the total glutamate in the brain. GABA is synthesised from a different glutamate pool than the one from which glutamine is preferentially formed. It is tempting though probably unrealistic to equate these different pools with different cellular or subcellular compartments.

The metabolic function of transmitter amino acids means that they are probably present in all neurons in the brain (this may not be the case for GABA), unlike for example ACh and monoamines which are only present in those neurons in which they function as a transmitter. Thus regional measuremerts of amino acid concentrations are not necessarily good indicators of transmitter function and measurements of the distribution of glutamate or aspartate is unlikely to help in the mapping of pathways.

Those amino acids with transmitter function are found in nerve endings (synaptosomes) following conventional subcellular fractionation, but typically only about 50% of the total brain content is associated with particulate fractions, the remainder being soluble. Under comparable conditions, 90% of ACh is associated with particulate fractions. This difference is partly a reflection of the metabolic function of amino acids and partly due to loss and redistribution during fractionation. Most of the amino acids present in synaptosomes can be released, unlike ACh (see Chapter 6), by hypo-osmotic treatment arguing against a predominant vesicular storage. The best evidence for a vesicular localisation is obtained from visualisation of GABA-like and glutamate-like immunoreactivity in fixed tissue and their concentration in what appears to be synaptic vesicles.

GABA

Distribution of GABA

In the rat, monkey and human brain, concentrations of GABA are highest in substantia nigra, globus pallidus and hypothalamus (4–10 μmol/g), intermediate in caudate, putamen and thalamus (3–4 μmol/g) and lowest in the medulla and pons. In the spinal cord, GABA concentrations are highest in laminae II to IV of the dorsal gray matter (2 μmol/g), intermediate in the ventral gray matter (1 μmol/g), low in the white matter and virtually absent from the nerve roots.

Synthesis

The synthesis and degradation of GABA is intimately related to the metabolism of glucose via the glycolytic and tricarboxylic acid pathways. The synthesis of GABA from α-oxoglutarate and its metabolism to succinate is termed the 'GABA shunt' since it bypasses the normal tricarboxylic acid pathway from α-oxoglutarate to succinate via succinyl CoA (Fig. 11.1). About 8% of the flux of intermediates through the tricarboxylic acid cycle is via the GABA shunt.

GABA is formed by the irreversible decarboxylation of glutamate, catalysed by the enzyme glutamic acid decarboxylase (GAD). Alternative routes for the synthesis of GABA, e.g. from putrescine have been demonstrated but are thought to be quantitatively insignificant under

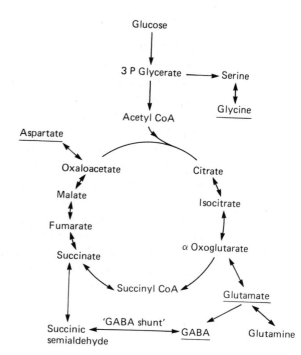

Fig. 11.1. The metabolic relationship between putative amino acid neurotransmitters (underlined) and the glycolytic and tricarboxylic acid cycles.

normal circumstances. GAD activity is concentrated in nerve endings and antibodies raised against the purified enzyme are used as immunocytochemical markers of GABAergic nerve endings.

Control of GABA synthesis

The rate of synthesis of GABA is probably controlled by the activity of GAD. It is not clear which of the many factors that influence GAD activity are involved in physiological regulation. Substrate availability is unlikely to influence activity directly since the glutamate concentration in presynaptic terminals is sufficient for maximal enzymic activity. The mammalian enzyme is not subject to feed back inhibition by GABA. GAD, in common with other decarboxylases and transaminases, requires pyridoxal phosphate as a cofactor. During catalytic activity, pyridoxal phosphate undergoes cycles of dissociation and reassociation with GAD. Glutamate promotes dissociation and adenine nucleotides block reassociation of cofactor and enzyme. Thus, physiological changes in the concentrations of these endogenous substances could alter GAD activity. Factors influencing the binding of pyridoxal phosphate seem to be important since *in vivo* the enzyme is only about 35% saturated with coenzyme, despite the brain concentration being sufficient to fully saturate the enzyme. GAD undergoes Ca^{2+} dependent binding to brain membranes and is inhibited by Cl^-, Zn^{2+} and sulphydryl agents. The significance of these findings to the physiological control of GAD activity is unclear.

Inhibitors of GAD

Drugs which inhibit GAD activity reduce GABA synthesis and invariably induce seizures in experimental animals. Many drugs inhibit GAD by interfering with the coenzymic function of pyridoxal phosphate. Thiosemicarbazide and isoniazid act by forming a Schiff's base complex with the carbonyl group of pyridoxal phosphate. Structural analogues of pyridoxal phosphate (e.g. 4-deoxypyridoxine or 3-methoxypyridoxine) may also act partially in this way and partially by competing with pyridoxal for the phosphorylation reaction catalysed by pyridoxal kinase, hence decreasing the synthesis of pyridoxal phosphate. Unfortunately drugs which interfere with pyridoxal phosphate are not specific for GAD, since other pyridoxal phosphate requiring enzymes will be inhibited. Some drugs inhibit GAD via mechanisms unrelated to pyridoxal phosphate. Thus, 3-mercaptopropionic acid is a competitive inhibitor of GAD with respect to glutamate and allylglycine is metabolised *in vivo* to 2-keto-4-pentenoic acid, which is a potent inhibitor of GAD.

GABA release

In vivo release of GABA has been demonstrated from the exposed surface of the mammalian cerebral cortex, in response to local or remote electrical stimulation, that produced mainly prolonged inhibition of synaptic activity in the cortex. Only amino acids of putative transmitter function were released. GABA release was abolished if the cortex was perfused with Ca^{2+} free medium. Clearly the exact site of GABA release is difficult to define in such *in vivo* preparations. GABA release from defined anatomical pathways (see synapses using GABA as a transmitter) *in vivo* has been demonstrated and has contributed to the establishment of their GABA-ergic nature. For example, stimulation of the striatum causes a several fold increase in the release of GABA from the perfused substantia nigra — supporting the GABAergic nature of the strio-nigral pathway in the rat. Stimulation of the cerebellar cortex causes an increase of GABA concentration in the fourth ventricle as a result of increased release from Purkinje cell endings in the nuclei surrounding the ventricle.

Endogenous or preloaded radiolabelled GABA is released from brain slices and synaptosomes *in vitro* by depolarising electrical or K^+ stimulation. Release is calcium dependent and blocked by tetanus toxin.

The K^+ evoked release of GABA from synaptosomes is inhibited by GABA and GABA agonists, e.g. muscimol and such inhibition is antagonised by bicuculline and picrotoxin. This suggests the presence of autoreceptors on GABA nerve terminals, which are able to regulate GABA release. These receptors have a pharmacological profile similar to $GABA_A$ receptors except that δ aminolevulinic acid is a weak agonist showing some selectivity at autoreceptors.

GABA uptake

Synaptosomes and brain slices rapidly accumulate exogenous GABA by a structurally specific high affinity ($Km \sim 10^{-5}$ M) carrier-mediated uptake process. This is temperature dependent, requires the presence of sodium ions in the external medium and mediates net inward transport rather than just exchange between intra-and extracellular compartments. This specific mechanism for GABA uptake contrasts with the broad specificity low affinity (Km 10^{-3} M) uptake system associated with the uptake of neuroactive and non-neuroactive amino acids. GABA is taken up into both nerve terminals and glial cells by the high affinity uptake process, although the relative contributions of the two sites are difficult to assess. Autoradiographic studies show that not all nerve terminals accumulate [^{3}H] GABA, but there is a high correlation between GABA uptake and GAD activity supporting the view that uptake is specifically into those nerve terminals which release GABA. The physiological function of the uptake process is presumably to limit the life time of synaptically released GABA and prevent its accumulation within the synaptic cleft.

Inhibitors of GABA uptake

Various drugs inhibit GABA uptake in a relatively non-specific manner, e.g. haloperidol, imipramine, chlorpromazine. Close structural analogues of GABA, e.g. 2-chloro-GABA, 4-methyl-GABA are competitive inhibitors of GABA uptake. It is clear that the structural configuration for binding to the uptake carrier differs from that required for GABA receptor binding or binding to the enzyme GABA-transaminase. Consequently some GABA analogues (Fig. 11.2) are able to interact relatively specifically with GABA uptake sites. The neuronal and glial carriers also differ in their structural requirements since L 2,4-diaminobutyric acid and cis-aminocyclohexane carboxylic acid selectively inhibit neuronal uptake while THPO (see Fig. 11.2 legend for full name) and β-alanine selectively inhibit glial uptake. GABA uptake inhibitors have been shown to potentiate the effects of iontophoretically applied GABA on neuronal firing and the behavioural effects of focally injected GABA. However, some of the inhibitors are themselves substrates for the uptake carrier, cause displacement of GABA from nerve terminals and may be released as 'false neurotransmitters'. This may be the basis of the convulsions induced in mice by intracerebroventricular administration of neuronal selective GABA uptake inhibitors.

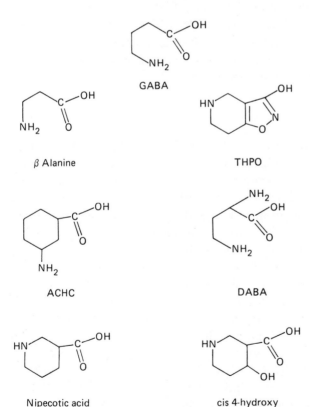

Fig. 11.2. The structure of some GABA uptake inhibitors. β alanine and THPO (4, 5, 6, 7 tetrahydroisoxazolo [4, 5c] pyridin-3-ol) are glial selective and ACHC (aminocyclohexane carboxylic acid) and DABA (L diamino butyric acid) are neuronal selective. GABA is shown in a folded conformation.

GABA metabolism

The principle route of GABA metabolism is to succinic semialdehyde (SSA) and succinate, catalysed by the enzymes GABA-transaminase (GABA-T) and succinic semialdehyde dehydrogenase (SSADH) (Fig. 11.1). Although the GABA-T reaction is reversible, it normally proceeds in the direction of GABA breakdown, the high activity and irreversibility of SSADH ensuring a low brain concentration of succinic semialdehyde. The distribution of brain GABA-T and SSADH do not correlate with the distribution of GABA concentration and thus are not considered as markers for GABA neurons. GABA-T is a mitochondrial enzyme present in nerve endings and glial cells. It requires pyridoxal phosphate but the cofactor is more firmly bound than to GAD.

Inhibitors of GABA metabolism

A number of drugs inhibit GABA-T with varying specificity. Since GABA-T and GAD both require pyridoxal phosphate as cofactor, drugs which interfere with pyridoxal phosphate have complex and often unpredictable effects on the two enzymes and consequently on the concentration of GABA. For example, amino-oxyacetic acid, hydroxylamine and L glutamate γ hydrazide preferentially (although not specifically) inhibit GABA-T *in vivo*, although they are potent GAD inhibitors *in vitro*. Amino-oxyacetic acid was used in research for a number of years as the most specific GABA-T inhibitor, causing several fold increase in brain GABA concentration when administered systemically.

A number of inhibitors of GABA-T do not interfere with pyridoxal phosphate function. They are analogues of GABA which act as false substrates and are catalytically converted by GABA-T to an intermediate which binds tightly to the active site of the enzyme causing irreversible inactivation. They are known as 'suicide substrates' and some are shown structurally in Fig. 11.3. Ethanolamine O-sulphate (EOS) and γ-vinyl GABA (GVG) do not have direct effects upon GAD and are thus the most selective inhibitors whereas γ-acetylenic GABA is also an inhibitor of GAD *in vitro* and *in vivo*. EOS and GVG have only weak effects on GABA uptake and GABA receptor binding. EOS and GVG do not cross the blood–brain barrier very readily but both cause several fold increases in brain GABA concentration when administered systemically in large doses. At least 50% inhibition of GABA-T is required before an increase in GABA concentration is seen, since the enzyme capacity is greatly in excess of that required for GABA breakdown. The site of the increase in brain GABA is not known with certainty but would be expected to occur in both nerve ending and glial compartments.

Administration of EOS and GVG to animals protects against various forms of experimentally induced epilepsy, causes a reduction in food consumption, moderate antinociception and, with higher doses, causes

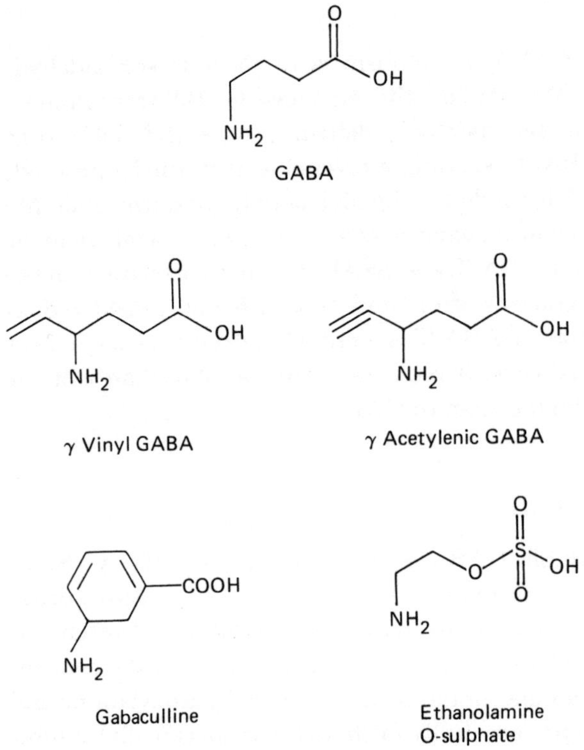

Fig. 11.3. The structure of some 'suicide substrate' inhibitors of GABA-transaminase. GABA is shown in an extended conformation.

reduction in locomotor activity, hunched posture, piloerection and ptosis. These behavioural effects are attributed to enhancement of GABA mediated neurotransmission, presumably as a result of an increased neuronal pool of releasable GABA.

Administration of GABA-T inhibitors has been suggested as a possible therapeutic strategy for enhancing GABA mediated neurotransmission in the treatment of various neurological and psychiatric disorders. A number of encouraging trials of GVG in the treatment of clinical epilepsy have been reported.

Repeated administration of EOS to animals for one month causes a progressive reduction in GAD activity. This is thought to be due to the elevated concentration of GABA causing a feedback suppression of new enzyme synthesis and not due to an effect upon pre-existing enzyme.

Sodium valproate causes an increase in brain GABA concentration in rodents. The mechanism is contentious but has been attributed to GABA-T inhibition. However, valproate is a rather weak inhibitor of GABA-T *in vitro*. It is a more potent inhibitor of SSADH and aldehyde reductase (see alternative pathways). The inhibition of SSA metabolism could drive the GABA-T reaction in reverse and increase brain GABA concentrations. The relationship of such effects to the anticonvulsant action of valproate are not established (see Chapter 17).

Alternative metabolic pathways of GABA

Many alternative pathways other than oxidation to succinate for the metabolism of GABA have been shown or postulated to exist in mammalian brain. Two peptides homocarnosine (GABA-histidine) and homoanserine (GABA-1-methyl histidine) are present in brain and CSF. Other GABA peptides include GABA-lysine and GABA-cystathionine. The biological significance of these peptides is unknown. Other metabolites include γ-guanidinobutyric acid, γ-butyrobetaine, γ-aminobutyrylcholine and γ-amino-β-hydroxybutyric acid. The conversion of GABA to γ-hydroxybutyric acid (GHB) by the reduction of SSA (rather than the normal oxidation) has been demonstrated *in vivo* and *in vitro*. GHB has anaesthetic properties when administered to animals and may have implications for sleep, has been advocated as a neurotransmitter and causes an increase in brain dopamine by blocking impulse traffic in dopaminergic neurons.

Figure 11.4 shows a diagrammatic representation of a GABA synapse.

GABA turnover

The turnover of GABA has been estimated by radioisotope incorporation and by measuring GABA accumulation after inhibition of GABA-T. Turnover rates of GABA with these techniques are about 10 times faster than acetylcholine and 100–1000 times faster than catecholamines.

GABA turnover has been shown to be reduced by benzodiazepines, valproate and other anticonvulsant drugs, and to be increased during bicuculline induced seizures and administration of morphine.

Synapses using GABA as transmitter

There are few well described pathways in which 'long' GABAergic neurons mediate postsynaptic inhibition from one brain centre to another. The best documented is in the dorsal part of the lateral vestibular nucleus (Deiter's nucleus) of the brainstem where cerebellar Purkinje cells mediate monosynaptic inhibition, mediated by GABA. The evidence includes:

1 Inhibitory hyperpolarising synaptic potentials recorded in a Deiter's neuron following cerebellar stimulation are mimicked by local iontophoretic application of GABA. The iontophoretically and electrically induced hyperpolarisations have the same reversal potential and both are antagonised by bicuculline and picrotoxin (GABA$_A$ antagonists) but not strychnine.

2 High concentrations of GABA and GAD are found in the dorsal but not the ventral part of Deiter's nucleus. Lesions of the cerebellar cortex causing degeneration of Purkinje axons reduced GABA and GAD in the dorsal, but not ventral, part of the nucleus, indicating an enrichment of

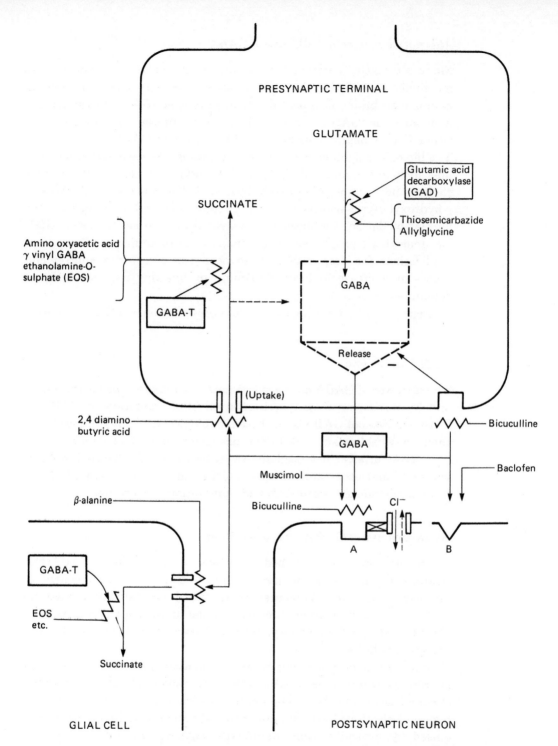

Fig. 11.4. A diagrammatic representation of a GABA synapse. Synthesis of GABA from glutamate is catalysed by glutamic acid decarboxylase (GAD) before incorporation of GABA into vesicles and release by nerve terminal depolarisation. It interacts with postsynaptic receptors — shown are GABA$_A$ receptors which are linked to Cl$^-$ channels and GABA$_B$ receptors where the effector mechanisms are not fully established (see Chapter 12). It also interacts with presynaptic autoreceptors. There is a carrier mediated uptake of GABA into nerve terminals and glial cells and then metabolism to succinic semialdehyde and succinate catalysed by GABA-transminase (GABA-T) and succinic semialdehyde dehydrogenase. Drugs blocking GABA synthesis, action, uptake and metabolism (∿) are shown.

GABA and GAD in synaptic endings rather than cell bodies within the nucleus.

3 Repeated electrical stimulation of the cerebellum causes an increase in CSF GABA concentration in the fourth ventricle, probably as a result of increased liberation from Purkinje nerve endings in nearby Deiter's nucleus.

A second well documented 'long' GABAergic pathway has cell bodies in the striatum and projects to the dopamine cells of substantia nigra (strionigral pathway). Other pathways utilising GABA as a neurotransmitter have been proposed in dopamine rich areas of the brain, e.g. striatum to globus pallidus, and pathways projecting from the nucleus accumbens to substantia nigra, ventral tegmentum, entopeduncular nucleus and globus pallidus, although the evidence for the GABAergic nature of these pathways is less complete than for the other examples cited.

However, the majority of GABA releasing neurons are short interneurons mediating local inhibition in many brain areas including the cerebellar and cerebral cortex, hippocampus, thalamus and brainstem.

In the cerebellar cortex, four of the five types of neurons are inhibitory and thought to use GABA as a neurotransmitter. These are: the Purkinje cells which synapse with Deiter's nucleus (discussed above) and deep cerebellar nuclei (fastigial, dentate, interposed nuclei), the stellate cells and basket cells which synapse on the dendrites and cell bodies of the Purkinje cells, and the Golgi cells which mediate feed forward and feedback inhibition of the excitatory granule cells. In the cerebral cortex, the inhibition of pyramidal tract neurons by basket cells is GABA mediated. Basket cells are activated by recurrent collaterals of the pyramidal cell axons and by extrinsic afferents and so mediate feedback and feedforward inhibition of pyramidal cells. The inhibition of hippocampal pyramidal and granule cells is mediated by local negative feedback circuits via GABA utilising basket cells.

Stimulation of muscle or cutaneous afferent fibres entering the spinal cord is followed by a long-latency prolonged inhibition of motoneurons, associated with prolonged depolarisation of afferent terminals. GABAergic interneurons mediate this depolarisation at axo-axonal synapses with the primary afferent fibres. This results in reduced release of excitatory neurotransmitter from the primary afferent endings and is termed presynaptic inhibition. GABA mediated presynaptic inhibition is not restricted to the spinal cord but occurs throughout the brain.

Glycine

Distribution

There is a uniformity of glycine concentration in the gray matter of the forebrain and the basal ganglia (2μmol/g). Only in the medulla and spinal cord does the concentration exceed 3μmol/g. In the spinal cord, glycine concentration is higher in the ventral than dorsal gray matter.

Synthesis of glycine

Serine is the major metabolic precursor of glycine in the CNS. Serine is converted to glycine by serine hydroxymethyl transferase (SHMT), an enzyme which requires tetrahydrofolate as a cofactor. Serine is derived from glucose by alternate pathways, with 3-phosphoglycerate acting as the branch point (Fig. 11.5), with the non-phosphorylated pathway via glycerate being the more important. Another biosynthetic route to glycine is via transamination of glyoxylate catalysed by glycine aminotransferase. Isotope incorporation suggests that serine is the main precursor and there is a good correlation between SHMT activity and glycine concentrations in the spinal cord. SHMT and D-glycerate dehydrogenase (which is

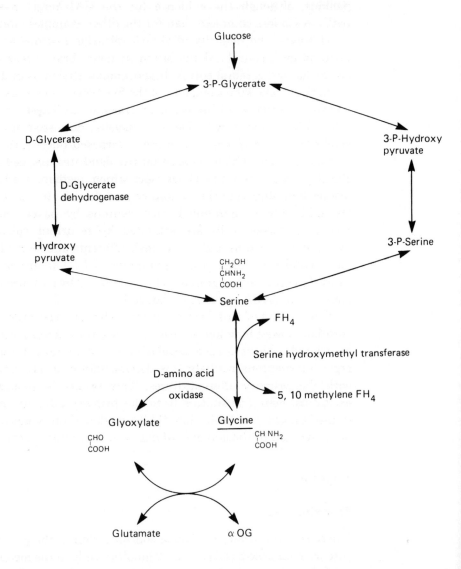

Fig. 11.5. The synthesis and metabolism of glycine.

inhibited non-competitively by glycine) are the rate controlling enzymes in biosynthesis of transmitter glycine.

Release and inactivation

Although release of glycine by stimulation of specific pathways has not been established, glycine is released in a Ca^{2+} dependent manner from slices of spinal cord and synaptosomes prepared from spinal cord by electrical and K^+ stimulation.

A sodium dependent high affinity uptake mechanism for glycine has been demonstrated in spinal, medullary and pontine tissue but not elsewhere in the brain. Autoradiographic evidence suggests that uptake is primarily into nerve terminals clustered around motor neuron cell bodies in the ventral horn of spinal cord. Biochemical studies show that uptake in spinal cord is into a population of terminals separate from those which accumulate GABA and glutamate. There are no agents which specifically influence high affinity glycine uptake.

Actions

Glycine produces a reversible inhibition of neuronal firing, particularly of spinal neurons, by hyperpolarising the nerve membrane by increasing the permeability to Cl^-. The glycine receptor has not been as well studied as other amino acid receptors but is distinct from the receptor by which GABA mediates increasing Cl^- permeability. The action of glycine is selectively antagonised by strychnine and [^{3}H]-strychnine has been used as a radioligand to quantitate glycine receptors and visualise them autoradiographically.

Glycine catabolism

Glycine is converted to serine via SMHT, and to glyoxylate by glycine aminotransferase and D-amino acid oxidase (an enzyme only present in the hind brain and spinal cord). Thus as with other amino acids, there is no distinct end product of glycine metabolism.

Synapses using glycine as transmitter

The main action of glycine is to mediate interneuron inhibition in the spinal cord and brainstem. The best example is the Renshaw cell. This is activated by recurrent collaterals of spinal motor neurons and in turn synapses on the motor neuron cell body to inhibit firing. Glycine mediated inhibition has also been reported in higher brain centres, for example substantia nigra and ventral tegmentum, cerebellum (Golgi cells) and cortex and a glycinergic pathway from the frontal cortex to the hypothalamus proposed.

Glutamate and aspartate

Distribution

Glutamate and aspartate show less variation in concentration in brain areas than GABA. Highest concentrations of glutamate and aspartate are found in cerebellar and cerebral cortices, caudate nucleus and hippocampus. Concentrations in some predominantly gray structures (hypothalamus, substantia nigra, red nucleus) are the same as white matter. In the spinal cord, glutamate is present in higher concentrations in the dorsal gray matter and dorsal roots than the ventral gray matter and ventral roots, whereas the opposite is true of aspartate.

Synthesis

Both these putative excitatory amino acid neurotransmitter are intimately related to intermediates of the tricarboxylic acid cycle (Fig. 11.1). Aspartate is formed by transamination of oxaloacetate, catalysed by aspartate aminotransferase. Aspartate may also be formed from pyruvate by CO_2 fixation.

Glutamate is formed by transamination from α-oxoglutarate (with GABA or aspartate acting as the NH_2 donor), direct amination of α-oxoglutarate by ammonia catalysed by glutamate dehydrogenase and by the deamination of glutamine, catalysed by glutaminase.

The relative contributions of these pathways to the synthesis of transmitter glutamate has been studied in slices of the dentate gyrus of the hippocampal formation, where there is strong evidence for a transmitter role of glutamate. Most of the glutamate available for release by depolarising stimuli was derived from glutamine, while most of the glutamate derived from glucose served a different, presumably metabolic, function. The importance of glutamine as a precursor for releasable glutamate has also been demonstrated with synaptosomal preparations (see section on metabolism).

Release

The release of glutamate (and aspartate) has been demonstrated from the cortical surface, slices of brain and synaptosomal preparations. Glutamate release shares many characteristics with GABA release. It is released by electrical or potassium depolarisation, is Ca^{2+} dependent and Mg^{2+} inhibits release. Because of the lack of a unique synthesising enzyme or other specific markers for glutamate or aspartate using pathways, the demonstration of Ca^{2+} dependent release and its reduction by selective lesions has played an important role in the identification of such pathways.

Uptake

Enzymic inactivation is not important in terminating the synaptic actions of glutamate and aspartate. Rapid removal is thought to take place via a high affinity, sodium dependent uptake system (K_m in low μM range) present in glia and nerve endings. A low affinity uptake system (K_M high μM-low mM range) also exists in neurons and glia. The relative contributions of nerve terminal and glial uptake is not clear. A number of compounds are able to inhibit carrier-mediated glutamate and aspartate uptake, two of the most specific are threo-3-hydroxy D aspartate and dihydrokainate. These uptake inhibitors potentiate the excitant effects of iontophoretically applied L-glutamate and L-aspartate. The role of low affinity uptake should not be discounted since the effects of excitatory amino acids are potentiated by compounds which compete only for the low affinity carrier, e.g. L-histidine.

D-aspartate has proved a particularly useful compound. It inhibits glutamate uptake but is also itself a substrate for the carrier and is not metabolised. [^{3}H]-D-aspartate autoradiography has been used for anterograde and retrograde tracing of excitatory amino acid pathways. Material transported from cell bodies to nerve terminals is releasable by high K^+ in a Ca^{2+} dependent manner.

The similar kinetics of glutamate and aspartate uptake, their mutual inhibition and their parallel inhibition by structural analogues indicates that the two amino acids are transported by a common carrier, rather than two separate carriers. SITS (4 acetamido-4'-isothiocyano-2,2' disulphonic acid stilbene) is claimed to be a more potent inhibitor of glial than neuronal uptake of glutamate.

Figure 11.6 shows a diagrammatic representation of synapse using glutamate as a transmitter.

Pathways

A combination of techniques (including [^{3}H]-D-aspartate autoradiography, the effects of lesions on release, uptake and amino acid content and electophysiological comparisons of iontophoretic application of amino acids, stimulation of fibre tracts and their pharmacological antagonism) have lead to a number of pathways being proposed with excitatory amino acids as transmitters. In most cases no definitive distinction has been made between glutamate and aspartate.

A number of corticofugal pathways have been proposed; such as those from frontal cortex to dopamine rich areas of the brain (striatum, tuberculum olfactorium, nucleus accumbens and substantia nigra); from the sensorimotor cortex to red nucleus, pontine nuclei, cuneate nucleus and spinal cord; medio-frontal, pyriform and entorhinal cortices to the amygdala; from the entire cortex, but particularly the pyriform cortex, to the thalamus; visual cortex to lateral geniculate nucleus and superior

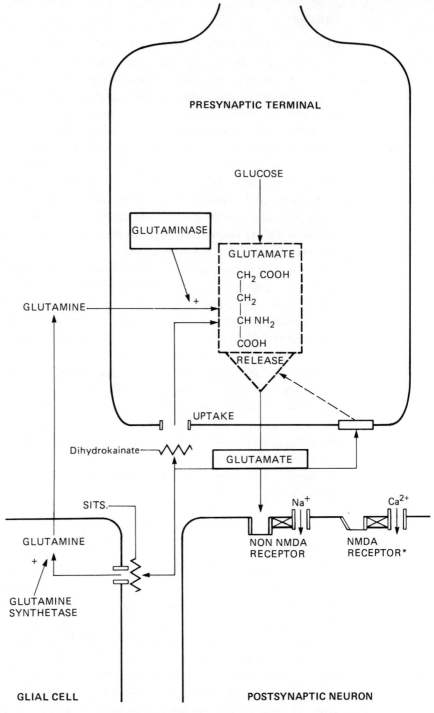

Fig. 11.6. A diagrammatic representation of a glutamate synapse. The synthesis of glutamate is from glucose or glutamine. It is incorporated into vesicles and released by nerve terminal depolarisation to interact with postsynaptic receptors — three classes have been advocated and termed N-methyl-D-aspartate (N), quisqualate (Q) and kainate (K) after selective agonists (see Chapter 13). Interaction with presynaptic autoreceptors may regulate release. There is a carrier mediated uptake into neurons and glia where conversion of glutamate to glutamine is catalysed by glutamine synthetase. Part of the glial glutamine is transferred to neurons and acts as a precursor for transmitter glutamate ('the glutamine cycle'). SITS = 4 acetamido-4'-isothiocyano-2,2' disulphonic acid stilbene. Drugs stopping synthesis and uptake are shown ($\approx$).

colliculus and from entorhinal cortex to the dentate gyrus of the hippocampal formation (perforant path). Allocortical projections include projections from hippocampal pyramidal cells to the lateral septum and from the hippocampus-subiculum to nucleus accumbens, the nucleus of the diagonal band, the bed nucleus of stria terminals, the mediobasal hypothalamus and mammillary bodies.

In the cerebellum, glutamate is proposed to be the transmitter released by granule cells and aspartate by the climbing fibres. In the hippocampus, glutamate/aspartate have been suggested as the transmitters of the Schaffer collateral and commissural fibres.

Excitatory transmitters have been proposed in several sensory pathways; the auditory nerve terminating in the cochlear nucleus, the fibres of the lateral olfactory cortex, the retina and in primary afferent fibres synapsing in the spinal cord.

Further metabolism of glutamate

Glutamate released by nerve ending is taken up into nerve terminals and glia, where it is converted to glutamine, catalysed by glutamine synthetase. Glutamine is proposed to be transferred from glia via the interstitial fluid to neurons, where it is an important precursor of transmitter glutamate and GABA. Glutaminase, the enzyme which catalyses the conversion of glutamine to glutamate is particularly active in the mitochondria of nerve endings. This proposed recycling of neuronal glutamate via glial glutamine is termed the 'glutamine cycle' and is shown diagrammatically in Fig. 11.6.

References and further reading

Di Chiara G & Gessa GL (eds) (1981) *Glutamate as a Neurotransmitter*. Raven Press, New York.

De Feudis FV & Mandel P (eds) *Amino Acid Neurotransmitters*. Raven Press, New York.

Fogg GE & Foster AC (1983) Amino acid neurotransmitters and their pathways in the mammalian central nervous system. *Neuroscience* **9**, 701-19.

Johnston GAR (1978) Neuropharmacology of amino acid inhibitory transmitters. *Ann. Rev. Pharmacol. Toxicol* **18**, 269-89.

Krogsgaard-Larsen P (1980) Inhibitors of GABA uptake systems. *Molec. Cell. Biochem.* **31**, 105-21.

Metcalf BW (1979) Inhibitors of GABA metabolism. *Biochem. Pharmacol.* **28**, 1705-12.

Okada Y & Roberts E (eds) (1982) *Problems in GABA Research. From Brain to Bacteria.* Excerpta Medica, Amsterdam.

Palfreyman MG, Schechter PJ, Buckett WR, Tell GP & Kochweser J (1981) The pharmacology of GABA-transaminase inhibitors. *Biochem. Pharmacol.* **30**, 817-24.

Puil E (1981) S-glutamate: its interactions with spinal neurons. *Brain Res. Rev.* **3**, 229-22.

Roberts E Chase TN & Tower DB (eds) (1976) *GABA in Nervous System Function*. Raven Press, New York.

Roberts PJ, Storm-Mathisen J & Johnston GAR (eds) (1981) *Glutamate: Transmitter in the Central Nervous System*. John Wiley, Chichester.

Otterser OP & Storm-Mathisen J (1984) Neurons containing or accumulating transmitter amino acids. In: Björklund A, Hökfelt T & Kuhar MJ (eds) *Handbook of Chemical Neuroanatomy*, Vol 3, Part II. Elsevier, Amsterdam.

Walker JE (1983) Glutamate, GABA and CNS disease. A review. *Neurochem. Res.* **8**, 521-50.

12   GABA receptors

N.G. BOWERY

The observation that γ-aminobutyric acid (GABA) will depress neuronal activity within the mammalian central nervous system was originally described by Hayashi in 1954. On administering GABA through micro-tubes inserted into the feline cerebral cortex it was noticed that neuronal activity decreased in the vicinity of the injection. Subsequent investigations in which microiontophoretic techniques were employed confirmed this observation not only in the cortex but elsewhere. However the role of GABA in synaptic inhibitory processing was not readily accepted until the end of the 1960s. Using intracellular recording techniques Krnjevic & Schwartz (1967) showed that the decrease in neuronal firing produced by GABA is concomitant with an increase in membrane potential and conductance. This effect of GABA mimics synaptic inhibition. For example, cathodal stimulation of the cerebral cortex where the neurons are much more sensitive to GABA than to glycine produces synaptic inhibition which is qualitatively imitated by iontophoretically-applied GABA. The generation of an inhibitory postsynaptic potential can be reversed by increasing the intraneuronal chloride ion concentration. The action of applied GABA can be similarly reversed. It would seem that the increase in membrane potential produced by synaptic inhibition or GABA results from an increased conductance to chloride ions. In both cases the effect is mediated by GABA acting at receptors on the cell surface since intracellular injections of GABA produce no change in membrane potential. Activation of the receptor causes the associated chloride ion channels to open allowing a net inward movement of the ion resulting in hyperpolarisation. When chloride ions are injected into the cells, the chloride gradient is reversed and GABA then produces a depolarisation.

So what are the characteristics of this receptor for GABA controlling chloride ion movement? How specific are the structural requirements for activation and blockade and is it an homogenous population or are there different receptors which may be classified as a group under the single title 'GABA receptor'?

Agonists

GABA is a 4-carbon, straight chain amino acid (Fig. 12.1). Numerous modifications have been made to the GABA structure. These include

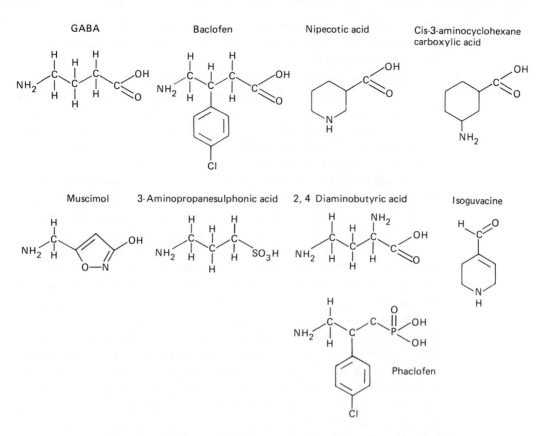

Fig. 12.1. Structures of GABA, muscimol, baclofen, nipecotic acid, cis-3-aminocyclohexane carboxylic acid (ACHC), 2, 4, diaminobutyric acid, isoguvacine and phaclofen.

lengthening and shortening of the carbon chain, removal and replacement of the terminal amino and carboxylic functions and additions to the chain. The effects of such changes on GABA-mimetic activity at central sites *in vivo* have been studied quite extensively using iontophoretic or surface application (on the cerebral cortex) of each analogue and comparing its ability to inhibit neuronal firing with that of GABA. Briefly, increasing the chain length to 5 carbon atoms (γ-aminovaleric acid) and beyond sequentially decreases activity as does a stepwise reduction in length. The neuronal depressant activity of the 2 and 3 carbon compounds (glycine and β-alanine respectively) however, can be equal to or more than GABA but this is due to an action at a separate receptor sensitive to the antagonist strychnine. Strychnine is ineffective as a GABA antagonist at concentrations which block responses to glycine. Although the receptors for GABA and glycine are distinct they may be linked to the same mechanism governing membrane conductance.

Removal or displacement of the terminal amino function in GABA abolishes activity. Substitution of the carboxylic acid moiety by other than sulphinic or sulphonic acid groups reduces activity. The sulphonic acid derivative 3-aminopropane sulphonic acid (3-APS) is as active if not more active than GABA.

A guanidino group can be inserted into the straight chain provided the methylene chain is reduced accordingly. Thus β-guanidinopropionic acid and guanidoacetic acid are effective though weak agonists. Additions to the side chain, e.g. β-hydroxyl depress activity. Notable in this group is the analogue β-chlorophenyl GABA (baclofen, Fig. 12.1) which appears to be devoid of activity at the postsynaptic GABA receptor.

The relative activity of some of these analogues in a variety of test systems is shown in the upper part of Table 12.1. Whilst data obtained with these simple analogues provide some information about the requirements for attachment and activation at the receptor, their structural flexibility does not facilitate the determination of the active conformation. Crystallographic studies have indicated that GABA adopts a partially folded conformation in the solid state although this does not necessarily reflect the conformation interacting at the recognition site. The discovery of active analogues with more restricted conformations has begun to provide us with more positive, though indirect, evidence that GABA interacts with its receptor in a 'partially extended and almost planar conformation.' Examples of these more 'rigid' analogues are listed in the lower part of Table 12.1. Among these is the naturally-occurring alkaloid muscimol (Fig. 12.1) which was first shown to be a GABA-like depressant in 1968 by Johnston *et al.* This substance is particularly interesting since it is more active than GABA as a postsynaptic GABA receptor agonist and there was some suggestion that this compound might penetrate the brain. However, after systemic administration the observed effects differ from those obtained following intracerebroventricular injection and also differ from the expected actions of a GABA-mimetic. This may arise from the rapid production of active metabolites.

Antagonists

It is widely accepted that bicuculline (and its methohalide salts) (Fig. 12.2) is a GABA receptor antagonist. It appears to compete with GABA for the same recognition site although there may be different classes of bicuculline-sensitive receptors and/or different conformational states of the GABA receptor binding agonist or antagonist preferentially. Certainly structural similarities between bicuculline and GABA, muscimol and other analogues have been noted (e.g. Johnston 1976). By contrast, picrotoxin (active moiety picrotoxinin, Fig. 12.2) which is also a selective GABA antagonist in the mammalian CNS has no obvious structural similarity to GABA and does not appear to compete for the same recognition site. Instead, it may interfere with the mechanism(s) distal to the receptor, i.e. increase in ion flux. If this is so then presumably a site exists juxtaposed to the chloride ion channel which, when 'activated'

Table 12.1.

The last two data columns are grouped under the spanning heading **Inhibition of ^{3}[H]-GABA uptake**.

Analogue	Cat motoneurons	Cat cortical inhibition	Inhibition of cat spinal interneurons	Rat brain radiolabelled GABA binding	Rat sympathetic ganglion depolarisation	Decrease in evoked transmitter output from rat atria	Neuronal (rat cerebral cortex)	Glial (rat sympathetic ganglia)
GABA	− − −	+ + + +	1	ne	1	1	1	1
Glycine	− −	+ +			0.01	ne	ne	ne
β-alanine	− − − −	+ + + +		0.008	0.048	ne	0.001	0.12
δ-amino valeric acid	− −	+ +		0.07	0.001	ne	0.1	ne
3-aminopropane sulphonic acid		ne		0.008	3.4	ne	0.02	0.007
β-guanidinopropionic acid		+ + + +		1	0.12		0.1	0.2
γ-amino β-hydroxy-n-butyric acid	− −	+ + + +		0.2	0.27	0.03	0.2	0.44
β-amino-n-butyric acid	ne	ne		0.1	ne	ne		0.2
α-amino-n-butyric acid	ne	ne			ne			0.12
(±)baclofen (β-p-chlorophenyl GABA)		Depressant effect not blocked by bicuculline	Depressant effect not blocked by bicuculline	<0.003 (0.01 bicuculline)	ne	0.93	ne	ne
Imidazole acetic acid				0.38	0.1	ne	0.002	~0.01
Trans-4-aminocrotonic acid				0.8	1.48		1	~0.5
4-aminotetrolic acid			0.2–0.5		0.0028		0.05, 0.07	ne
Trans-3-aminocyclopentane carboxylic acid				1.3	ne	ne	0.85	ne
Isonipecotic acid			1	0.023	0.011	ne	0.004	ne
Isoguvacine			2–4	0.024	0.23	ne	0.004	ne
Muscimol			2–4	11.3	5.08	0.02	0.2	ne
2,4 diamino-n-butyric acid		+		<0.003	0.0012	ne	0.3	
(±) cis-3-aminocyclohexane carboxylic acid (ACHC)		0.2		0.00045	ne	ne	0.4	0.03
(±) nipecotic acid				<0.003	ne	ne	1.8	
Effect of:								
Bicuculline		Blocks	Blocks	Displaces label	Blocks	ne	ne	ne
Picrotoxin		Blocks		No displacement	Blocks	ne	ne	ne

Values in each column give molar potencies (GABA = 1) except in the first three columns where relative activities are given in the arbitrary units employed by the original investigators. In the first column the number of − signs is inversely related to the amount of current required to discharge an effective amount of drug iontophoretically; in the second column the number of + signs is proportional to the depression of evoked responses on topical application of the compounds in 0.1–1% solution. In the third column the values cited refer to relative potencies determined by comparing the iontophoretic currents required to produce a comparable depression in neuronal firing. (ne = indicates no observable effect.)

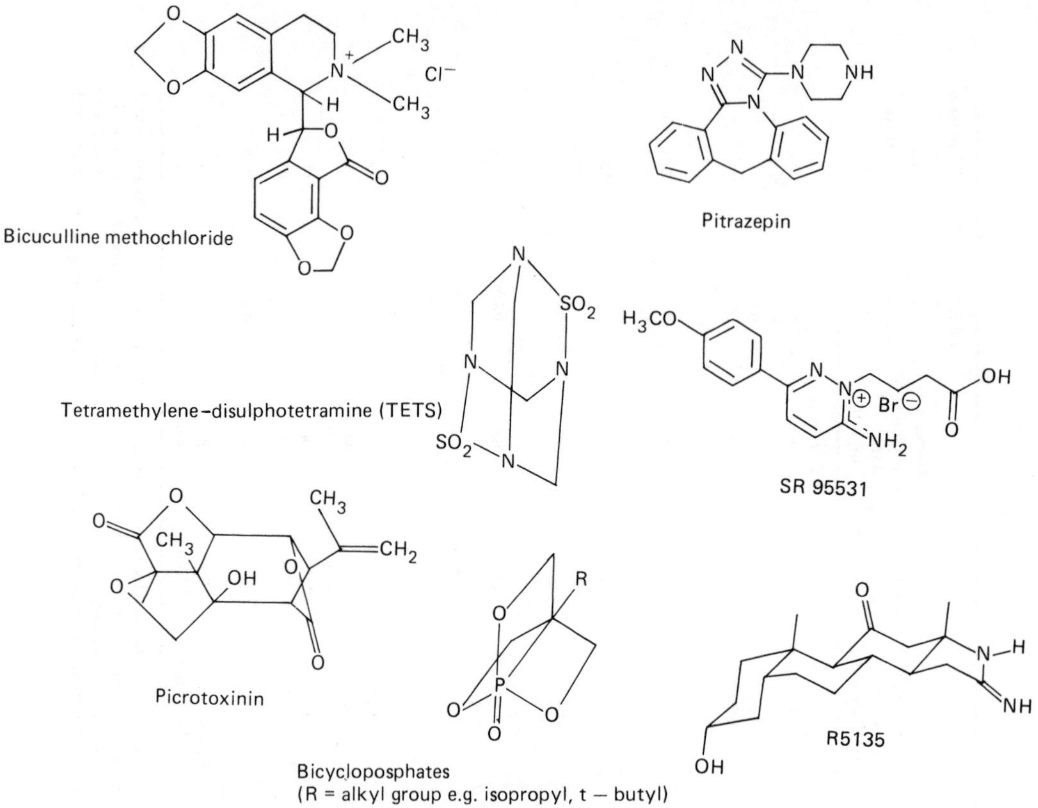

Fig. 12.2. Structures of certain compounds which prevent the action of GABA.

by picrotoxin, decreases chloride movement. Other GABA antagonists have been described (Fig. 12.2), all of which are convulsants but many, like picrotoxin, do not appear to compete for the GABA recognition site. These substances include tetramethylene-disulphotetramine (TETS), d-tubocurarine, penicillin, alkyl bicyclophosphates, bemegride, leptazol and the convulsant benzodiazepine Ro5–3663. Among these the convulsants (TETS and bicyclophosphates) have been shown to interact with the picrotoxin site. Quantitative comparison within the CNS between bicuculline and other antagonists such as picrotoxin have never been clearly defined and this may be in part due to their different sites of action.

Methods for studying mammalian GABA receptors

In vivo studies

Considerable information about the structural requirements of the bicuculline-sensitive GABA receptor has been obtained from iontophoretic studies, within the CNS in which the activity of various analogues is compared with that of GABA on the same firing unit by ejection of test substances from adjacent barrels of a multibarrelled pipette. Activity is estimated on the basis of the currents required to eject sufficient GABA and analogue to slow down the cell firing to the same extent and with the same time course. However, information obtained in this way is rather more qualitative than quantitative since it is virtually impossible to determine the concentration of GABA or analogue achieved in the vicinity of the receptors. Measurements of the amount released from the pipettes in relation to the applied current can facilitate comparisons but even then the extracellular volume of distribution must be assumed to be constant. A further problem is the contribution of other factors which may influence the action of an analogue at the receptor but which are difficult to control under these conditions. For example, if a substance is not a substrate for the transport processes thought to be responsible for the synaptic inactivation of GABA, its potency relative to GABA may be spuriously high. Also the frequent need to apply an excitant to increase cell-firing before depressant activity can be observed may complicate the analysis. Of course, information obtained in this way is essential for our understanding of the GABA receptor on central neurons. However, the possible use of *in vitro* model systems is an attractive idea since these overcome the problems of quantitation and modifying factors can be controlled more readily.

Binding studies

A model system frequently employed is that of specific radiolabelled ligand binding to brain membrane fractions (see Chapter 4). The radiolabelled ligands usually employed for studies at the GABA receptor are [³H]-GABA and [³H]-muscimol and the antagonist [³H]-bicuculline methiodide. Displacement of specifically bound ligand by non-radioactive analogues appears to occur in proportion to their relative potencies as GABA-mimetics determined iontophoretically. The recognition site(s) for GABA detected in this way is (are) sensitive to bicuculline but not picrotoxin. Although it can be argued that the specific binding of labelled GABA or muscimol occurs at sites which might not be the functional receptor(s) the rank order of potency of agonists in this system compares favourably with qualitative data obtained iontophoretically. This rank order, however, can alter marginally depending on the manner in which the membrane fractions are treated.

Sympathetic ganglion model

An alternative *in vitro* approach to receptor *in vivo* analysis which still measures responses to a drug rather than its binding characteristics is the use of whole tissue in isolation. For example, thin slices of brain or tissue cultures from a variety of brain regions such as olfactory cortex, hippocampus, cerebellum, spinal cord, cuneate nucleus or hypothalamus can be maintained *in vitro* to allow stable intracellular or extracellular recording whilst being able to control the external environment.

Perhaps an even simpler approach is to use a model system obtained from peripheral nerve tissue. De Groat (1970) first noted that following close intra-arterial injection of GABA to the feline superior cervical ganglion there was a transient shift in the potential recorded from the sur-

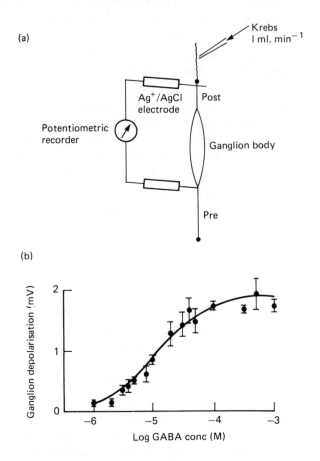

Fig. 12.3. Diagrammatic representation of the ganglion superfusion system. Desheathed sympathetic ganglia are suspended vertically (post-ganglionic trunk uppermost) and superfused with Krebs-Henseleit solution at ambient temperature. Surface potential is recorded with respect to the post-ganglionic trunk using Ag/AgCl electrodes connected across a potentiometric recorder. (b) Mean log concentration-response curve of ganglia surface potential changes produced by GABA (1–100 μM). Data compiled from 10 ganglia. Each concentration of GABA was applied for 3 min at intervals of at least 15 min. Each point and vertical bar gives the mean and standard error of at least three measurements in separate experiments. The curve is drawn according to the equation:

$$\frac{y}{y_{max}} = \frac{x^n}{x^n + k},$$

where y is the observed response in millivolts, y max is the asymptotic response (1.9 mV), x is the concentration of GABA, $n = 1$ (Hill coefficient), k is a constant (ED_{50}) = 12.5 μM. (From Bowery & Brown 1974.)

face of the ganglion. This depolarising effect of GABA could be mimicked by recognised GABA-like agonists and antagonised by picrotoxin. Similar results can be obtained *in vitro* using the superior cervical ganglion of the rat. The neuronal depolarisation produced by GABA in this tissue can be detected on the ganglion surface (Bowery & Brown 1974) (Fig 12.3(a)). The magnitude of the response to GABA is dose-dependent between 0.3–300 μM (ED$_{50}$ = 12.5 μM) (Fig 12.3(b)). A detailed study of the receptor in this tissue has provided sufficient evidence to accept it as a model for the central receptor.

Direct and indirect agonist effects at GABA receptors

If one compares the relative potencies of selected GABA analogues in the different systems referred to above, i.e. central iontophoretic application *in vivo*, ligand binding to membrane fractions and ganglion depolarisation; it is very similar, particularly between the flexible analogues (see Table 12.1). However, on closer examination of the effects of diaminobutyric acid (DABA) and cis-3-aminocyclohexane carboxylic acid (ACHC) there is a clear distinction between their iontophoretic potencies and their potencies on the ganglion model and in ligand binding studies. The explanation for this became apparent on examining the affinity of these compounds for the neuronal transport system for GABA. The inactivation system for GABA following its synaptic release is thought to depend on removal by active transport back into the nerve terminals and/or into surrounding glial cells. The recognition site associated with the uptake of GABA appears to differ from the postsynaptic site such that certain analogues of GABA, e.g. nipecotic acid and ACHC have considerable affinity for the uptake site but are virtually inactive at the postsynaptic receptor. Conversely, receptor agonists such as muscimol and isoguvacine have very low affinity for the transport sites. The recognition sites associated with neuronal and glial GABA transport also exhibit different structural requirements. β-alanine is a selective inhibitor/substrate for glial transport whereas DABA and ACHC are selective for neuronal processes. The apparent GABA-mimetic activity of ACHC and, at least in part, DABA observed in the CNS *in vivo* is probably due to an indirect effect on GABA nerve terminals displacing or preventing the reuptake of GABA. In sympathetic ganglia there are no neuronal stores of GABA to displace so that ACHC and DABA are inactive in this system. However, if the glial concentration of GABA is raised in sympathetic ganglia, the GABA-mimetic effect of β-alanine is enhanced.

What emerges from this is that drugs may influence the GABA receptor indirectly. They may augment the synaptic action by prevention of reuptake or they may displace GABA from neuronal (or glial) stores, like imipramine and tyramine respectively at adrenergic synapses.

Postsynaptic influences on GABA receptor function

GABA receptor activation can be influenced by drugs which in themselves do not act at the GABA recognition site but at an associated site instead. Reference has already been made to picrotoxin acting distal to the receptor but yet in an apparently selective manner. There is now evidence indicating the presence of endogenous substances closely associated with GABA nerve terminals or the GABA site. These compounds, which may be proteins or phospholipids, appear to influence GABA receptor function by modulation through an allosteric site(s). The benzodiazepines are ligands for these sites and act to increase GABA binding and function. Conversely inverse agonists for these sites, e.g. β-carboline methyl ester decrease GABA function. Neither the benzodiazepines nor the inverse agonists are GABA receptor agonists since they do not bind to the GABA recognition site. Evidence for the existence of such receptors derives from binding studies with radiolabelled benzodiazepines and more recently from photo-affinity and receptor antibody labelling techniques.

Whilst the benzodiazepines can facilitate GABA receptor mechanisms the reverse also appears to occur, i.e. GABA enhances specific benzodiazepine binding. The enhancement in [^{3}H]-diazepam binding to brain membrane fractions produced by GABA is controlled by a bicuculline-sensitive receptor. The action of GABA is mimicked by a variety of accepted GABA-mimetics but at low (4°C) incubation temperatures 3-APS and isoguvacine are only partial agonists and piperidine-4-sulphonic acid and 4,5,6,7-tetrahydroisoxazolo 5,4-c pyridin-3-ol (THIP) are competitive antagonists. Only at higher temperatures (~37°C) are these compounds effective GABA-mimetics.

In the light of these GABA-benzodiazepine interactions it is possible that different classes or functional states of GABA receptors exist within the CNS. Kinetic analysis of GABA binding to synaptic membranes can show the presence of more than one site. Benzodiazepines appear to facilitate GABA binding to a high rather than low affinity site whereas treatment of the membranes with detergent increases the affinity and binding capacity of the high and low affinity components. These apparently distinct sites have not been differentiated on the basis of structural requirements. However, they all appear to be susceptible to the GABA antagonist bicuculline.

The existence of bicuculline-insensitive GABA receptors has been suggested since certain GABA analogues such as cis-4-aminocrotonic acid can inhibit neuronal firing yet their action is not blocked by bicuculline. There are also a number of reports where GABA has been shown to inhibit neuronal activity in a bicuculline-resistant manner.

A bicuculline-insensitive GABA receptor

The presence of GABA receptors on peripheral neuronal cell bodies (ganglia) and on unmyelinated axons suggested that they may also be present on the axon terminals of post-ganglionic fibres. Since recording from these terminals was not possible, the assumption was made that if GABA depolarises them in the same manner as the cell bodies this could lead to a decrease in the evoked output of transmitter. The same mechanism may account for the suggested inhibitory role of GABA at presynaptic terminals within the central nervous system. Depolarisation of primary afferent terminals within the spinal cord can be induced by GABA and this has been linked with a decrease in transmitter output from these sensory endings.

A system suitable for testing our assumption on peripheral terminals was the efflux of $[^3H]$-NA from isolated superfused atria of the rat. Atria incubated in low concentrations of radioactive NA accumulate the label into terminal stores and subsequent transmural stimulation gives rise to an increased efflux of catecholamine detected as an increase in the tritium content of the effluent. GABA (0.3–300 μM) decreases the evoked output without affecting the basal level in accordance with the original hypothesis. This decrease in transmitter output can also be detected as a decrease in the postsynaptic response to nerve stimulation. GABA reduces the twitch response of the vas deferens (mouse and guinea-pig) to coaxial stimulation. In both systems, i.e. atria and vas deferens, the effect of GABA is dose dependent with identical ED_{50} values (3–4 μM).

At first it was assumed that the reduction in evoked transmitter outflow was due, as expected, to the presence of Cl^- dependent GABA receptors on the terminals. However, this is not the case. GABA probably depolarises the terminals but this does not appear to be associated with the decrease in transmitter outflow. In fact, GABA appears to act on a receptor quite different from that mediating depolarisation of the nerve cell body or hyperpolarisation within the CNS. This conclusion stems from studies with numerous GABA analogues and antagonists.

None of the recognised GABA antagonists such as bicuculline or picrotoxin prevents the reduction in transmitter release produced by GABA and by far the majority of accepted GABA agonists fail to mimic the action of GABA at this site (Table 12.1). Of particular importance in this connection are 3-APS and isoguvacine: these are inactive at the novel site but yet are potent agonists at bicuculline sensitive sites (Table 12.1). By contrast, baclofen which is very weak or inactive at bicuculline-sensitive sites mimics GABA in a potent and stereospecific manner in the atria and vas deferens. The ($-$) isomer is more active than the ($+$) form. The response to baclofen, like GABA, is unaffected by pretreatment with bicuculline methobromide (Fig. 12.4).

We chose to designate these novel receptors by the term 'GABA$_B$' to contrast with the term 'GABA$_A$' representing the classical bicuculline-sensitive receptors (Hill & Bowery 1981). GABA$_A$ covers all types of bicuculline-sensitive sites irrespective of their anatomical location or association with benzodiazepine binding sites although further subdivision of the GABA$_A$ classification may prove to be necessary.

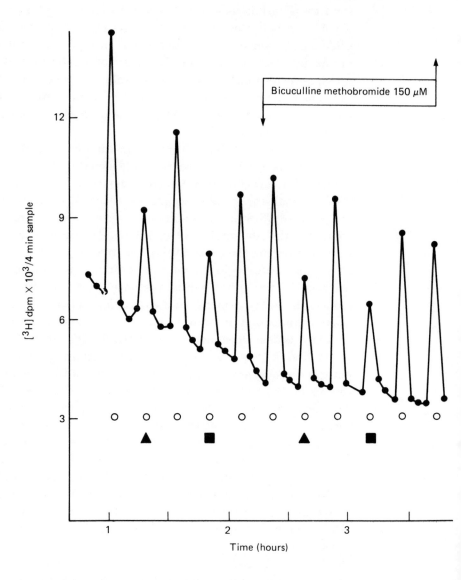

Fig. 12.4. The effect of GABA and baclofen on the evoked release of [³H]-noradrenaline from rat atria: lack of antagonism by bicuculline methobromide. Atria from a single rat were incubated in 0.4 μM [³H]-NA for 40 min at 32°C followed by a further 30 min incubation in radioactive-free Krebs-Henseleit solution. The tissue was then superfused with fresh solution containing 2.5 μM yohimbine and the superfusate collected for 4 min periods consecutively. The tritium content of each sample was then assayed by scintillation spectrometry and the values (dpm/sample) plotted against time. Transmural stimulation (10 V, 3 Hz, 0.5 ms for 1 min) indicated by the open dots (○) increased the tritium content of samples collected during these periods. The addition of GABA (10^{-4} M ▲) or (±) baclofen (10^{-4} M ■) 30s before and during stimulation reduced the evoked release but neither compound affected basal release. The continuous presence of bicuculline methobromide (150 μM) in the superfusion solution failed to alter the reduction by either GABA or baclofen. All solutions contained 0.1 mM ascorbic acid and 0.5 mM iproniazid to reduce noradrenaline catabolism. (From Bowery *et al.* 1981.)

By making use of results obtained with various GABA agonists and antagonists in peripheral preparations it has been possible to demonstrate the presence of GABA$_B$ receptors within the CNS. Baclofen and GABA but not 3-APS reduce the K$^+$ (25 mM)-evoked efflux of [^{3}H]-NA from cerebellar cortex slices without producing any change in basal efflux. This reduction is not prevented by bicuculline and the effect of baclofen is again stereospecific.

The reduction produced by GABA is only apparent when the release of [^{3}H]-NA is evoked with 25 mM or higher concentrations of K$^+$. In the presence of 15 mM GABA enhances the evoked output by approximately 40%. However, this is converted to a reduction in the presence of bicuculline. This may partly account for the disparity in results obtained with GABA on release of transmitters from CNS slices. For example, it has previously been noted by others that GABA only enhances the K$^+$-evoked release of [^{3}H]-NA from slices of rat cerebral cortex. It has also been shown that GABA can inhibit the evoked release of [^{3}H]-DA from rat striatal slices but yet other groups have observed the opposite effect.

A variety of other techniques have been employed to demonstrate the presence of GABA$_B$ sites in mammalian brain including radiolabelled receptor binding to neuronal membranes, receptor autoradiography, neurochemistry and electrophysiological measurements *in vitro* and *in vivo*. One of the overall features to emerge from these studies is the pharmacological similarity of the receptor irrespective of the system (see Bowery *et al.* 1984). Furthermore, the similarity extends to the receptor characteristics described in peripheral tissue, and thus differ markedly from those GABA$_A$ sites. A summary of the differences between GABA$_A$ and GABA$_B$ sites is given in Table 12.2. This not only highlights some of the agonist and antagonist specificities but also the distinguishing features. For example, there is an absolute dependence on divalent cations for ligands to bind to GABA$_B$ sites whereas no such dependence occurs at GABA$_A$ sites. Barbiturates and benzodiazepines exert no effect on either the response to GABA$_B$ site activation or the binding of ligands to these sites.

Receptor mechanisms

Two of the preliminary observations made on intact rat atria and whole brain membranes led us to the view that the mechanism(s) associated with GABA$_B$ sites might well differ from the Cl$^-$ dependent process activated by bicuculline-sensitive GABA$_A$ sites. Firstly, the inhibition of evoked [^{3}H]-NA release produced by GABA and baclofen was still evident in the absence of chloride ions and secondly, the binding of ligands to GABA$_B$ sites was diminished by GTP and other guanyl nucleotides whereas that to GABA$_A$ sites was unaffected.

The lack of any association of GABA$_B$ sites with Cl$^-$ channels has now been observed at the cellular level by many groups who have instead

Table 12.2. The different pharmacological characteristics of $GABA_A$ and $GABA_B$ receptors

		$GABA_A$	$GABA_B$
Ligand			
Agonists	Muscimol	√√√√	√
	Isoguvacine	√√	X
	Piperidine-4-sulphonic acid	√√	X
	(−) Baclofen	X	√√√
	GABA	√√√	√√√
Agonists/antagonists	3-Aminopropane sulphonic acid	Potent agonist	Very weak antagonist
	5-Amino valeric acid	Agonist	Very weak antagonist
Antagonists	Bicuculline	√	X
	Picrotoxin	√	X
	Bicyclophosphates	√	X
	Ro 5135	√	X
	Pitrazepin	√	X
	SR 95531	√	X
	Phaclofen	X	Weak antagonist
Consequences of receptor activation			
		Increase in Cl^- conductance	Increase in K^+ conductance and decrease in Ca^{2+} conductance
			Adenylate cyclase activation or inhibition
Influences of chemical factors on receptor binding			
Ca^{2+}/Mg^{2+}		No significant dependence	Absolute dependence
Triton detergent		Increase in high affinity binding capacity	Decrease in binding capacity
Benzodiazepines and barbiturates		Enhancement of ligand binding and functional response	No effect
Guanyl nucleotides		No effect	Decrease in binding affinity

Number of √ indicates potency; X = inactive.

implicated Ca^{2+} and K^+ channels in $GABA_B$-mediated effects. There is certainly a decrease in inward Ca^{2+} transport, which may result either directly or indirectly from an increase in K^+ conductance. Such a blockade of Ca^{2+} movement would readily account for the diminution in transmitter output produced by the activation of $GABA_B$ sites on presynaptic terminals. However, an increase in K^+ conductance alone may be important at postsynaptic $GABA_B$ sites. Orthodromic activation of CA_I pyramidal cells produces a biphasic i.p.s.p. both phases of which may be mediated solely by GABA. Whilst the initial i.p.s.p. is bicuculline-sensitive and mediated by an increase in Cl^- conductance the slower i.p.s.p. appears to result from an increase in K^+ conductance, and $(-)$ baclofen only mimics this secondary event.

The influence of guanyl nucleotides, in particular GTP, on the binding of radiolabelled ligands to their receptors can often be considered as an indicator of a link with adenylate cyclase and both inhibitory and excitatory connections with this enzyme may be reflected in the attenuation of ligand binding by GTP. In fact GTP depressed the binding of $[^3H]$-GABA and $[^3H]$-baclofen to $GABA_B$ sites on rat brain membranes but had no effect on the binding properties of $GABA_A$ sites. Saturation analysis indicated that the observed changes at $GABA_B$ sites result from a decrease in binding affinities.

The subsequent step was to examine whether $GABA_B$ agonists could influence the formation of cyclic AMP in rat brain slices. Under our incubation conditions $GABA_B$ site activation in slices of cerebellar and cerebral cortex produced no change in basal cyclic AMP formation. We therefore considered the possibility that the GTP dependence may reflect an inhibitory action on the cyclase enzyme. To examine this we first activated the enzyme by β-adrenoceptor stimulation and compared this with the combination of adrenoceptor stimulant plus $GABA_B$ agonist. Surprisingly the formation of cyclic AMP was enhanced rather than inhibited even in the presence of a phosphodiesterase inhibitor. However, it has been reported that $GABA_B$ activation can depress basal cyclic formation in membranes prepared from rat cerebellum. $GABA_B$ site activation can also decrease the stimulant action of forskolin on adenylate cyclase. Since forskolin acts directly on the catalytic subunit of the enzyme whilst β-stimulants act through membrane receptors, further studies are obviously needed to clarify the nature of the association between $GABA_B$ sites and cyclase and to discern whether this is fundamental to the mechanism of $GABA_B$-mediated effects.

Location of $GABA_B$ sites in brain

Evidence is accruing for both pre- and postsynaptic locations for $GABA_B$ sites in the brain. Thus although most of the information obtained so far indicates a preponderance of presynaptic sites, binding studies on rat cerebellar tissue and electrophysiological experiments on CA_1, pyramidal cells of the rat hippocampus point towards a postsynaptic locus. Certainly binding studies on membranes prepared from lesioned brain tissue indicated that $GABA_B$ sites are present on presynaptic terminals of the cerebral cortex and striatum. A presynaptic location concurs with conclusions obtained in neurochemical release experiments performed on cerebral cortex and striatal slices. To determine the location more precisely we have employed the technique of dry-mounting autoradiography in brain slices from normal and lesioned tissues. In brief, sections mounted on glass slides were incubated with radiolabelled GABA or baclofen in Tris-buffer solution containing Ca^{2+} (2.5 mM) and sucrose to maintain isotonicity. The distribution of radioactivity over the section was then determined by placing the dry section in close apposition to tritium-sensitive film or emulsion-coated coverslips. After a period of up to 4 weeks the photographic emulsion was developed and the grain pattern analysed under the light microscope. The patterns of distribution of $GABA_A$ and $GABA_B$ sites differ significantly. Whilst a similar pattern occurs in, for example, the cerebral cortex and superior colliculus, the distributions in many other regions differ. For example, $GABA_B$ sites in the spinal cord are highly concentrated in the laminae of the dorsal horns, in particular laminae II and III. After neonatal capsaicin administration the number of grains detectable over sections of cord obtained from adult rats was reduced by about 50%. Capsaicin causes degeneration of small diameter afferents to the cord. This was evidenced in our study by reductions in substance P and fluoride-resistant acid phosphatase, both of which are considered to be markers for primary afferent terminals. We can conclude therefore that $GABA_B$ sites are likely to be present on the small diameter fibres entering the dorsal horn. In the dorsal horn intrinsic GABA neurons which impinge on the terminals of the dorsal root afferents have been described. It seems likely therefore, that $GABA_B$ sites on these afferents are innervated.

Note added in proof

Two significant observations have been sequencing of the $GABA_A$ receptor by Barnard's and Seeburg's groups (Schofield *et al.* 1987) and the evidence of Dutar and Nicoll (1988) for a physiological role of $GABA_B$ receptors in mammalian hippocampus.

The sequence of the $GABA_A$ site was achieved following the solublisation and purification of the $GABA_A$ receptor complex in bovine brain by tagging with a benzodiazepine ligand. Since the $GABA_A$ recognition site coexists on the same macromolecule this has provided the basis for generating peptide sequences, allowing the isolation of cloned cDNAs encoding two subunits which comprise the $GABA_A$ receptor. One subunit (α) appears to carry the GABA recognition site whereas the other (β) carries the benzodiazepine binding site. The molecular masses of these subunits are 49 and 51 K Daltons respectively. Interestingly there appears to be a similarity between parts of these subunit sequences and the subunits of the nicotinic acetylcholine receptor and the strychnine-sensitive glycine receptor. This has prompted Schofield *et al.* (1987) to propose the existence of a superfamily of chemically-gated ion channel receptors which may also include excitatory amino acid receptors. An important feature of this study was the expression of $GABA_A$ receptors in xenopus oöcytes by injection by α-subunit and β-subunit RNAs prepared by inserting cloned cDNAs into plasmids and performing *in vitro* transcription. Only when both RNAs were injected together was GABA able to produce an increase in membrane conductance analogous to that produced by injection of total rat brain mRNA. However, current indications are that the reported sequence is still incomplete and, moreover, the active sites or amino acid residues responsible for attachment of GABA and its antagonists are not known. Presumably this will be ascertained by traditional structure/activity studies.

Studies reported by Dutar and Nicoll (1988) employed the GABA$_B$ antagonist, phaclofen, to antagonise a synaptically-mediated hyperpolarisation recorded in CA1 pyramidal cells of the rat hippocampus *in vitro*. Following stimulation of the stratum radiatum a biphasic IPSP occurs of which only the initial response can be blocked by bicuculline. The late response is, however, blocked by phaclofen, a weak but selective antagonist for GABA$_B$ sites, indicating that GABA may mediate both phases of the response through separate receptors. Evidence for a similar physiological role for GABA receptors in the neocortex, lateral geniculate and septum has since been noted by other groups.

References and further reading

Bowery NG & Brown DA (1974) Depolarizing actions of γ-aminobutyric acid and related compounds on rat superior cervical ganglia *in vitro*. *Br. J. Pharmac.* **50**, 205–18.

Bowery NG, Doble A, Hill DR, Hudson AL, Shaw JS, Turnbull MJ & Warrington R (1981) Bicuculline-insensitive GABA receptors on peripheral autonomic nerve terminals. *Eur. J. Pharmacol.* **71**, 53–70.

Bowery NG, Hill DR, Hudson AL, Doble A, Middlemiss DN, Shaw J & Turnball MJ (1980) (−)Baclofen decreases neurotransmitter release in the mammalian CNS by an action at a novel GABA receptor. *Nature* **283**, 92–4.

Bowery NG, Hudson AL, Hill DR & Price GW (1984) Bicuculline-insensitive GABA$_B$ receptors. In: Paton W, Mitchell J & Turner P (eds) *Proc. 9th IUPHAR Congress.* MacMillan, London. pp. 159–170.

Curtis DR & Watkins JC (1965) The pharmacology of amino acids related to gamma-aminobutyric acid. *Pharmacol. Rev.* **17**, 347–91.

De Groat WC (1970) The actions of γ-aminobutyric acid and related amino acids on mammalian autonomic ganglia. *J. Pharmac. Exp. Ther.* **172**, 348–96.

Dutar P & Nicoll RA (1988) A physiological role for GABA$_B$ receptors in the central nervous system. *Nature* **332**, 156–8.

Haefely W, Kyburz E, Gerecke M & Mohler H (1985) Recent advances in the molecular pharmacology of benzodiazepine receptors and in the structure-activity relationships of their agonists and antagonists. *Advances in Drug Research* **14**, 165–22.

Hill DR & Bowery NG (1981) ^{3}H-baclofen and ^{3}H-GABA bind to bicuculline-insensitive GABA$_B$ sites in rat brain. *Nature* **209**, 149–52.

Iversen LL & Kelly JS (1975) Uptake and metabolism of γ-aminobutyric acid by neurones and glial cells. *Biochem. Pharmacol.* **24**, 933–8.

Johnston GAR (1976) In: Roberts E, Chase TN & Tower DB (eds) *GABA in Nervous System Function.* Raven Press, New York.

Johnston GAR, Curtis DR, de Groat WC & Duggan AW (1968) Central actions of ibotenic acid and muscimol. *Biochem. Pharmacol.* **17**, 2488–9.

Kerr DIB, Ong J, Prager RH, Gynther BD & Curtis DR (1987) Phaclofen: a peripheral and central baclofen antagonist. *Brain Res.* **405**, 150–4.

Krnjevic K & Schwartz S (1967) The action of γ-aminobutyric acid on cortical neurones. *Exp. Brain Res.* **3**, 320–36.

Schofield PR, Darlison MG, Fujita N, Bart DR, Stephenson FA, Rodriguez H, Rhee LM, Ramachandran J, Reale V, Glencorse TA, Seeburg PH & Barnard EA (1987) Sequence and functional expression of the GABA$_A$ receptor shows a ligand-gates receptor superfamily. *Nature* **328**, 221–9.

Zukin SR, Young AB & Snyder SH (1974) Gamma-aminobutyric acid binding to receptor sites in rat central nervous system. *Proc. Natl. Acad. Sci. USA.* **71**, 4802–7.

13 Excitatory amino acid receptors

J. DAVIES

The depolarising action of the dicarboxylic acids, L-glutamate and L-aspartate, on neurons in the mammalian central nervous system (CNS) was first reported more than 25 years ago. Recently, significant progress has been achieved in characterising the receptors with which excitatory amino acids interact and it is now clear that some of these receptors are transmitter receptors. However, the identity of the transmitter(s) acting at these receptors is still not known.

It has long been recognised that specific pharmacological antagonists of the actions of excitatory amino acids would aid the identification of excitatory synaptic pathways utilising amino acids as transmitters. Such antagonists have now been developed and have led to the characterisation of multiple receptors for excitatory amino acids and in renewed interest in the role of these agents in physiological and pathological processes in the CNS. Electrophysiological investigations *in vivo* (employing the iono-phoretic method of drug application near single neurons) and *in vitro* (using slices and cultures of CNS tissue) have been particularly important in providing evidence for the existence of different excitatory amino acid receptors and in elucidating their role in synaptic transmission. More recently, ligand binding studies have also yielded data consistent with the presence of multiple excitatory amino acid receptors in CNS tissue. This chapter summarises some of the more significant advances in excitatory amino acid receptor research.

Electrophysiological classification of excitatory amino acid receptors

The major breakthrough in the characterisation of excitatory amino acid receptors followed the discovery that the higher homologue of glutamic acid, α-aminodipic acid (αAA), antagonised the excitatory actions of L-aspartate and L-glutamate but not those of non-amino acid excitants such as ACh on CNS neurons when administered into their vicinity by ionophoresis (McLennan & Hall 1978; Davies & Watkins 1979). However, since αAA did not clearly distinguish between the excitatory actions of L-aspartate as opposed to those of L-glutamate, it was hypothesised that these agonists may act on a mixed population of receptors. This led researchers to study the effects of αAA on a series of excitatory amino acid agonists with more rigid conformations than either aspartate or

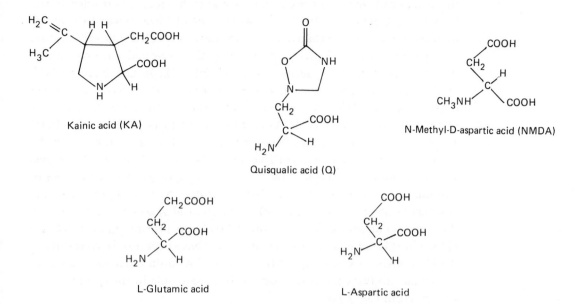

Fig. 13.1. Structures of selective agonists for the different excitatory amino acid receptors (top row) and structures of L-glutamic and L-aspartic acids.

glutamate on the basis that they may be more selective agonists at specific receptor sites, if such existed. The agonists chosen were N-methyl-D-aspartic acid (NMDA), an analogue of aspartic acid, and kainic and quisqualic acid, both analogues of glutamic acid (Fig. 13.1). These three agonists are more potent excitants of CNS neurons than either glutamate or aspartate. It was rapidly shown that αAA antagonised the excitatory effects of NMDA but not those of kainate or quisqualate, and this led to the conclusion that at least two different excitatory amino acid receptors existed which were referred to as NMDA- and non-NMDA-receptors. Subsequently, many other excitatory amino acid antagonists were synthesised and tested, and it is now generally agreed that there are probably at least three subtypes of excitatory amino acid receptor that have been named NMDA, kainate and quisqualate receptors after the three selective agonists (Watkins & Evans 1981). However, the division of receptors into the kainate and quisqualate subtypes is far from clear, and it is currently advisable to confine the division to NMDA and non-NMDA receptors.

NMDA receptors

These are the most clearly defined receptors on electrophysiological grounds. Subsequent to the discovery that αAA selectively antagonised the excitatory action of NMDA it was shown that divalent cations such as magnesium and cobalt (but not calcium) and several higher homologues of αAA exhibited similar selective antagonist properties. Furthermore, the antagonist acivity of αAA and its higher homologues resided in the D-isomers (Davis *et al.* 1978). However, none of these newer antagonists was any more effective than αAA. Later studies revealed that substitution of a phosphonic acid group in place of the terminal carboxyl group in this homologous series (i.e. H_2O_3P-$(CH_2)n$-$CH(NH_2)$-$COOH$, ω-phosphono-α-carboxylic acids) considerably enhanced antagonist potency against NMDA compared with that against the dicarboxylic acids. The most active NMDA-receptor antagonists in this series (AP5 and AP7; n = 5 and 7 in the above structure) are indicated in Fig. 13.2. All these substances are competitive antagonists of NMDA. None has significant effects on the actions of kainate and quisqualate, or on those of non-amino acid excitants on CNS neurons. Nor do they have any observable effects on resting membrane potential or conductance. As with the α-amino dicarboxylic acids, the NMDA-receptor antagonist activity of the phosphonate antagonists (where they have been resolved) resides in the D-isomers. An example of the action of AP5 on chemically-induced and synaptically-evoked excitation of Renshaw cells in the spinal cord is illustrated in Fig. 13.3.

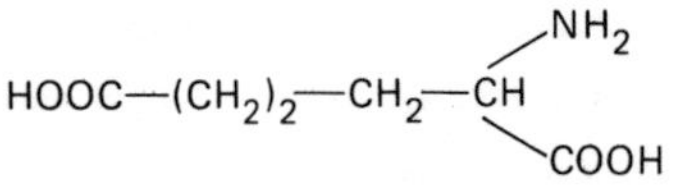

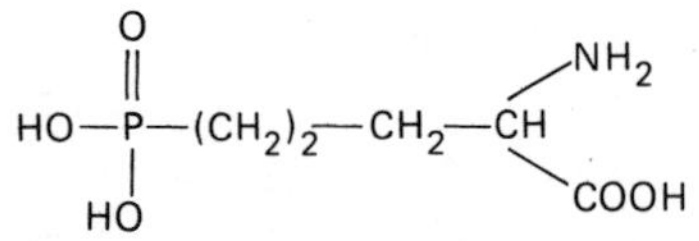

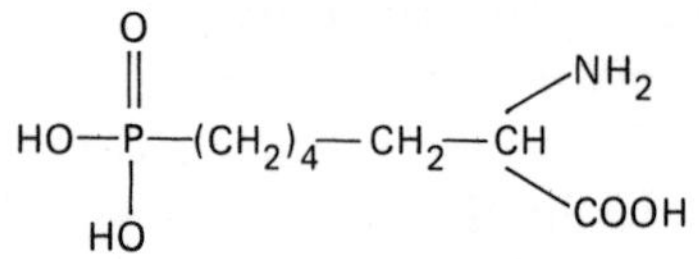

Fig. 13.2. Chemical structure of some selective NMDA receptor antagonists. αAA, D-α-aminoadipic acid; AP5 (APV), D-2-amino-5-phosphono-pentanoic acid (D-2-amino-5-phosphono-valeric acid); AP7, D-2-amino-7-phosphono-heptanoic acid; CPP, 3-(2-carboxypiperazine-4-yl) propyl-1-phosphonic acid. The D-(-) isomers of αAA, AP5 and AP7 carry NMDA antagonist activity, the isomers of CPP have not been resolved.

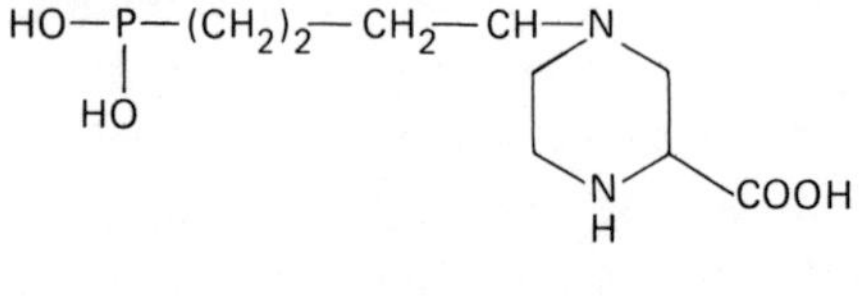

Non-NMDA (kainate/quisqualate) receptors

Several compounds have been developed which antagonise the actions of kainate and quisqualate in addition to those of NMDA and are thus broad spectrum excitatory amino acid antagonists (Watkins & Evans 1981). While agents that selectively antagonise the actions of kainate or quisqualate are not yet available, some of the broad spectrum antagonists do display certain differential effects on responses to kainate and quisqualate that suggest that these two excitants act at different receptors. The more useful and interesting broad spectrum excitatory amino acid antagonists are illustrated in Fig. 13.4. They have been divided into three groups; those that depress responses to NMDA, kainate and quisqualate with little differential effect against any particular agonist, those where the order of sensitivity of the agonist response to the antagonist is NMDA > kainate > quisqualate and others where the order of agonist sensitivity to the antagonist is kainate > quisqualate > NMDA. As already mentioned, it is partly on the basis of the differential sensitivity of agonist responses to some of the broad spectrum antagonists that non-NMDA-receptors have been subdivided into the kainate and quisqualate class of receptors. For instance, in studies on some CNS neurons low doses of GAMS (Fig. 13.4) depress responses to kainate but not those to quisqualate or NMDA indicating that kainate may act at a different site from the other two agonists. However, it must be stressed that more potent and selective antagonists for the excitatory actions of either kainate or quisqualate, are required to confirm this subdivision of the non-NMDA receptors.

Receptors mediating the excitatory actions of glutamic and aspartic acids

It appears that the endogenous excitatory amino acids, L-glutamate and L-aspartate, are capable of interacting with both NMDA and non-NMDA receptors to some extent (Watkins & Evans 1981). This conclusion stems from the observation that ionophoretic administration of NMDA-receptor antagonists in amounts sufficient to depress responses to NMDA also reduce, but generally do not abolish, excitation induced by glutamate and aspartate. The residual response to these excitatory amino acids can often be completely depressed by addition of the broad spectrum antagonists at concentrations which also depress responses to kainate and quisqualate. However, responses to L-aspartate are frequently more sensitive to selective NMDA antagonists than responses to L-glutamate (e.g. Fig. 13.3(B), whereas depression of responses to the latter tends to be correlated (at least in some instances) with depression of responses to quisqualate. It has been suggested therefore that NMDA receptors may make a major contribution to the composite response induced by L-aspartate, while quisqualate receptors perhaps contribute more to the

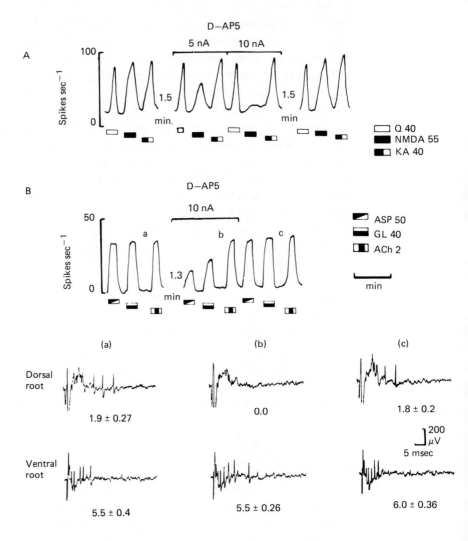

Fig. 13.3. Selective antagonist action of the D-isomer of AP5 on amino acid-induced and synaptically-evoked excitation of spinal neurons. Records A and B are from a dorsal horn neuron and Renshaw cell respectively. A is a ratemeter record of cell firing illustrating the reversible depression of responses to NMDA (55 nA) but not those to quisqualate (Q, 40 nA) or kainate (KA, 40 nA) following the ionophoretic ejection of 5 nA, then 10 nA of AP5. In B the ejection of 10 nA of AP5 reduces excitation induced by L-aspartate (ASP, 50 nA) and L-glutamate (GL, 40 nA) but not that to acetylcholine (ACh, 2 nA). Note, responses to L-aspartate are depressed more than responses to L-glutamate. The lower two records (a–c) are representative oscilloscope-sweeps of the synaptic responses evoked in the same cell by stimulating the dorsal and ventral roots (a) before, (b) during the ejection of 10 nA AP5, and (c) 3 min after terminating the AP5 ejection. The numbers below each record a–c indicate the mean ±s.e. number of action potentials in 20 trials. Note, the polysynaptic response evoked from the dorsal root is reduced by AP5 whereas the cholinergic response evoked from recurrent motor axon collaterals in the ventral root is unaffected.

overall response induced by L-glutamate. Unfortunately, there are several instances where responses to NMDA, kainate and quisqualate are markedly reduced or even abolished in the absence of significant effects on responses to L-glutamate. Hence, it remains to be seen whether or not this interpretation of the data is correct.

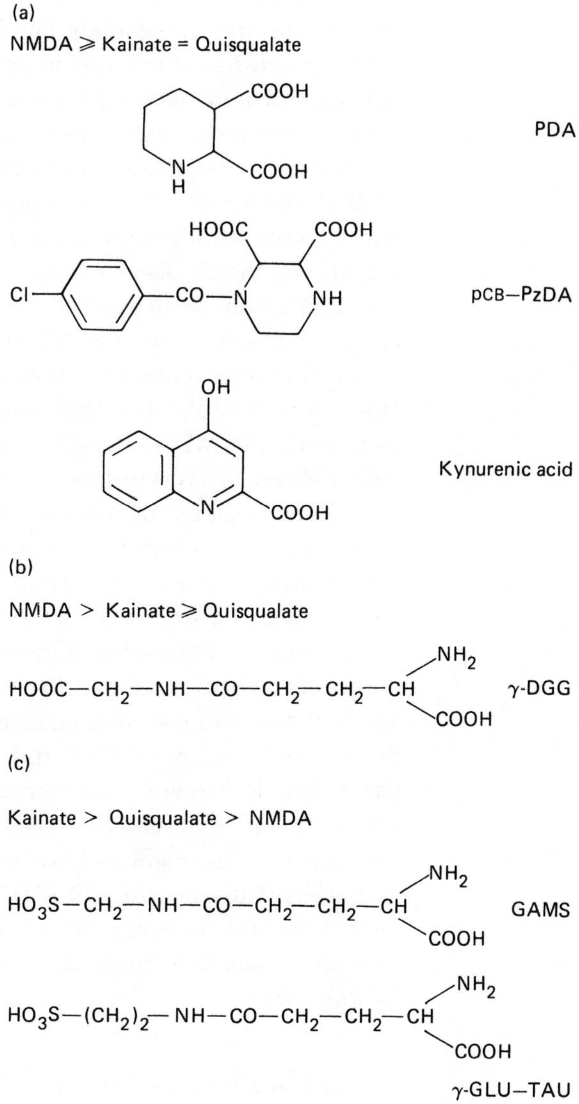

(a)

NMDA $\geqslant$ Kainate = Quisqualate

PDA

pCB–PzDA

Kynurenic acid

(b)

NMDA > Kainate $\geqslant$ Quisqualate

γ-DGG

(c)

Kainate > Quisqualate > NMDA

GAMS

γ-GLU–TAU

Fig. 13.4. Structure of broad spectrum excitatory amino acid antagonists that interact with NMDA, kainate and quisqualate receptors. (a) PDA, (±)-*cis*-2,3-piperidine dicarboxylic acid; pCB-PzDA, p-chlorobenzoyl-2,3-piperazine dicarboxylic acid; kynurenic acid; (b) γDGG, γ-D-glutamylglycine; (c) GAMS, γ-D-glutamylaminomethyl sulphonic acid; γ-GLU-TAU, γ-D-glutamyltaurine.

Intracellular studies

Intracellular studies, particularly *in vitro* on cultured CNS neurons employing the voltage clamp and patch clamp techniques have provided additional evidence supporting the existence of NMDA and non-NMDA receptors. In some studies the membrane potential was clamped at various holding potentials and the current resulting from the application of a constant amount of each of kainate, quisqualate and NMDA was determined. These showed that the current/voltage curves obtained with kainate and quisqualate were similar and exhibited little voltage dependency, whereas that for NMDA was highly voltage dependent at negative membrane potentials (Mayer & Westbrook 1985). The current/voltage curve for L-glutamate was intermediate between that for NMDA and that for kainate and quisqualate but in the presence of a selective NMDA-receptor antagonist it was converted to one that resembled the curves for kainate and quisqualate (Mayer & Westbrook 1984). The differing voltage sensitivities of the responses induced by NMDA on the one hand, and by kainate and quisqualate on the other, is consistent with the existence of NMDA and non-NMDA subtypes of excitatory amino acid receptors and supports the notion that L-glutamate may be an agonist at both receptors. A more significant discovery emanating from these studies was that when magnesium ions were omitted from the extracellular bathing medium the current-voltage curves for NMDA and L-glutamate were converted to curves that were similar to those obtained with kainate and quisqualate. It is now well established that magnesium blocks the ion channels opened as a result of NMDA—receptor activation at negative membrane potentials (Mayer & Westbrook 1985; Nowak *et al.* 1984). This voltage-dependent block by magnesium readily explains the ability of this ion to antagonise the excitatory effects of NMDA when it is administrated near CNS neurons by microionophoresis. Since this voltage-dependent magnesium block occurs with concentrations of the ion normally present in extracellular fluid this has important implications for the modulation of excitatory events mediated by NMDA receptors (Mayer & Westbrook 1987). Patch-clamp studies on cultured CNS cells have also revealed other differences between NMDA and non-NMDA receptors. Whilst the ion channels linked to both receptors are permeable to sodium and potassium ions those linked to NMDA receptors are also permeable to calcium ions and seem to be regulated by low concentrations of glycine. Glycine potentiates the response to NMDA and is thought to act at allosteric sites on the NMDA receptor complex that are distinct from the classical strychnine-sensitive sites involved in synaptic inhibition (Ascher & Nowak 1987).

Ligand binding studies and amino acid receptor classification

Neurochemical studies involving ligand binding techniques provide additional evidence that multiple excitatory amino receptors are present in the CNS. The most widely used ligand in these studies is [^{3}H]-L-glutamate although recently more selective ligands such as D-[^{3}H]-AP5, [^{3}H]-kainate and [^{3}H]-AMPA (a quisqualate receptor agonist) have been employed. Binding studies have been performed on purified synaptic plasma membranes and crude synaptic membranes obtained from various brain regions (Foster & Fagg 1984).

[^{3}H]-L-Glutamate binding

At least three distinct types of binding have been differentiated for [^{3}H]-L-glutamate (see Foster & Fagg 1984). One is the Na^+-dependent binding site thought to be responsible for inactivating synaptically released excitatory amino acids. Binding of L-glutamate to the other two sites is independent of Na^+ ions in the bathing medium. One of these Na^+-independent sites is dependent on the presence of Cl^- and Ca^{2+} ions in the assay medium whereas the other is independent of these two ions. A proportion of the binding of [^{3}H]-L-glutamate to the Na^+-independent and Cl^-/Ca^{2+}-independent site is displaced most readily by excitatory amino acid agonists and antagonists that are selective for the NMDA receptor in electrophysiological studies. The remainder of the [^{3}H]-L-glutamate binding to this site is displaced most readily by quisqualate. Thus a subpopulation of NMDA and quisqualate sites appears to have been identified in binding studies. Kainate is an extremely weak displacer of L-glutamate binding from all sites in isolated membranes, yet this substance itself binds to brain membranes with an affinity in the nanomolar range indicating that a separate subset of receptors may exist for this amino acid. Indeed, recent quantitative autoradiographic analysis of the distribution of Cl^-/Ca^{2+}-independent L-glutamate binding sites in the rat hippocampus revealed that NMDA, kainate and quisqualate each displace L-glutamate binding from different anatomical locations (Monaghan et al. 1985). These data are thus consistent with the notion that three distinct L-glutamate binding sites exist that coincide with NMDA, kainate and quisqualate receptors identified electrophysiologically.

Binding of other amino acid ligands

Data on the binding of other amino acid ligands to brain membranes is sparse compared with that for L-glutamate. NMDA does not have sufficient affinity to yield acceptable ratios of specific to non-specific binding. [^{3}H]-D-AP5 and [^{3}H]-CPP binding is displaced by excitatory amino acid agonists and antagonists with potencies parallelling their relative potencies as NMDA agonists or antagonists in electrophysiological studies. This suggests that AP5 and CPP are binding at NMDA-receptor sites (Monaghan et al. 1984; Olverman et al. 1986). The heterocyclic analogue of L-glutamate, α-amino-3hydroxyl-5methyl-4isoxazolepropionic acid (AMPA) binds to a subpopulation of Cl^-/Ca^{2+}-independent sites and is more effectively displaced from these sites by quisqualate than by compounds active at NMDA-receptors (Foster & Fagg 1984). Hence, binding sites for AMPA may represent quisqualate receptors.

Non-amino acids acting as NMDA-antagonists

In addition to the amino acid antagonists already mentioned several compounds which are not amino acid analogues have been demonstrated to selectively antagonise the actions of NMDA. These include the dissociative anaesthetics ketamine and phencyclidine (PCP), sigma opioid benzomorphans such as cyclazocine, the morphinan derivative, dextrorphan, and most recently, the dibenzocyclohepteneimine, MK801. These substances readily cross the blood–brain barrier unlike the amino acid analogues and are thus active as antagonists when administered systemically. However, they are non-competitive antagonists of NMDA and electrophysiological and binding studies indicate that they act at the ion channel associated with the NMDA receptor but at a different site from Mg^{2+}. Their site of action correlates with the high affinity binding site for $^3[H]$-PCP and its thienyl analogue $^3[H]$-TCP (Kemp et al. 1987; Lodge et al. 1987).

Excitatory amino acid receptors and synaptic excitation

The more potent and selective NMDA-receptor antagonists and broad spectrum excitatory amino acid antagonists have been used to determine whether excitatory transmission in particular neuronal pathways is mediated by an amino acid, and also to characterise the synaptic receptors involved. For example, in the spinal cord it has been demonstrated that selective NMDA-receptor antagonists, such as AP5 and αAA, depress the polysynaptic excitation of spinal interneurons evoked by stimulation of low threshold muscle and cutaneous sensory afferents in the hind limb when applied with ionophoretic currents [doses] that selectively depress excitatory responses of the same cells to NMDA. In contrast, spinal neurons excited monosynaptically by the same stimuli were unaffected by selective NMDA antagonists, but were depressed by ionophoresis of broad spectrum antagonists in conjunction with the depression of responses of the neurons to kainate and quisqualate in addition to those of NMDA (Davies & Watkins 1983). These data suggest that excitatory amino acids are likely to be released as transmitters by both the terminals of primary afferent fibres and excitatory interneurons in the spinal cord, and that the synaptic receptors involved are of the non-NMDA and NMDA types respectively. Similar studies have been conducted in many other regions of the CNS. Some of the excitatory pathways examined and the subtype of amino acid receptor mediating the synaptic response are summarised in Table 13.1.

Reference to Table 13.1 shows that the transmitter involved in all the pathways studied is probably an amino acid and that the transmitter receptor in most instances is the non-NMDA type receptor. However, several factors suggest that NMDA receptors play a more important role in excitatory synaptic transmission than is indicated by the data in

Table 13.1. Amino acid receptors involved in some excitatory pathways in the CNS (see text for NMDA effects in hippocampus).

CNS region	Afferent pathway*	Synaptic response**	Receptor	Reference
Spinal cord	Primary afferent	MS	Non-NMDA	Davies & Watkins (1983)
	Primary afferent	PS	NMDA	Davies & Watkins (1983)
Caudate nucleus	Corticofugal	MS	Non-NMDA	Herrling (1985)
Cuneate nucleus	Pyramidal tract	MS	Non-NMDA	Davies et al. (1987)
	Primary afferent	MS	Non-NMDA	Davies et al (1987)
Cochlear nucleus	Auditory nerve	MS	NMDA	Martin (1980)
Cerebral cortex	Corpus callosum	MS	NMDA/non-NMDA	Thomson (1986)
Cerebellum	Climbing fibre-Purkinje cell	MS	Non-NMDA	Davies et al. (1987)
	Parallel fibre-interneuron	MS	NMDA	Davies et al. (1987)
Hippocampus				
CA1	Schaffer collateral-commissural	MS	Non-NMDA	Collingridge et al. (1987)
Dentate gyrus	Lateral perforant path	MS	Non-NMDA	Collingridge et al. (1987)
	Medial perforant path	MS	Non-NMDA	Collingridge et al. (1987)
CA3	Perforant path	MS	Non-NMDA	Collingridge et al. (1987)
	Mossy fibre path	MS	Non-NMDA	Collingridge et al. (1987)
	Commissural fibre	MS	Non-NMDA	Collingridge et al. (1987)
Red nucleus	Corticorubral	MS	NMDA	Davies et al. (1987)
	Interpositorubral	MS	Non-NMDA	Davies et al. (1987)
Thalamus	Corticofugal	MS	Non-NMDA	Davies et al. (1987)
	Interposito-thalamic	MS	Non-NMDA	Davies et al. (1987)
	Facial cutaneous afferents	MS	Non-NMDA	Salt (1986)

*All pathways stimulated electrically with single stimuli.
**MS = monosynaptic pathway, PS = polysynaptic pathway.

Table 13.1. For instance, in the hippocampus the synaptic excitation evoked by single pulse stimulation of the principal pathways is insensitive to selective NMDA-receptor antagonists. However, when a brief period of tetanic stimulation is applied to these pathways the synaptic response evoked by subsequent single pulse stimulation produces an enhanced synaptic response that can last for days. This enhanced synaptic response is attenuated, and its initiation by tetanic stimuli prevented, by selective NMDA-receptor antagonists indicating the involvement of NMDA receptors in this phenomenon (Collingridge et al. 1987). This potentiation has been termed long-term potentiation (LTP) and is considered to be a useful model of learning and memory. The ability of NMDA antagonists to block LTP suggests that NMDA receptors mediate this form of synaptic plasticity in the hippocampus. Further evidence that NMDA receptors play a significant role in excitatory synaptic events derives from studies in the rat ventrobasal thalamus (Salt 1986). Here it has been demonstrated that the synaptic excitation of neurons evoked by single pulse electrical stimulation of sensory afferents is insensitive to antagonism by selective NMDA antagonists, but these antagonists reduced synaptic responses evoked by trains of stimuli. This has led to the suggestion that it is the pattern of afferent activity that governs the recruitment of the NMDA-receptor mediated response. This is an important consideration since, under physiological conditions neurons are more likely to be subjected to asynchronous synaptic bombardment rather than the synchronous pattern of excitation induced by electrical stimulation of afferent pathways. To explain this phenomenon it has been proposed that prolonged synaptic activation evoked by trains of stimuli could result in relieving the voltage-dependent block by Mg^{2+} of the NMDA-linked ion channels, thus unmasking the NMDA receptor-mediated events. In support of this hypothesis an NMDA receptor-mediated excitatory synaptic potential (EPSP) that is voltage-dependent can be demonstrated in neurons in the cortical slice when Mg^{2+} ions are absent from the bathing medium (Thomson 1986). Furthermore, a short latency non-NMDA and longer latency NMDA component of the EPSP has been demonstrated in spinal neurons in Xenopus (Dale & Roberts 1985). Thus, it could be argued that, in addition to non-NMDA receptors, NMDA receptors play an important role in regulating excitability of the CNS. Such a role is also indicated by recent reports that NMDA-receptor antagonists have powerful anticonvulsant actions in a variety of animal models (Meldrum 1987).

Concluding remarks

The identification of different types of receptor for excitatory amino acids and the clear demonstration of their involvement in synaptic transmission provides compelling support for the long postulated transmitter role for acidic amino acids in the vertebrate CNS. While in most CNS pathways studied to date non-NMDA (kainate and quisqualate) receptors appear to be the main transmitter receptors involved in fast monosynaptic excitatory events, NMDA receptors seeming to mediate slower excitatory events, accumulating evidence suggests that synaptic excitation may be a consequence of transmitter interaction with both NMDA and non-NMDA type receptors. However, the identity of the transmitter acting at the different subtypes of excitatory amino acid receptor is not known. Interestingly, the endogenous amino acids L-glutamate and L-aspartate interact with NMDA and non-NMDA receptors. Thus, either of these agents or some similar endogenous amino acid could be the synaptic transmitter in amino acid utilising pathways.

Finally, research in progress indicates that, in addition to being useful aids for analysing amino acid mediated excitatory synaptic events, selective NMDA-receptor antagonists may have potential as antiepileptic drugs, centrally acting muscle relaxants and as neuro-protective agents in cerebrovascular accidents and some neurodegenerative disorders such as Alzheimer's and Huntington's disease (Greenamyre 1986; Meldrum 1985; Rothman & Olney 1987).

References and further reading

Ascher P & Novak L (1987) Electrophysiological studies of NMDA receptors. *Trends Neurosci.* **10**, 284-8.

Cavalheiro EA, Lehmann J & Turski L (eds) (1988) *Excitatory amino acids 1988. An International Symposium.* Alan R. Liss, New York.

Collingridge GL, Coan EJ, Herron C E & Lester RAJ (1987) Role of excitatory amino acid receptors in synaptic transmission and plasticity in hippocampal pathways. In: Hicks TP, Lodge D & McLennan H (eds) *Neurology and Neurobiology, Excitatory Amino Acid Transmission* vol. 24. AR Liss, New York. pp. 317-24.

Dale N & Roberts A (1985) Dual-component amino-acid-mediated synaptic potentials. Excitatory drive for swimming in xenopus embryos. *J. Physiol.* **363**, 35-59.

Davies J, Evans RH, Francis AA & Watkins JC (1978) Excitatory amino acid receptor differentiation by selective antagonists and role in synaptic excitation. In: Simons P (ed) *Advances in Pharmacology and Therapeutics* vol. 12. *Neurotransmitters.* Pergamon Press, Oxford. pp. 161-70.

Davies J, Quinlan JE & Sheardown MJ (1987) Mediation of excitatory transmission in specific brain pathways by amino acids acting at NMDA and non-NMDA receptors. In: Hicks TP, Lodge D & McLennan H (eds) *Excitatory Amino Acid Transmission. Neurology & Neurobiology* vol. 24. AR Liss, New York. pp. 277-84.

Davies J & Watkins JC (1979) Selective antagonism of amino acid-induced and synaptic excitation in the cat spinal cord. *J. Physiol.* **297**, 621-35.

Davies J & Watkins JC (1983) Role of excitatory amino acid receptors in mono and polysynaptic excitation in the cat spinal cord. *Exp. Brain Res.* **49**, 280-90.

Foster AC & Fagg GE (1984) Acidic amino acid binding sites in mammalian neuronal membranes. Their characteristics and relationship to synaptic receptors. *Brain Res. Rev.* **7**, 103-64.

Greenamyre JT (1986) The role of glutamate in neurotransmission and in neurologic disease. *Archiv. Neurol.* **43**, 1058-63.

Herrling PL (1985) Pharmacology of the corticocaudate excitatory postsynaptic potential in the cat: evidence for its mediation by quisqualate or kainate receptors. *Neuroscience* **14**, 417-26.

Kemp JA, Forster AC & Wong EHF (1987) Non-competitive antagonists of excitatory amino-acid receptors. *Trends Neurosci.* **10**, 294-8.

Lodge D (ed) (1988) *Excitatory Amino Acids in Health and Disease.* John Wiley, London.

Lodge D, Aram JA, Church J, Davies SN, Martin D, O'Saughnessy CJ & Zeman S (1987) Excitatory amino acids and phencyclidine-like drugs. In: Hicks TP, Lodge D & McLennan H (eds) *Excitatory Amino Acid Transmission, Neurology and Neurobiology* vol. 24. AR Liss, New York. pp. 83-90.

Martin MR (1980) The effects of iontophoretically applied antagonists on auditory nerve and amino acid evoked excitation of antereoventral cochlear nucleus neurons. *Neuropharmacology* **19**, 519-28.

Mayer ML & Westbrook GL (1984) Mixed-agonist action of excitatory amino acids on mouse spinal cord neurons under voltage clamp. *J. Physiol.* **354**, 29-53.

Mayer ML & Westbrook GL (1985) The action of N-methyl-D-aspartic acid on mouse spinal neurons in culture. *J. Physiol.* **361**, 65-90.

Mayer ML & Westbrook GL (1987) The physiology of excitatory amino acids in the vertebrate central nervous system. *Prog. in Neurobiol.* **28**, 192-276.

McLennan H & Hall JG (1978) The actions of D-α-aminoadipate on excitatory amino acid receptors of rat thalamic neurons. *Brain Research* **149**, 541-5.

Meldrum B (1985) Possible therapeutic applications of antagonists of excitatory amino acid neurotransmitters. *Clin. Sci.* **68**, 113-22.

Meldrum B (1987) Excitatory amino acids and epilepsy. In: Hicks TP, Lodge D & McLennan H (eds) *Excitatory Amino Acid Transmission, Neurology & Neurobiology* vol. 24. A.R. Liss, New York. pp. 189–96.

Monaghan DT, Yao D & Cotman CW (1985) L-[^{3}H]-Glutamate binds to kainate-, NMDA- and AMPA-sensitive binding sites: An autoradiographic analysis. *Brain Res.* **340**, 378–83.

Monaghan DT, Yao D, Olverman HJ, Watkins JC & Cotman CW (1984) Autoradiography of D-2-[^{3}H]amino-5-phosphopentanoate binding sites in rat brain. *Neurosci. Lett.* **52**, 253–8.

Nowak L, Bregestovski P, Ascher P, Herbet H & Prochiantz A (1984) Magnesium gates glutamate activated channels in mouse central neurons. *Nature* **307**, 462–5.

Olverman HJ, Monaghan DT, Cotman CW & Watkins JC (1986) [3H]CPP, a new competitive ligand for NMDA receptors. *Eur. J. Pharmacol.* **131**, 161–2.

Rothman SM & Olney JW (1987) Excitotoxicity and the NMDA receptor. *Trends Neurosci.* **10**, 299–302.

Salt TE (1986) Mediation of thalamic sensory input by both NMDA receptors and non-NMDA receptors. *Nature* **322**, 263–5.

Thomson AM (1986) A magnesium sensitive postsynaptic potential in rat cerebral cortex resembles neuronal responses to N-methylaspartate. *J. Physiol.* **370**, 531–49.

Watkins JC & Evans RH (1981) Excitatory amino acid transmitters. *Ann. Rev. Pharmacol. Toxicol.* **21**, 165–204.

14   Peptides

C.C. JORDAN

Potential neurotransmitter function of peptides

Most of the neurotransmitter substances discussed in this volume are relatively simple molecules (amino acids, catecholamines, 5-hydroxytryptamine, etc.) with molecular weights of less than 200. Their identity, if not their function, has been known for many years and, in the majority of cases, the mechanisms of synthesis, release, actions and degradation are known in some detail. In the last 10 to 15 years it has become apparent that these small molecules are not the only chemical signalling agents utilised by neurons. A vast range of peptides has been shown to occur in the nervous system: many of these appear to be associated with discrete neuronal pathways and some occur in the same neurons as established neurotransmitters such as dopamine and 5-HT (i.e. they are co-stored).

It is fair to say that little is known of the exact function of these peptides in the majority of cases. Nevertheless, it is clear that peptides do serve an important role either as neurotransmitters in the established sense or as more subtle short- or long-term modulators of neuronal firing. For example, a peptide released from a nerve terminal may facilitate the actions of a fast neurotransmitter thereby providing a low resistance pathway for rapid transfer of information. Alternatively, it could be envisaged that peptides are continuously released by certain neurons as an index of their general level of activity. This, in turn might determine whether or not other neurons are active (e.g. in diurnal rhythms). An extension of this concept has been advanced by Wall and his colleagues (see Fitzgerald & Woolf 1984) for C-fibre primary afferent neurons. They suggest that peptides may be transported by axonal flow as an alternative (or rather, in addition to) electrical signalling. By this means, it is suggested that a long-term 'view' of the local environment surrounding the peripheral terminals of sensory fibres is conveyed to their central connections in the spinal cord. This, in turn, may influence receptive fields within the dorsal horn.

Of course, the concept of neurons utilising peptides as chemical signals is not new. It is well established that neurons of the hypothalamus release regulatory hormones or releasing factors which pass via the hypothalamico-adenohypophyseal portal system to control the secretion of hormones by the adenohypophysis. Such factors include thyrotropin regulatory hormone (TRH), luteinising hormone-regulatory hormone

(LH-RH) and growth hormone-release inhibitory hormone (GH-RIH). Each of these has been shown to occur in other regions of the nervous system and so may serve some function other than that recognised for the pituitary gland.

Other peptides which may have a role in the CNS have established roles in the periphery. An example here is the gastrin family of peptides which are major determinants of digestive processes.

Approaches to studying neuropeptides

Two factors may be identified as generating the rapid expansion of interest in neuropeptides in recent years. The first is the discovery by Hughes *et al.* (1975) of the endogenous opioid peptides methionine- and leucine-enkephalin. The search for an endogenous opioid was prompted by the knowledge that (a) there were specific opioid receptors for which there were selective agonists (e.g. morphine) and antagonists (e.g. naloxone) and (b) electrical stimulation of the periaqueductal grey area of the brain in rats produced an antinociceptive effect which could be blocked by naloxone (Reynolds 1969). The discovery of the opioid peptides has given credence to the view that peptides may be neurotransmitters (see also Chapter 22).

The second major influence has been the development of radioimmunoassay and immunohistochemical techniques, especially those involving monoclonal antibodies. It is now a relatively straightforward procedure to raise antibodies to small peptides. Various techniques have evolved to label these antibodies with fluorescent or other markers and so provide a means of visualising those areas of high concentration of individual peptides in the nervous system. These techniques have been so successful that there is now a vast literature on the distribution of perhaps 30 peptides but very little other information to support it. Thus, the functional role (if any) of a peptide in a given pathway remains unknown in the majority of cases. The reader should be warned also that antibodies used in many of these studies may not have sufficient specificity to distinguish between related peptides.

The synthesis and metabolism of most neuropeptides remains largely unknown although the techniques of molecular biology are proving valuable in predicting potential precursor sequences. It is not clear whether peptides are stored in the form in which they are released from the neuron or whether they are cleaved from the precursor on demand. In this respect, a peptide functioning as a fast neurotransmitter may demand a different kind of processing to a long-term neuromodulator.

Degradation of neuropeptides is likely to involve peptidases (there is little evidence for reuptake mechanisms) but it remains to be established whether enzymes specific to a given peptide are involved.

Peptides present a challenge to the pharmacologist and medicinal chemist. They require care in handling (many are absorbed onto glass) and invariably they are expensive to buy. The flexible backbone of many neuropeptides means that the molecule can adopt a large number of low energy conformations and so structure-activity relationships become extremely complex. In the literature, most attempts at modifying the biological activities of peptides have involved:

1 Studying fragments of the parent molecule;

2 The empirical substitution of single or multiple amino acid residues;

3 A combination of **1** and **2**.

Whilst these approaches have brought some success, the development of sophisticated molecular graphics facilities on computer promises to revolutionise future studies of peptide structure-activity relationships.

Standard abbreviations for amino acid residues used in the text are given in Table 14.1.

Table 14.1. Abbreviations for amino acid residues used in the text

Abbreviation	Amino acid	Abbreviation	Amino acid
Ala	Alanine	Leu	Leucine
Arg	Arginine	Lys	Lysine
Asn	Asparagine	Met	Methionine
Asp	Aspartate	Nle	Norleucine
Cys	Cysteine	Phe	Phenylalanine
Cys Cys	Cystine	Pro	Proline
Gln	Glutamine	Ser	Serine
Glu	Glutamate	Thr	Threonine
pGlu	Pyroglutamate	Trp	Tryptophan
Gly	Glycine	Tyr	Tyrosine
Ile	Isoleucine	Val	Valine

Evidence for the roles of some of the best-studied peptides in the nervous system is discussed in the following sections. The opioid peptides are considered separately in Chapters 15 and 22.

Cholecystokinin

Identification and distribution

The peptide now recognised as cholecystokinin (CCK) was identified originally as two separate active principles responsible for causing contraction of the gallbladder and stimulation of pancreatic enzyme secretion. However, Jorpes and Mutt (1966) found that both activities reside in a single 33 amino acid peptide, cholecystokinin (CCK-33), extracted from porcine intestine. CCK-39, an N-terminal extended form may serve as a precursor for CCK-33. CCK and related peptides may have neurotransmitter/neuromodulator roles in the CNS. Whilst CCK-33 and CCK-39 are both found in mammalian brain, they may act simply as precursors for the predominant form which is the C-terminal octapeptide, CCK-8.

Table 14.2. Structures of peptides related to cholecystokinin

CCK-33 (Porcine)	Lys-Ala-Pro-Ser-Gly-Arg-Val- Ser-Met-Ile-Lys-Asn-Leu-Gln-Ser- Leu-Asp-Pro-Ser-His-Arg-Ile-Ser- Asp-Tyr-Met-Gly-Trp-Met-Asp-Phe.NH$_2$ $\mid$ SO$_3$
CCK-8	Asp-Tyr-Met-Gly-Trp-Met-Asp-Phe.NH$_2$ $\mid$ SO$_3$
Caerulein	pGlu-Gln- Asp-Tyr-Thr-Gly-Trp-Met-Asp-Phe.NH$_2$ $\mid$ SO$_3$
Pentagastrin	tBoc-β.Ala-Trp-Met-Asp-Phe.NH$_2$
Big gastrin-1	pGlu-Leu- Gly-Pro-Gln-Gly-Pro-Pro-His-Leu- Val-Ala-Asp-Pro-Ser-Lys-Lys-Gln- Gly-Pro-Trp-Leu-Glu-Glu-Glu-Glu- Glu-Ala-Tyr-Gly-Trp-Met-Asp-Phe.NH$_2$ $\mid$ SO$_3$

Note the highly conserved C-terminal region. In the cholecystokinin group of peptides, the (sulphated) tyrosine residue is seventh from the C-terminus. In the gastrin group, the tyrosine residue is sixth from the C-terminus. Sulphated and non-sulphated forms are found in the CNS but the presence of the tyrosyl sulphate is important for some biological activities (see text).

Cholecystokinin is a member of the gastrin family of peptides which are characterised by a highly conserved C-terminal sequence — Gly-Trp-Met-Asp-Phe. NH$_2$ (Table 14.2). This means that studies of distribution in the CNS by radio-immunoassay or immunohistochemistry require qualification in that there may be extensive cross-reactivity between antibodies for related peptides. The problems are highlighted by the discrepancies between the reported effects of capsaicin treatment on levels of CCK in the spinal cord as measured by immunohistochemistry or radio-immunoassay. This may be because some 'CCK' antibodies recognise calcitonin gene-related peptide (Ju *et al.* 1986). However, gel filtration and HPLC analyses suggest that the main form of CCK-LI in the brain is CCK-8.

In the brain, CCK and gastrin occur in different forms which vary between species but the C-terminus of CCK appears to be conserved throughout the species. Nevertheless, variations in other parts of the molecule may render identification and quantification by immunohisto-chemistry or radio-immunoassay unreliable.

An unusual feature of these peptides is that the tyrosine residue in the C-terminal sequence is sulphated (Table 14.2). This has an important bearing on their biological activities (see below).

The following conclusions have been drawn from experiments in which the identity of the peptides was checked rigorously (Rehfeld *et al.* 1985):

Sulphated CCK-8 (Table 14.2) is the major component in the cerebral cortex although it may exist in three forms which vary in their charge characteristics.

There are also *large molecular forms* (e.g. CCK-58, CCK-33 and *C-terminal amidated fragments* of CCK-8 (CCK-7, CCK-5, CCK-4). The latter compound is potentially of interest since it binds with much higher affinity to CCK binding sites in the brain than the periphery.

N-terminal fragments are thought to be biologically inactive and probably occur as biproducts.

True gastrin has been found in only two areas of the CNS — the hypothalamo-neurohypophyseal neurons and the medulla. Gastrins in the pituitary are identical with those in antral gastrin cells, namely gastrin component 1, gastrin-34 and gastrin-17. These may be present in sulphated or non-sulphated form.

Distribution of cholecystokinin-related peptides in the CNS

Cholecystokinin is present in exceptionally high concentrations in several areas of the CNS (Fig. 14.1) and, in some of these (e.g. cerebral cortex, hippocampus, septum) it far exceeds the level of any other peptide

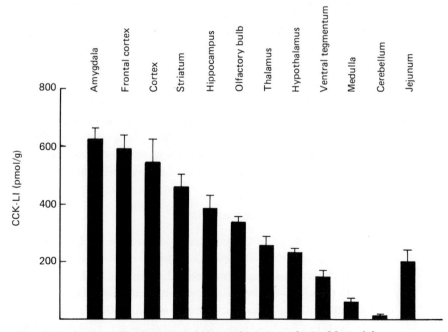

Fig. 14.1. Regional distribution of cholecystokinin in rat brain. Most of the immunoreactivity was shown to be present as CCK-8. The cholecystokinin content of rat jejunum is shown for comparison. (Redrawn from Dockray 1982.)

(Crawley 1985). There are various reports of coexistence of CCK with established neurotransmitters. For example, within the A10 group of dopamine-containing neurons, CCK is present in almost half of the cell bodies. CCK also appears to coexist with substance P in the spinal cord and with vasopressin in the hypothalamus.

In the forebrain of the rat, CCK-containing neurons are most prominent in the cerebral cortex (Fallon & Seroogy 1985), cell bodies being found especially in the piriform, anterior cingulate, entorhinal and pre-frontal areas. Most of the CCK-containing cells are local circuit neurons although some have longer projections also. Within the basal forebrain, there are CCK-LI cell bodies distributed throughout the olfactory and limbic areas and CCK is in several hypothalamic nuclei and is co-localised with other peptides in magnocellular neurons which project to the posterior pituitary. Cells in the parvocellular paraventricular nucleus project to the median eminence and to the brainstem.

Of particular interest is a group of CCK-LI neurons which overlap the A8, A9 and A10 dopaminergic cell body areas and the B6 and B8 5-HT-containing cell bodies of the raphe nuclei. CCK-containing cells in the pars compacta of the substantia nigra and the ventral tegmental area have numerous projections including those to the caudate-putamen, nucleus accumbens, olfactory tubercle, lateral septum and amygdala. Those in the caudal-dorsal and median raphe also project to the lateral caudate-putamen, septum and amygdala. Whilst, in the rat, dopamine and CCK coexist in neurons of the meso-limbic projections, in the nigrostriatal pathway they may be located entirely in separate neurons.

CCK-LI cells bodies form a sub-population of dorsal root ganglion cells and some intrinsic spinal neurons, notably in the substantia gelatinosa, contain CCK-LI also. A number of pathways exhibiting positive CCK-LI are associated with sensory systems (visual, auditory, olfactory, gustatory and visceral).

Approximately 90% of the CCK-related peptides (predominantly CCK-8) in rat hypothalamus and cerebral cortex are associated with the crude particulate fraction in tissue homogenates (Emson 1980). A high concentration of CCK-8 is present in the vesicular component, suggesting that the peptide may be stored in synaptic vesicles.

Synthesis and metabolism

Deschenes *et al.* (1984) have sequenced a cDNA encoding for prepro-cholecystokinin in the rat. This is a 95 residue peptide in which the various cholecystokinin sequences are embedded but the tyrosine at the C-terminal region is not sulphated: sulphation appears to be a post-translational process. Vargas *et al.* (1985) have identified an enzyme system (3′-phosphoadenyl 5′-phosphoro sulphate: CCK sulphotransferase) in rat brain capable of sulphating the tyrosine residue of various CCK-related peptides. Although it is associated with microsomal and synaptosomal fractions it has a rather low pH optimum for a physiologically important enzyme system. Also no marked regional differences in tissue content of the enzyme were detected and levels did not correlate with the large variations in CCK content. Furthermore, the enzyme is present in non-neuronal tissue such as liver and spleen.

The importance of the C-terminal tyrosyl sulphate group for most of the biological activities of the CCK group of peptides suggests that its removal could be a crucial step in terminating their biological actions. However, there was little evidence of desulphation of CCK-8 following release and most of the products suggested metabolism by peptidases (Vargas *et al.* 1985). The nature of these peptidases remains to be established although CCK-8, in common with some other neuropeptides, is known to be a substrate for endopeptidase-24.11 which cleaves sulphated CCK-8 at the Gly^4-Trp^5 and Asp^7-$Phe^8.NH_2$ bonds. Pig striatal membranes have the capacity to hydrolyse the same bonds and this activity is inhibited by phosphoramidon. However, phosphoramidon-insensitive capacity is present also (Matsas *et al.* 1984). It is not clear whether there are any CCK-specific degrading enzymes present.

Release from neurons

In response to depolarising stimuli, CCK-related peptides (principally CCK-8) are released from synaptosomes and slice preparations from

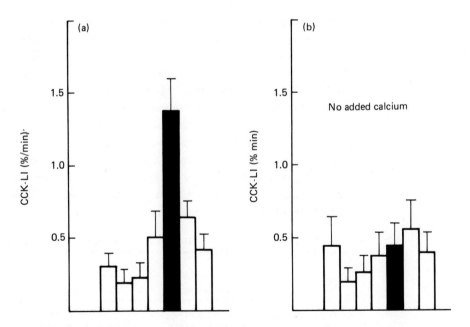

Fig. 14.2. Release of cholecystokinin-like immunoreactivity (predominantly CCK-8) from slices of rat cerebral cortex. Each column represents the release of CCK-LI (expressed as a rate constant) during a three minute collection period. Solid columns indicate presence of high potassium ion concentration (44 mM) as depolarising stimulus. Left hand panel — normal Krebs' solution: right hand panel — Krebs' solution with no added calcium. (Adapted from Emson *et al.* 1980.)

several brain areas including cerebral cortex, hypothalamus and periaque-ductal grey (see Fig. 14.2).

Electrophysiological actions

CCK-8 has excitatory effects when applied by iontophoresis to neurons in the cerebral cortex, hippocampus or dorsal horn of the spinal cord — that is, areas of the CNS which have high concentrations of CCK-LI. In common with glutamate, CCK increased the excitability and decreased the membrane resistance of pyramidal cells in the hippocampus (Dodd & Kelly 1981). The co-existence of CCK-LI and dopamine in mesolimbic neurons, prompted the determination of the effects of CCK-8 applied to the A10 dopamine cell body area of the ventral tegmental area (although recent autoradiographic evidence suggests that CCK binding sites may not be present on dopaminergic neurons). CCK-8 caused burst firing of these neurons and, surprisingly, a similar effect was observed following systemic administration of the peptide (see Emson & Marley 1983). However, when CCK is co-administered with apomorphine it potentiates the inhibitory effects of the dopamine agonist on neurons in the substantia nigra (Hommer & Skirboll 1983).

CCK receptors

Cholecystokinin is a rare example of a neuropeptide for which there is not only a potent antagonist available, but it is non-peptide in structure. Early work had shown proglumide and benzpotript (Fig. 14.3) to be weak antagonists against CCK in peripheral tissues such as guinea-pig gall-bladder (Hahne *et al.* 1981). However, their low potency (Table 14.3) rendered them of limited value and there was little convincing evidence of activity at CCK receptors in the CNS. A substantial improvement in potency was made in a systematic study of extracts of fermentation broths in a CCK-binding assay. This yielded a novel compound, asperlicin (Fig. 14.3), which had higher affinity for CCK-binding sites and was a se-lective antagonist against CCK in peripheral tissues (Table 14.3). Further improvements in potency and pharmacokinetic properties were achieved

Table 14.3. Displacement of $[^{125}I]$-CCK-8 binding in rat pancreas and guinea-pig brain

Displacing agent	IC_{50}(nM)		Ratio brain: pancreas
	Rat pancreas	Guinea-pig brain	
CCK-8	0.17 ± 0.01	0.39 ± 0.06	2.3
Proglumide	$250\,000 \pm 60\,000$	$800\,000 \pm 42\,000$	3.2
Asperlicin	184 ± 64	$>100\,000$	>543
L-364, 718	0.08 ± 0.02	245 ± 97	3063

Values quoted are IC_{50}s and so do not represent true estimates of apparent affinity. The ratio of IC_{50} values is given to demonstrate the increased selectivity obtained with asperlicin and L-364, 718. Data from Chang & Lotti (1986).

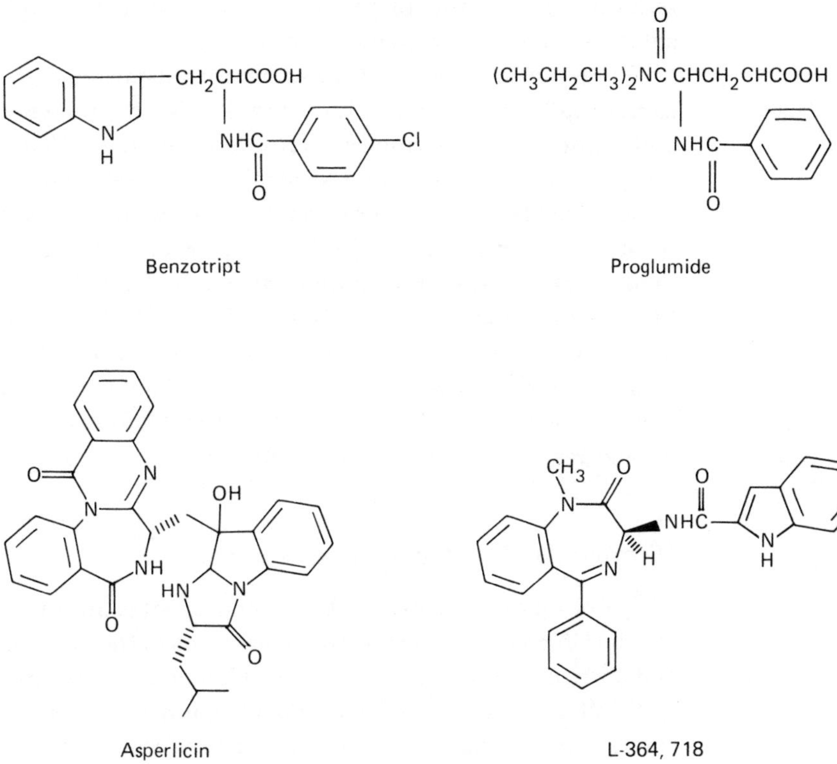

Fig. 14.3. Structures of some CCK antagonists.

through leads provided by this compound culminating in L-364, 718, which has a very high affinity ($K_i = 0.1$ nM) for CCK binding sites in the rat pancreas (Evans *et al.* 1986). Furthermore, it is a competitive antagonist against CCK-induced contractions of the guinea-pig ileum *in vitro* (pA$_2$ = 9.9) and of the guinea-pig gall-bladder *in vivo* (0.1 mg/kg, i.v.) and is active orally.

CCK antagonists identified in the rat pancreatic tissue binding assay have relatively low affinity for the CNS CCK binding site (Table 14.3) (see Chang & Lotti 1986). Assuming that CCK binding sites may be equated with functional receptors, it is becoming increasingly apparent that there are two sub-types of CCK receptor: those associated with the pancreas are designated 'Type A' whereas those widely distributed in the CNS are 'Type B' (Moran *et al.* 1986). The affinity of [125I]-CCK-33 for both sites is of the order of 1 nM but they are distinguished by the displacement profiles of related peptides. In particular, binding to sites in the brain, but not the pancreas, is displaced by peptides of the gastrin family (Innis & Snyder 1980). A further distinction is that cyclic GMP inhibits CCK binding in the pancreas but not in the brain. Whilst most of the *effects* of CCK-related peptides in the CNS depend on the presence of the tyrosyl sulphate group, this does not seem to apply to *binding sites* in the brain which show little discrimination between sulphated and non-sulphated forms.

From our knowledge of other neurotransmitter systems, it would be surprising to find an absolute distinction between receptors in the CNS and those in the periphery. The description of CCK-A and CCK-B receptors as 'peripheral' and 'central' respectively thus seems unlikely to be sustainable. Indeed, recent analyses of binding sites in brain sections by autoradiography using [³H]-L-364,718 has revealed 'peripheral' type binding sites in the brain (Hill *et al.* 1987). Thus, in confirmation of the findings of Moran *et al.* (1986), [³H]-L-364,718 binding sites were found in the area postrema, nucleus tractus solitarius and interpeduncular nucleus. CCK-A sites in the area postrema and nucleus tractus solitarius may be associated with vagal afferent projections involved in cardiovascular and respiratory control mechanisms.

Distribution of CCK-binding sites in the CNS

[¹²⁵I]-Bolton and Hunter-CCK-33 binding sites are distributed throughout the CNS with particular concentrations in the olfactory, visual, limbic and cortical areas. The presence of high concentrations in the olfactory bulb, olfactory tract and superficial laminae of the primary olfactory cortex suggests that CCK may have an important controlling influence on olfactory inputs. In particular, the established effects of CCK on feeding behaviour (see below) could be exerted in part through the olfactory system (Innis & Aghajanian 1985).

In the visual system, binding sites are present on retinal ganglion cells, their axons and in their central projection areas in the nucleus of the optic tract, ventrolateral nucleus of the geniculate and the superior colliculus. In the limbic system, CCK binding sites are found in the mamillary nuclei, the hippocampus and amygdala whilst, in the cerebral cortex, they are present in high concentrations in layers II–IV and V. In layers II and III, these sites may be involved in transmission between intrinsic interneurons. The localisation of CCK binding sites in the mesolimbic and nigrostriatal systems has been studied in more detail (Gaudreau *et al.* 1987). It appears that CCK binding sites are localised mainly on intrinsic neuron cell bodies and/or interneurons in the striatum and substantia nigra rather than dopamine-containing neurons of the nigrostriatal and mesolimbic pathways.

CCK binding sites are associated with fibre tracts in a number of locations. This may reflect transport of receptors along the neuron rather than a functional role on axons. Ligation of the vagus nerve in the rat results in an accumulation of binding sites proximal to the ligature (Innis & Aghajanian 1985) but it remains possible that CCK receptors are functionally linked on axons or nerve terminals.

Functional roles of cholecystokinin

The peripheral involvement of CCK-related peptides in normal digestion is well-established. In the CNS, their roles are far less clear but at least three possibilities are under consideration.

Modulation of activity in dopamine pathways

The co-existence of CCK-8 and dopamine in neurons of the mesolimbic system has prompted speculation that there may be a functional interaction between them. However, there are conflicting reports on such interactions. CCK-8 has been claimed to inhibit or to enhance the actions of dopamine in electrophysiological, biochemical and behavioural studies and there is similar uncertainty as regards interactions at the level of their release, although this may be explained in part by the doses used in each study. Crawley (1985b) has reported that CCK-8, when administered bilaterally into the nucleus accumbens of the conscious rat, potentiates the locomotor response to dopamine, administered simultaneously by the same route, or the stereotopy induced by apomorphine administered subcutaneously. A similar potentiation was not observed when CCK-8 was co-administered with dopamine into the caudate nucleus. It was concluded that, where the peptide and catecholamine were co-stored, CCK may have a modulating influence on dopamine-mediated transmission.

Notwithstanding the lack of unanimity on the interaction between CCK and dopamine systems, the CCK agonist analogue, ceruletide, has been tested in the clinical management of schizophrenia, but again, no clear-cut result was obtained.

Satiety

CCK and related peptides, administered by a peripheral or central route, cause inhibition of feeding in a variety of species (Dockray 1982). In man, satiety has been observed following intravenous administration of CCK. There is considerable debate as to whether this involves a peripheral or central action. A major difficulty in establishing the locus of action is that it is not clear how readily the peptide crosses the blood-brain barrier, although there are reports that $[^{125}I]$-CCK-8 administered to rabbits intracerebroventricularly appears in the plasma quite rapidly.

In the rat, bilateral vagotomy (abdominal level) abolishes the satiety effects of CCK as do bilateral lesions of the nucleus of the solitary tract, midbrain and paraventricular nucleus of the hypothalamus. This suggests a predominantly peripheral action of CCK which leads to activation of vagal afferent pathways. However, central sites of action may be important under certain conditions and there is considerable evidence implicating a central role for CCK in the control of feeding. It is interesting to note that there is a reduced level of CCK in the brains of obese mice compared to their lean littermates (see Baile *et al.* 1986).

Analgesia

CCK-8 and caerulein produce antinociceptive effects when administered systemically or centrally (i.c.v. or intrathecally) in rodents. In some cases, CCK-8 appears more potent than morphine (see Sheehan & De Belleroche 1984). Curiously, though, CCK-8 is reported to antagonise the antinociceptive effects of morphine and opioid peptides. Conversely, the weak CCK antagonist, proglumide, potentiates the effects of morphine whilst the opioid antagonist, naloxone, potentiates CCK-induced antinociception (see Pittaway *et al.* 1987).

Administered intrathecally in the rat, CCK-8 produces antinociceptive effects but, at higher doses, a hyperalgesic effect may result (Pittaway *et al.* 1987). CCK-4 and pentagastrin are ineffective as antinociceptive agents, suggesting that a CCK-A type receptor may be involved in the mechanism for CCK-8 and caerulein.

Bombesin

Identification

Bombesin was first isolated from the skin of amphibia (Bombina) by Erspamer and colleagues. It is a tetradecapeptide having a considerable

Table 14.4. Structures of some peptides related to bombesin

Bombesin	pGlu-Gln-Arg- Leu-Gly-Asn-Gln-Trp-Ala-Val-Gly-His-Leu-Met.NH$_2$
Alytesin	pGlu-Gly-Arg- Leu-Gly-Thr-Gln-Trp-Ala-Val-Gly-His-Leu-Met.NH$_2$
Litorin	pGlu-Gln-Trp-Ala-Val-Gly-His-Phe-Met.NH$_2$
Ranatensin	pGlu-Val-Pro-Gln-Trp-Ala-Val-Gly-His-Phe-Met.NH$_2$
Neuromedin C	Gly-Asn-His-Trp-Ala-Val-Gly-His-Leu-Met.NH$_2$
Gastrin-releasing peptide	Ala-Pro-Val-Ser-Val-Gly- Gly-Gly-Thr-Val-Leu-Ala-Lys-Met-Tyr-Pro- Arg-Gly-Asn-His-Trp-Ala-Val-Gly-His-Leu-Met.NH$_2$
Neuromedin B	Gly-Asn-Leu-Trp-Ala-Thr-Gly-His-Phe-Met.NH$_2$
Neuromedin B32	Ala- Pro-Leu-Ser-Trp-Asp-Leu-Pro-Glu-Pro-Arg- Ser-Arg-Ala-Gly-Lys-Ile-Arg-Val-His-Pro- Arg-Gly-Asn-Leu-Trp-Ala-Thr-Gly-His-Phe-Met.NH$_2$

Bombesin, alytesin, litorin and ranatensin are amphibian peptides. Note the high degree of conservation of C-terminal residues but that the penultimate residue may be leucine or phenylalanine. Neuromedin B-30 lacks the N-terminal pair of residues in neuromedin B-32.

degree of sequence homology with other amphibian peptides (alytesin, litorin and ranatensin) — see Table 14.4. Bombesin has some pharmacological characteristics in common with CCK and substance P and has some structural features in common with the latter.

In mammals, bombesin-like immunoreactivity has been identified in the CNS and in the stomach. Peptides extracted from CNS tissue, in particular the spinal cord, include the decapeptide, neuromedin B and two extended forms (B-30 and B32) plus another decapeptide, neuromedin C (Minamino et al. 1985; Roth et al. 1983) whilst a 27 amino acid peptide, gastric gastrin-releasing peptide (GRP) has been isolated from porcine stomach (Table 14.4). All of these peptides have much of the C-terminal sequence in common and it is here that the key elements for biological activity appear to be located.

Distribution of bombesin-like peptides

Bombesin-like immunoreactivity may represent one or more of the several related peptides depicted in Table 14.4 or indeed, as yet unidentified peptides. In peripheral tissues of the rat, the gastrointestinal tract has some of the highest levels where the immunoreactivity appears to be associated with nerve fibres, especially in the myenteric plexus, but also in the sub-mucosal plexus and mucosa (Dockray et al. 1979). However, in man it is present in endocrine-like cells.

In the rat CNS, the highest levels of bombesin-like immunoreactivity are present in the substantia gelatinosa and nucleus tractus solitarius and also in the interpeduncular nucleus and arcuate nucleus. Mesolimbic areas (amygdala, nucleus accumbens and stria terminalis) also contain bombesin-like immunoreactivity.

Highest levels of neuromedin C-LI were found in the pituitary gland with somewhat lower levels in the olfactory bulbs, hippocampus, striatum, cortex and hypothalamus (Minamino et al. 1984), the tissue content of neuromedin B being greater than that of neuromedin C. The two peptides may be representatives of two families of bombesin-like peptides — the neuromedin B group and the neuromedin C/gastrin-releasing peptide group (Minamino et al. 1985).

Pharmacological effects

Bombesin has a stimulant action on gastrointestinal and uterine smooth muscle, and on the release of gastrin and cholecystokinin in the gastrointestinal tract, amylase and trypsinogen from the pancreas and growth hormone from the pituitary gland. In most species, bombesin causes renin secretion, a slow onset hypertensive action and an antidiuretic effect.

Among the reported central actions of bombesin are inhibition of gastric acid secretion, increased sympathetic outflow, antinociceptive effects, hyperglycaemia and stereotyped scratching behaviour and, in common with CCK, bombesin causes satiety. Bombesin has been implicated in the induction or maintenance of certain tumours.

Generally, bombesin appears to have an excitatory action on central neurons (Dreifuss & Raggenbass 1986). In the hemisected spinal cord of the frog, bombesin causes a tetrodotoxin-sensitive depolarisation of motoneurons (Nicoll 1978).

Receptor sub-types

On the basis of relative activities of bombesin-like peptide agonists in a range of bioassay preparations, it appears that there may be two sub-types of receptor which have different C- and N-terminal structural requirements. However, this remains to be confirmed with selective antagonists.

A number of neurokinin antagonists have been shown to block the effects of bombesin in functional pharmacological test systems. For example, Jensen et al. (1984) found that, in the guinea-pig pancreas, [D.Arg^1,D.Pro^2,D.Trp^{7,9},Leu^{11}]-SP(1–11) inhibited the stimulatory action of bombesin-related peptides (and of substance P but not CCK-8, carbachol or VIP) on amylase secretion. Binding of [^{125}I]-[Tyr^4]-bombesin in the pancreas was displaced by the antagonist but not by substance P itself. In brain slice preparations, Yachnis et al. (1984) found that three substance P antagonists (each having D.Trp substitutions at positions 7 and 9 of substance P) inhibited the binding of [^{125}I]-[Tyr^4]-bombesin and, one of them ([D.Arg^1,D.Trp^{7,9},Leu^{11}]-SP(1–11), spantide (see p. 231) antagonised the actions of bombesin in promoting hypothermia or grooming following i.c.v. injection in the rat. However, other studies have not confirmed this (see Pappas et al. 1985).

Antagonism of the effects of bombesin by some 'substance P antagonists' is perhaps not surprising in view of (a) the similarity in C-terminal sequences of bombesin and the tachykinins (see Tables 14.4, 14.5) and (b) the low affinity of substance P antagonists compared to substance P itself, suggesting that the compounds available are a less than perfect 'fit' at neurokinin (substance P) receptors.

A series of [D.Phe^{12}]-bombesin analogues is reported to have selective antagonist activity against bombesin-induced amylase release in the guinea-pig pancreas (Heinz-Erian et al. 1987). Each had an apparent affinity constant of about 5 μM in functional tests and they may provide useful leads to establish whether there are sub-classes of bombesin receptor.

Functional roles

Although no physiological role has been established for bombesin-like peptides, comparison of their relative distributions and pharmacological actions draws attention to some areas of interest.

Gastric secretion

Bombesin or GRP, when injected i.c.v. or into specific hypothalamic nuclei, inhibit stimulated gastric acid secretion in several species (Tache *et al.* 1986). Conversely, peripheral administration of bombesin in dog, cat or man produces increased secretion. It is known that sympathetic outflow increases following central administration of bombesin, and it is likely that the inhibitory effects on gastric secretion are mediated through the sympathetic rather than the parasympathetic system.

Satiety

In common with cholecystokinin, bombesin-like peptides, administered centrally or peripherally, reduce food intake in the rat (see Negri 1986) but it is not clear whether similar mechanisms are involved.

Hyperglycaemia

Administered i.c.v., bombesin produces a powerful hyperglycaemic effect; in order to achieve the same response to systemic administration, a dose 10 000 times greater than that effective centrally is required. The probable mechanism of action is an increase in sympathetic outflow leading to raised plasma adrenaline concentrations and hence decreased plasma insulin and increased glucagon (see Nemeroff *et al.* 1982).

Sensory transmission in the spinal cord

In the spinal cord of the cat and rat, levels of bombesin-like immunoreactivity are substantially higher in the dorsal than the ventral horn. In common with CCK and substance P, the highest concentrations are in the superficial layers of the dorsal horn (O'Donohue *et al.* 1984). Autoradiographic localisation of $[^{125}I]$-$[Tyr^4]$-bombesin binding revealed a similar pattern of distribution. Most of the bombesin-like immunoreactivity in the spinal cord appears to be contained in primary afferent neurons since it is present in dorsal root ganglion cells and levels are reduced following dorsal root section. Nevertheless, some bombesin-containing cells seem to be intrinsic spinal neurons (Massari *et al.* 1983). $[^{125}I]$-$[Tyr^4]$-bombesin binding in the spinal cord is unaffected by dorsal root section suggesting that bombesin receptors may be located postsynaptically.

When injected intrathecally into the conscious mouse, bombesin and GRP cause biting and scratching behaviour — an effect again shared by substance P, although the duration of the response to the bombesin group of peptides is considerably longer (O'Donohue *et al.* 1984).

The increased locomotor activity which follows administration of bombesin i.c.v. appears dependent on dopamine pathways since it is antagonised by the dopamine antagonist/neuroleptic, fluphenazine, or by prior treatment with the dopamine neurotoxin, 6-hydroxydopamine (Merali *et al.* 1985).

Hypothermia

Administered i.c.v., bombesin produces a profound fall in body temperature in animals placed in a cold environment but, in a warm environment, a hyperthermic response is observed. Thus, the animals become truly poikilothermic (see Nemeroff *et al.* 1982).

The tachykinins

Introduction

In 1931, von Euler and Gaddum reported that extracts of equine intestine contained a smooth muscle spasmogen which was not antagonised by atropine. The active principle was given the name 'substance P': this derives from the powdered form in which the laboratory standard (against which extracts were assayed) was held. Substance P was subsequently shown to be peptide in nature but its sequence remained unresolved until 1971 when the structure of a sialogogic peptide in the hypothalamus was fully characterised and then synthesised by Chang and Leeman.

Substance P is but one member of a family of peptides (the

Table 14.5. Structures of some naturally-occurring tachykinins

	1	2	3	4	5	6	7	8	9	10	11
Substance P	Arg-	Pro-	Lys-	Pro-	Gln-	Gln-	Phe-	Phe-	Gly-	Leu-	Met.NH$_2$
Physalaemin	pGlu-	Ala-	Asp-	Pro-	Asn-	Lys-	Phe-	Tyr-	Gly-	Leu-	Met.NH$_2$
Uperolein	pGlu-	Pro-	Asp-	Pro-	Asn-	Ala-	Phe-	Tyr-	Gly-	Leu-	Met.NH$_2$
Phyllomedusin		pGlu-	Asn-	Pro-	Asn-	Arg-	Phe-	Ile-	Gly-	Leu-	Met.NH$_2$
Eledoisin		pGlu-	Pro-	Ser-	Lys-	Asp-	Ala-	Phe-	Ile-	Gly-	Leu-Met.NH$_2$
Kassinin	Asp-	Val-	Pro-	Lys-	Ser-	Asp-	Gln-	Phe-	Val-	Gly-	Leu-Met.NH$_2$
Neurokinin A			His-	Lys-	Thr-	Asp-	Ser-	Phe-	Val-	Gly-	Leu-Met.NH$_2$
Neurokinin B			Asp-	Met-	His-	Asp-	Phe-	Phe-	Val-	Gly-	Leu-Met.NH$_2$
Neuropeptide K	Asp-Ala-Asp-Ser-Ser-Ile- Glu- Lys- Gln-Val-Ala-Leu- Leu-Lys-Ala-Leu-Tyr-Gly- His- Gly- Gln-Ile-Ser-His- Lys-Arg-His-Lys-Thr-Asp-Ser- Phe-Gly-Leu-Met.NH$_2$										

Solid bars indicate highly conserved residues in the C-terminus. Neuropeptide K may be the immediate precursor of neurokinin A.

tachykinins) which occur widely in the animal kingdom. Quite recently, groups working independently in Japan and the United Kingdom isolated two novel mammalian tachykinins which are referred to in the literature by several names. This has now been resolved with the general acceptance of the terms 'neurokinin A' and 'neurokinin B'. Structures of some tachykinins are given in Table 14.5.

Note that the family is characterised by the highly conserved C-terminal sequence Phe-X-Gly-Leu-Met.NH$_2$ (where X is an aromatic (Phe, Tyr) or aliphatic (Ile, Val) residue. The residue at X may confer some receptor selectivity on the molecule. The N-terminus is more variable although there are points of similarity in a number of the peptides.

Distribution

The most detailed distribution studies have been directed towards substance P-like immunoreactivity (SPLI) (Cuello *et al.* 1982; Hökfelt *et al.* 1982) although it may be that some reports in the literature involve antibodies which do not distinguish between the three mammalian tachykinins. Nevertheless, antibodies directed towards neurokinin A or neurokinin B have revealed different distribution patterns suggesting that much of the SP-LI does indeed represent authentic substance P.

There is a large number of substance P-immunoreactive cell bodies in the central nervous system of the rat (Ljungdahl *et al.* 1978). There is an important substance P-containing projection from the caudate putamen to the substantia nigra pars reticulata and compacta. There are high concentrations of neurokinin A and neurokinin B in the substantia nigra also; indeed, this area has the highest concentration of neurokinin B described (Kimura *et al.* 1985). From the medial habenula, SPLI-containing neurons project to the lateral habenula, the ventral tegmental area and the interpeduncular nucleus and to the dorsal raphe nucleus. At least some of the raphe projections to the spinal trigeminal nucleus and to the dorsal and ventral horns of the spinal cord contain SPLI and thyrotropin-releasing hormone in addition to 5-HT.

Substance P-containing neurons in the medial amygdala have connections with the central amygdala and, via the stria terminalis, with the hypothalamus. Some cells arising in the brainstem project to the frontal cortex but, in general, concentrations of neurokinin B exceed cortical levels of substance P and neurokinin A (Table 14.6).

The nucleus of the tractus solitarius receives substance P-immunoreactive fibres which probably arise from the sensory ganglia of the VII, IX and X cranial nerves. The nucleus spinalis of the trigeminal nerve has a heavy innervation from the trigeminal ganglia. Peripheral branches of these and of cells in the dorsal root ganglia project to blood vessels, glands and epidermis of the skin and adventitia of the gastrointestinal tract.

Table 14.6. Gross distribution of substance P, neurokinin A and neurokinin B in the CNS of the rat

Region of CNS	Immunoreactivity (pmol/g wet weight)			Molar ratio	
	Neurokinin A	Neurokinin B	Substance P	SP : NKA	SP : NKB
Substantia nigra	277.9 ± 42.5	37.2 ± 5.9	840.3 ± 78.9	3.0	22.6
Striatum	38.6 ± 3.5	13.9 ± 2.1	155.9 ± 18.3	4.0	11.2
Spinal cord	45.8 ± 0.3	18.8 ± 1.3	127.7 ± 11.0	2.8	6.8
Cerebral cortex	2.6 ± 0.3	14.5 ± 1.5	10.8 ± 0.8	4.2	0.7
Cerebellum	1.6 ± 0.5	1.6 ± 0.4	4.7 ± 0.4	2.9	2.9

Values are mean ± S.D. obtained from six animals. Tachykinin levels were measured by radio-immunoassay and HPLC. From Kimura *et al.* (1985).

Synthesis and metabolism

Two tachykinin precursors have been identified in bovine brain (Nawa *et al.* 1983). α-preprotachykinin contains the substance P sequence whilst β-preprotachykinin contains both the substance P and neurokinin A sequence. It is not clear to what extent substance P and neurokinin A may be processed separately nor whether their release from neurons is linked. The precursor for neurokinin B has yet to be reported. The 35 residue peptide, neuropeptide K, which has neurokinin A as its C-terminal sequence may be an immediate precursor for the latter peptide (Tatemoto *et al.* 1985).

The principal means of terminating the actions of tachykinins is believed to be metabolism and several enzyme systems having the capacity to metabolise substance P have been identified (see Krause 1985). These include:

Substance P endopeptidase — a membrane bound neutral metalloendopeptidase. This cleaves substance P at the Gln^6-Phe^7, Phe^7-Phe^8 and Phe^8-Gly^9 bonds. Its K_m value with substance P as substrate is 29 μM and it is not inhibited by phosphoramidon.

Endopeptidase 24.11 — this is found widely in tissues such as kidney, heart, pancreas, pituitary and brain. It cleaves substance P at the Gln^6-Phe^7, Phe^7-Phe^8 and Gly^9-Leu^{10} bonds and is inhibited by phosphoramidon.

Post-proline cleaving enzyme — this is a cytoplasmic enzyme which cleaves at the carboxyl side of l-prolyl residues (positions 2 and 4 in substance P) and has high catalytic efficiency with substance P as substrate. It has been suggested that this enzyme may be involved in the generation of N- and C-terminal fragments which have different biological functions (see p. 229). If this were the case, and post-proline cleaving enzyme has access to substance P in nerve terminals or in the synaptic cleft, then this enzyme could be considered the final step in the expression of this neuropeptide.

Undoubtedly, other possibilities exist for the metabolism of tachykinins. Indeed, Chubb *et al.* (1980) have noted the parallel distribution of substance P and acetylcholinesterase in several areas of the CNS. Furthermore, they report that substance P is cleaved by this enzyme at the Gln^6–Phe^7, Phe^7-Phe^8 and Leu^{10}–Met^{11}.NH^2 bonds through a mechanism which is blocked by acetylcholine and diisopropylphosphofluoridate but not eserine or edrophonium. Whilst the rate of metabolism is slow compared to that of acetylcholine, it points to the fact that acetylcholinesterase may have roles other than those associated with cholinergic transmission.

Release of tachykinins

Release of tachykinins from the peripheral and central nervous systems has been demonstrated *in vitro* and *in vivo*. Substance P levels (measured by radio-immunoassay and, in many cases, characterised by HPLC as being authentic substance P) are elevated by high potassium concentrations or electrical stimulation in perfusates from neonatal rat isolated spinal cord, dorsal root ganglion cells in culture and slices of spinal cord. Yaksh *et al.* (1980) perfused the intrathecal space around the spinal cord of the anaesthetised cat and demonstrated a release of SPLI in response to electrical stimulation of the sciatic nerve at Aδ/C fibre strengths but not Aα/Aβ strengths. The release was reduced by morphine via a naloxone-sensitive mechanism and this has a bearing on the roles of substance P and opioid systems in nociception (see Chapter 22).

A marked increase in the release of endogenous substance P from the substantia nigra was noted following depolarisation of cell bodies in the caudate nucleus of the anaesthetised cat (Michelot *et al.* 1979).

Release of SPLI from peripheral terminals of sensory neurons has been demonstrated following antidromic stimulation of trigeminal afferents in the tooth pulp and eye of the cat and rabbit and the sciatic nerve afferents to the skin of the hindlimb footpad in the rat. Neurokinin A and substance P are released from vagal afferent nerves in the respiratory tract of the guinea-pig when challenged with the irritant substance capsaicin.

Receptor sub-types

Most of the biological actions of the tachykinins are dependent on the essential integrity of the conserved C-terminal region. However, there are actions peculiar to substance P itself which are dependent on the charged basic residues (Arg^1 and Lys^3) of the N-terminus. Particular examples of this are the release of histamine from mast cells and chemotactic effects. These latter effects are shared by other non-tachykinin basic peptides and so it is not clear whether a tachykinin receptor is involved (see Foreman & Jordan 1983).

Pioneering work by Erspamer and colleagues in which a range of naturally-occurring tachykinins were tested on a great variety of

Table 14.7. Classification of functional neurokinin receptors

NK-1	*Example tissues:*
	Guinea-pig ileum, longitudinal smooth muscle — direct contractile response
	Rabbit thoracic aorta — endothelium-dependent relaxation
	Rat salivary gland — stimulation of secretion
	Activities of naturally-occurring tachykinins:
	Physalaemin = Substance P > Eledoisin > Neurokinin A > Neurokinin B
	Selective agonists:
	Substance P methyl ester, [pGlu^6, Pro^9]-SP (6–11)
NK-2	*Example tissues*:
	Rat vas deferens — potentiation of twitch response to field stimulation
	Rat colon muscularis mucosae — contraction
	Rabbit pulmonary artery — endothelium independent contraction
	Activities of naturally-occurring tachykinins:
	Neurokinin A > Neurokinin B > Substance P > Physalaemin
	Selective agonists:
	[pGlu^6, D.Pro^9]-SP (6–11), [Nle^{10}]-NKA (4–10)
NK-3	*Example tissues:*
	Rat portal vein — contraction
	Guinea-pig ileum — atropine-sensitive, indirect contractile response of longitudinal smooth muscle
	Activities of naturally-occurring tachykinins:
	Neurokinin B > Neurokinin A > Substance P > Physalaemin
	Selective agonist:
	Succcinyl-[Asp^6, MePhe^8]-SP (6–11) ('senktide')

preparations *in vitro* and *in vivo* revealed marked differences in rank orders of agonist activities. Lee *et al.* (1982) extended these observations and they proposed a two-receptor classification with the sub-types denoted SP-P and SP-E. 'P' and 'E' refer to physalaemin and eledoisin as potent agonists in each case. Subsequent work, especially that of Regoli and co-workers and Laufer and co-workers indicated the existence of a third receptor sub-type (NKB or SP-N respectively). Confusion has arisen in the literature because of the proliferation of nomenclature for receptor sub-types defined by functional or binding studies but this was resolved at an international symposium in 1986. The agreed nomenclature for the three receptor sub-types is NK-1, NK-2 and NK-3 (NK = neurokinin) (see Henry *et al.* 1987). The basis of the classification derived from functional tests is outlined in Table 14.7.

Note that in Table 14.7 the receptor types are defined solely in terms of agonist activities. Whilst many compounds have been claimed to be competitive tachykinin antagonists, they have shortcomings in terms of potency and selectivity which limits their usefulness for receptor characterisation. Most of the compounds have followed the leads established by Folkers' and Regoli's groups in which positions seven and nine in the substance P sequence are substituted with D.trytophan. Two examples are as follows:

Arg-Pro-Lys-Pro-Gln-Gln-Phe-Phe-Gly-Leu-Met.NH$_2$
(substance P)
D.Arg-Pro-Lys-Pro-Gln-Gln-D.Trp-Phe-D.Trp-Leu-Leu.NH$_2$ (Spantide)
Pro-Gln-Gln-D.Trp-D.Trp-D.Trp-Leu-Met.NH$_2$

These latter two compounds have pA$_2$ values of approximately 6.5 against substance P on the guinea-pig ileum in the presence of atropine to block NK-3-mediated events.

Neurokinin receptors in the CNS have proved difficult to characterise. Technical difficulties associated with electrophysiological techniques (low transport numbers in iontophoresis, adsorption to glass, etc.) are a considerable obstacle. There are few reports in which neurokinin receptor antagonists have been shown to block the effects of neurokinin agonists and, indeed, there are numerous examples of antagonists having apparent agonist (i.e. depolarising/excitatory) effects (see Brown *et al.* 1985).

When using brief (0.1–2.0 seconds) applications of substance P to produce depolarisation responses in ventral roots of the neonatal rat spinal cord *in vitro*, Akagi *et al.* (1985) have demonstrated an antagonist effect of [D.Arg^1,D.Pro^2,D.Trp^{7,9}]-SP(1-11). Furthermore, this group has devised a remarkable technique whereby the spinal cord, sensory roots and tail are dissected out intact. Ventral root potentials can be recorded in response to pinching the tail and these responses are blocked by opioid agonists and enhanced by bicuculline but they are unaffected by [D.Arg^1,-D.Pro^2,Trp^{7,9}]-SP(1–11). However, when ventral root potentials are evoked by perfusion of the tail with a solution containing capsaicin as an irritant, opioids and the substance P antagonist are both effective. The authors concluded that substance P may be involved in chemosensitive rather than mechanosensitive processes (Otsuka *et al.* 1985).

Binding studies

Radioligand binding studies have used [^{3}H]- or [^{125}I]-Bolton and Hunter labelled tachykinins since the antagonists so far described have relatively low affinities.

Autoradiographic visualisation of binding sites for substance P shows a similar distribution pattern irrespective of whether [^{125}I]-physalaemin, [^{125}I]-Bolton and Hunter substance P or [^{3}H]-substance P is used as labelled ligand (Quirion & Dam 1985). In the CNS of the rat, high densities of binding sites are observed in the olfactory bulb, caudate-putamen, septum, amygdalo-hippocampal area, superior colliculus, locus coeruleus, nucleus tractus solitarius and in laminae I, II and X of the spinal cord. These sites, although not characterised at each location, are likely to be equivalent to NK-1 functional receptors.

If [^{125}I]-Bolton and Hunter neurokinin A is used as labelled ligand, a

Table 14.8. Comparative distribution of substance P and neurokinin A binding sites in the central nervous system of the rat

Area	Binding sites	
	*SP	*NKA
Olfactory bulb	+ + + +	+ + +
Cingulate cortex (layer 3–4)	+ +	+ + + +
Frontal cortex (layer 3–4)	+	+ + + +
Caudate putamen	+ + + +	+
Nucleus accumbens	+ + + +	+
Cortical nucleus of amygdala	+ + +	−
Hippocampus	+ +	+
Thalamus	+	−
Interpeduncular nucleus	+	−
Substantia nigra	−	+
Dorsal raphe	+ +	−
Superior colliculus	+ + + +	−
Nucleus tractus solitarius	+ + +	+ + + +
Trigeminal nucleus	+ + +	+
Cerebellum	+ + +	−
Spinal cord (laminae I, II, X)	+ + + +	+
Spinal cord (intermediolateral column)	+ + +	−

Distribution of binding sites as defined by autoradiographic analysis of radiolabelled substance P (*SP) or neurokinin A (*NKA) binding.
+ + + + very high; + + + high; + + moderate; + low; − very low densities of binding sites.
Modified from Quirion & Dam (1985).

different pattern is obtained. The binding sites are more localised and high densities are found in some areas where there are low densities of substance P binding sites (e.g. in the cerebral cortex) (see Table 14.8).

Overall, the distribution of binding sites does not always correlate well with the distribution of endogenous tachykinins. For example, areas such as the substantia nigra and ventral tegmental area, which have high levels of endogenous tachykinins, have low levels of substance P and neurokinin A binding.

Binding sites which, almost certainly, correspond to the functional NK-3 receptor have been identified in the CNS either with the relatively non-selective naturally-occurring tachykinins or, more recently, with the selective NK-3 agonist, senktide (see Table 14.7) as [^{125}I]-Bolton & Hunter-senktide (Laufer *et al.* 1986). Highest levels of binding were found in cerebral cortex followed by the olfactory bulb, hypothalamus and hippocampus, with somewhat lower levels in the striatum, midbrain, cerebellum and brainstem.

Post-receptor mechanisms

In the gastrointestinal tract, tachykinins cause contraction directly via an action on smooth muscle and indirectly through the release of other mediators, principally acetylcholine. Depolarising actions on myenteric neurons appear to be the result of a decrease in the resting potassium conductance (Katayama *et al.* 1979). Similarly, on smooth muscle there is a decrease in resting potassium conductance which increases the rate of phasic contractions. In certain tissues, NK-1, NK-2 and NK-3 receptors appear to be linked to inositol phospholipid hydrolysis (see Guard *et al.* 1987).

Functional roles of tachykinins

Sensory neurons

Most of the interest in the tachykinins has centred on their possible association with primary afferent neurons, especially those believed to be involved in nociception. If substance P or a related peptide does indeed function as a neurotransmitter at the first sensory synapse, then a drug which inhibited its release or blocked its postsynaptic action would be expected to produce analgesia (Cutting & Jordan 1974).

The central terminals of these sensory neurons are not the only points of interest. These are bipolar neurons, having cell bodies in the dorsal root ganglia, and axons projecting both to the spinal cord, via the dorsal roots, and to the periphery, where their terminals form the sensory endings. From experiments in which [^{35}S]-methionine was incorporated into substance P, it appears that only 20% of the total substance P synthesised in dorsal root ganglia is transported to the central terminals, the balance being transported to the periphery (Keen *et al.* 1982). Furthermore, SP-LI has been demonstrated in free nerve endings in the skin and viscera where it is probably involved in the control of the vasculature and perhaps other functions. Dale suggested that the chemical transmitter released at the peripheral terminals of the nerve to cause vasodilatation would be released at its central terminals also. Is substance P an example of such a compound? Certainly it is a potent vasodilator and a series of experiments involving measurement of vasodilatation and plasma extravasation in animals, intradermal injection of peptides in man and measurement of the release of histamine from mast cells suggests that substance P could play a key role in neurogenic vascular responses. In man, intradermal injection of substance P produces a spreading flare around the site of the injection and a slowly-developing wheal at the site of injection. The flare, but not the wheal response, is prevented by prior intradermal administration of a local anaesthetic or by systemic administration of a histamine H_1 antagonist. Tachykinin analogues which produce a flare response are effective histamine releasing agents *in vitro.*

Antidromic stimulation of the distal end of the saphenous nerve of the rat causes plasma extravasation in the skin of the hind-limb and this is mimicked by intra-arterial infusion of substance P at very low concentrations. The neurogenic effect is reduced in animals pre-treated with the sensory neuron toxin, capsaicin, or during infusion of a neurokinin receptor antagonist (Lembeck & Gamse 1982).

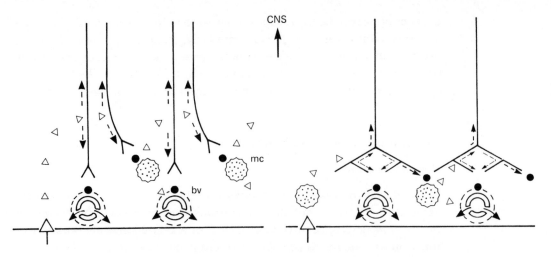

Fig. 14.4. Schematic representation of two possible models of the mechanism of the spreading flare and plasma extravasation response to injury in the skin. Left hand panel (after Lembeck & Gamse 1982) — injury (bold arrow) causes local release of chemical mediators (histamine, prostaglandins, bradykinin, potassium ions) which depolarise unmyelinated sensory neurons. The resulting action potentials (--→) spread both ortho- and antidromically causing release of substance P at their peripheral terminals which, in turn acts on blood vessels and mast cells to produce vasodilatation and histamine release respectively. Histamine may contribute to the vasodilatation but also serves to activate adjacent neurons so promoting the spread of the response. Right hand panel (after Foreman & Jordan 1983) — similar mechanism but the limits of the flare response are determined by the disposition of the terminal arborisations of neurons activated by the cascade mechanism. In both cases, histamine and substance P could be involved in vasodilatation but there is some evidence to suggest that histamine may play only a minor role. ▷, Histamine; •, substance P; bv, blood vessel; mc, Mast cell.

sensory neuron toxin, capsaicin, or during infusion of a neurokinin receptor antagonist (Lembeck & Gamse 1982).

The results of these and other studies have suggested a mechanism for the local control of the vasculature in the skin and viscera in normal physiological mechanisms (e.g. vasodilatation in response to local heating, as in a hot bath) and the response to injury, although the extent to which chronic inflammation has a neurogenic basis remains a matter of debate. Two suggested mechanisms are illustrated in Fig. 14.4. A similar mechanism may operate in intra- and extra-cranial blood vessels (Moskowitz & Barley 1985) and it has been suggested that a disturbance of the interaction of the substance P-containing neurons of the trigeminal system with their target organs (cerebral blood vessels) may contribute to the pathogenesis of migraine.

Yet another role of tachykinins in sensory nerves is suggested by the presence of SP-LI in axon collaterals which project to autonomic ganglia. Anatomical studies by Cuello and Hökfelt and their respective co-workers and electrophysiological experiments by Otsuka and his colleagues suggest that these collaterals synapse with postganglionic neurons and are, at least in part, responsible for slow EPSPs in the postganglionic

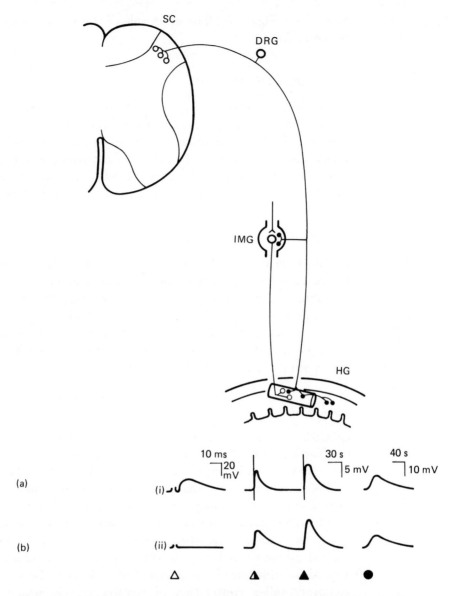

Fig. 14.5. (a) Schematic representation of organisation of substance P-containing sensory neuron innervating the hind gut. The central branch of its axon projects to the substantia gelatinosa of the spinal cord (SC) whilst its peripheral branch projects to the hind gut (HG) by way of the splanchnic nerves, inferior mesenteric ganglion (IMG) and colonic nerves. In the colon, it forms peri-and paravascular nerves and has links to the submucous plexus. In the IMG, collaterals branch extensively and form axo-dendritic synapses with sympathetic neurons. DRG — dorsal root ganglion. (b) Schematic representation of synaptic potentials and responses to pressure application of substance P in the inferior mesenteric ganglion of the guinea-pig. (i) Cholinergic fast responses to stimulation of lumbar splanchnic nerves at 0.5 Hz (△); cholinergic fast and non-cholinergic slow EPSPs in response to repetitive stimulation of the lumbar splanchnic nerves (30 (▲) or 60 (▲) stimuli at 20 Hz); depolarisation produced by pressure application of substance P (●). In (ii), responses at (△), (▲), (▲) are in the presence of hexamethonium and atropine: that at (●) is in the presence of the nicotinic antagonist dihydro-β-erythroidine and atropine. Note the difference in time scales for the various recordings. (After Cuello *et al.* 1982 and Konishi *et al.* 1985 respectively.)

neuron (see Fig. 14.5). The exact role of these axon collaterals has not been established.

Gastrointestinal tract

In the gastrointestinal tract, many of the sensory neurons having their origins in the dorsal root ganglia and sensory ganglia of the vagus nerve contain SP-LI. In addition to these extrinsic neurons, there is a population of intrinsic SP-LI neurons contained entirely within the gut wall. The distribution and functional roles of these groups of neurons have been reviewed by Pernow (1983) and Costa *et al.* (1985).

INTRINSIC NEURONS

1 *Myenteric plexus.* SP-LI positive cells in the myenteric ganglia project to local myenteric ganglia, to the longitudinal and circular muscle layers, the submucous ganglia and the mucosa. Substance P-containing cells may represent as many as 20% of myenteric neurons.
2 *Submucous plexus.* About 11% of cell bodies in the submucous plexus contain substance P and these project to the mucosa. All of these appear to contain the enzyme cholineacetyltransferase also.

EXTRINSIC NEURONS

Extrinsic substance P-containing neurons are present in smaller numbers than intrinsic SP-LI positive cells. Unlike the intrinsic neurons, these are sensitive to the substance P-depleting action of capsaicin.

Thus, substance P-containing neurons are well placed to influence gastrointestinal physiology. Release of substance P from an isolated loop of guinea-pig small intestine has been demonstrated by Donnerer *et al.* (1984) and this was increased when peristalsis was induced by raising luminal pressure and was blocked by hexamethonium, as was the peristalsis. Substance P antagonists block the non-cholinergic ascending excitatory reflex contraction of circular muscle which results from localised distension of guinea-pig small intestine (Costa *et al.* 1985).

Respiratory tract

Lundberg and colleagues have demonstrated that antidromic activation of vagal afferents in the guinea-pig respiratory tract cause an atropine-resistant bronchoconstriction and plasma extravasation response. Substance P and neurokinin A released from vagus nerve terminals appear to contribute to these responses and to the increased mucus secretion provoked by exposure to irritants such as cigarette smoke (see Lundberg *et al.* 1985). Barnes (1986) has reviewed evidence for the involvement of peptides, especially tachykinins, in the symptoms (bronchoconstriction, oedema and increased mucus secretion) associated with asthma.

Tachykinins may exert a regulatory influence over dopamine-containing neurons in the basal ganglia. The release of dopamine from the caudate nucleus in the anaesthetised cat is increased by infusion of substance P into the substantia nigra (see Glowinski *et al.* 1982), whilst a substance P blocking antibody reduces dopamine release. Substance P-containing fibres are present in the substantia nigra in close apposition to cell bodies and dendrites of tyrosine hydroxylase-positive (i.e. presumed dopaminergic) neurons, although it is not clear whether they make synaptic contact. Iontophoretic application of substance P increases the firing rate of neurons of the pars compacta in the rat and unilateral local injection of substance P into this area in the conscious rat is reported to cause contralateral turning.

Dopaminergic cell bodies in the ventral tegmental area are activated by local bilateral injection of substance P or the stable analogue [pGlu^5,MePhe^8,Sar^9]-SP(5–11) resulting in an increase in locomotor activity. This effect is blocked by haloperidol, presumably acting as a dopamine antagonist at mesolimbic dopamine-mediated synapses (Eison *et al.* 1982) (see Fig. 14.6).

In the absence of suitable neurokinin receptor antagonists, micro-injection of a monoclonal antibody against substance P has been used to block the actions of endogenous tachykinins in discrete areas of the brain (see Elliott *et al.* 1986). Injection of the antibody into the nucleus accumbens produced an apparent reduction in the turnover of dopamine and prevented the hyperlocomotor response to amphetamine, again suggesting that there is a tonic facilitatory influence of substance P on dopamine-containing neurons in the nucleus accumbens.

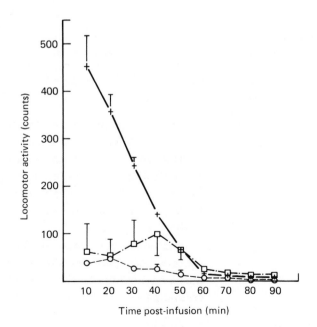

Fig. 14.6. Effect of haloperidol on the locomotor response to local injection of [pGlu^5, MePhe^8, Sar^9]-SP(5–11) (DiMeC7) into the ventral tegmental area (VTA) of the rat. + —— +, DiMeC7 (2.5 μg) + saline i.p. □ — · — □, DiMeC7 (2.5 μg) + haloperidol (0.2 mg/kg, i.p.). ○ ---- ○, Saline (2 μl) + haloperidol (0.2 mg/kg, i.p.). Haloperidol was administered 30 min prior to VTA injection of DiMeC7. Redrawn from Eison *et al.* (1982).

Calcitonin gene-derived peptides
(calcitonin and calcitonin gene-related peptide)

Occurrence and distribution

The existence of the hormone, calcitonin, and in particular, its involvement in the control of plasma calcium levels has been known for some time. The existence of calcitonin gene-related peptide (CGRP) was a recent prediction arising from a study of the calcitonin gene. This was found to encode two related but distinct mRNAs — one for the calcitonin precursor and the other for the CGRP precursor (Rosenfeld *et al.* 1983). One or other of the two peptides is expressed preferentially depending on the tissue. In the rat, CGRP is the main product in the nervous system and calcitonin in the thyroid C-cells. Slight variants on the first established α-CGRPs found in rat and human have been described. These differ by one or three amino acids respectively. Structures are illustrated in Table 14.9.

Table 14.9. Structures of some calcitonin gene-derived peptides

Calcitonin (Human)	Cys- Gly- Asn-Leu-Ser- Thr-Cys-Met-Leu-Gly- Thr-Tyr-Thr-Gln- Asp-Phe-Asn-Lys- Phe-His- Thr-Phe-Pro- Gln- Thr-Ala- Ile- Gly- Val- Gly- Ala- Pro.NH$_2$

α-CGRP (Human)

1	2	3	4	5	6	7	8	9	10
Ala-	Cys-	Asp-	Thr-	Ala-	Thr-	Cys-	Val-	Thr-	His-
11	12	13	14	15	16	17	18	19	20
Arg-	Leu-	Ala-	Gly-	Leu-	Leu-	Ser-	Arg-	Ser-	Gly-
21	22	23	24	25	26	27	28	29	30
Gly-	Val-	Val-	Lys-	Asn-	Asn-	Phe-	Val-	Pro-	Thr-
31	32	33	34	35	36	37	38	39	40
Asn-	Val-	Gly-	Ser-	Lys-	Ala-	Phe.NH$_2$			

Human β-CGRP has Asn at position 3, Met at position 22 and Ser at position 26.

Since the principal calcitonin gene peptide expressed in the nervous system is CGRP, most distribution studies have concentrated on this peptide. In common with several neuropeptides, CGRP occurs in high concentrations in the dorsal horn of the spinal cord and appears to be associated with primary afferent neurons (Skofitsch & Jacobowitz 1985). In the dorsal horn of the human spinal cord, there is a marked overlap of CGRP- and substance P-like immunoreactivity and, in the rat, there is immunohistochemical evidence that some primary sensory neurons contain both peptides (Wiesenfeld-Hallin *et al.* 1984). Other sensory nuclei having high levels of CGRP-like immunoreactivity are those of the cranial nerves such as the nucleus tractus solitarius.

Areas of the brain rich in CGRP-like immunoreactive cell bodies include the preoptic area and hypothalamus, medial amygdala, hippocampus and dentate gyrus, central grey and the ventromedial nucleus of the thalamus and the ventral tegmental nucleus. Thus, the peptide could be involved in a range of physiological functions (Skofitsch & Jacobowitz 1985).

CGRP is also widespread in the peripheral nervous system. It is present in the peripheral terminals of sensory neurons (e.g. in the skin), in neurons supplying blood vessels, the respiratory tract and throughout the gastrointestinal tract where it may be present in neurons of intrinsic or extrinsic origin (see Goodman & Iversen 1986).

Release

CGRP-like immunoreactivity is released from the isolated perfused guinea-pig lung in response to challenge with high potassium concentration or the irritant, capsaicin, or to electrical stimulation of the vagus nerve (Saria *et al.* 1987). The metabolic fate of CGRP or calcitonin once released is unknown. Their long duration of action in some tests suggests that they may be relatively stable to peptidase activity although this is not the only possible explanation.

Electrophysiological effects

In the rat forebrain, CGRP and calcitonin tend to reduce the excitability of neurons. However, when applied to myenteric neurons in the guinea-pig ileum CGRP (but not calcitonin) was a potent depolarising agent in all cells examined ($ED_{50} = 50$ nM). The reversal potential was close to that expected for a mechanism involving calcium-dependent potassium channels (Palmer *et al.* 1986). Calcitonin had no effect at concentrations up to 100 μM. This marked distinction between the two peptides contrasts with the reported similarity of effects in other systems and mutual displacement in binding studies. However, it is premature to conclude that a novel receptor for CGRP is present in myenteric neurons.

Binding studies

There are numerous reports of the occurrence and distribution of high affinity binding sites (K_D approximately 0.2 nM) for [125I]-CGRP in nervous and other tissues. Analogues lacking the disulphide bridge have substantially reduced affinity and, taken together with the similar distribution patterns in rat and human brain, provides some corroboration of the authenticity of these sites as receptors (see Inagahi *et al.* 1986).

High densities of [125I]-human- CGRP binding sites are present in several areas of the CNS including the caudal neostriatum, amygdaloid nuclei, inferior colliculus, vagal complex, dorsal periaqueductal grey, locus coeruleus and the molecular and Purkinje layers of the cerebellum. The substantia gelatinosa of the nucleus of the spinal tract has high densities of binding sites in human brain but not in the rat. Thus, high densities of [^{125}I]-CGRP binding sites are generally associated with areas high in CGRP content. In the rat, Skofitsch & Jacobowitz (1985) found dense binding in the spinal trigeminal tract and the dorsal horn of the spinal cord. These authors noted the association of high densities of binding sites with CNS areas involved in a variety of sensory functions.

Goltzman & Mitchell (1985) have reported that there appear to be distinct populations of binding sites for which either rat CGRP (rCGRP) or salmon calcitonin (sCT) has higher affinity. Thus, the hypothalamus, kidney and bone have high relative densities of sCT binding sites whilst in the spinal cord, adrenal and pituitary, there is preferential binding of rCGRP. Furthermore, they argue that, whereas sCT-preferring sites are associated with adenylate cyclase, rCGRP-preferring sites are not so linked. However, other reports suggest that this distinction is not clear and CGRP-preferring sites may be linked to adenylate cyclase in some tissues.

Pharmacological actions

CGRP has effects on a wide range of smooth muscle preparations, endocrine glands, the cardiovascular system and the CNS. In gastrointestinal smooth muscle, CGRP produces mainly contractile effects whilst, in blood vessels, it causes dilatation. In some cases, this latter effect has been shown to involve an endothelium-dependent mechanism (see Goodman & Iversen 1986).

CGRP inhibits secretion in the gastrointestinal tract and reduces feeding. In the endocrine system, the peptide reduces growth hormone secretion and it has similar effects to calcitonin in reducing plasma calcium.

Functional roles

Much of the interest in CGRP has centred on its association with primary sensory neurons. When administered directly into the spinal cerebrospinal fluid by intrathecal injection in the conscious rat, CGRP (10 or 20 μg) had little behavioural effect in its own right whereas substance P, administered by the same route, produced a pronounced caudally-directed scratching and biting behaviour. However, when CGRP and substance P were co-administered, an enhanced and prolonged scratching response was observed (Wiesenfeld-Hallin *et al.* 1984). Whether this reflects a true physiological synergism of the peptides or, for example, competition for degradative enzymes is not known. Despite these effects which follow intrathecal administration, CGRP administered i.c.v. has an antinociceptive effect in the acetic acid-induced abdominal constriction test in the mouse (Bates *et al.* 1984). In this respect, the actions of CGRP parallel those of calcitonin.

In human skin the intradermal injection of CGRP produces a local wheal and spreading flare. It is less potent than substance P but produces a third component which is a slowly-developing but intense erythema persisting for several hours (see Foreman 1987). This does not involve a neurogenic mechanism nor the release of histamine but is associated with an infiltration of granulocytes. In the rat, plasma extravasation from blood vessels in the skin is unaffected by CGRP but it potentiates the protein leakage induced by various tachykinins (Gamse & Saria 1985).

Analgesic activity

As a hormone, calcitonin is involved in calcium and phosphate metabolism. However, it has effects on the CNS including antinociception following administration i.c.v. in animals or by subarachnoid infusion in man (Pecile *et al.* 1975; Fraoli *et al.* 1982). This effect is blocked by low doses of naloxone (see Braga *et al.* 1978) but it is dependent on the integrity of central 5-HT containing neurons (Clementi *et al.* 1985). Local injections of salmon calcitonin into the periaqueductal grey area of the rat brain (an area rich in calcitonin binding sites) caused marked increases in latencies in the hot-plate test (see Fabbri *et al.* 1985).

An interesting feature of the analgesic effect produced by calcitonin is its long duration of action. However, its use in man is limited by the need to administer the peptide directly into the cerebrospinal fluid.

Calcium metabolism

Calcitonin is secreted into the general circulation by 'C'–cells of the mammalian thyroid and possibly by cells of the hypophyseal pars intermedia. It lowers raised plasma calcium concentrations by suppressing resorption of bone. Whilst CGRP has similar effects on plasma calcium, it is not clear whether this represents a normal physiological action. Nevertheless, calcium may play a key role in the overall effects of both peptides. For example, the antinociceptive effects of calcitonin are blocked by raising the extracellular calcium concentration or by co-administration of the calcium ionophore, A23187 (Bates *et al.* 1981b).

Growth hormone release

In the freely-moving conscious rat, plasma concentrations of growth hormone follow a pulsatile pattern. Intraventricular administration of rat CGRP or salmon calcitonin via indwelling cannulae suppressed the peaks of growth hormone release (Tannenbaum & Goltzman 1985). The mechanism of action and physiological significance remain to be established.

Satiety

The doses of rat CGRP and salmon calcitonin which, when administered i.c.v., inhibit growth hormone release, also cause satiety in the rat (Tannenbaum & Goltzman 1985). CGRP is located in brain areas subserving taste and appetite modulation and so it may have some functional role in this respect.

Neurotensin

Identification and distribution

The discovery of neurotensin closely followed the structural characterisation of substance P, being identified as a vasodilator principle in bovine hypothalamus (see Leeman & Carraway 1982). The sequence of the 13 residue peptide proved to be identical in bovine hypothalamus and intestine (see Table 14.10).

Neurotensin appears to have a highly conserved structure throughout mammalian species but variants and shorter analogues occur in some species (Table 14.10). One such peptide, neuromedin N, is a hexapeptide isolated from porcine spinal cord. It shows close homology with the C-terminus of neurotensin and has similar pharmacological activities (Minamino *et al.* 1984).

Table 14.10. Structures of some petides related to neurotensin

	1	2	3	4	5	6	7	8	9	10	11	12	13
Neurotensin (Bovine)	pGlu-	Leu-	Tyr-	Glu-	Asn-	Lys-	Pro-	Arg-	Arg-	Pro-	Tyr-	Ile-	Leu
Neuromedin N (Porcine)								Lys-	Ile-	Pro-	Tyr-	Ile-	Leu
LANT-6 (Chicken)								Lys-	Asn-	Pro-	Tyr-	Ile-	Leu
Xenopsin							pGlu-	Gly-	Lys-	Arg-	Pro-	Trp-	Ile-Leu

Neurotensin-like immunoreactivity is found in many areas of the CNS in several species including man. However, the brain content probably represents no more than 10% of the total body neurotensin-like immunoreactivity. Neurotensin is present in perikarya and neuronal processes and appears to be concentrated in axon terminals. In the human brain, the predominant areas of neurotensin-like immunoreactive cell groups are located in the central hypothalamus and several limbic areas (Polak & Bloom 1982; Mai *et al.* 1987). Rat brain has similarly high levels in these areas. A second group of cell bodies is located in the bed of the stria terminalis, the septal region and the amygdaloid complex.

There are some discrepancies between reports of neurotensin distribution in various species but this is perhaps most apparent in human tissue where post-mortem delay may be considerable. In most species there are high concentrations of neurotensin in the caudate nucleus, globus pallidus and putamen and in limbic areas — especially the nucleus accumbens, together with the septal area and amygdala.

In the spinal cord, along with several other neuropeptides, neurotensin is concentrated in the substantia gelatinosa where fibres run in a rostrocaudal direction. These cells appear to be intrinsic spinal neurons rather than primary afferents (Yaksh *et al.* 1982).

In the gastrointestinal tract, neurotensin is concentrated in the ileum of many species but in mammals, including man, this appears to be located in mucosal endocrine cells rather than neurons (Polak & Bloom 1982).

Other tissues with high neurotensin content in mammals are the thymus gland and, at least in the cat, the adrenal medulla. In the latter case, it is associated with a sub-population of noradrenaline-containing cells.

Synthesis and release

Cloned cDNAs encoding neurotensin have been derived from canine enteric mucosal cells and nucleotide sequencing has revealed the structure of a 170 amino acid potential precursor for neurotensin and the related peptide neuromedin N (Dobner *et al.* 1987). The precursor structure includes a further sequence: Lys-Phe-Pro-Thr-Ala-Leu, which is related to neuromedin N (Fig. 14.7), but this is bound by paired basic amino acids

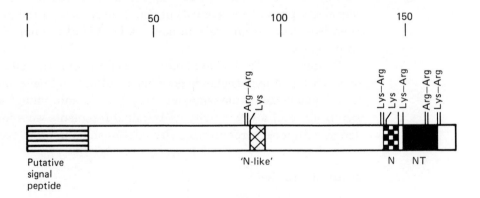

Fig. 14.7. Schematic representation of proposed preproneurotensin/neuromedin N. Numbers above figure indicate amino acid residues and the positions of the three neurotensin sequences are indicated as shaded areas ('N-like' = neuromedin N-like peptide; N = neuromedin N; NT = neurotensin). Positions of paired basic residues where cleavage is likely to occur are indicated also. (After Dobner *et al.* 1987.)

only at the N-terminus. Cleavage just prior to the neuromedin N sequence would yield a 53 amino acid peptide. Whether this is of physiological significance remains to be determined.

The release of endogenous neurotensin-like immunoreactivity has been demonstrated *in vitro* using slices of hypothalamus — an area rich in neurotensin. The potassium-evoked release is calcium-dependent and the released material has been confirmed as authentic neurotensin, although it is rapidly degraded by peptidases (Maeda & Frohman 1981). Release was also evoked by dopamine. In the decerebrate cat in which the spinal intrathecal space is perfused, electrical stimulation of the sciatic nerve causes an increase in neurotensin-like immunoreactivity appearing in the perfusate (Yaksh *et al.* 1982). Plasma neurotensin levels rise following a meal and, whilst most components appear to stimulate neurotensin release, fat is the strongest stimulus. The origin of this neurotensin is the ileum (see Bloom & Polak 1982).

Electrophysiological effects

Neurotensin is variously reported to produce excitatory, inhibitory or no effects on the firing of spontaneously firing or glutamate-driven neurons in the CNS (see Nemeroff *et al.* 1982; Baldino *et al.* 1985). Excitatory responses to neurotensin (which often outlast the duration of application) have been observed in the frontal cortex, hippocampus, striatum, lateral thalamus, preoptic/anterior hypothalamic areas and laminae I–III of the dorsal horn of the spinal cord. In the gastrointestinal tract, neurotensin causes depolarisation of myenteric neurons. Inhibitory effects have been reported in the locus coeruleus, on dopaminergic neurons in the nucleus accumbens and Purkinje cells of the rat cerebellum. In the lateral hypothalamus, the excitatory response to peripheral administration of insulin or 2-deoxyglucose was suppressed by neurotensin. An absence of any electrophysiological effects of neurotensin is reported for some locus coeruleus neurons and cells in laminae IV–VII of the dorsal horn of the spinal cord.

Baldino *et al.* (1985) have studied the effects of neurotensin fragments on the firing of hypothalamic neurons in culture and have found that the C-terminal hexapeptide sequence (NT_{8-13}) is the minimum fragment with significant excitatory activity. N-terminal fragments were inactive. This agrees with most structure-activity relationships in other tissues.

Binding studies

Specific binding sites for neurotensin have been characterised by autoradiography on brain sections using [^{125}I]-neurotensin or [^{3}H]-neurotensin. An alternative approach has been to use a photoaffinity label [^{125}I]-azidobenzoyl-[Trp^{11}]-neurotensin. ([^{125}IAB]-NT). With this technique, a similar distribution of binding has been observed with particular concentrations of label found in dopamine-containing areas such as the substantia nigra and ventral tegmental area (Rostène *et al.* 1986).

Other areas with high concentrations of binding sites include the substantia gelatinosa of the spinal cord and trigeminal nuclear complex, median raphe nucleus, hypothalamus, thalamus and stria terminalis. The cerebral cortex has only moderate levels of binding (Uhl 1982).

Pharmacological effects

Neurotensin has a wide range of pharmacological effects. On the cardiovascular system, administered peripherally or centrally, neurotensin has a hypotensive effect in most species. It causes marked vasodilatation and an increase in vascular permeability although, in some vascular beds, it causes vasoconstriction (especially in the gastrointestinal tract, subcutaneous adipose tissue and skin). Some of the actions of neurotensin on the cardiovascular system may be mediated through release of histamine.

On gastrointestinal smooth muscle, neurotensin may have a contractile (guinea-pig ileum or taenia coli) or relaxant (rat ileum) effect. Gastric acid secretion is variously reported to be increased or decreased. Neurotensin has a marked hyperglycaemic effect in some species but its mechanism is a matter of debate.

Actions on the central nervous system

When administered i.c.v. (but not i.v.) in mice, a few picomoles of neurotensin has an antinociceptive effect in the hot-plate test. Even lower doses proved effective in the acetic acid-induced abdominal writhing test (Clineschmidt *et al.* 1979). The effects seem to be independent of an action on locomotor activity although the doses used are known to reduce body temperature (Fig. 14.8). The antinociceptive effects were not blocked by the opioid antagonist, naloxone, but they were reduced by TRH administered centrally or peripherally. The mechanism of this antagonism is not known but it is worth noting that the hypothermic effect of neurotensin is also blocked (Nemeroff *et al.* 1982).

Discrete injections of neurotensin into the brain have located several sites where antinociceptive effects result. These include the medial thalamus, medial preoptic area, periaqueductal grey and central amygdaloid nucleus. Bilateral transection of the stria terminalis blocks the antinociceptive effect of intra-amygdaloid neurotensin (Bodnar *et al.* 1982).

Administration of neurotensin by the intrathecal route in the rat, at relatively high doses, causes a dose-dependent increase in the hot-plate latency but no effect in the tail-flick test. It is effective, however, in the acetic acid-induced abdominal constriction test (Yaksh *et al.* 1982). Thus, neurotensin may have an additional spinal locus of action.

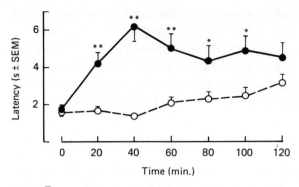

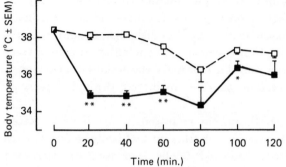

Fig 14.8 Effect of intracisternal injection of saline (open symbols) or neurotensin (1 μg) (filled symbols) in the mouse. *Upper panel*: latency of response to noxious stimulus (tail immersion in water bath at 48°C); *lower panel*: colonic temperature (ambient temperature 23°C). *$P < 0.01$; **$P < 0.001$ compared to controls. (Redrawn from Nemeroff *et al.* 1982.)

An interesting observation is that administration of a neurotensin antiserum via an indwelling cannula into the lateral ventricle of the rat causes a small, but significant decrease in response latency in the tail-flick test when using a high or moderate intensity stimulus but it has no effect on thermoregulation or locomotor activity (Bodnar *et al.* 1982). This suggests that neurotensin may have a physiological role in the control of responses to noxious stimuli.

Interaction with dopamine neurons

Administered by the i.c.v. route, neurotensin, in relatively high doses (1–15 nmol) causes a marked decrease in locomotor activity. In contrast, [D.Tyr[11]]-NT and [D.Phe[11]]-NT, whilst producing a hypothermic effect, cause an increase in locomotor activity.

The locomotor response to peripherally-administered d-amphetamine, cocaine or methylphenidate (which act, at least in part, indirectly through central dopamine pathways), is reduced by neurotensin administered i.c.v., but the response to directly-acting dopamine agonists, such as apomorphine and lergotrile, is unaffected by neurotensin. It was concluded that this effect on dopamine mechanisms is mediated through a presynaptic action on neurons in the meso-limbic system. Direct injection of neurotensin into the nucleus accumbens blocked amphetamine-induced locomotor activity without producing hypothermia. Furthermore, neurotensin appeared to be selective for the mesolimbic system since there was no effect on the stereotyped behaviours induced by amphetamine through an action on the nigrostriatal pathway (Nemeroff *et al.* 1982).

Whilst neurotensin appears to inhibit dopamine-mediated transmission in mesolimbic terminal areas, it increases activity when injected into the A10 (ventral tegmental area) cell body area. This is seen as an increase in locomotor activity and a parallel increase in dopamine turnover in the nucleus accumbens. Finally, following administration of single or chronic doses of haloperidol, there is an increase in the neurotensin content of the nucleus accumbens in the rat (see Nemeroff *et al.* 1982).

Thus, neurotensin appears to have a complex modulating effect on dopamine neurons in the mesolimbic system.

Hypothermia

Central, but not peripheral, administration of neurotensin produces a profound hypothermic effect in the rat in a cold or normal ambient temperature. At higher temperatures, no effect is seen (compare with the effects of bombesin, p. 226). This effect is dependent on the essential integrity of the C-terminus of the peptide and may be mediated in part through dopamine pathways since depletion of dopamine with 6-hydroxy-dopamine augments its action (see Nemeroff *et al.* 1982).

Somatostatin

Identification

Somatostatin was isolated from ovine hypothalamus in the course of a search for factors controlling growth hormone release. The active principle proved to be a tetradecapeptide and was sequenced and synthesised by Brazeau *et al.* (1973). In addition an N-terminal extended form has been identified (somatostatin-28 - see Table 14.11) and fragments of this not including the somatostatin-14 sequence (e.g. somatostatin-28(1–12) may occur independently. In somatostatin-28, the somatostatin-14 sequence is preceded at its N-terminus by a pair of basic residues which would facilitate 'trypsin-like' conversion to the tetradecapeptide.

Table 14.11. Structures of somatostatin-14 and somatostatin 28

1	2	3	4	5	6	7	8	9	10	11	12	13	14

Ser-Ala-Asn-Ser-Asn-Pro-Ala-Met-Ala-Pro-Arg-Glu-Arg-Lys-

15	16	17	18	19	20	21	22	23	24	25	26	27	28

Ala-Gly-Cys-Lys-Asn-Phe-Phe-Trp-Lys-Thr-Phe-Thr-Ser-Cys

Note that somatostatin-14 is identical with the sequence somatostatin-28(15–28) shown above.

Synthesis, distribution and release

The pre-prosomatostatins have been deduced for a number of species and, whereas there is a high degree of sequence homology between species, post-translational processing of a peptide may lead to important differences being introduced. For example, in the anglerfish, a large fraction of somatostatin-28 is hydroxylated at position 23 (lysine) whereas, in the catfish, (which has an atypical somatostatin-22) threonine at position 5 is O-glycosylated (see Andrews & Dixon 1986). Whilst this has no direct bearing on known mammalian forms of somatostatin, it is worth noting that such post-translational modifications could not be predicted from knowledge of the primary structure of the pre-prohormone and it remains essential to characterise the final product.

Somatostatin has a widespread distribution throughout the CNS. In the cerebral cortex and hippocampus it is believed to be present mainly in intrinsic neurons. The peptide is present in high levels in several areas of the limbic system including the amygdala, stria terminalis, habenula, septum and olfactory tubercles. Much of this somatostatin-like immunoreactivity appears to be associated with long projection neurons emanating from the periventricular hypothalamus and passing through the median forebrain bundle to the olfactory tubercle, lateral septum, habenula and also to the hippocampus. Caudally, there are projections to the locus coeruleus and substantia nigra.

Somatostatin-immunoreactive nerve fibres and terminals are present throughout the entire length of the spinal cord with the greatest concentrations in lamina II of the dorsal horn, the dorsolateral funiculus and the area adjacent to the central canal (lamina X). Some fibres are present in the ventral horn around somatic motor nuclei. The dorsal horn content is derived in part from small capsaicin-sensitive primary sensory neurons but a substantial proportion is associated with intrinsic neurons having their cell bodies in lamina II (Polak & Bloom 1986). In agreement with the suggestion that some primary sensory neurons contain somatostatin, nerve endings containing somatostatin-like immunoreactivity are found beneath the epidermis.

Most authors agree that somatostatin-14 is the predominant form of the peptide in the CNS although there are suggestions that, in rat brain, somatostatin-28 predominates in cell bodies and even that, in man, the 28 residue peptide is the major component overall.

In some peripheral neurons, somatostatin and noradrenaline are co-localised whereas, in the CNS, it may co-exist with another peptide, neuropeptide Y (NPY) or with gamma-aminobutyric acid (GABA) (see Epelbaum 1986). At all levels of the gastrointestinal tract, somatostatin-28 is the main component of somatostatin-LI in endocrine cells of the mucosa but somatostatin-14 in neurons of the non-mucosal layers. In the pancreatic islets, somatostatin is present in the 'D-cells'.

Basal plasma levels of somatostatin are the result of its secretion from the splanchnic organs. Ingestion of a mixed meal causes a rise in peripheral vein plasma levels of the peptide largely because of its increased secretion from the pancreas and stomach.

Electrical stimulation of the preoptic area of the hypothalamus *in vivo* produces an increase in portal blood levels of somatostatin. A similar but more marked effect is achieved through stimulation of the median eminence (Millar *et al.* 1983). Release from the median eminence in the conscious rat has been detected by means of a push-pull cannula system (see Epelbaum 1986). In the spinal cord of the decerebrate rabbit, somatostatin can be measured in perfusates obtained from a push-pull cannula inserted into the dorsal horn. Levels of somatostatin are increased when noxious thermal (but not non-noxious thermal or noxious mechanical) stimuli are applied to the skin. This contrasts with effects on substance P release in the same experiments since this is released only by noxious mechanical stimuli.

In vitro, somatostatin-14,-28 and somatostatin-28(1–12) are released from rat hypothalamus (as well as the cortex and amygdala) by depolarising stimuli via a calcium-dependent mechanism.

Binding studies

Radioligand binding studies employing a range of iodinated somatostatin analogues have revealed an uneven distribution of binding sites in the brain. Saturation studies suggest that there is a single population of high affinity (K_D in the low nanomolar range) binding sites but there are discrepancies in the apparent receptor numbers in different brain areas depending on the radioligand employed. This, together with the biphasic displacement profile of a cyclic somatostatin analogue have been interpreted by some authors as evidence for sub-types of somatostatin receptor (Tran *et al.* 1985) designated types 'A' (nanomolar affinity for somatostatin) and 'B' (micromolar affinity for somatostatin). Whether this is a genuine sub-class of functional receptor is not clear. It should be noted that some somatostatin analogues having complex displacement profiles are quite potent μ-opioid receptor antagonists (Maurer *et al.* 1982) and so some of their binding properties may relate to opioid rather than somatostatin binding sites.

Autoradiographic analysis of the distribution of binding sites reveals further discrepancies in that the highest densities of binding sites are not always in those areas with the highest concentrations of somatostatin. Binding sites are particularly concentrated in limbic areas such as the hippocampus, amygdaloid nuclei, bed nucleus of the stria terminalis, olfactory tubercle and septum, but the mediobasal hypothalamus and upper layers of the cortex (which have high concentrations of endogenous peptide) have relatively low densities of binding sites.

In the pituitary gland, binding sites are restricted to the adenohypophysis.

Electrophysiological effects

When applied to myenteric neurons in the guinea-pig ileum, somatostatin causes hyperpolarisation and inhibition of cell firing although depolarisation is seen occasionally. A marked degree of tachyphylaxis occurs (see North & Egan 1982).

In the CNS, again somatostatin generally has a hyperpolarising/inhibitory action. This effect has been reported in the cerebral cortex, hypothalamus, hippocampus, cerebellar cortex and spinal cord. However, as with myenteric neurons, excitatory responses have been observed in the same areas (see Kelly 1982; Kuraishi *et al.* 1985). It is possible that, in many cases, indirect effects of somatostatin are being observed and that excitatory responses are the result of disinhibition of the neuron from which recordings are being made.

Functional roles

The changes in neurotransmitter levels associated with degenerative diseases are not necessarily indicative of an important causal relationship with the symptoms of the particular disease state. However, in the case of Alzheimer's disease, there may be a more specific association of somatostatin since, along with cholineacetyltransferase activity, it has been found quite consistently to be depleted in the cerebral cortex (Davis *et al.* 1980). In Parkinsonian patients having dementia, there are also reduced levels of somatostatin in frontal cortex whereas, in non-demented patients, somatostatin levels appear normal.

Sensory mechanisms

The presence of somatostatin in some primary sensory neurons suggests that it may have a role in sensory perception. Somatostatin is known to inhibit the release of a number of neurotransmitter substances and, of particular interest in this regard is the observation that it inhibits substance P release in the dental pulp in response to electrical stimulation of the inferior alveolar nerve. If substance P or a related peptide is an important neurotransmitter at central and peripheral terminals of sensory neurons, then inhibition of its release would be expected to produce analgesia or block neurogenic vasodilatation and plasma extravasation. Somatostatin has been tested for such effects. In the rat, when administered intrathecally, it produces antinociceptive effects and, when administered intra-arterially, it blocks the vasodilator and plasma extravasation response to stimulation of the saphenous nerve (see Lembeck *et al.* 1982). However, other experiments have demonstrated that somatostatin produces a biting and scratching response which is enhanced by concurrent administration of CGRP (Wiesenfeld-Hallin 1986). Nevertheless, the antinociceptive effects of somatostatin have been extended to man in that intrathecal infusions of somatostatin in patients suffering from severe pain associated with cancer are reported to produce powerful analgesic effects. Furthermore, cluster headache (Sicuteri *et al.* 1984) and headache associated with pituitary tumours (Williams *et al.* 1987) have shown some improvement when treated with infusions of somatostatin or subcutaneous injections of the cyclic analogue SMS 201-995 respectively.

Convulsions

Szabo and Reichlin (1981) noted that the severe duodenal ulcers caused by cysteamine (β-mercaptoethylamine), due to increased gastrin and gastric acid secretion, can be prevented by administration of somatostatin. They considered the possibility that cysteamine depletes somatostatin and this they confirmed to be the case in the hypothalamus and gastrointestinal tract of the rat. The effect is quite rapid in onset but reversible and is relatively selective for somatostatin although prolactin

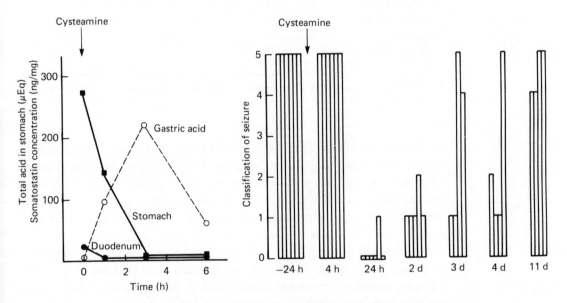

Fig. 14.9 Effect of cysteamine on gastric acid secretion and kindled seizures in the rat. *Left hand panel*: time course of changes in somatostatin content of stomach (■) and duodenum (●) and in gastric acid secretion (○) following administration of cysteamine (at arrow). (After Szabo & Reichlin 1985.) *Right hand panel*: bilateral electrodes were implanted stereotaxically into the amygdala of adult rats. Two weeks after surgery, electrical stimulation (160 μA, 60 Hz, a.c. for 1 s) was applied and the bipolar EEG recorded. Kindling was observed as an increase in the post-stimulus after discharge and this resulted in an increased susceptibility to seizure activity. For the experiment, electrical stimulation was applied to the left amygdala at sufficient strength to induce Class 5 seizures (characterised by rearing and falling). Animals were tested 24 hours before and at intervals after administration of cysteamine (200 mg/kg, i.p. at arrow) and seizures were classified on a scale from 0 (no seizures), 1 (least severe — mouth and facial movements) to 5 (most severe — see above). Each vertical bar represents a single animal: six animals were entered into the experiment but only four were followed for the entire 11 day post-cysteamine observation period. (Adapted from Higuchi *et al.* 1983.)

Table 14.12. Levels of some neuropeptides in brain nuclei and posterior pituitary following treatment with cysteamine

	Control	Cysteamine
LH-RH		
Median eminence	18.6 ± 3.3	18.1 ± 2.4
Medial preoptic nucleus	0.20 ± 0.05	0.16 ± 0.01
Vasopressin		
Median eminence	55.6 ± 12.3	47.5 ± 4.5
Anterior hypothalamus	6.05 ± 0.34	7.36 ± 0.97
Posterior pituitary	18.2 ± 0.0027	18.4 ± 0.0024
Enkephalin		
Globus pallidus	38.3 ± 7.9	53.9 ± 5.6
Middle hypothalamus	12.1 ± 1.9	11.2 ± 0.8
VIP		
Cerebral cortex	1.77 ± 0.09	1.44 ± 0.20
Suprachiasmatic nucleus	2.67 ± 0.25	2.49 ± 0.42
Nucleus accumbens	0.50 ± 0.13	0.37 ± 0.10
Cholecystokinin		
Cerebral cortex	11.9 ± 1.5	10.9 ± 1.7
Caudate nucleus	5.47 ± 1.09	4.46 ± 0.42
Somatostatin		
Median eminence	85.0 ± 8.7	26.7 ± 3.4*
Periventricular nucleus	4.3 ± 0.6	0.9 ± 0.2*

Peptide levels are expressed in ng/mg protein. Measurements were made four hours after injection of cysteamine (300 mg/kg, s.c.). Data from Palkovits *et al.* (1982). *$P < 0.05$.

levels are reduced also (Fig. 14.9 and Table 14.12). In fact, the ulcerogenic effects of cysteamine appear to be independent of depletion of somatostatin since vagotomy prevents cysteamine-induced duodenal ulceration but not the depletion of gastric somatostatin. Nevertheless, the ulcerogenic potency of cysteamine analogues is correlated with their ability to deplete somatostatin (Szabo & Reichlin 1985).

In the rat, epileptiform activity can be generated by very brief electrical stimulation of the amygdala each day (kindling). In these animals, somatostatin levels were found to be increased. Administered directly into the cerebral ventricles, somatostatin causes generalised tonic-clonic seizures. Conversely, the kindled seizure activity can be suppressed by injection of somatostatin antibodies into the lateral ventricle or by intraperitoneal administration of cysteamine (Higuchi *et al.* 1983). Taken together, these results suggest that somatostatin may have a role in the genesis of epileptiform activity.

Control of growth hormone secretion

The somatostatin-containing neurons which project from the anterior hypothalamus to the median eminence appear to be the final common pathway for inhibition of growth hormone release. Lesions of this

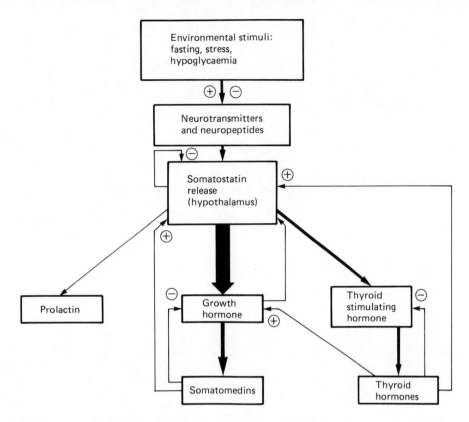

Fig. 14.10. Schematic representation of the various interactions between somatostatin release and other hormones. (Adapted from Epelbaum 1986.)

pathway lead to increased growth hormone secretion. However, this is but one component of a highly complex feedback control of the secretion of growth hormone and, indeed, thyroid stimulating hormone and prolactin. Some of the components of this system are represented in Fig. 14.10.

Acromegaly arises through excessive secretion of growth hormone from a pituitary adenoma consisting almost entirely of growth hormone secreting cells (somatotrophs). Somatostatin administered to acromegalic patients reduces growth hormone secretion but its effects are rather variable. A synthetic cyclic analogue of somatostatin (SMS 201-995) (Fig. 14.11) is a potent and long-acting somatostatin mimetic even when administered subcutaneously and has been used successfully in preliminary trials in the treatment of acromegaly (see Lamberts & del Pozo 1986).

Behavioural effects

Somatostatin administered i.c.v. or by direct injection into discrete brain areas produces behavioural changes which can be of an overall stimulant or depressant nature. Excitatory effects include barrel rotations and

Somatostatin

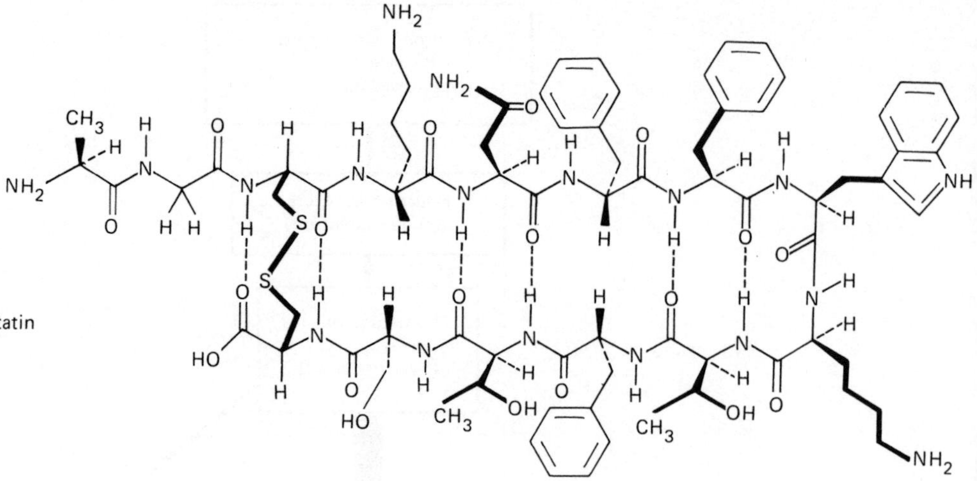

SMS 201-995

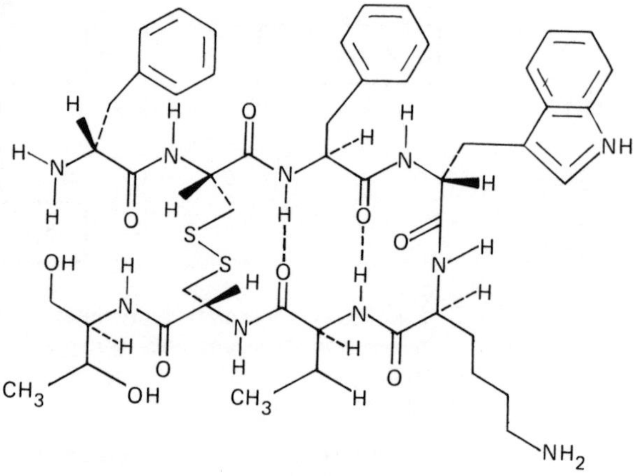

Fig. 14.11. Proposed conformations for somatostatin (*top*) and the cyclic analogue, SMS 201-995. (From Pless *et al.* 1986.)

tremor and even generalised tonic/clonic seizures in the rat. Conversely, decreased motor activity has been observed in the monkey and rat (see Epelbaum 1986).

Growth hormone is secreted during slow wave sleep and there are reports that when administered to rat, cat or man it causes an increase in paradoxical sleep. Growth hormone also increases somatostatin secretion. The possibility that somatostatin may also influence sleep has been investigated. Chronic infusion of somatostatin in the rat caused an increase in paradoxical sleep whereas cysteamine reduced paradoxical sleep. Neither treatment modified slow wave sleep (Danguir 1986). Thus, it is possible that somatostatin is one of the components of the complex processes that control sleep.

Vasoactive intestinal polypeptide

Occurrence and distribution

Vasoactive intestinal polypeptide (VIP) is a highly basic 28-amino acid peptide originally isolated from porcine intestine by Said and Mutt. As with many gut/brain peptides, VIP is related to other naturally-occurring peptides — in particular, secretin, but also pancreatic glucagon, gastric inhibitory peptide (GIP) and histidine-isoleucine-containing peptide (PHI) (see Table 14.13). VIP has a high degree of homology between mammalian species.

VIP-like peptides are found in the CNS of a wide range of mammalian species and, in the pig at least, the peptide in the brain is identical with that in the intestine. In the periphery, VIP occurs in neurons of the gastrointestinal tract, respiratory tract, urogenital tract, exocrine glands and some autonomic ganglia. In the various locations described,

Table 14.13. Structures of some peptides related to vasoactive intestinal polypeptide (VIP)

	1	2	3	4	5	6	7	8	9	10	11	12
Porcine VIP	His-	Ser-	Asp-	Ala-	Val-	Phe-	Thr-	Asp-	Asn-	Tyr-	Thr-	Arg-
PHI	His-	Ala-	Asp-	Gly-	Val-	Phe-	Thr-	Ser-	Asp-	Phe-	Ser-	Arg-
Secretin	His-	Ser-	Asp-	Gly-	Thr-	Phe-	Thr-	Ser-	Glu-	Leu-	Ser-	Arg-
Glucagon	His-	Ser-	Gln-	Gly-	Thr-	Phe-	Thr-	Ser-	Asp-	Tyr-	Ser-	Lys-
Helodermin	His-	Ser-	Asp-	Ala-	Ile-	Phe-	Thr-	Gln-	Gln-	Tyr-	Ser-	Lys-
GIP	Tyr-	Ala-	Glu-	Gly-	Thr-	Phe-	Ile-	Ser-	Asp-	Tyr-	Ser-	Ile

	13	14	15	16	17	18	19	20	21	22	23	24
Porcine VIP	Leu-	Arg-	Lys-	Gln-	Met-	Ala-	Val-	Lys-	Lys-	Tyr-	Leu-	Asn-
PHI	Leu-	Leu-	Gly-	Gln-	Leu-	Ser-	Ala-	Lys-	Lys-	Tyr-	Leu-	Glu-
Secretin	Leu-	Arg-	Asp-	Ser-	Ala-	Arg-	Leu-	Gln-	Arg-	Leu-	Leu-	Gln-
Glucagon	Tyr-	Leu-	Asp-	Ser-	Arg-	Arg-	Ala-	Gln-	Asp-	Phe-	Val-	Gln
Helodermin	Leu-	Leu-	Ala-	Lys-	Leu-	Ala-	Leu-	Gln-	Lys-	Tyr-	Leu-	Ala-
GIP	Ala-	Met-	Asp-	Lys-	Ile-	Arg-	Gln-	Gln-	Asp-	Phe-	Val-	Asn-

	25	26	27	28	29	30	31	32	33	34	35	36
Porcine VIP	Ser-	Ile-	Leu-	Asn.NH$_2$								
PHI	Ser-	Leu-	Ile.	NH$_2$								
Secretin	Gly-	Leu-	Val.	NH$_2$								
Glucagon	Trp-	Leu-	Met-	Asn-	Thr-							
Helodermin	Ser-	Ile-	Leu-	Gly-	Ser-	Arg-	Thr-	Ser-	Pro-	Pro-	Pro.	NH$_2$
GIP	Trp-	Leu-	Leu-	Ala-	Gln-	Lys-	Gly-	Lys-	Lys-	Ser-	Asp-	Trp-

	37	38	39	40	41	42
GIP	Lys-	His-	Asn-	Ile-	Thr-	Gln

The sequences are given for porcine peptides with the exception of helodermin which is derived from Gila monster venom.

VIP-immunoreactive neurons are associated with smooth muscle, blood vessels and secretory cells and this is reflected in the pharmacological actions of the peptide which include smooth muscle relaxation, vasodilatation and facilitation of secretion.

In the CNS, highest concentrations of VIP-like immunoreactivity are found in the cerebral cortex, hippocampus, amygdala and hypothalamus (Loren *et al.* 1979). Although its actual concentration is considerably lower than many other peptides, it has been suggested that more than 1% of cortical neuron cell bodies may contain VIP. In these areas of highest concentration, VIP-containing cells appear to be local interneurons but some fibres may innervate pial blood vessels. VIP-like immunoreactive cells are found also in the periaqueductal grey area, thalamus and superior colliculus and in a sub-population of primary afferent neurons projecting to the spinal cord.

Ultrastructural examination of the cat submandibular gland revealed that VIP-positive terminals appear identical with those considered to be cholinergic. These terminals contain large numbers of small clear vesicles and a limited number of large, dense core vesicles in which VIP seems to be localised (Johansson & Lundberg 1981). Studies of acetylcholinesterase or cholinacetyltransferase content of neurons supports the view that VIP and acetylcholine are co-stored in some neurons.

Release and degradation

VIP-like immunoreactivity is released into the perfusate following exposure to depolarising stimuli in slices of hypothalamus or synaptosomal preparations obtained from rat brain and there are several examples of release being demonstrated in peripheral tissues.

In common with other neuropeptides, VIP is degraded by peptidases in brain homogenates but it is not known whether there is a specific degrading enzyme.

Electrophysiological studies

VIP has a potent excitatory action on neurons in several areas of the CNS including the cerebral cortex, hippocampus and spinal cord. The depolarising effect is associated with a decrease in membrane resistance but the ionic basis of the response remains to be established (Kelly 1982).

Binding studies

Binding sites for radiolabelled VIP are widely distributed in the CNS and in peripheral organs. In rat brain slice or synaptosome preparations, saturation analyses suggest there are two binding sites: a high affinity site with a K_D of approximately 2–5 nM and a lower affinity site with a K_D of about 30–60 nM. The related peptides secretin, PHI and GIP are poor displacers of VIP binding.

Autoradiographic analysis of the distribution of binding sites indicates that the highest densities are found in the supraoptic and suprachiasmatic nuclei, the superior colliculus, pineal gland and area postrema. Moderate densities are found in the cerebral cortex, limbic areas, thalamus and hypothalamus. Because of the lack of a range of compounds having well-defined pharmacological actions at VIP receptors it is difficult to establish whether these radioligand binding sites are indeed functional receptors. However, there are indications that sub-types of receptor for the VIP family of peptides may be distinguishable. Many of the actions of VIP appear to be linked to activation of adenylate cyclase. If the relative activities of VIP- and secretin-like peptides on stimulation of adenylate cyclase are compared in a range of tissues, it is possible to distinguish between VIP-preferring and secretin-preferring systems. Thus, in rat lung, liver, brain and anterior pituitary, VIP is more potent than secretin whereas in rat pancreas and heart, the converse is true (Christophe & Waelbroeck 1982).

Further support for this subdivision of receptors comes from recent reports of the development of selective VIP antagonists. It was found that an analogue of the related peptide, growth hormone releasing factor (GRF) [N-acetyl-Tyr^1,D.Phe^2]-GRF(1–29)NH$_2$ antagonised the stimulatory effects of VIP and GRF, but not secretin, on adenylate cyclase activity in the rat pancreas. In a further extension of this observation, Pandol et al. (1986) synthesised another compound, [4Cl-D.Phe^6,Leu^{17}]-VIP, which proved to be a competitive and relatively selective antagonist against VIP-induced amylase release and VIP-stimulated short circuit current in colonic tumour cells. The availability of such compounds should allow a more detailed study of the receptor populations for this group of peptides.

Pharmacological actions and functional roles

VIP has effects on the release of several hormones. These include a stimulant effect on prolactin, growth hormone, adrenocorticotrophic hormone (ACTH) and luteinising hormone-releasing hormone (LH-RH) and an inhibitory effect on the release of somatostatin.

On smooth muscle of the genito-urinary tract, VIP generally has a relaxant effect and it is a powerful vasodilator in the heart, lungs and exocrine glands. There is particular interest in the possible roles of VIP in the respiratory tract (Barnes 1986). Here, VIP-immunoreactive neurons are present in the smooth muscle layer, around sub-mucosal glands in the walls of blood vessels and in ganglion-like structures. VIP itself has a potent relaxant effect on bronchial smooth muscle, it causes vasodilatation and, in some species, stimulation of mucus secretion.

Synergistic effects of VIP with other neurotransmitters

In postganglionic neurons innervating certain exocrine glands, such as sweat glands and those in the nasal mucosa and salivary glands, VIP coexists with acetylcholine. Both substances are released in response to electrical stimulation of the postganglionic nerve supplying the submandibular gland. Nerve stimulation causes both vasodilatation and increased secretion but only the latter is blocked by atropine. When administered by local intra-arterial injection, acetylcholine produces an increase in salivary secretion through an action on muscarinic receptors whereas VIP produces vasodilatation. Administered together, the two compounds act synergistically to cause enhanced vasodilatation and secretion (Lundberg *et al.*). The interaction between VIP and acetylcholine extends further to an enhancement of muscarinic receptor binding in the cat submandibular gland. In addition, VIP enchances the stimulant effects of low concentrations of acetylcholine on phosphoinositide turnover in rat cerebral cortex (see Raiteri *et al.* 1987).

References and further reading

Akagi H, Konishi S, Otsuka M & Yanagisawa M (1985) The role of substance P as a neurotransmitter in the reflexes of slow time courses in the neonatal rat spinal cord. *Br. J. Pharmac.* **84**, 663–73.

Andrews PC & Dixon JE (1986) Biosynthesis and processing of the somatostatin family of peptide hormones. *Scand. J. Gastroenterol.* **21** (Suppl. 119), 22–8.

Baile CF, McLaughlin CL & Della-Fera MA (1986) Role of cholecystokinin and opioid peptides in control of food intake. *Physiol. Rev.* **66**, 172–234.

Baldino F, Davis LG & Wolfson B (1985) Structure-activity studies with carboxy- and amino-terminal fragments of neurotensin on hypothalamic neurons in vitro. *Brain Res.* **342**, 266–72.

Barnes PJ (1986) Airway neuropeptides and asthma. *Trends in Pharmacological Sciences* **8**, 24–7.

Bates RFL, Buckley GA, Eglen RM & Strettle RJ (1981a) Hyperalgesia induced by chronic subcutaneous injection of calcitonin. *Br. J. Pharmac.* **74**, 280P.

Bates RFL, Buckley GA, Eglen RM & Strettle RJ (1981b) Antagonism of calcitonin induced analgesia by ionophore A23187. *Br. J. Pharmac.* **74**, 857P.

Bates RFL, Buckley GA & McArdle CA (1984) Comparison of the antinociceptive effects of centrally administered calcitonin and calcitonin gene-related peptide. *Br. J. Pharmac.* **82** (Proc. Suppl.), 295P.

Bishop JF, Moody TW & O'Donohue TL (1986) Peptide transmitters of primary sensory neurons: similar actions of tachykinins and bombesin-like peptides. *Peptides* **7**, 835–42.

Bodnar RJ, Wallace MM, Nilaver G & Zimmerman EA (1982) The effects of centrally administered antisera to neurotensin and related peptides upon nociception and related behaviours. *Ann. N.Y. Acad. Sci.* **400**, 244–57.

Braga P C, Ferri S, Santagostino A, Olgiati V R & Pecile A (1978) Lack of opiate receptor involvement in centrally induced calcitonin analgesia. *Life Sci.* **22**, 971–8.

Brazeau P, Vale W L, Burgus R, Ling N, Butcher M, Rivier J & Guillemin R (1973) Hypothalamic polypeptide that inhibits the secretion of immunoreactive pituitary growth hormone. *Science* **179**, 77–9.

Brown JR, Calthrop JG, Hawcock AB & Jordan CC (1985) Studies with tachykinin antagonists on neuronal preparations in vitro. In: Håkanson R & Sundler F (eds) *Tachykinin Antagonists.* Elsevier, Amsterdam. pp. 335–65.

Chang RSL & Lotti VJ (1986) Biochemical and pharmacological characterization of an extremely potent and selective nonpeptide cholecystokinin antagonist. *Proc. Natl. Acad. Sci. U.S.A.* **83**, 4923–6.

Christophe J & Waelbroeck M (1982) Heterogeneity of neurotransmitter receptors: A comparison of beta-adrenergic, muscarininc cholinergic and VIP receptors. In: Bloom S R, Polak JM & Lindenlaub E (eds) *Systemic Role of Regulatory Peptides.* FK Schattauer Verlag, Stuttgart. pp. 55–75.

Chubb IW, Hodgson AJ & White G H (1980) Acetylcholinesterase hydrolyses substance P. *Neuroscience* **5**, 2065–72.

Clementi G, Amico-Roxas M, Rapisardra E, Caruso A, Prato A, Trombadore S, Priolo G & Scapagnini U (1985) The analgesic activity of calcitonin and the central serotoninergic system. *Eur. J. Pharmac.* **108**, 71–5.

Clineschmidt BV, McGuffin JC & Bunting PB (1979) Neurotensin: antinocisponsive action in rodents. *Eur. J. Pharmac.* **54**, 129–39.

Costa M, Furness JB, Llewellyn-Smith IJ, Murphy R, Bornstein JC & Keast JR (1985) Functional roles for substance P-containing neurones in the gastrointestinal tract. In: Jordan CC & Oehme P (eds) *Substance P: Metabolism & Biological Actions.* Taylor & Francis, London. pp. 99–119.

Crawley JN (1985a) Comparative distribution of cholecystokinin and other neuropeptides. *Ann. N.Y. Acad. Sci.* **448**, 1–8.

Crawley JN (1985b) Behavioural evidence for cholecystokinin modulation of dopamine in the mesolimbic pathway. *Prog. Clin. Biol. Res.* **192**, 131–8.

Cuello AC, Priestley JV & Matthews MR (1982) Localization of substance P in neuronal pathways. In: Porter R & O'Connor M (eds) *Substance P in the Nervous System,* Ciba Symposium 91. Pitman Press, London. pp. 59–79.

Cutting DA & Jordan CC (1974) Alternative approaches to analgesia: baclofen as a model compound. *Br. J. Pharmac.* **54**, 171–9.

Danguir J (1986) Intracerebroventricular infusion of somatostatin selectively increases paradoxical sleep in rats. *Brain Res* **367**, 26–30.

Davis P. Katzman R & Terry RD (1980) Reduced somatostatin-like immunoreactivity in cerebral cortex from cases of Alzheimer's disease and Alzheimer senile dementia. *Nature* **288**, 279–80.

Deschenes RJ, Lorenz LJ, Haun RS, Roos BA, Collier KJ & Dixon JE (1984) Cloning and sequence analysis of a cDNA encoding rat preprocholecystokinin. *Proc. Natl. Acad. Sci. U.S.A.* **81**, 726–30.

Dobner PR, Barber DL, Villa-Komaroff L & McKiernan C (1987) Cloning and sequence analysis of cDNA for the canine neurotensin/neuromedin N precursor. *Proc. Natl. Acad. Sci. USA.* **84**, 3516–20.

Dockray GJ (1982) The physiology of cholecystokinin in brain and gut. *Br. Med. Bull.* **38**, 253–8.

Dockray GJ, Vaillant C & Walsh JH (1979) The neuronal origin of bombesin-like immunoreactivity in the rat gastrointestinal tract. *Neuroscience* **4**, 1561–8.

Dodd J & Kelly JS (1981) The actions of cholecystokinin and related peptides on pyramidal neurones of the mammalian hippocampus. *Brain Res.* **205**, 337–50.

Donnerer J, Barthó L, Holzer P & Lembeck F (1984) Intestinal peristalsis associated with release of immunoreactive substance P. *Neuroscience* **11**, 913–8.

Dreifuss JJ & Raggenbass M (1986) Tachykinins and bombesin excite non-pyramidal neurones in rat hippocampus. *J. Physiol.* **379**, 417–28.

Eison AS, Eison MS & Iversen SD (1982) The behavioural effects of a novel substance P analogue following infusion into the ventral tegmental area or substantia nigra of rat brain. *Brain Res.* **238**, 137–52.

Elliott PJ, Nemeroff CB & Kilts CD (1986) Evidence for a tonic facilitatory influence of substance P on dopamine release in the nucleus accumbens. *Brain Res.* **385**, 379–82.

Emson PC, Lee CM & Rehfeld JF (1980) Cholecystokinin octapeptide: vesicular localisation and calcium-dependent release from rat brain in vitro. *Life Sci.* **26**, 2157–63.

Emson PC & Marley PD (1982) Cholecystokinin and vasoactive intestinal polypeptide. In: Iversen LL, Iversen SD & Snyder SH (eds) *Handbook of Psychopharmacology.* Plenum Press, New York. pp.255–306.

Epelbaum J (1986) Somatostatin in the central nervous system: physiology and pathological implications. *Prog. Neurobiol.* **27**, 63–100.

Evans BE, Bock MG, Rittle KE, DiPardo RM, Whitter WL, Veber DF, Anderson PS & Freidinger RM (1986) Design of potent, orally effective, nonpeptidal antagonists of the peptide hormone cholecystokinin. *Proc. Natl. Acad. Sci. USA* **83**, 4918–22.

Fabbri A, Fraioli F, Pert CB & Pert A (1985) Calcitonin receptors in the rat mesencephalon mediate its analgesic actions: autoradiographic and behavioural analyses. *Brain Res.* **343**, 205–15.

Fallon JH & Seroogy KB (1985) The distribution and some connections of cholecystokinin neurons in the rat brain. *Ann. N.Y. Acad. Sci.* **448**, 121–32.

Fitzgerald M & Woolf CJ (1984) Axon transport and sensory nerve function. In: Chahl LA, Szolcsányi J & Lembeck F (eds) *Antidromic Vasodilatation and Neurogenic Inflammation.* Akademiai Kiado, Budapest. pp. 119–37.

Foreman JC (1987) Substance P and calcitonin gene-related peptide: effects on mast cells and in human skin. *Int. Arch. Allergy Appl. Immunol.* **82**, 366–71.

Foreman JC & Jordan CC (1983) Histamine release and vascular changes induced by neuropeptides. *Agents and Actions* **13**, 105–16.

Fraioli F, Fabbri A, Gnessi L, Moretti C, Santoro C & Felici M (1982) Subarachnoid injection of calcitonin induces analgesia in man. *Eur. J. Pharmac.* **78**, 381–2.

Gamse R & Saria A (1985) Potentiation of tachykinin-induced plasma protein extravasation by calcitonin gene-related peptide. *Eur. J. Pharmac.* **114**, 61–6.

Gaudreau P, Quirion R, St-Pierre S, Chiueh CC & Pert A (1987) Localisation of cholecystokinin receptors in relation to the nigrostriatal and mesolimbic dopaminergic pathways. *Neuropeptides* **9**, 283–93.

Glowinski J, Torrens Y & Beaujouan JC (1982) The striatonigral substance P pathway and dopaminergic mechanisms. In: Porter R & O'Connor M (ed) *Substance P in the Nervous System.* Pitman Press, London. pp. 281–91.

Goltzman D & Mitchell J (1985) Interaction of calcitonin and calcitonin gene-related peptide at receptor sites in target tissue. *Science* **227**, 1343–5.

Goodman EC & Iversen LL (1986) Calcitonin gene-related peptide: novel neuropeptide. *Life Sci.* **38**, 2169–78.

Guard S, Watling KJ & Watson SP (1988) Neurokinin-3 receptors are linked to inositol phospholipid hydrolysis in the guinea-pig ileum longitudinal muscle-myenteric plexus preparation. *Br. J. Pharmac.* **94**, 148–54.

Hahne WF, Jensen RT, Lemp GF & Gardner JD (1981) Proglumide and benzotript: members of a different class of cholecystokinin receptor antagonists. *Proc. Natl. Acad. Sci. USA* **78**, 6304–8.

Heinz-Erian P, Coy DH, Tamura MM Jones SW, Gardner JD & Jensen RT (1987) [D.Phe^{12}]-bombesin analogues: a new class of bombesin receptor antagonists. *Am. J. Physiol.* **252**, G439–42.

Henry JL, Couture R, Cuello AC, Pelletier G & Regoli D (1987). *Proceedings of "Substance P and Neurokinins".* Springer Verlag in press.

Higuchi T, Sikand GS, Kato N, Wada JA & Friesen HG (1983) Profound suppression of kindled seizures by cysteamine: a possible role of somatostatin to kindled seizures. *Brain Res.* **288**, 359–62.

Hill DR, Campbell NJ, Shaw TM & Woodruff GN (1987) Autoradiographic localization and biochemical characterization of peripheral type CCK receptors in rat CNS using highly selective nonpeptide CCK antagonists. *J. Neurosci.* **7**, 2967–76.

Hökfelt T, Vincent S, Dalsgaard C-J, Skirboll L, Johansson O, Schultzberg M, Lundberg JM, Rosell S, Pernow B & Janscó G (1982) Distribution of substance P in brain and periphery and its possible role as a co-transmitter. In: Porter R & O'Connor M (eds) *Substance P in the Nervous System,* Ciba Symposium 91. Pitman Press, London. pp. 84–100.

Hommer DW & Skirboll LR (1983) Cholecystokinin-like peptides potentiate apomorphine-induced inhibition of dopamine neurones. *Eur. J. Pharmac.* **91**, 151–2.

Hughes J, Smith TW, Kosterlitz HW, Fothergill LA, Morgan BA & Morris HR (1975) Identification of two related pentapeptides from the brain with potent opiate agonist activity. *Nature* **258**, 577–9.

Innis RB & Aghajanian G (1985) Cholecystokinin acts as an excitatory neuromodulator in rat amygdala. *Soc. Neurosci. Abstr.* **11** Pt 2, 285–6.

Innis R B & Snyder S H (1980) Distinct cholecystokinin receptors in brain and pancreas. *Proc. Natl Acad. Sci. USA,* **77**, 6917–21.

Jensen RT, Jones SW, Folkers K & Gardner JD (1984) A synthetic peptide that is a bombesin receptor antagonist. *Nature* **309**, 61–3.

Johansson O & Lundberg JM (1981) Ultrastructural localisation of VIP-like immunoreactivity in large dense-core vesicles of 'cholinergic-type' nerve terminals in cat exocrine glands. *Neuroscience* **6**, 847–62.

Jorpes E & Mutt V (1966) Cholecystokinin and pancreozymin: one single hormone? *Acta. Physiol. Scand.* **66**, 196–202.

Ju G, Hökfelt T, Fischer JA *et al.* (1986) Does cholecystokinin-like immunoreactivity in rat primary sensory neurons represent calcitonin gene-related peptide? *Neurosci. Lett* **56**, 257–63.

Katayama Y, North RA & Williams JT (1979) The action of substance P on neurones of the myenteric plexus of the guinea-pig small intestine. *Proc. Roy. Soc. London, Ser. B.* **206**, 191–208.

Keen P, Harmar AJ, Spears F & Winter E (1982) Biosynthesis and axonal transport and turnover of neuronal substance P. In: Porter R & O'Connor M (eds) *Substance P in the Nervous System.* Pitman Press, London. pp. 145–64.

Kelly JS (1982) Electrophysiology of peptides in the central nervous system. *Br. Med. Bull.* **38**, 283–90.

Kimura S, Ogawa T, Goto K, Sugita Y, Munekata E & Kanazawa I. (1985) Endogenous ligands for tachykinin receptors in mammals. In: Jordan CC & Oehme P (eds) *Substance P: Metabolism and Biological Actions.* Taylor & Francis, London. pp. 33–43.

Konishi S, Okamoto T & Otsuka M (1985) Substance P as a neurotransmitter released from peripheral branches of primary afferent neurones producing slow synaptic excitation in autonomic ganglion cells. In: Jordan CC & Oehme P (eds) *Substance P: Metabolism and Biological Actions.* Taylor & Francis, London. pp. 121–36.

Krause JE (1985) On the physiological metabolism of substance P. In: Jordan CC & Oehme P (eds) *Substance P: Metabolism and Biological Actions.* Taylor & Francis, London. pp. 13–31.

Kuraishi Y, Hirota N, Sato Y, Hino Y, Satoh M & Takagi H (1985) Evidence that substance P and somatostatin transmit separate information related to pain in the spinal dorsal horn. *Brain Res.* **325**, 294–8.

Lamberts SWJ & del Pozo E (1986) Acute and long-term effects of SMS 201-995 in acromegaly. *Scand. J. Gastroenterol.* **21**, (Suppl. 119), 141–8.

Laufer R, Gilon C, Chorev M & Selinger Z (1986) Characterization of a neurokinin B receptor site in rat brain using a highly selective radioligand. *J. Biol. Chem.* **261**, 10257–63.

Lee C-M, Iversen LL, Hanley MR & Sandberg BEB (1982) The possible existence of multiple receptors for substance P. *Naunyn-Schmiedeberg's Arch. Pharmac.* **318**, 281–7.

Leeman SE & Carraway RE (1982) Neurotensin: discovery, isolation, characterization, synthesis and possible physiological roles. *Ann. N. Y. Acad. Sci.* **400**, 1–16.

Lembeck F (1985) Substance P and sensory neurones. In: Jordan CC & Oehe P (eds) *Substance P: Metabolism and Biological Actions.* Taylor & Francis, London. pp. 137–51.

Lembeck F, Donnerer J & Barthó L (1982) Inhibition of neurogenic vasodilatation and plasma extravasation by substance P antagonists, somatostatin and [D.Met^2,Pro^5]-enkephalinamide. *Eur. J. Pharmac.* **85**, 171–6.

Lembeck F & Gamse R (1982) Substance P in peripheral sensory neurones. In: Porter R & O'Connor (eds) *Substance P in the Nervous System.* Pitman Press, London. pp. 35–54.

Ljungdahl Å, Hökfelt T & Nilsson G (1978) Distribution of substance P-like immunoreactivity in the central nervous system of the rat. I. Cell bodies and nerve terminals. *Neuroscience* **3**, 861–943.

Loren I, Alumets J, Håkanson R *et al.* (1979) Distribution of vasoactive intestinal polypeptide in the rat and mouse brain. *Neuroscience* **4**, 1953–76.

Lundberg JM, Ängaard A, Fahrenburg J, Hökfelt T & Mutt V (1980) Vasoactive intestinal polypeptide in cholinergic neurons of exocrine glands: Functional significance of coexisting transmitters for vasodilation and secretion. *Proc. Natl Acad. Sci. USA* **77**, 1651–5.

Lundberg JM, Saria A, Theodorsson-Norheim E, Brodin E, Hua X, Martling C-R, Gamse R & Hökfelt T (1985) Multiple tachykinins in capsaicin-sensitive afferents: occurrence, release and biological effects with special reference to irritation of the airways. In: Håkanson R & Sundler F (eds) *Tachykinin Antagonists.* Elsevier, Amsterdam. pp. 159–69.

Maeda K & Frohman LA (1981) Neurotensin release by rat hypothalamic fragments in vitro. *Brain Res.* **210**, 261–9.

Mai JK, Triepel J & Metz J (1987) Neurotensin in the human brain. *Neuroscience* **22**, 499–524.

Massari VJ, Tizabi Y, Park CH, Moody TW, Helke CJ & O'Donohue TL (1983) Distribution and origin of bombesin, substance P and somatostatin in rat spinal cord. *Peptides* **4**, 673–81.

Matsas R, Turner AJ & Kenny AJ (1984) Endopeptidase-24.11 and aminopeptidase activity in brain synaptic membranes are jointly responsible for the hydrolysis of cholecysto-kinin octapeptide (CCK-8). *FEBS Lett.* **175**, 124–8.

Maurer R, Gaehwiler BH, Buescher HH, Hill RC & Roemer D (1982) Opiate antagonistic properties of an octapeptide somatostatin analog. *Proc. Natl Acad. Sci.* **79**, 4815–7.

Merali Z, Johnston S & Sisteh J (1985) Role of dopaminergic system (s) in mediation of the behavioural effects of bombesin. *Pharmac. Biochem. Behav.* **23**, 243–8.

Michelot R, Levielv, Giorguieff-Chesselet MF, Cherémy A & Glowinski J (1979) Effects of the unilateral nigral modulation of substance P transmission on the activity of the two nigro-striatal dopaminergic pathways. *Life Sci.* **24**, 715–24.

Millar R, Sheward W, Wegener I & Fink G (1983) Somatostatin-28 is a hormonally active peptide secreted into hypophyseal portal vessel blood. *Brain Res.* **260**, 334–7.

Minamino N, Kangawa K & Matsuo H (1984) Neuromedin N: a novel neurotensin-like peptide identified in pig spinal cord. *Biochem. Biophys. Res. Commun.* **122**, 542–9.

Minamino N, Sudoh T, Kangawa K & Matsuo H (1985) Neuromedin B-23 and B-30: Two "big" neuromedin B identified in porcine brain and spinal cord. *Biochem. Biophys. Res. Commun.* **130**, 685–91.

Moran TH, Robinson PH, Goldrich MS & McHugh PR (1986) Two brain cholecystokinin receptors: Implication for behavioural actions. *Brain Res.* **362**, 175–9.

Moskowitz MA & Barley PE (1985) The trigeminovascular system and vascular head pain: a role for substance P. In: Jordan CC & Oehme P (eds) *Substance P: Metabolism and Biological Actions.* Taylor & Francis, London. pp. 153–63.

Nawa H, Hirose T, Takashima H, Inayama S & Nakanishi S (1983) Nucleotide sequences of cloned cDNAs for two types of bovine brain substance P precursor. *Nature* **306**, 32–6.

Negri S (1986) Satiety and scratching: effects of bombesin-like peptides. *Eur. J. Pharmac.* **132**, 207–12.

Nemeroff CB, Luttinger D & Prange AJ (1982) Neurotensin and bombesin. In: Iversen LL, Iversen SD & Snyder SH (eds), *Handbook of Psychopharmacology,* Vol. 16. Plenum Press, New York. pp. 363–466.

Nicoll RA (1978) The action of thyrotropin-releasing hormone, substance P and related peptides on frog spinal motoneurones. *J. Pharmac. Exp. Ther.* **207**, 817–24.

North RA & Egan TM (1982) Electrophysiology of peptides in the peripheral nervous system. *Br. Med. Bull.* **38**, 291–6.

O'Donohue TL, Massari VJ, Pazoles CJ, Chronwall BM, Schults CW, Quirion R, Chase TN & Moody TW (1984) A role for bombesin in sensory processing in the spinal cord. *J. Neurosci.* **4**, 2956–62.

Otsuka M, Yanagisawa M & Akagi H (1985) The effects of a substance P antagonist on the isolated spinal cord of the newborn rat. In: Kobayashi H *et al.* (eds) *Neurosecretion and the Biology of Neuropeptides.* Japan Sci. Soc. Press Tokyo/ Springer Verlag, Berlin. pp. 302–07.

Palkovits M, Brownstein MJ, Eiden LE, Beinfeld MC, Russell J & Arimura A (1982) Selective depletion of somatostatin in rat brain by cysteamine. *Brain Res.* **240**, 178–80.

Palmer JM, Schemann, M, Tamura K & Wood JD (1986) Calcitonin gene-related peptide excites myenteric neurons. *Eur. J. Pharmac.* **132**, 163–70.

Pandol SJ, Dharmsmathaphorn K, Schoeffield MS, Vale W & Rivier J (1986) Vasoactive intestinal polypeptide receptor antagonist [4Cl-D.Phe^6,Leu^{17}]-VIP. *Am. J. Physiol.* **250**, G553–G557.

Pappas T, Hamel D, Debas H, Walsh J & Tache Y (1985) Spantide: failure to antagonize bombesin-induced stimulation of gastrin secretion in dogs. *Peptides* **6**, 1001–3.

Pecile A, Ferri S, Brage PC & Olgiati VR (1975) Effects of intracerebroventricular calcitonin in the conscious rabbit. *Experientia* **31**, 332–3.

Pernow B (1983). Substance P. *Pharmac. Rev.* **35**, 85–141.

Pittaway KM, Rodriguez RE, Hughes J & Hill RG (1987) CCK-8 analgesia and hyperalgesia after intrathecal administration in the rat: comparison with CCK-related peptides, *Neuropeptides* **10**, 87–108.

Pless J, Bauer W, Briner U, Doepfner W, Marbach P, Maurer R, Petcher TJ, Reubi J-C & Vonderscher J (1986) Chemistry and pharmacology of SMS 201-955, a long-acting octapeptide analogue of somatostatin. *Scand J. Gastroenterol.* **21**, (Suppl. 119), 54–64.

Polak JM & Bloom SR (1982) The central and peripheral distribution of neurotensin. *Ann. N.Y. Acad. Sci.* **400**, 75–93.

Polak JM & Bloom SR (1986) Somatostatin localization in tissues. *Scand. J. Gastroenterol.* **21** (Suppl. 119), 11–21.

Quirion R & Dam T-V (1985) Multiple tachykinin receptors. In: Jordan CC & Oehme P (eds) *Substance P: Metabolism and Biological Actions.* Taylor & Francis, London. pp. 45–81.

Raiteri M, Marchi M & Paudice P (1987) Vasoactive intestinal polypeptide (VIP) potentiates the muscarininc stimulation of phosphoinositide turnover in the rat cerebral cortex. *Eur. J. Pharmac.* **133**, 127–8.

Rehfeld JF, Hansen HF, Marley PD & Stengaard-Pedersen K (1985) Molecular forms of cholecystokinin in the brain and the relationship to neuronal gastrins. *Ann. N. Y. Acad Sci.* **448**, 11–23.

Reynolds DV (1969) Surgery in the cat during electrical analgesia induced by focal brain stimulation. *Science* **164**, 444–8.

Rosenfeld MG, Mermod JJ, Amara SG, Swanson LW, Sawchenko PE, Rivier J, Vale W W & Evans RM (1983) Production of a novel neuropeptide encoded by the calcitonin gene via tissue-specific RNA processing. *Nature* **304**, 129–35.

Rostène WH, Mazella J, Dussaillant M & Vincent J-P (1986) Photoaffinity labelling of neurotensin binding sites on rat brain sections. *Eur. J. Pharmac.* **130**, 337–40.

Roth KA, Evans CJ, Lorenz RG, Weber E, Barchas JD & Chang JK (1983) Identification of gastrin releasing peptide-related substances in guinea-pig and rat brain. *Biochem. Biophys. Res. Commun.* **112**, 528–36.

Saria A, Gamse R, Yan Z, Wolf G, Loidolt D, Martling C-R & Lundberg JM (1987) Tachykinins and calcitonin gene-related peptide in the respiratory system. In: Sicuteri F *et al.* (eds) *Trends in Cluster Headache.* Elsevier Amsterdam. pp. 231–9.

Sheehan MJ & de Belleroche J (1984) Central actions of CCK: behavioural and release studies. In: de Belleroche J & Dockray GJ (eds), *CCK in the Nervous System.* Ellis Harwood, Chichester. pp.110–127.

Sicuteri F, Gepetti P, Marabinin S & Lembeck F (1984) Pain relief by somatostatin in attacks of cluster headache. *Pain* **18**, 359–65.

Skofitsch G & Jacobowitz DM (1985) Calcitonin gene-related peptide: Detailed immuno-histochemical distribution in the central nervous system. *Peptides* **6**, 721–45.

Szabo S & Reichlin S (1981) Somatostatin in rat tissues is depleted by cysteamine administration. *Endocrinology* **109**, 2255–7.

Szabo S & Reichlin S (1985) Somatostatin depletion by cysteamine: mechanism and implication for duodenal ulceration. *Fed. Proc.* **44**, 2540–5.

Tache Y, Lesiege D & Goto Y (1986) Neural pathways involved in intracisternal bombesin-induced inhibition of gastric secretion in rats. *Dig. Dis. Sci.* **31**, 412–17.

Tannebaum GS & Goltzman D (1985) Calcitonin gene-related peptide mimics calcitonin actions in brain on growth hormone release and feeding. *Endocrinology* **116**, 2685–7.

Tatemoto K, Lundberg, JM, Jornvall H & Mutt V (1985) Neuropeptide K: isolation, structure and biological activities of a novel brain peptide. *Biochem. Biophys. Res. Commun.* **128**, 947–53.

Tran V, Flint-Beal M & Martin J (1985) Two types of somatostatin receptor differentiated by cyclic somatostatin analogs. *Science* **228**, 492–5.

Uhl GR (1982) Distribution of neurotensin and its receptor in the central nervous system. *Ann. N.Y. Acad. Sci.* **400**, 132–49.

Vargas F, Frerot O, Tuong MD, Zuzel K, Rose C & Schwartz J-C (1985) Sulfation and desul-fation of cholecystokinin. *Ann. N.Y. Acad. Sci.* **448**, 110–20.

Wiesenfeld-Hallin Z (1985) Intrathecal somatostatin modulates spinal sensory and reflex mechanisms: behavioural and electrophysiological studies in the rat. *Neurosci. Lett.* **62**, 69–74.

Wiesenfeld-Hallin Z, Hökfelt T, Lundberg JM, Forssmann WG, Reinecke M, Tschopp FA &

Fischer JA (1984) Immunoreactive calcitonin gene-related peptide and substance P coexist in sensory neurones to the spinal cord and interact in spinal behavioural responses of the rat. *Neurosci. Lett.* **52**, 199–204.

Williams G, Ball JA, Lawson RA, Maskill MR, Joplin GF & Bloom SR (1987) Analgesic effects of the somatostatin analogue SMS 205–995 in headache associated with pituitary tumour. *Clin. Sci.* **73** (Suppl. 17), 25p.

Yachnis AT, Crawley JN, Jensen RT, McGrane MM & Moody TW (1984) The antagonism of bombesin in the CNS by substance P analogues. *Life Sci* **35**, 1963–9.

Yaksh TL, Schmauss C, Micevych PE, Abay EO & Go VLW (1982) Pharmacological studies on the application, disposition and release of neurotensin in the spinal cord. *Ann. N.Y. Acad. Sci.* **400**, 228–42.

15   Opioid receptors

A.H. DICKENSON

The concept of receptors in pharmacology has a central role in explaining both drug effects and the actions of endogenous neurotransmitter function. In the case of opioids the evidence for the existence of a specific receptor was available long before biochemical studies pinned down the endogenous entity.

Synthesis of an enormous variety of compounds based on the structure of morphine clearly showed structural requirements for opioid effects and sterochemical specificity was also established. Similarly the ability of naloxone to act as an antagonist and the availability of isolated tissues, notably guinea-pig ileum, allowed specific dose dependent effects of opioids to be demonstrated. The work of Martin on dependence and tolerance, and indeed cross tolerance between opioids but not non-opioids established a framework for the search for the opiate receptor. Martin's work in the spinal dog clearly showed that the actions of morphine, two benzomorphan derivatives (cyclazocine and pentazocine) and allylnormetazocine (SKF 10047) were attributable to three distinct receptor sites, designated mu(μ), kappa(κ) and sigma (σ) where morphine, ketocylazocine and SKF 10047 were prototypical agonists. The effects of these agents were gauged on a variety of physiological measures such as respiration, heart rate, temperature, state of the pupils and nociceptive reflexes. Subsequently many other drugs were incorporated into this schema so that agonists, antagonists and partial agonists at these sites could be identified.

Identification of an opioid receptor, or specific binding site in neural tissue, in the early seventies by three independent groups was one stimulus to a search for the endogenous ligands and the discovery of the enkephalins. When the activity effects of the endogenous enkephalins was compared with that of morphine on guinea-pig ileum and mouse vas deferens and their relative resistance to antagonism by naloxone observed, the results produced evidence for a further distinct (fourth) receptor, the delta (δ) site, for which the enkephalins had highest affinity. In retrospect it was perhaps somewhat fortuitous that Hughes and Kosterlitz discovered the enkephalins in extracts of pig brain since they were first tested on guinea-pig ileum which is low in delta receptors. Soon after the isolation of the enkephalins a larger opioid, β-endorphin, was reported in bovine pituitary by Goldstein and colleagues and subsequently many other opioid peptides have been isolated, notably dynorphin, again

Table 15.1. Opioid receptors and their ligands. The relative affinity of naloxone for the μ, δ and κ sites is 0.85, 0.06 and 0.09 respectively (Kosterlitz 1985)

	Receptors			
	Mu (μ)	Delta (δ)	Kappa (κ)	
Endogenous	β-endorphin	Methionine enkephalin	Dynorphin A1–13	Little δ but some
Agonist	Metorphamide	Leucine enkephalin	Dynorphin A1–8	μ affinity
Ligands	Enkephalins	β-endorphin	Dynorphin B	
Synthetic	Morphine	DPDPE	U50488H	
Agonist	DAGO	DADLE	Bremazocine (μ & δ also)	
Ligands		DTLET	Pentazocine	
Antagonists	Naloxone	ICI 174864	MR 2266	
		Naloxone	Naloxone	
Location in	Guinea-pig ileum		Guinea-pig ileum	
peripheral	Mouse vas deferens	Mouse vas deferens	Mouse vas deferens	
tissues		Hamster vas deferens	Rabbit vas deferens	

first reported by Goldstein and his group. These endogenous opioids have now been purified and their amino acid sequences established (see Chapter 22).

Such studies have now led to the generally accepted proposal that there are three distinct opioid receptors and that a variety of peptides constitute the endogenous ligands. (Table 15.1). In addition, a number of synthetic peptides and non-peptides have been produced which have high selectivity for the receptors and so are useful tools for studying physiological function at these sites. The reader may have noted that three rather than four sites have now been cited. The reason is that the sigma site is likely to represent a site associated with the NMDA type of excitatory amino acid receptor (Chapter 13).

There are several pitfalls in the study of opioid peptides and their receptors which relate to the inability of some of these compounds to cross the blood–brain barrier, their rapid degradation by peptidases, the influence of ions in the bathing media on ligand binding and cross-selectivity of some of the opioids used. However, the use of peptidase inhibitors, selective agonists and combinations of isolated peripheral tissues containing one or more receptor types can circumvent many of these problems.

Endogenous opioids and receptors

The endogenous opioids fall into three main groups. They are peptides derived from larger precursor molecules and can be termed β-endorphin and related fragments, enkephalins and dynorphins. The larger endorphin (31 amino acids) and dynorphins (13 and 18 amino acids) (Fig. 15.1 and 22.2) are reasonably stable to peptidase activity but since the opioid activity of all these peptides depends on tyrosine at the N terminus, both non-opioid and smaller opioid peptides may occur following clipping, either as a result of processing of the precursor or peptidase effects on the final released peptide. A good example is the dynorphin family where some actions of dynorphin A (non-opioid) are not reversed by naloxone although the leucine enkephalin sequence occurs within the dynorphins (it is, however, unknown as to whether any leucine enkephalin is released).

Table 15. 1 lists the three main types of opioid receptor together with the putative endogenous ligands for the receptors and examples of selective synthetic agonists and antagonists for the three receptors. It should be noted that the synthetic ligands have considerably higher affinities for the receptor subtypes than the endogenous ligands.

Table 15.2. Opioid precursors and their products

Proenkephalin	→	Methionine enkephalin
		Leucine enkephalin
		Octapeptide
		Heptapeptide
		Peptide F
		Peptide E
		BAM 12
		BAM 18
		BAM 22
Proopiocortin	→	β-endorphin 1–31
		ACTH
		α-endorphin (βend 1–17)
		γ-endorphin (βend 1–16)
		β-endorphin 2–17
Prodynorphin	→	Dynorphin$_A$ 1–17
		Dynorphin$_A$ 1–8
		α-neoendorphin
		β-neoendorphin
		Dynorphin β
		Leucine enkephalin

μ receptor and ligands

The μ receptor is widely distributed in the CNS and PNS and this reflects the wide spectrum of effects produced by morphine and other related opiates such as heroin, methadone, pethidine etc. a full account of which is given in Chapter 22. Whilst synthetic opioids and derivatives from opium have high affinity for this receptor together with a good selectivity, morphine and Tyr-D.Ala-Me.Phe-Gly-ol (DAGO) being useful ligands to probe μ receptor activation, the endogenous ligands for this receptor are less clearly defined. Thus although β-endorphin has high affinity for this receptor it has affinity for the δ receptor also. The argument that the endogenous ligand for the μ receptor is β-endorphin may hold for certain areas of the nervous system but in the spinal cord, where μ receptors are found in high concentrations in dorsal horns, β-endorphin is not present in adult animals. Nevertheless the spinal actions of morphine, following intrathecal or epidural application, in many species including man, have been sufficiently well characterised by clinical, behavioural and electrophysiological approaches to lend testament to the functional coupling of the μ receptor. Perhaps some of the fragments from pro-opiocortin such as metorphamide are μ ligands at this level of the CNS but this requires confirmation.

The μ receptor has a wide distribution in PNS and CNS and highest densities are found in superficial spinal cord and trigeminal nucleus caudalis, brainstem nuclei such as the chemoreceptor trigger zone, nucleus of the solitary tract, respiratory nuclei, cough centre and related areas, as well as periaqueductal and periventricular zones of the midbrain, the striatum, amygdala and cortical regions. In the PNS the myenteric plexus contains high concentrations of μ receptor binding sites and various peripheral tissues contain μ receptors.

The coupling of the μ receptor has received much attention and two systems are clearly involved. Its activation produces an inhibition of adenylate cyclase so that reduced cyclic AMP levels have been observed in many systems. Electrophysiological studies have shown that μ opioids open potassium channels so hyperpolarising neurons, reducing action potential duration and hence reducing calcium fluxes. Whether this coupling to K^+ channels is direct or via adenylate cyclase or calcium (calcium activated K^+ channels) is as yet unclear. Nevertheless, the inhibitory effects of μ receptor activation, the reduced neuronal activity or inhibitions and reduced release of other neurotransmitters (demonstrated for most candidates such as ACh, NA, 5-HT, DA, peptides etc.) are explicable in terms of these mechanisms. A predominant effect of opioids acting via the μ-receptor is the presynaptic inhibition of neurotransmitter release, two examples being presynaptic μ receptors on striatal dopamine neurons and on primary afferent sensory fibres in spinal cord and trigeminal areas. There is evidence for a postsynaptic hyperpolarisation of neurons, some of which may well be local interneurons, whilst others may be projection or output cells. In certain areas of the CNS, in particular hippocampus and spinal cord, activation of the μ receptor can lead to excitatory effects. In the hippocampus the mechanisms of opioid excitation appears to be via a disinhibition of GABA neurons, since bicuculline-sensitive IPSPs recorded in hippocampal neurons are abolished by opioids (see Duggan & North 1984). In the spinal cord, particularly in the substantia gelatinosa zone, opioids applied directly can cause neuronal excitations which may be due to a similar mechanism.

Delta receptors and ligands

In the case of the δ receptor the endogenous ligands are now much more clearly defined and the two enkephalins, methionine- and leucine-enkephalin are endogenous ligands for the δ receptor although it should not be forgotten that they also have appreciable affinity for the μ receptor. The distribution in nervous tissues of the enkephalins parallels that of the delta receptor, and indeed the μ receptor since these two receptor subtypes are closely associated. However, despite some early suggestions that the μ and δ receptors might be allosterically coupled there is now evidence showing that selective μ and δ opioids produce only additive effects and there is no evidence as yet for the two receptors being found on the same neuron. The δ receptor nevertheless is coupled to K^+ channels with the net effect being similar to μ activation, namely channel opening. Although less thoroughly studied, due mainly to their relatively recent characterisation and the lack of selective ligands, δ receptor induced inhibition of neuronal activity and reduced transmitter release parallel the effects of μ receptor activation.

Two problems have arisen from studies of δ mediated events which may lead to some misinterpretation of results. Firstly, several ligands claimed to be selective for the δ receptor, such as D.Ala-D.Leu-enkephalin (DADLE), unlike enkephalin dimers such as DPDPE (see below) are not very selective and have effects which are μ mediated. A tactic to circumvent this is to either block μ (and/or κ) receptors with compounds such as β-funaltrexamine, an irreversible μ ligand or, in the case of binding studies, to use excess unlabelled μ ligands in the incubation medium. Secondly, the enkephalins are rapidly degraded by at least three types of peptidase; aminopeptidases, enkephalinase and dipeptidylamino-peptidase and this can alter their apparent activity in a given tissue preparation. Inhibitors of these metallo-enzymes have been designed which are all mono- or bidendate chelating agents based on enkephalin and have been shown *in vitro* and *in vivo* to protect either exogenous or endogenous enkephalins. The enzyme inhibitor, kelatorphan, which is a mixed inhibitor of all three enzymes is worthy of note both as a research tool and as a compound of possible therapeutic potential.

A stable, peptidase resistant δ agonist is D-penicillamine, D-penicilla-mine enkephalin (DPDPE) which, due to the bridge formed between the penicillamine residues, becomes conformationally restricted and imparts high δ selectivity to the enkephalin analogue compared to the native peptide. The fact that modified enkephalins such as DAGO have high μ selectivity would indicate that small differences exist between the conformational requirements for μ and δ receptor activity. Furthermore, the ability of the native enkephalins to act on the μ as well as the δ receptor, albeit with lower affinity, and the fact that various modified enkephalins such as D.Ala-D.Leu enkephalin, (DADLE),Tyr-D.Thr-Gly-Phe-Leu-Thr (DTLET) and Tyr-D.Ser-Gly-Phe-Leu-descarboxy-Thr produce δ mediated effects at low concentrations and μ binding at higher concentrations supports the close parallels between μ and δ receptors. However, a word of caution is appropriate here since the above agonists have been cited in various publications as δ agonists and their effects on various physiological events as evidence for an involvement of δ receptors in these functions. Their selectivity is not sufficient for these conclusions to be drawn unless differential δ and δ/μ effects can be shown dependent on the dose used.

An intriguing point arises in respect of the functional role of the enkephalins, for although they have most effect at the δ receptor, their affinity for them is quite low. Since the density of δ receptors is also generally lower than that of μ receptors, it may be that before the enkephalins can produce effective transmission in terms of receptor binding they will need very high efficacy or the amounts released would have to be high. This latter possibility might be the case since not only do the enkephalinases have low affinity for their substrate but high efficacy and low affinity of peptide agonists is not common.

Kappa receptors

The kappa (κ) receptor was originally characterised by biossay techniques by Martin and colleagues in the dog and was so named because ketocyclazocine was a selective agonist. The ethyl derivative (EKC) has been widely employed as a prototypical κ ligand but has μ affinity approaching that for the κ site and, as with some of the δ ligands, caution is needed in interpreting the effects of EKC as purely κ mediated. Selective agonists do exist. Synthetic compounds such as U50488H and U69503 are good probes for the κ site and various dynorphin fragments are reasonably selective. The endogenous ligand for the receptor is presumably derived from dynorphin and the Al-13 fragment is a likely candidate. However, some κ agonists do have a residual μ affinity which now appears to be expressed as μ antagonist activity. This has been illustrated in various peripheral and central tissues. Hence, bremazocine, a compound with κ agonist activity, reverses the inhibition of the field-stimulated contractile response produced by morphine in rat vas deferens and guinea-pig ileum. Furthermore other κ agonists have been shown to antagonise both morphine analgesia and μ receptor mediated neuronal inhibitions.

Activation of the κ receptor reduces calcium channel opening, which would be expected to reduce transmitter release and lead to neuronal inhibition. Although this occurs in some areas of the CNS, such as the locus coeruleus, neuronal excitations have also been observed in the spinal cord, hippocampus and striatum, all areas where μ agonists produce consistent inhibitions. Few studies as yet have looked at neurotransmitter release but efflux of substance P from the spinal cord, elicited by peripheral stimuli, is inhibited by μ and δ agonists but not by κ agonists and the spontaneous release is, in fact, elevated by a κ ligand. Other differences between κ mediated effects and those of μ and δ agonists are:
1 κ agonists being aversive in behavioural self administration experiments whereas most opiates produce reinforcement,

2 marked motor effects of some κ agonists on spinal application, again an effect not seen for μ and δ agonists

3 a lack of gastrointestinal function changes after κ opioids.

Whether these are κ agonist effects or due to μ antagonism remains to be clarified and a problem in this regard is the lack of any useful κ antagonist. Naloxone has low affinity for the κ receptor so reversal of κ effects requires high doses of this antagonist. This requirement may explain some purported non-opioid effects of κ ligands but it must also be noted that some dynorphin fragments, e.g. dynorphin 2-17, lacking opioid activity, do produce observable effects in some tissues.

References and further reading

Dickenson A (1986) A new approach to pain relief. *Nature* **320**, 681–2.

Duggan A & North A (1984) Electrophysiology of opioids. *Pharmac. Rev.* **35**, 219–81.

Kosterlitz HW (1985) Opioid peptides and their receptors. *Proc. Roy. Soc. London. Ser B* **225**, 27–40.

Martin WR (1984) Pharmacology of opioids. *Pharmac. Rev.* **35**, 283–323.

North A (1986) Opioid receptors types and membrane ion channels. *Trends Neurosci.* **9**, 114–7.

III   Applied neuropharmacology

16 Parkinsonism and other movement disorders

R.J. HARDIE

The precise role of those subcortical structures known as the basal ganglia is not known. They comprise the caudate nucleus and putamen (together termed the corpus striatum), the globus pallidus and the substantia nigra. Together they receive afferent inputs from virtually all areas of the cerebral cortex and so could conceivably play a part in almost any cerebral activity.

They constitute the extra-pyramidal motor system, in contrast to the direct cortico-spinal neurons which traverse the pyramidal tracts so conspicuous in the medulla. From a knowledge of human diseases involving the basal ganglia, it becomes clear that they have a fundamental role in the control of movement. Paradoxically, movement may either become slow and diminished, as is seen in Parkinson's disease, or it may become rapid, excessive and involuntary, for example in Huntington's chorea, depending on the exact site of pathology.

It was only in 1960 that Parkinson's disease became the first neurological condition in which a specific and focal abnormality of a cerebral transmitter substance was identified. Since that time a pivotal role for dopamine (DA) has been firmly established, as much by clinical research into that distressing malady as by more basic experimentation using rather unsatisfactory animal models of extrapyramidal disturbances. Indeed despite the subsequent discovery of numerous other, currently more fashionable, peptides and neurotransmitters that are concentrated within the basal ganglia and deficient in diseases of that region, the functional significance of these other substances is completely enigmatic.

This chapter will therefore concentrate on the clinical neuropharmacology of DA systems in Parkinson's disease. Much less, of practical benefit at least, is known about Huntington's chorea, which is at the opposite end of the range of diseases known clinically as movement disorders.

Rather more common, however, and illustrating the whole spectrum of movement disorders are those iatrogenic conditions induced by neuroleptic drugs, including drug-induced Parkinsonism and tardive dyskinesia. Only under these circumstances, or during therapeutic attempts to manipulate central DA transmission in Parkinson's or Huntington's disease, are both Parkinsonism and chorea seen simultaneously. Any study of the pharmacology of the basal ganglia must

Table 16.1. Comparison of clinical movement disorders

	Diminshed movement	Excessive movement
Disease	Parkinson's disease	Huntington's chorea
Drugs	Dopamine-depleting agents Dopamine receptor antagonists	Levodopa Dopamine receptor agonists Dopamine receptor antagonists (chronic exposure only)

examine this remarkable co-existence of two apparently contradictory states (Table 16.1).

Parkinson's disease

Clinical aspects

In 1817 a General Practitioner from Shoreditch first drew attention to a condition which now universally bears his name. The cardinal features of James Parkinson's disease include:

1 slowness and poverty of all movements (bradykinesia, akinesia)
2 muscle stiffness of a particular type known as 'cogwheel' rigidity
3 tremor of the limbs present mainly at rest.

When fully developed, these features together with the typical shuffling festinant gait comprise a clinical syndrome that is easily recognisable even to those with no medical training. Parkinson's disease (PD) is a progressive degenerative condition of the central nervous system (CNS) of unknown cause. It is one of the commonest CNS diseases, with prevalence rates which increase with age; it occurs predominantly in those over 55 years, affecting at least 1% of that population.

As discussed later in this chapter, the administration of neuroleptic drugs can cause an almost identical syndrome, and PD is referred to as primary, or idiopathic, Parkinsonism to distinguish it from secondary, drug-induced cases. Many people developed Parkinsonism following a worldwide pandemic of encephalitis lethargica around 1920. The causative agent, presumably a virus, was never identified however, and cases of post-encephalitic Parkinsonism due to a variety of infections are today fortunately rare. Other rare causes of secondary Parkinsonism include manganese and carbon monoxide poisoning.

Neuropathology

It has been known for more than half a century that the brains of patients with PD lacked the dark pigment that gives rise to the name substantia nigra. This 'black substance' is situated at the junction of the tectum and tegmentum of the human midbrain and is normally visible to the naked eye. It is now known that this pigment represents melanin granules contained within the cell bodies of neurons that project rostrally to the striatum, and that it is these cells which are lost in PD. Similar but less marked loss of other catecholamine-producing pigmented neurons also occurs, for example in the locus coeruleus (noradrenaline) and nucleus paranigralis (DA).

The exact significance of the pigment is still a mystery. For example, it is unclear whether its accumulation might accelerate the normal rate of degeneration of nigro-striatal neurons that occurs with ageing. Alternatively, it has been suggested that neuromelanin is simply a cytoplasmic 'slag heap' of metabolic waste material, whose build-up is symptomatic of an effete cell that is about to die. Furthermore midbrain pigment is not found in rodents, being confined to higher mammalian species and in particular primates. It is of great interest that diseases resembling Parkinsonism have not been described in veterinary practice and apparently do not occur in any species other than man.

The other histological hallmark of PD is an eosinophilic intra-neuronal inclusion body known as a Lewy body. This equally enigmatic structure is found scattered throughout all those areas of Parkinsonian brains that exhibit cell loss. These areas include not only substantia nigra and locus coeruleus but also dorsal raphe nucleus, hypothalamus and sympathetic paravertebral ganglia. Thus Lewy bodies are not confined exclusively to melanin-containing regions.

Neurochemistry

Reserpine, a substance which depletes brain monoamines, causes a striking state of inhibition of locomotor activity in rodents known as catalepsy. When reserpine first became available clinically for the treatment of hypertension, it was soon recognised as causing Parkinsonism in humans. It was subsequently shown that levodopa reversed the catalepsy of reserpinised animals, an effect potentiated by MAO inhibitors.

It was then pointed out by Carlsson that 70% of brain DA is localised in the basal ganglia, and he suggested (Carlsson 1959) that DA might play a role in extrapyramidal function and basal ganglia disorders.

In a seminal paper the following year, Ehringer and Hornykiewicz (1960) first reported markedly diminished DA concentrations in the basal ganglia of brains from patients with both post-encephalitic and idiopathic Parkinsonism. Their original observations have since been fully confirmed and accordingly various means were explored in attempts to augment central DA formation.

As might be anticipated from the distribution of Lewy bodies, neurochemical abnormalities have since been found much more widely (Hornykiewicz & Kish 1987). Indeed they are restricted neither to the basal ganglia nor even to those pigmented neuronal systems that utilise catecholamine transmitters. Unfortunately, as will be discussed later in this chapter, the functional significance of these wider deficits is unknown.

Early trials of levodopa

Orally administered DA is destroyed by MAO in gut wall and liver and does not pass from the systemic circulation into the brain, across the blood–brain barrier (BBB). Thus the next step was to examine the effects of racemic dihydroxy-phenylalanine (DL-DOPA) in Parkinsonian patients. Encouraging early reports of both oral and intravenous DL-DOPA were not confirmed by subsequent double-blind clinical trials, and equally disappointing results were obtained with its own natural precursor, tyrosine.

Using very large doses, 3–16 g, of oral DL-DOPA however, Cotzias and his colleagues in 1967 were able to describe impressive and unequivocal improvement, which was soon to be reproduced using half the quantity of the L-isomer alone, L-DOPA or levodopa. This then was the first successful experiment in manipulating central DA systems to ameliorate PD.

Current drug treatments

It must be emphasised that PD is an incurable, progressive condition. All existing forms of drug treatment provide only symptomatic relief and probably do not alter the course of the underlying disease process.

Nevertheless, the efficacy of levodopa has led to a revolution in patient management. Previous treatments, such as anti-cholinergic drugs, had very little effect on symptoms and no impact at all on the inexorable downhill course of the disease. Patients can now look forward to many years of improved quality of life. Levodopa is regarded with little hesitation by most authorities as the treatment of choice. Indeed response to it is usually so good as to be regarded as diagnostic for the disease. For these reasons levodopa will be considered first and in greatest detail.

There are drawbacks associated with levodopa treatment however, particularly over the course of several years, and various alternative strategies have been employed in attempts to manipulate central DA systems. These are summarised in Fig. 16.1. One option is to develop direct agonists of postsynaptic striatal DA receptors, such as apomorphine and bromocriptine. Another is to try to inhibit catabolism of the endogenous transmitter, carried out mainly by intra-neuronal MAO type B. Finally there are some compounds that are believed to alter the release and/or re-uptake of DA from the presynaptic membrane.

It is important to appreciate that the neurochemical substrate retains a dynamic capacity to respond to changes until very late in the course of the disease. For example, it is estimated that about 80% of nigro-striatal neurons, and of striatal DA, must be lost before symptoms appear. Thus considerable functional reserve capacity must exist within this system, to compensate for reduced cell numbers by increased DA turnover in the surviving neurons. This is reflected by an increase in the ratio of the main

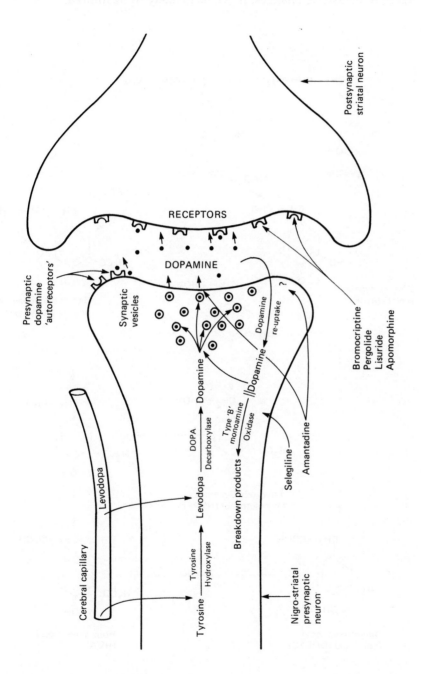

Fig. 16.1. The nigro-striatal dopaminergic synapse. Site of action of various anti-Parkinsonism drugs.

metabolite, homovanillic acid (HVA), to DA itself by 2 or 3 times the normal value of unity. Later adaptive changes may also occur postsynaptically, including a state of denervation supersensitivity to DA. Since any effective treatment that augments striatal DA function may well reverse these homeostatic changes, its value is likely to be limited.

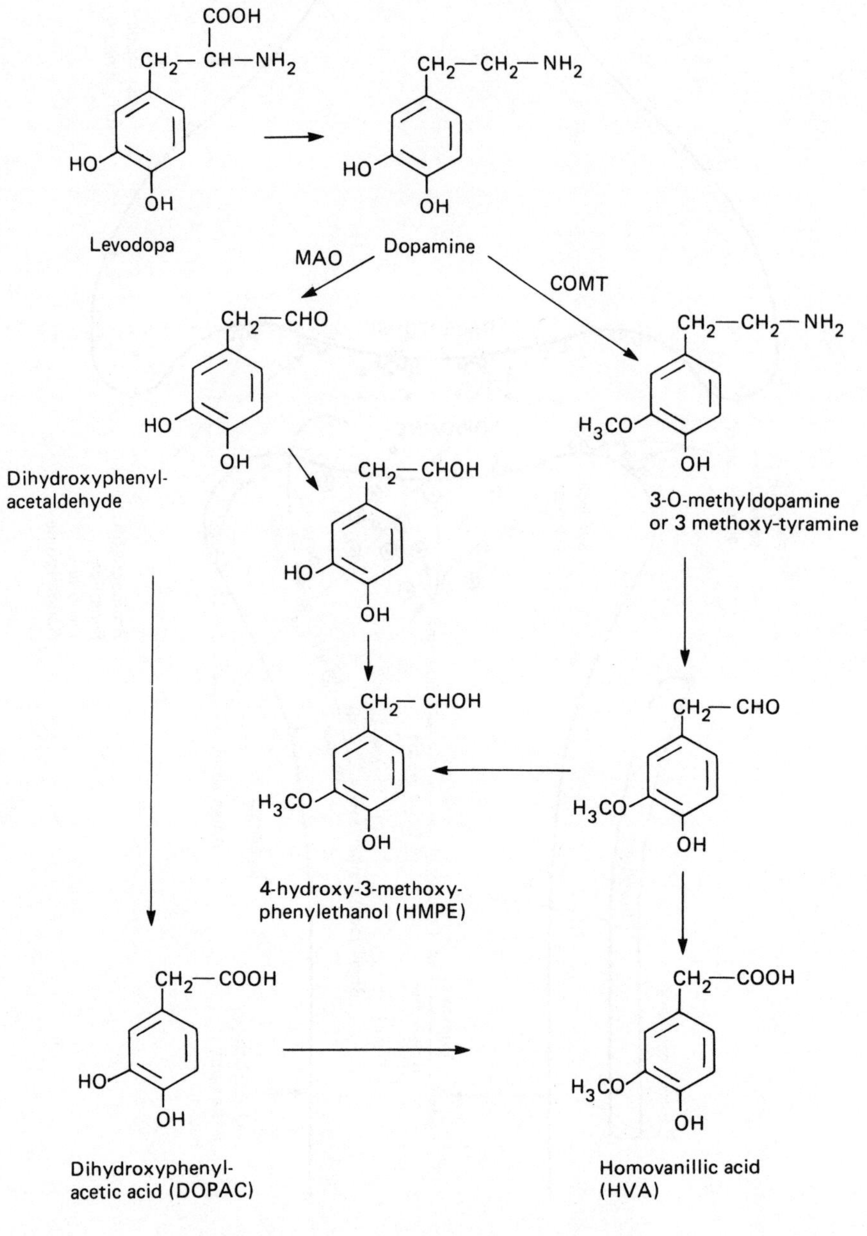

Fig. 16.2. Metabolism of levodopa — decarboxylated derivatives.

Levodopa

Pharmacokinetics

L-DOPA or levodopa is a naturally occurring amino acid which is found only in trace amounts in the normal diet. It is absorbed, mainly in the duodenum and jejunum, via a stereospecific active transport mechanism for which other large neutral amino acids (e.g. leucine, isoleucine and valine) are also substrates. The compound is avidly decarboxylated to DA by the ubiquitous enzyme aromatic amino acid decarboxylase (AADC) whose activity is particularly high in liver, kidney, heart and lungs. Thus considerable pre-systemic metabolism in the gastrointestinal wall and liver prevents 60–80% of an oral dose from reaching the systemic circulation. Indeed less than 1% reaches the brain unchanged. The major urinary metabolites of levodopa are DA itself and its decarboxylated derivatives HVA and dihydroxy-phenyl-acetic acid, DOPAC (Fig. 16.2).

The formation of DA in the circulation causes two main adverse effects: postural hypotension, because of effects on vasomotor control; and nausea and vomiting by stimulation of the chemoreceptor trigger zone in the brainstem. These effects caused very high drop-out rates from the early clinical trials of levodopa, often at dosages below those necessary to produce a therapeutic response. Fortunately sufficient patients were able to tolerate levodopa for the treatment quickly to be acknowledged as a major advance. For an account of the original development of levodopa therapy, see Brogden *et al.* (1971).

Decarboxylase inhibitors

The introduction a few years later of combination therapy using levodopa with either benserazide or carbidopa reduced considerably the incidence of dose-limiting emesis and hypotension. Both hydrazine derivatives, these compounds only inhibit peripheral AADC and so DA is not formed in the circulation. Neither compound enters the brain to any significant extent hence the term extracerebral dopa decarboxylase inhibitor, ExCDDI.

Levodopa itself still crosses the BBB, via a stereospecific carrier mechanism very similar to that in the gut, and is converted to DA by uninhibited central decarboxylation at its site of action. Absolute bioavailability of levodopa is increased approximately fivefold and so much lower doses are required for a similar clinical response. Because this strategy is so advantageous, levodopa is now seldom prescribed alone.

In the presence of ExCDDIs, a high proportion of oral levodopa is converted to 3-methoxy-tyrosine or 0-methyl dopa (OMD) by the enzyme COMT. In patients on chronic oral therapy, the plasma OMD concentration is often ten times that of levodopa. This represents a very significant loss and an inhibitor of COMT could be of great potential value, but

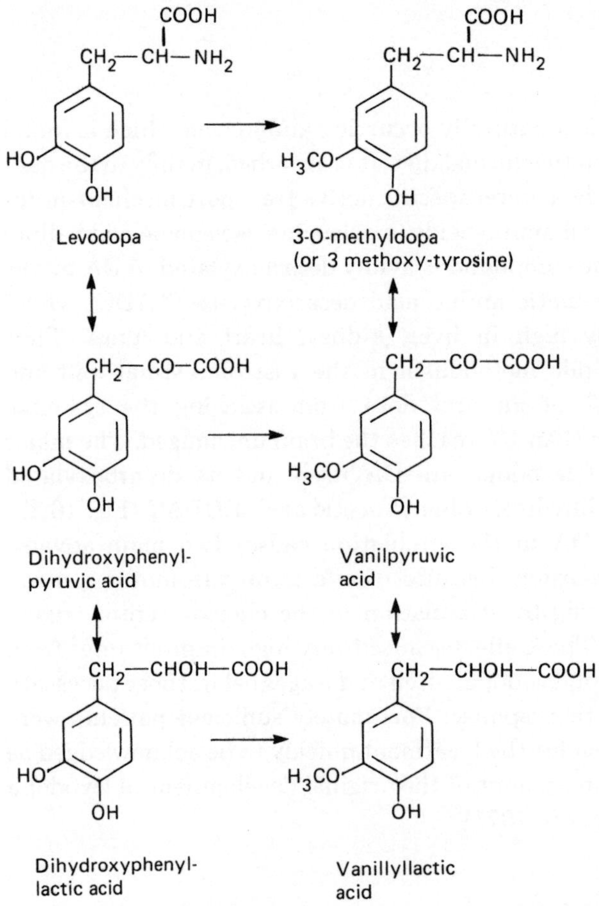

Fig. 16.3. Metabolism of levodopa — non-decarboxylated derivatives.

unfortunately one suitable for use in humans has not so far been developed. Non-decarboxylated metabolites appear in the urine such as vanillyllactic acid and dihydroxy phenyl-lactic acid (Fig. 16.3), together with much smaller amounts of HVA and DOPAC than would be present without an ExCDDI.

Pharmacodynamics

It is generally assumed that levodopa requires enzymatic decarboxylation within the striatum in order to exert its anti-Parkinsonian effect. There remains some doubt about this, since it would be hard to prove *in vivo*, but the evidence is broadly consistent with this assumption.

AADC within the brain is found in highest concentration in striatal neurons. Following acute and chronic administration of levodopa to experimental animals there is a dose-dependent rise in striatal DA and HVA levels, whilst brain NA concentration does not change and 5-HT levels fall.

It is known that the degeneration of nigro-striatal neurons in PD accounts for the loss of about 90% of normal basal ganglia AADC. It has therefore been suggested that the residual activity is insufficient to convert large amounts of exogenous levodopa to DA, particularly in the advanced stages of the disease when the efficacy of the drug declines markedly. Decarboxylation might then take place in 5-HT neurons or possibly glial cells and DA arrive simply by diffusion. Non-neuronal decarboxylation might also occur.

The technique of positron emission tomography, PET, has recently provided important new evidence. A positron-emitting isotope, [18]fluoro-dopa, is administered intravenously to subjects pre-treated with an ExCDDI and is taken up specifically by the human striatum, where its metabolites (presumably mainly $[^{18}F]$-DA) remain concentrated for hours. This suggests that storage does occur, although other metabolites may be present as well and would be indistinguishable. The main difference from healthy subjects is that in patients with PD, labelled dopa is taken up less completely by the striatum and its concentration falls more quickly.

The same technique is also being used to examine another important pharmacodynamic factor, namely changes at DA receptor sites. Experimental models of Parkinsonism can never satisfactorily reproduce the gradual denervation and DA depletion within the striatum that probably takes decades to develop in PD. It is clear that postsynaptic structures remain relatively intact, otherwise levodopa treatment would not be so effective, but it is also likely that gradual compensatory adjustments in receptor density and affinity would be reversed by levodopa administration.

Unfortunately there is insufficient evidence from post-mortem neurochemical studies on the brains of PD victims upon which to base any firm conclusions about receptor changes associated with long-term levodopa therapy. The available evidence has been reviewed by Calne and Stoessl (1987). It is to be hoped that PET studies using suitably labelled DA receptor ligands such as $[^{11}C]$-spiperone will soon provide valuable additional information in this area.

Although as we have seen levodopa is thought to exert its anti-Parkinsonian actions following conversion to DA, the possible role of other metabolites or endogenous compounds cannot be dismissed. For example, OMD concentrations far exceed those of levodopa in plasma and both compete for transport across the BBB by the carrier system. There is conflicting evidence about whether OMD or O-methoxy-tyramine (the O-methylated metabolite of DA) may have partial agonist, or indeed antagonist, properties at postsynaptic receptor sites. Part of this conflict arises because of alterations in distribution of each compound when both are present, but some interference seems inevitable.

Apart from small molecules resulting from simple metabolic transformations, more complex derivatives known to have partial agonist properties, such as tetrahydro-isoquinolines, have also been identified in trace amounts in the urine of PD patients receiving levodopa. Their significance is not known, but it has even been suggested that these compounds may have toxic effects which limit the benefits of treatment.

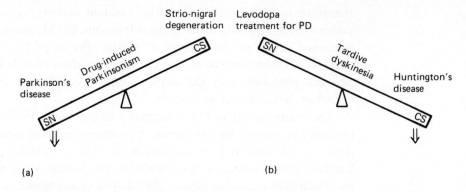

Fig. 16.4. Neuronal imbalances causing Parkinsonism and chorea. Normally there is a fine balance between output from substantia nigra (SN) and the corpus striatum (CS), at the fulcrum of which is the dopamine synapse. (a) Imbalance causing Parkinsonism. If the effective SN output is reduced relative to CS output, Parkinsonism results. This may occur because of SN cell loss alone (PD) or with additional but less marked CS loss (strio-nigral degeneration), and also following pharmacological impairment of dopamine transmission (depleting agents, receptor antagonists). (b) Imbalance causing chorea. If the effective CS output is reduced relative to SN output, chorea results. This may occur because of CS cell loss alone (HD), or following chronic neuroleptic blockade at the synapse (TD). Chorea is also provoked by levodopa treatment in PD.

Clinical experience

As already mentioned, the response to levodopa is usually invariable, striking and almost diagnostic. Those patients who do not respond to adequate doses often later develop additional clinical features of a more widespread degenerative condition known to be resistant to levodopa therapy. Such conditions may mimic idiopathic Parkinsonism in their early stages and are sometimes known as Parkinsonism-plus syndromes. They include striato-nigral degeneration (in which postsynaptic striatal neurons are lost, see Fig. 16.4), progressive supranuclear palsy and other multiple system atrophies.

Even if the diagnosis of PD is correct, the therapeutic effect is not always well sustained. After between 5 and 8 years of treatment most patients have deteriorated to their pre-treatment level of disability and some are significantly worse despite appropriate increments in dosage (Fig. 16.5). This is assumed to correlate with continued nigral cell loss as the underlying disease advances. Furthermore, a series of distressing complications gradually emerge that present major management problems. Most of these take the form of fluctuations in motor response to the drug.

For example, abnormal involuntary movements (AIMs) frequently develop and may gradually become more severe with increasing duration of therapy. Thus up to 75% of patients may be affected after 5 years. Fidgeting that is initially imperceptible to the untrained eye slowly becomes more obvious. Some unfortunate victims may ultimately experience violent and exhausting AIMs in responses to relatively low doses.

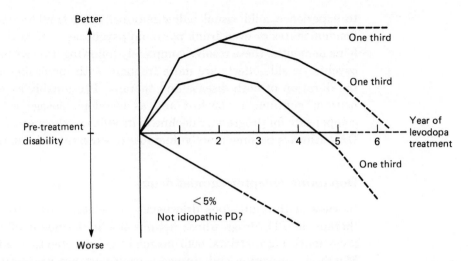

Fig. 16.5 The decline in therapeutic benefit of levodopa. (Redrawn from *Lancet* (1977), i, 345–9.)

Such drug-induced movement usually coincides with high brain concentrations of levodopa and is known as peak-dose dyskinesia. It is exactly analogous to the stereotypy provoked in experimental animals by DA receptor agonists. Indeed identical AIMs are seen when apomorphine is given to such patients. Levodopa-induced dyskinesia has only ever been reported in patients with basal ganglia disease. It is believed to reflect the state of denervation hypersensitivity of the central DA receptors exposed to chronic but intermittent excitation, although certain facts do not fit this simple explanation (see DA receptor agonists below).

Also after about 5 years of treatment about two-thirds of patients experience a wearing-off of the response 2 or 3 hours after each oral dose, when AIMs disappear and Parkinsonian disability re-emerges. This phenomenon is almost certainly due to declining capacity to store newly synthesised DA in presynaptic vesicles as nigro-striatal neurons continue to be lost.

A small group of patients experience abrupt and spectacular transformations from AIMs with acceptable mobility to profound Parkinsonism and vice versa. Such changes in clinical state are so rapid that victims liken them to the operation of an internal switch, and the term 'on-off syndrome' is used. These subjects appear to be hardly able to store any transmitter, and their motor response closely follows changes in levodopa concentration in plasma (and more closely those in brain) during conventional intermittent oral therapy. Continuous intravenous administration is able to smooth out their response, however (Hardie *et al.* 1984), and therefore attempts are being made to develop a sustained-release oral formulation.

In the advanced stages of PD, other distressing complications of levodopa therapy may also be encountered. Susceptible patients begin to experience mild visual hallucinations, more troublesome toxic confusional states or even frank paranoid psychoses. Unless there is underlying dementia, these resolve completely following drug withdrawal. Such psychiatric side-effects are more frequent with increasing age and with the duration of both disease and therapy. Presumably as nigro-striatal neurons continue to be lost and as levodopa dosage is increased to compensate for progressive decline in its efficacy, the meso-cortico-limbic DA pathways become more vulnerable to excessive stimulation.

Dopamine receptor agonist drugs

In view of the numerous drawbacks associated with chronic levodopa therapy in PD, drugs whose actions are independent of the diseased presynaptic nigro-striatal neurons might be expected to be advantageous. Metabolic activation and storage capacity are not necessary. Moreover, although the physiological role of the D_1 receptor subtype is uncertain, drugs that selectively stimulate D_2 sites might have fewer undesirable actions. Agonists with a long duration of action would be particularly suited to oral administration.

Unfortunately so far, the limited clinical experience with DA receptor agonists has failed to confirm in practice their theoretical advantages. This is partly because of potent adverse reactions which are of course those seen following systemic formation of DA when levodopa is given without a ExCDDI. Nausea and vomiting can occur at very low dosage and prevent further absorption, and psychiatric reactions and troublesome postural hypotension are also encountered.

Within the last few years, however, domperidone has become available for clinical use. This compound is a DA receptor antagonist that does not cross the BBB but which reduces significantly the incidence of emesis and hypotension associated with agonist drugs. Its value is thus analogous to that of ExCDDIs, since both are confined to the systemic circulation and used in combination with a centrally acting drug to reduce unwanted peripheral actions. Indeed domperidone could be given with levodopa to reduce the unwanted effects of systemic DA formation, but unlike ExCDDIs it would not improve the bioavailability of levodopa.

Even when administered with domperidone, the results of using DA receptor agonists have been disappointing. The risk of psychiatric complications such as hallucinations, confusion and psychosis is greater than when used alone because larger doses can be employed. Furthermore, although these agents possess unequivocal anti-Parkinsonian activity, their maximal effect is only ever equal to, and usually less than, that achieved with levodopa in the same subjects.

Most of the agonists that have been used belong to the ergolene family derived from ergot alkaloids. They include bromocriptine, pergolide and lisuride. None is a pure D_2 agonist and each has a slightly different spectrum of properties. Much of their toxicity may be related to the ergot nucleus (lysergic acid is another member of this class of compounds), and agonists of other classes are currently being developed.

Bromocriptine

The only substantial clinical experience with a DA receptor agonist in PD is with bromocriptine, the first such agent to become available for use in humans. Its value has already been established in the management of pituitary tumours which secrete high concentrations of prolactin and require DA inhibitory control. However, since the first report in 1974 of its use as an adjuvant to levodopa, more than a decade of clinical experience has failed to establish a clear role for it in PD and the issue remains controversial (Hardie 1987).

Despite the disadvantages, most physicians still prefer to employ combination therapy with levodopa and ExCDDI. Occasionally the addition of bromocriptine later may be helpful because of its longer duration of response (4–8 hours) in patients with 'wearing-off' effects, but such polypharmacy is usually best avoided.

Experience with sustained bromocriptine therapy as first-line treatment in newly-diagnosed cases is even more limited. Unacceptable adverse reactions are frequent and the response in those patients able to tolerate effective doses tends to decline rapidly. This may in part be due to true tachyphylaxis mediated by receptor changes, although patients usually remain responsive to the introduction of levodopa.

One intriguing and so far unexplained fact that has emerged from these trials, in direct contrast with levodopa, is that AIMs are almost never seen. This may be related to the differential actions of bromocriptine at various receptor sub-types. There is experimental evidence that the drug, as well as being a D_2 agonist, has partial agonist activity at D_1 sites and may actually require the presence of presynaptic striatal structures (autoreceptors?) to exert its full anti-Parkinsonian effect.

Clearly it would be desirable to examine a pure D_2 agonist in man, but such an agent is not yet available. Perhaps it is not possible in the diseased striatum to separate anti-Parkinsonian effect from drug-induced AIMs, but this remains one of the most desirable goals sought by clinical neuropharmacologists (see also tardive dyskinesia below).

Other agents modifying dopamine function

Selegiline

Formerly known as (−)-deprenyl, selegiline (phenyl-isopropyl-methyl-propinylamine hydrochloride) is a novel and selective inhibitor of the MAO isoenzyme type B, MAO_B, found in platelets and in the striatum and for which DA is the preferred substrate. Unlike conventional MAOIs, selegiline therapy requires no dietary restrictions and can safely be given with levodopa.

A single 10 mg dose of selegiline is easily sufficient to inhibit platelet MAO for more than 24 hours. Because it is itself metabolised by MAO_B to form a product which combines irreversibly and lethally with the active centre of the enzyme, it is known as a 'suicide' inhibitor. Indeed it has recently been shown *in vivo* by PET using a positron-emitting ^{11}C label that when given to human volunteers the compound remains fixed in the basal ganglia for several months.

Selegiline is itself metabolised partly to a mixture of amphetamine and metamphetamine, which may explain occasional complaints of euphoria, insomnia and hallucinations in patients receiving it, and raises the possibility of indirect DA-releasing properties. Inhibition of neuronal uptake of certain amines including DA can also be demonstrated in experimental animals.

Given all these possible actions, it is perhaps surprising that in clinical trials selegiline has no appreciable anti-Parkinsonian effects when given alone. Even when given to patients already receiving combination therapy with levodopa plus ExCDDI, significant clinical benefit is seen in only about one third of subjects, particularly those with fluctuations in motor response to levodopa. Nevertheless it has been suggested that long-term 'triple therapy' with levodopa, ExCDDI and selegiline could be advantageous and might reduce the dosage requirement for levodopa itself. This issue is considered further at the end of this chapter (see 'Prevention' p. 292).

Amantadine

This anti-viral agent was discovered by chance to be of mild benefit in PD. It is a primary amine whose mechanism of action remains uncertain. Increased synthesis, enhanced release and inhibited re-uptake of DA have all been demonstrated *in vitro*, and the drug also has anti-cholinergic properties. In patients the benefits are usually only modest and tolerance often develops, so it is now seldom used.

Anti-cholinergic drugs

The usefulness of natural belladonna alkaloids in PD has been known for more than 100 years. Moreover, physostigmine makes the symptoms worse, a property not shared by quarternary compounds which inhibit cholinesterase without crossing the BBB.

The striatum contains the highest concentration of acetyl choline (ACh) found in any region of the brain. Systemic physostigmine, intra-caudate injection of ACh and oxotremorine or arecoline given by either route all cause tremor in experimental animals. This has been used as a rather imperfect model for the screening of anti-PD drugs, particularly since direct injection of ACh into the pallidum of Parkinsonian patients undergoing stereotaxic surgery also produces tremor.

However, cholinomimetic agents have little effect on overall motor activity apart from slight general inhibition in some species which may be partly mediated by alterations in arousal, and physostigmine does not cause tremor or other motor effects in healthy human subjects. It is only in animals with nigro-striatal lesions or exposed to neuroleptics, or in humans with PD, that there is clear evidence of antagonism between DA and ACh.

Generally it is believed that the dopaminergic nigro-striatal tract inhibits cholinergic striatal interneurons, and that a functional balance exists between these two systems. In PD this balance is lost and the cholinergic system effectively becomes over-active, hence the response to atropine-like drugs. Cholinergic neurons are now known to comprise less than 5% of the total striatal cell population, so the importance of such an interaction is much less certain. The response may be more directly related to effects on the output systems from the striatum and also on the efferent neurons of the pars reticulata of the substantia nigra.

In the last 40 years a wide variety of semi-synthetic anti-cholinergic compounds have been developed for their central selectivity, but all are associated to some degree with the typical peripheral anti-muscarinic effects of constipation, dry mouth, blurred vision and urinary retention. Some, like benzhexol, are thought to have an additional effect in inhibiting striatal DA re-uptake.

None of these agents is entirely satisfactory, however, and their role is rather uncertain. They exert a modest effect in attenuating Parkinsonian tremor and relieving muscular rigidity, but it is doubtful whether they improve functional disability in patients because they do not reverse akinesia. This observation suggests that the so-called positive features of increased tremor and rigidity are the result of disinhibited cholinergic efferent activity, whereas the negative symptom of reduced and slowed motor activity correlates directly with the extent of DA deficiency. The beneficial effects are often hard to demonstrate after a few years of treatment suggesting that tolerance develops, perhaps as cholinergic activity reverts to normal.

Since PD patients are usually elderly, they are particularly susceptible to central as well as peripheral adverse reactions. Thus anti-cholinergic drugs may cause unpleasant toxic confusional states and there is some evidence that they impair intellectual functions especially during long-term treatment. For these reasons, drugs of this class are now no longer used routinely by many specialists.

Theoretical treatment strategies

Manipulation of central dopamine systems

Tyrosine. The effects of the immediate precursor of levodopa, tyrosine, are disappointing. The response is not at all comparable to that seen with levodopa and of no practical benefit. Presumably this is because only very small quantities reach the CNS unchanged and its conversion to levodopa is slow.

Tetrahydrobiopterin. The hydroxylation of both tyrosine to levodopa and of 5-HTP to 5-HT requires the presence of the co-factor biopterin in its reduced form, tetrahydrobiopterin or BH_4. Clinical trials of this agent are currently in progress but preliminary results have not been encouraging.

Antidepressants. There is a high incidence of depression among PD patients, up to 30% in some studies, and it is tempting to speculate that this may reflect DA deficiency in other pathways such as the meso-cortico-limbic system. This matter is rather controversial, since many of the clinical studies have not used appropriate control subjects with matched degrees of physical disability. Also Parkinsonian patients may appear to be depressed when this is not the case because poverty of movement reduces non-verbal communication. It is estimated that about 5 or 10% of patients are truly depressed.

In practice, tricyclic antidepressants are quite often prescribed in combination with anti-Parkinsonian agents and a therapeutic trial may certainly be worthwhile. Although it has recently been withdrawn due to unacceptable toxicity, nomifensine has been shown to have weak anti-Parkinsonian efficacy and like members of the imipramine class it inhibits re-uptake of DA and NA (see Chapter 19). Moreover, many tricyclic antidepressant drugs also have anti-cholinergic properties. However, it is hard to distinguish selective improvement in motor function from an effect due to mood elevation, and benefit should be critically evaluated.

Manipulation of other neurotransmitter systems

Over the last 20 years the concept of a selective and focal DA deficiency in PD has had to be revised. This is particularly so since the discovery of many novel neuropeptides, some of which are highly localised within the basal ganglia such as cholecystokinin, neurotensin and vasoactive inhibitory peptide. As already discussed, more than 90% of striatal cells are not cholinergic. The medium spiny neurons represent the efferent projections to the pallidum and to the pars reticulata of the substantia nigra and use GABA, substance P and enkephalins as neurotransmitters (Pasik *et al.* 1987).

Post-mortem neurochemical analysis has identified decreased concentrations in certain brain areas of NA, 5-HT, glutamic acid decarboxylase (responsible for the synthesis of GABA), substance P, somatostatin and methionine enkephalin (Hornykiewicz & Kish 1987). Whether any of these additional abnormalities are primary, or whether they are epiphenomena secondary to nigro-striatal degeneration, is simply not known but the therapeutic implications are clear: correcting DA deficiency alone may be of limited benefit, especially in the long term. For these reasons, many attempts have been made to improve patients using alternative strategies.

Noradrenaline and 5-HT. NA can be derived directly not only from DA but also from L-threo-dihydroxy-phenylserine (L-threo-DOPS). It has been claimed by Narabayashi *et al.* (1987) that this substance may have useful effects in PD, particularly for patients with 'freezing' of gait. Trials of 5-HTP have not demonstrated any benefit.

GABA. Unfortunately, various attempts to augment GABA transmission have all failed to demonstrate benefit. These include inhibition of GABA metabolism using sodium valproate, and trials of GABA-mimetic drugs such as baclofen and muscimol.

Prevention

The ultimate altruistic aim of medical science in any disease is prevention rather than cure. Unfortunately the aetiology of PD remains as much a mystery now as when James Parkinson in 1817 wrote: 'Uncertainty existing as to the nature of the proximate cause of this disease, its remote causes must necessarily be referred to with indecision.' Although the 'proximate cause' is now believed to be degeneration of the nigro-striatal pathway, the 'remote cause' of this degeneration is still not known. By analogy with cases of secondary Parkinsonism, infective agents such as viruses and toxic substances seem the most likely culprits, but all known plausible candidates have been excluded.

An outbreak of Parkinsonism in 1982 among Californian heroin addicts has re-awakened interest in a search for a possible environmental toxin. The discovery of the effects of MPTP was a chance consequence of illegal attempts to synthesise heroin-like compounds for sale to American addicts (Langston *et al.* 1983).

MPTP is a piperidine derivative (1-methyl-4-phenyl-1,2,3,6-tetrahydro-pyridine) that shows selective toxicity for pigmented nigro-striatal neurons. Exposure to this substance, even in trace amounts and via cutaneous and inhalation routes, results in symptoms and signs identical to those of idiopathic Parkinsonism. This irreversible behavioural syndrome is only seen in humans and other primate species, but not in lower mammals which do not possess neuromelanin. In laboratory primates it has provided a unique experimental tool, both for studying aetiology of PD and for screening drugs with possible therapeutic activity.

The exact mechanism of MPTP toxicity is still not fully understood. It is known that MPTP itself is in fact an inert 'protoxin', and that it is conversion *in vivo* to a charged pyridinium species MPP^+, via another intermediate compound MPDP, which accounts for its lethal effects upon

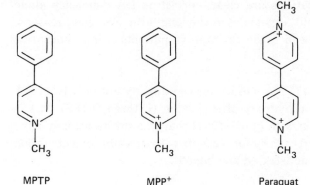

Fig. 16.6. Structure of MPTP, MPP$^+$ and paraquat.

MPTP   MPP$^+$ Paraquat

nigro-striatal neurons. The charge leads to trapping of the toxic species within the intraneuronal compartment (Snyder and d'Amato 1986).

The biotransformation of MPTP to MPP$^+$ is catalysed in mitochondria by the enzyme MAO and occurs in almost every tissue in the body that has been studied. Quite why the toxic effects should be confined to the cells of the zona compacta of the substantia nigra remains a mystery. Other DA-producing cells remain unaffected, including the adrenal medulla and the hypothalamus. It has been suggested that the DA re-uptake mechanisms or the neuromelanin of the target neurons may hold the key.

As yet, no naturally occurring substance with comparable toxicity has been identified, although the similarity between the molecular structures of MPTP and paraquat, a widely used herbicide, has excited speculation about a causal link between PD and industrial chemicals (Fig. 16.6). Such speculation has been encouraged by the demonstration that inhibitors of MAO$_B$ such as selegiline completely prevent both clinical Parkinsonism and nigral cell death in primates exposed to MPTP.

Another hypothesis concerns the toxic effects of free radicals and peroxide which are natural by-products of DA oxidation by MAO to form dopa quinone, the essential constituent of neuromelanin. A gradual cumulative action could account for the steady loss of nigro-striatal neurons seen with normal ageing, whereupon the additional insult from a putative environmental toxin might be enough to result some years later in the manifestation of PD.

It has also recently been claimed that treatment with selegiline may retard the course of the underlying disease process in PD. If so, it would represent a completely new therapeutic strategy. Early introduction or indeed prophylactic pre-symptomatic treatment for all at-risk (i.e. over 50 years of age) individuals has been advocated by some. However, it has also recently been found that, under certain experimental conditions, selegiline potentiates MPTP toxicity. Clinical trials currently under way may provide the answer, but only over the course of 5 or 10 years of follow-up. Meanwhile, this indication for the drug remains controversial.

Brain transplants — a cure?

The extreme specificity which characterises the neurons of the CNS also results in vulnerability to all sorts of degenerative processes because they cannot be replaced. Notwithstanding enormous compensatory changes which occur amongst surviving cells in the Parkinsonian brain, once 70-80% of the nigro-striatal neurons are lost clinical deficits become apparent and further decline is inexorable. Part of this decline may result from the increased metabolic demands placed by such compensation upon the remaining but ailing cells.

The recent refinement of procedures to transplant suspensions of DA-rich cell groups to certain sites within the CNS has now for the first time raised the restoration of neural function as a real practical possibility. So far research has concentrated on using embryonic tissue in the hope of improving graft survival and, in behavioural models of Parkinsonism, dopaminergic synaptic function can be restored (Bjorklund *et al.* 1983; Olson *et al.* 1987).

Further intensive work is in progress to study possible therapeutic applications, and a very small number of pioneer operations have been carried out in human patients. The ethical and technical problems are formidable, but progress is eagerly awaited by all those involved in the care of PD victims

Neuroleptic-induced movement disorders

Clinical trials of chlorpromazine for mental illness in the early 1950s demonstrated that, as well as sedation, it caused a state of apparent indifference and slowing of responses to external stimuli, together with diminution of initiative and of anxiety. These behavioural characteristics were referred to as the 'neuroleptic syndrome' and are now known to be shared by all clinically useful anti-psychotic agents, hence the term neuroleptic drugs.

In addition, all such drugs induce extrapyramidal features that are indistinguishable from idiopathic PD. Indeed during neuroleptic treatment a great variety of clinical movement disorders have been observed whose mechanisms are poorly understood. The same movement disorders can be induced by metoclopramide and prochlorperazine, drugs of the same class but used widely as anti-emetics and in the treatment of dizziness rather than as psychotropic drugs. Since these drugs are all DA receptor antagonists, it is assumed that alterations of central DA transmission are responsible.

Acute dystonic reactions, i.e. involuntary sustained contractions of skeletal muscle such as in torticollis or oculo-gyric crises, may occur within the first few days of treatment. In contrast, a general state of motor restlessness known as akathisia usually takes one or two months to develop. The most commonly seen disorders, neuroleptic-induced Parkinsonism and tardive dyskinesia, typically emerge even later.

Neuroleptic-induced Parkinsonism

Although there remains some uncertainty regarding the relevance of DA antagonism to the therapeutic efficacy of neuroleptic drugs in psychotic patients, there is no doubt that their capacity to cause Parkinsonism is directly related to their potency *in vitro* as DA receptor antagonists, and presumably also *in vivo* at the postsynaptic receptors of the nigro-striatal tract.

So far it has not proved possible to dissociate completely anti-psychotic properties from extrapyramidal side-effects. Indeed it was originally believed that mild Parkinsonian features were inevitable in patients receiving effective dosage, although this belief has now been discredited. Some agents do have rather more favourable profiles than others, but those that are said to be relatively free from this complication (e.g. thioridazine) tend to be the least potent.

Within individuals, Parkinsonian features appear in proportion to neuroleptic dosage, usually after some weeks or months of treatment but high doses can have effects within days. Tolerance to extrapyramidal actions may gradually develop later without any loss of anti-psychotic benefit. It has therefore been suggested that differential adaptive changes in DA turnover and receptor sensitivity may occur in different regions of the brain (see Chapter 7).

There is a remarkable variation in individual susceptibility to those unwanted effects. This probably correlates with pre-treatment loss of nigro-striatal neurons, since younger patients are in general more resistant. A few patients, usually elderly, develop apparently irreversible Parkinsonism which fails to improve after discontinuation of the offending drug. These may have underlying idiopathic PD which had originally been of pre-symptomatic severity.

Similarly the speed with which Parkinsonism resolves after drug withdrawal is very variable. Although the syndrome usually resolves within 3 months, some elderly patients may take 12 months or more before normal motor function is restored. Pharmacokinetic factors, particularly when using long-acting depot formulations, account for some of this variability, but the presence of subclinical impairment of basal ganglia function must also be important.

Treatment

The best treatment for drug-induced Parkinsonism is obviously withdrawal of the offending drug. Many patients continue to receive long-term neuroleptic medication inappropriately, and in others maintenance dose requirements may be considerably lower than the initial dosage needed to control an acute psychosis.

The value of anti-cholinergic drugs such as benzhexol is disputed. In the 1960s it became common practice to prescribe them routinely in the hope of preventing Parkinsonism or at least permitting the use of higher neuroleptic dosage. More recently doubt has been cast on the wisdom of this prophylactic strategy, and controlled trials have suggested that anticholinergic agents are actually of little or no benefit.

The use of levodopa has been limited by fears of precipitating further psychosis. Hence it has often been reported to be of no value. However, it is now recognised that levodopa may be effective in some patients if given in sufficient dosage.

Tardive dyskinesia

Clinical aspects

As its name implies, tardive dyskinesia (TD) usually takes many months or years to develop. In the adult it typically affects the oral region, with rapid repetitive and stereotyped involuntary movements of the face, tongue and jaw musculature. Choreiform dyskinesia may also affect the limbs and trunk. The involuntary movements are similar or identical to those that characterise Huntington's chorea (see below) or those provoked by levodopa in patients with PD.

Similar dyskinesia may occur spontaneously in patients who have never been exposed to drugs. It has been argued that the syndrome may just be a feature of institutionalised, usually elderly, chronic schizophrenics but there is strong epidemiological evidence to the contrary. Of those on long-term neuroleptic treatment, 20–40% exhibit orofacial dyskinesia, whereas it occurs much less frequently (5–8%) amongst comparable drug-free patients.

TD usually worsens during attempts to withdraw the cause by reducing neuroleptic dosage. Paradoxically, increasing the dose of the offending drug or substituting a more powerful DA receptor antagonist will temporarily suppress the movements. Ultimately however this strategy will lead to a 'breakthrough' of TD. Potentially the most serious feature of TD is that, following drug withdrawal, it usually persists and may get worse, or it may even appear for the first time. In some individuals, perhaps as many as 30%, the disorder is permanent and may be of distressing severity.

Pharmacology

Clinical studies indicate that despite the administration of DA antagonists there is over-stimulation of cerebral DA systems in TD. Thus DA agonists generally increase TD, whereas drugs that deplete DA (reserpine, tetrabenazine) or inhibit its synthesis (α-methyl-p-tyrosine) decrease it. There is, however, no direct clinical biochemical evidence of central DA overactivity, nor indeed of other neurotransmitter system disturbances.

In contrast, there is behavioural and biochemical evidence in rats that chronic administration of neuroleptic drugs gradually leads to a loss of

DA antagonism and, after about nine months, to the development of supersensitivity to DA. In this state animals show exaggerated stereotypy in response to apomorphine, and increases above pre-treatment values can be measured in striatal DA receptor numbers and affinity (see Chapter 7). These observations have naturally cast doubt on the DA hypothesis of schizophrenia, since similar tolerance and reversal of the acute actions of neuroleptics might be expected to occur in all cerebral DA systems.

Differential actions at D_1 and D_2 receptors may be important. It has been claimed that peri-oral movements in rats are mediated by D_1 stimulation (Rosengarten et al. 1983), since most neuroleptics have little (e.g. most phenothiazines) or virtually no (e.g. butyrophenones) affinity for D_1 receptors. Hence it has been argued that those compounds with a larger ratio of D_1/D_2 activity, such as thioridazine, produce less behavioural supersensitivity and so are less likely to provoke TD (Hyttel et al. 1985). Conversely, it has also been proposed that certain selective D_2 antagonists such as sulpiride, a substituted benzamide derivative, are associated with a lower risk of TD.

As yet, clinical experience with these newer agents is insufficient to resolve this matter, and extrapolation from data obtained in behavioural animal models is clearly of limited value. Not only are they very time-consuming and expensive, but also they cannot be directly comparable since actual abnormal movements are rarely if ever seen in neuroleptic-treated rodents. Spontaneous oral dyskinesia is elicited in primate species but only transiently and the movements may be decreased by anti-cholinergic drugs, a pattern not seen in TD in man.

In fact, anti-cholinergic drugs will exacerbate pre-existing TD. There is also evidence in both psychiatric patients and in animal models of TD that exposure to such drugs early in the course of neuroleptic treatment may increase the relative risk of developing TD later. Thus it is now even more difficult to justify using anti-cholinergic medication routinely to prevent drug-induced Parkinsonism.

Pathophysiology

It is not unusual to see patients on long-term neuroleptic treatment who display oro-facial dyskinesia simultaneously with the limb tremor, stooped posture and shuffling gait of drug-induced Parkinsonism. This certainly suggests that the acute actions and chronic adaptive changes following treatment with such drugs are not uniform in all regions of the brain. The effects may differ even within certain parts of the striatum, assuming that their distribution is uniform.

What remains puzzling is why TD only affects a certain proportion of patients exposed to similar prolonged treatment with high doses of neuroleptics. Even amongst susceptible individuals, the severity and anatomical distribution may differ widely. This is in direct contrast to animal models, in which biochemical and behavioural evidence of enhanced DA sensitivity is universal.

Age and the presence of minor extrapyramidal deficits are probably the keys. Since identical involuntary movements may occur spontaneously in the elderly and in patients with certain neurological or psychiatric conditions, neuroleptic drugs may be said to potentiate the underlying pathophysiological processes which are expressed as oro-facial dyskinesia. The ventro-lateral part of the striatum, somatotopically linked to cephalic movements, may be particularly vulnerable to, for example, ischaemic damage, whereas neuronal loss in other parts may account for the development of limb chorea.

The analogy between oro-facial dyskinesia and Parkinsonism is now apparent. Both are clinical syndromes that occur increasingly with age and to which neuroleptic drugs predispose. The exact and undoubtedly complex pharmacological consequences are not yet fully elucidated.

Huntington's disease

Huntington's disease (HD) is a rare genetic disorder of the CNS characterised by the progressive development of involuntary choreiform movements together with personality changes and dementia. It is particularly distressing because symptoms do not usually become apparent until the middle years of life, 30–50, by which time victims may already have raised a family of their own. Because the condition is autosomal dominant, there is a 50% chance that each child ultimately may be similarly afflicted.

Fine, almost imperceptible, chorea may first affect the fingers, where rhythmic flexion and extension movements are seen. Insidious onset of oro-facial, limb and trunk involvement soon follows, and exhausting dyskinesia may later affect the whole body. The involuntary movements always disappear during sleep. Psychological changes include early depression and concentration difficulties, followed by a gradual decline in ability to function at work and to manage domestic affairs and finally an apathetic state with frank dementia. Outbursts of excitement or temper, suicidal tendencies and paranoid delusions may also occur.

Pathophysiology

The pathology of HD is found mainly in the basal ganglia and cerebral cortex. There is severe atrophy and gliosis of the corpus striatum with relative sparing of neurons in the shrunken globus pallidus. There are correspondingly profound depletions in striatal GABA and ACh and in their neuronal enzyme markers GAD and ChAT. Peptides including substance P, methionine enkephalin and dynorphin, which are thought to co-exist with GABA in strio-nigral and strio-pallidal neurons, are also reduced, although their functional significance is not known. Moreover, there is thinning of the cortex with selective loss of efferent neurons in layers 3, 5 and 6 of the frontal and parietal regions. Cortical levels of glutamate, GAD and ChAT are generally normal however, and those systems containing DA and NA are also relatively spared.

The mechanism of neuronal loss in HD is unknown, but much attention has been focused on an animal model involving kainic acid. Direct intra-striatal injection of this substance, a rigid cyclic analogue of glutamic acid, causes extensive neuronal destruction and gliosis in rats with biochemical disturbances remarkably similar to those in HD. Administration of glutamate itself in high concentrations and another analogue, ibotenic acid, produces similar effects. For reasons that are unclear, chorea itself is not seen in animals thus treated.

Because there are widespread cortico-striatal projections which utilise glutamate as an excitatory transmitter, it has been postulated that an endogenous neurotoxin like kainic acid might be involved in the pathophysiology of HD. Alternatively, neuronal damage might be the result of normal glutamate release acting upon congenitally abnormal postsynaptic striatal membranes.

Treatment

There is no satisfactory treatment for this progressive, fatal condition. Drug management is confined to measures for symptomatic relief. Although striatal DA release is probably reduced in HD, loss of postsynaptic neurons bearing DA receptors is even greater. Thus net overactivity is thought to account for the beneficial actions of DA depleting agents and neuroleptic receptor antagonists. These remain the most widely used agents for the reduction of chorea, despite their potential hazards.

Unsuccessful therapeutic attempts have been made to overcome cholinergic deficits using precursors like choline and cholinomimetic agents such as pilocarpine and arecoline. This failure is probably because of loss of ACh receptors themselves. Similar experience with drugs aimed at augmenting GABA transmission, including muscimol, isoniazid and sodium valproate, has been disappointing. More encouraging preliminary results have been obtained with the $GABA_B$ agonist baclofen, beta-p-chlorphenyl-GABA, which appears to inhibit release of excitatory transmitters including glutamate.

Conclusions

Clinical disorders of the basal ganglia may give rise to either reductions or excesses in motor activity. In PD, loss of the nigrostriatal DA pathway results in characteristic slowness and poverty of spontaneous movement and failure to respond appropriately to environmental stimuli, i.e.

bradykinesia. The condition is ameliorated by the DA precursor levodopa or by DA receptor agonists such as bromocriptine.

By contrast, loss of neurons within the striatum itself occurs in HD. In this malady excessive spontaneous motor activity is seen, together with exaggerated and uncontrolled responses to external stimuli, i.e. chorea. The involuntary movements are generally reduced by neuroleptic drugs that simulate PD.

The full spectrum of movement disorders may be encountered during chronic administration of neuroleptic compounds, especially in elderly patients who perhaps have pre-existing basal ganglia damage. As well as Parkinsonism, a state of functional supersensitivity may develop. In this state, known as tardive dyskinesia, involuntary choreiform movements are also seen (Fig. 16.4). The same concatenation occurs in patients with PD in whom levodopa, but apparently not bromocriptine, may provoke dyskinesia. This suggests that certain pathways within the basal ganglia and possibly various DA receptor subtypes may have differential properties.

Finally it must be stressed that the causes of both these degenerative conditions, HD and PD, remain obscure. Manipulation of central DA systems provides only temporary symptomatic relief and it remains to be seen whether other neurotransmitters are of additional importance in the pathophysiology of basal ganglia disorders.

References and further reading

Bjorklund A, Dunnett SB, Gage FH, Iverson SD, Schmidt RH & Stenevi (1983) Intracerebral grafting of neuronal cell suspensions. *Acta Physiol. Scand.* Suppl 522, 1–75.

Brogden RN, Speight TM & Avery GS (1971) Levodopa: a review of its pharmacological properties and therapeutic uses with particular reference to Parkinsonism. *Drug* **2**, 262–400.

Calne DB & Stoessl AJ (1987) Transmitter receptor alterations in Parkinson's disease. *Adv. Neurol.* **45**, 45–9.

Carlsson A (1959) The occurrence, distribution and physiological role of catecholamines in the nervous system. *Pharmacol. Rev.* **11**, 490–3.

Casey DE, Chase TN, Christensen AV & Gerlach J (eds) (1985) *Dyskinesia: Research and Treatment.* Springer-Verlag, Berlin.

Cotzias GC, van Woert MH & Schiffer LM (1967) Aromatic amino acids and modification of Parkinsonism. *New Engl. J. Med.* **276**, 374–9.

Ehringer H & Hornykiewicz O (1960) Verteilung von Noradrenalin und Dopamin im Gehirn des Menschen und ihr Verhalten bei Erkrankungen des Extrapyramidalen Systems. *Klinische Wochenschrift* **38**, 1236–9.

Hardie RJ, Lees AJ & Stern GM (1984) On-off fluctuations in Parkinson's disease: a clinical and neuropharmacological study. *Brain* **107**, 487–506.

Hardie RJ (1987) The controversial role of dopamine receptor agonists. In: Rose FC (ed.) *Recent Advances in Parkinson's Disease.* John Libbey, London.

Hyttel J, Larsen JJ, Christensen AV & Arnt J (1985) Receptor-binding profiles of neuroleptics. In: Casey *et al.* (eds) *Dyskinesia: Research and Treatment.* Springer-Verlag, Berlin.

Hornykiewicz O & Kish SJ (1987) Biochemical pathophysiology of Parkinson's disease. *Adv. Neurol.* **45**, 19–34.

Langston JW, Ballard P, Tetrud JW & Irwin I (1983) Chronic Parkinsonism in humans due to a product of meperidine-analog synthesis. *Science* **219**, 979–80.

Marsden CD & Fahn S (1987) *Movement Disorders 2*. Butterworth, London.

Martin JB & Gusella JF (1986) Huntington's disease: pathogenesis and management. *New Engl. J. Med.* **315**, 1267–76.

Narabayashi H *et al.* (1987) Clinical effects of L-threo-3,4-dihydroxyphenylserine in cases of Parkinsonism and pure akinesia. *Adv. Neurol.* **45**, 593–602.

Olson L *et al.* (1987) Nigral and adrenal grafts in Parkinsonism: recent basic and clinical studies. *Adv. Neurol.* **45**, 85–94.

Pasik P *et al.* (1987) Ultrastructural chemoanatomy of the basal ganglia: an overview. *Adv. Neurol.* **45**, 59–66.

Quinn NP (1984) Anti-Parkinsonian drugs today. *Drugs* **28**, 236–62.

Rosengarten H, Schweitzer JW & Friedhoff AJ (1983) Induction of oral dyskinesias in naive rats by D-1 stimulation. *Life Sci.* **33**, 2479–82.

Snyder SH & d'Amato RJ (1986) MPTP: A neurotoxin relevant to the pathophysiology of Parkinson's disease. *Neurology* **36**, 250–8.

Yahr MD & Bergmann KJ (1987) *Parkinson's Disease*. Advances in Neurology vol 45. Raven Press, New York.

17   The epilepsies

B.S. MELDRUM

Clinical syndromes

Definition

Hughlings Jackson defined epilepsy as 'an episodic disorder of the nervous system arising from the excessively synchronous and sustained discharge of a group of neurons'. This definition successfully encompasses the diverse clinical manifestations of the disease, including disturbance of both motor and cognitive functions. It conforms to the precept that a single fit is not epilepsy. It does not exclude fits secondary to systemic metabolic disorders, although most authorities today do so. It has the great advantage of emphasising the crucial role of neuronal excitation and inhibition and, by implication, the neurotransmitter substances responsible for these processes.

Classification

Classifications based on aetiology, although logically desirable, at present create more problems than solutions. Thus most practical classifications are based on the clinical expression of the seizures. This is exemplified by the classification drawn up by the Commission on Terminology of the International League against Epilepsy (and subsequently revised, Commission 1981). The key factor is the *local* or *general* onset of the seizure, as evaluated from clinical observation and electroencephalography. Thus the major groups are:

1 *Partial (focal) seizures or seizures beginning locally*

   (a) *Simple partial seizures* (includes focal motor attacks and seizures with somatosensory signs or psychic symptoms).

   (b) *Complex partial seizures* (includes those forms of temporal lobe or 'psychomotor' seizures where consciousness is impaired — may begin with simple partial seizure).

   (c) *Secondary generalised* (seizures commencing as in (a) or (b) but evolving to generalised tonic-clonic, clonic or tonic seizures).

2 *Generalised seizures, bilateral symmetrical seizures, or seizures without local onset*

Includes:

(a) absence seizures and atypical absence;

(b) myoclonic seizures;

301   THE EPILEPSIES

(c) clonic seizures;

(d) tonic seizures;

(e) tonic-clonic seizures (TC);

(f) atonic seizures.

This classification ignores questions of frequency of seizures, duration of attacks, precipitating factors and any identifiable underlying pathology. Any type of attack maintained for more than 1 hour can be referred to as *status epilepticus*, although it may be qualified as *focal*, or *generalised*.

Specific pathological processes may themselves be either generalised or focal. Although there is a broad correspondence between partial seizures and focal pathology, this is by no means exact. Generalised pathologies may give rise to partial or focal seizures and vice versa.

Evidence that the underlying defect in cellular metabolism or neuro-humoral function differs between clinical categories of epilepsy is provided by the different pharmacological responsiveness of, for example, *absences*, myoclonic jerks, and partial seizures, to ethosuximide, benzo-diazepines and carbamazepine respectively.

Animal models of epilepsy

Animal models of epilepsy also show a differential effectiveness of anticonvulsant drugs. Additionally they permit the investigation of underlying biochemical changes.

Several animal syndromes of epilepsy appear to be genetically determined. In mice there are at least 12 single locus mutations that produce neurological syndromes with spontaneous seizures (Seyfried & Glaser 1985). One syndrome known as *'tottering'* has aroused much interest because the spontaneously-occurring seizures resemble absence attacks both behaviourally and electroencephalographically (Noebels & Sidman 1979). Among the syndromes showing seizures precipitated by sensory stimulation, sound-induced seizures in DBA/2 mice and posturally-induced seizures in EL (epilepsy-like) mice have been extensively studied biochemically and various abnormalities in ATPase and in monoamines and other neurotransmitter systems reported (see below).

Beagle dogs show a high incidence of epilepsy including secondary forms, and two types of primary convulsions resembling complex partial seizures and generalised tonic clonic seizures (Edmonds *et al.* 1979). Of the genetically-determined syndromes in animals the only one that has a precise counterpart in human epilepsy is the syndrome of photically-induced seizures in the Senegalese baboon, *Papio papio*. This shows similar genetic features and age and sex dependence in man and in the baboon (Meldrum 1980).

Syndromes of chronic focal epilepsy can be induced in mammals (rats, cats, monkeys) by topical application to the cortex of various metals, including cobalt, iron and alumina.

Focal electrical stimulations of certain brain areas at a strength sufficient to induce an after-discharge but not a seizure leads, when repeated a number of times at spaced (days) intervals, to the induction of a permanent tendency to readily triggered epileptic discharges. This process of epileptogenesis, referred to as 'kindling' (Goddard et al. 1969; McIntyre & Racine 1986) has provided an important model for evaluating the involvement of different neurotransmitters in epileptogenesis.

Electroshock or the acute administration of convulsant drugs such as pentylenetetrazol, picrotoxin and bicuculline, are frequently used to test anticonvulsant drugs.

Study of the biochemical or molecular mode of action of convulsant (and anticonvulsant) drugs has also indicated many ways in which disturbed neurotransmitter function can facilitate or provoke seizures.

Biochemical basis of epilepsy

The biochemical abnormalities that predispose to seizures in man are poorly understood and difficult to study. There is little opportunity to perform neurochemical studies in the primary syndromes of epilepsy, as they are chronic non-fatal syndromes that do not require neurosurgical intervention. The few reported studies of neurosurgical specimens are of necessity principally concerned with partial epilepsy (focal neo-cortical or temporal lobe seizures). Observations relating to neurotransmitters and their metabolites based on plasma, cerebrospinal fluid, or neurosurgical specimens from patients with epilepsy present problems that are discussed below.

Many inborn errors of metabolism are associated with seizures as a constant or variable feature of the neurological symptomatology. In a few such cases, particularly those involving disorders of amino acid metabolism, specific alterations in inhibitory or excitatory transmission can be proposed as explanations of the seizures.

Membrane-bound enzyme systems that hydrolyse ATP, and are probably related to ionic pumps for Na^+, K^+ and Ca^{++}, have frequently been reported to be abnormal in human epileptogenic material and in animal models of epilepsy (both induced and genetic). A reduction of Na-K dependent ATPase is reported in human focal epileptogenic tissue. This could be a result of drug therapy or of secondary cellular changes. However, a similar reduction in Na-K dependent ATPase activity has been described in experimental alumina foci. In DBA/2 mice, showing sound-induced seizures, a reduction in the activity of Na-K dependent ATPase was initially reported. Subsequently a selective reduction in the Ca^{++} activated ATPase in brain was described (see Palayoor et al. 1986). Other models of epilepsy, including chicks and gerbils with a genetic liability to reflex epilepsy, also show abnormalities in ATPase systems (Rosenblatt *et al.* 1977). Ouabain and other inhibitors of Na-K ATPase are potent convulsants when infused into the ventricles (Pedley *et al.* 1969). This is consistent with a defect in membrane ATPase contributing to epileptogenesis.

Many compounds occurring naturally in the brain have been found to be convulsant if injected intracerebroventricularly or intra-cortically. Among such compounds particular interest attaches to folic acid and its derivatives, and to the formaldehyde condensation products of catecholamines (tetrahydroisoquinolines) and of indoleamines (β-carbolines). There is a complex relationship between folates and both the synthesis and the further metabolism of monoamines. A metabolite of tryptophan, quinolinic acid, is a convulsant and excitotoxin. Enzymes for the synthesis and further metabolism of quinolinic acid are found in brain.

Different syndromes of epilepsy are likely to have different biochemical bases. Possibly also any one syndrome could be the end result of more than one pattern of metabolic abnormality. Metabolic abnormalities may be too general in nature to serve as a target for therapeutic modification. Genetically determined abnormalities in neurotransmitter systems (involving the receptor molecules or related ionophores, or the proteins involved in the synthesis or reuptake of neurotransmitters) may contribute to seizure susceptibility. Obviously, therapeutic benefit might be derived from correction of, or compensation for, a defect in neurotransmitter function. These possibilities will now be evaluated.

Neuropathology

The pathology found in the brains of patients with epilepsy is of three types (see Meldrum & Corsellis 1984).

1 *Focal lesions* that are themselves the primary causes of secondary epilepsy. These include congenital malformations (vascular), neoplasms, traumatic lesions, infarcts, abscesses, cysts and parasitic infestations (including cysticercosis). In general there is no clear pathological difference between such lesions whether they occur in patients with or without epilepsy.

2 *Diffuse infective or degenerative disease*, that is primary and has no specific relationship to epilepsy, but may be associated with epilepsy (including focal seizures and myoclonic syndromes). This group includes pathologies as diverse as the leucodystrophies, cerebral malaria, Huntington's chorea, and Alzheimer's disease.

3 *'Epileptic brain damage'*. This is a pathological syndrome which is found to varying degrees both in patients with primary or idiopathic epilepsy and in those in which epilepsy is clearly secondary to some focal or generalised disorder. It is characterised by a highly selective neuronal loss and by glial proliferation which is partly selective and partly diffuse. The lesions are either a consequence of seizure activity or of an episode

of diffuse cerebral hypoxia/ischaemia in the perinatal period or early childhood. In the hippocampus the neuronal loss involves selectively the pyramidal neurons in the endfolium and the Sommer sector. In the cerebellum the Purkinje and the basket cells are selectively involved, while in the neocortex, smaller pyramidal neurons, particularly in the 3rd cortical lamina, are most vulnerable. Glial proliferation is seen in all regions of selective neuronal loss, but also independently in the subpial region of the cortex.

The evidence that such pathological changes are secondary to epilepsy comes from both clinical observations and animal experiments. Pathology of recent origin but with a similar pattern of regional selectivity is found in children and adults dying acutely after *status epilepticus* (Meldrum & Corsellis 1984). Animal studies of drug induced *status epilepticus* (either generalised, due to bicuculline or allylglycine, or focal limbic due to kainic acid) also show neuronal loss, or its prodromal manifestation, 'ischaemic cell change', occurring with similar selectivity in the hippocampus, neocortex and cerebellum.

Cellular aetiology of epilepsy

The three types of pathology listed above do not give a clear indication of what cellular changes could be responsible for epileptic activity. It is necessary to look for changes that are common to all the pathological syndromes, and which could, on physiological grounds, be responsible for abnormal paroxysmal discharges. The following four possibilities are based on specific cytological immunochemical or neurophysiological findings but remain hypothetical as aetiological mechanisms.

Selective loss of inhibitory interneurons

Syndromes of spasticity following ischaemic lesions of the spinal cord are related to a selective loss of inhibitory (glycine) interneurons. A similar selective effect of ischaemia or hypoxia on GABA neurons in the neocortex, or hippocampus could be responsible for a lowered seizure threshold. There is animal experimental evidence that hypoxia in infancy can selectively damage GABA neurons in the cortex but the more familiar selective neuronal loss found in patients with epilepsy is not restricted to inhibitory interneurons. Thus, there is a reduction in hippocampal pyramidal neurons which are excitatory. There is a selective loss of GABA nerve terminals around an epileptic focus induced in the monkey cortex by the local application of alumina (Ribak *et al.* 1979).

Supersensitivity and sprouting following neuronal loss

These two secondary processes follow neuronal loss induced by local surgical or chemical lesions and could contribute to epileptogenesis.

Firstly, neurons that are postsynaptic to the degenerating neurons show supersensitivity to the transmitter concerned. Thus loss of excitatory pyramidal neurons in the cortex or hippocampus could be followed by supersensitivity to excitatory amino acid transmitters. Neocortex deafferented experimentally by undercutting shows an enhanced tendency to epileptiform 'afterdischarges' following electrical stimulation. Also, this supersensitivity of neurons to a particular transmitter could facilitate the spread and synchronisation of activity since they might respond to what would normally be a sub-threshold, non-stimulating, extracellular concentration of the appropriate neurotransmitter released from a nearby neuron. The time course of development of supersensitivity (1–4 weeks) is comparable to development of focal epilepsy in some animal models (alumina focus) but epileptogenesis following focal pathology in man has a much slower and more variable time-course.

Secondly, dendrites adjacent to regions of synaptic degeneration sometimes show 'sprouting', and grow to form new synapses occupying the sites left vacant. Such synapses are sometimes functionally inappropriate and could contribute to abnormal discharges.

Processes of the above two types will follow every pathological process involving neuronal degeneration, and could explain the relative lack of specificity in the primary pathologies of epilepsy.

Direct evidence for supersensitivity of excitatory amino acid receptors has been provided in hippocampal slices from 'kindled' rats and in human focal epileptic cortex. Responses to iontophoretically applied N-methyl-D-aspartate (NMDA) are enhanced in the CA_1 dendritic zones and in the dentate molecular layer in the rats (Mody & Heinemann 1987) and in superficial and intermediate laminae in the human cortex.

Dendritic degeneration and loss of spines

The use of Golgi and related silver staining techniques reveals a type of neuronal change that is seen in all three classes of epileptic pathology (**1–3**, p. 304). It consists of an apparently progressive simplification or degeneration of the complex dendritic trees of pyramidal neurons in the cortex and hippocampus, associated with a loss of the spinous processes (that are postsynaptic specialisations on the principal dendrites). This type of change was first reported in a variety of degenerative disorders including epilepsy. It is seen around experimental foci induced in the monkey cortex by alumina.

Loss of spines and dendritic simplification could be the ultrastructural correlate of an enhanced tendency to paroxysmal burst discharges, both because the degenerating dendrite might itself be more prone to burst firing and because such firing might more easily invade the soma because of electrotonic shortening. It may also reflect the supersensitivity of the NMDA receptor system observed in electrophysiological studies.

Glial proliferation

An increase in the number of fibrous or reactive astrocytes is seen characteristically in all three types of epileptic pathology, i.e. around a focal lesion, in diffuse degenerative disorders and in secondary epileptic pathology. It has been suggested that some failure in the capacity of astrocytes to regulate the extracellular environment could be responsible for locally enhanced epileptogenicity. However, direct experimental tests of the capacity of reactive astrocytes to regulate extracellular potassium concentration show enhanced rather than impaired function.

Cellular neurophysiology

The hypothesis of Hughlings Jackson that the critical abnormality responsible for epileptic phenomena is the excessive and synchronous discharge of groups of neurons has been amply confirmed. However, the related problems of which neurons are involved in paroxysmal discharges and what factors determine the initiation and spread of the abnormal discharges remain to be answered.

Some observations are almost universal. They are seen in acute *in vitro* models, as well as in chronic seizure foci in animals and man, both during seizures and as a feature of inter-ictal discharges. Generally single neurons show a characteristic pattern of burst firing, with action potentials occurring at a frequency higher than under normal circumstances (with an interspike interval of less than 5 msec). Such single cell bursts are commonly the concomitant of epileptic 'spikes' (duration less than 100 msec) recorded with macroelectrodes on the cortex or scalp.

Burst firing originates in two ways. It may arise 'spontaneously' as an intrinsic abnormality in an 'epileptic' neuron (variously called a 'Group I neuron' or a 'pacemaker' neuron) within a focus or it may occur in a normal neuron in response to an abnormal synaptic input. Evidence for the existence of 'epileptic' or 'Group I' neurons comes from studies in monkeys with chronic alumina foci in the parietal cortex in which the pattern of firing within bursts in some neurons is invariant during diverse patterns of motor behaviour or levels of alertness and stages of sleep. Antidromic activation of pyramidal tract neurons which show Group I type burst firing always results in a typical burst discharge, never a single action potential, indicating a persistent abnormality in membrane responsiveness. Within and around a focus some neurons show firing patterns that are sometimes normal and sometimes contain paroxysmal bursts. These have been called 'Group II neurons', and are thought to be rapidly recruited into burst firing by 'pacemaker' (Group I) neurons during spread of seizure activity.

This neurophysiological model of the epileptic focus, suggests that focal seizures may be prevented by two basic pharmacological approaches.

One would be to act directly on pacemaker neurons to stabilise membrane potential and decrease the occurrence of spontaneous bursts. The other would operate on synaptic mechanisms to prevent the recruitment, by 'pacemaker' neurons, of Group II or normal neurons into the paroxysmal discharge. Obvious mechanisms for achieving this include blockade of excessive excitatory synaptic action (by reducing the maximum rate of synthesis of excitatory transmitter, or its rate of release, or its postsynaptic action) and enhancement of inhibitory (feedback) systems to prevent recruitment into burst firing.

Intracellular recordings show that there is a distinctive and characteristic 'paroxysmal depolarisng shift' in membrane potential accompanying the burst firing of neurons (Prince 1968). Not surprisingly this depolarisation has some of the features of a giant excitatory synaptic potential but studies of burst firing induced by penicillin or bicuculline in hippocampal slices show that a failure of recurrent inhibition (due to impaired GABA function) is directly or indirectly responsible for the paroxysmal depolarising shift. Recurrent excitatory inputs are revealed when inhibition is impaired (Miles & Wong 1987). Repetitive excitatory (orthodromic) inputs can initiate dendritic burst firing. Hyperpolarisation of the soma by recurrent inhibitory systems normally prevents invasion of the soma by this bursting activity, but when this is inadequate, bursting and a paroxysmal depolarising shift are seen in soma records (Schwartzkroin & Wyler 1980). This process is probably facilitated in neurons in chronic foci in which the dendritic tree is shortened and denuded of spines, and in which antidromic impulses can trigger burst firing.

Thus, in studying neurotransmitter influences on epileptic activity it is necessary to consider excitatory and inhibitory influences on both soma and dendrites and their various interactions.

Neurohumoral dysfunction

The pathophysiology of epilepsy, as summarised above, indicates that abnormal neurotransmitter function or abnormal neuronal membrane properties are the major factors producing the paroxysmal manifestations of epilepsy.

Since studies of cellular electrophysiology in epilepsy indicate both impairment of postsynaptic inhibitory processes and facilitation of excitatory synaptic responses, as causes of paroxysmal depolarising responses, it will be necessary to consider appropriate features of excitatory and inhibitory transmission between central neurons and the neurotransmitters responsible for them. In fact pharmacological studies have provided convincing evidence that neurohumoral dysfunction can explain many forms of epilepsy. Several convulsant drugs have been shown to modify neurotransmission in highly specific ways. Analysis of the molecular basis of these phenomena has provided evidence for the importance of GABA in preventing epileptic discharges. Similarly the effects on seizure threshold of drugs having specific effects on monoaminergic transmission show that dopaminergic, noradrenergic and serotoninergic neurotransmission influence certain forms of epilepsy, especially syndromes of reflex epilepsy.

At the membrane level the magnitude and direction of induced potential changes is ultimately determined by the ratio of intracellular to extracellular ionic concentrations. Any disturbance in these concentrations will modify the relative efficacy of excitatory and inhibitory synaptic events. Thus faults in pumping mechanisms controlled by ATPase could be important. Also ionic redistribution, and the electrogenic action of some ionic pumps can contribute to changes in responsiveness during and after seizure activity.

Inhibitory amino acids

Amino acids found in the brain that inhibit neuronal firing include glycine, serine, GABA, taurine, L-α-alanine, β-alanine, imidazole-4-acetic acid, hypotaurine, L-cystathionine, 4-amino-3-hydroxybutyric acid, pipecolic acid and γ-amino-valeric acid (Curtis & Johnston 1974).

There is clear evidence that glycine and GABA are inhibitory transmitters in the spinal cord and brain. The physiological role of taurine is less well defined.

Glycine

In the spinal cord both physiological inhibitory action and that due to iontophoretically applied glycine can be blocked by strychnine and related alkaloids such as brucine and thebaine (Curtis & Johnston 1974) which can explain the convulsions that follow their systemic administration. However, there is no natural syndrome of epilepsy in animals or man that shows the same seizure pattern as that produced by alkaloids blocking inhibition induced glycine. Although ischaemic damage to the spinal cord results in a selective reduction in glycine content, and presumably of glycine containing interneurons. Such lesions both in man and experimental animals are associated with spasticity not seizures.

Epileptogenic foci in the human cortex and in the brains of experimental animals have either a normal or an elevated content of glycine. Infants with non-ketotic hyperglycinaemia, an inherited disorder of amino acid metabolsim, in which plasma and CSF glycine content is greatly elevated due to absence of the glycine cleavage enzyme, present with muscular hypotonia. This suggests that the raised CSF and brain glycine is enhancing physiological recurrent inhibition in the spinal cord. Such children also commonly show generalised myoclonic jerks, and spike and wave discharges on the EEG (Markand *et al.* 1982).

When tested in animal models of epilepsy glycine has little anticonvulsant action, but it can enhance the effect of some other anticonvulsants. Thus the effects of GABA-transaminase inhibitors, of diazepam and of barbiturates against chemically-induced (3-mercapto-propionic acid), reflex and kindled amygdaloid seizures in rodents are enhanced by the chronic oral administration of glycine (Seiler & Sarhan 1984; Peterson 1986).

GABA

In the cortex and hippocampus GABA is released by intrinsic neurons (aspinous stellate cells, basket cells) which are activated by output collaterals (from pyramidal neurons) and in turn act on pyramidal cell bodies, thus providing feedback inhibition. In the motor cortex these interneurons are also activated by collaterals of afferents from the thalamus. Thus these GABA releasing interneurons are well situated to suppress or prevent the excessive synchronous or sustained discharges of groups of neurons.

GABA neurons in focal epilepsy and in pathological conditions predisposing to epilepsy

Around an epileptogenic focus, induced experimentally by alumina in the monkey cortex, there is a selective loss of nerve terminals staining for the GABA synthesising enzyme glutamic acid decarboxylase (shown by light microscopy) and of symmetrical synapses (inhibitory) when compared with asymmetrical synapses (excitatory) (seen by electron microscopy) (Ribak *et al.* 1979). In human temporal lobe cortex, removed during neurosurgery for focal seizures, some samples show a reduced content of glutamic acid decarboxylase (GAD). In infant monkeys, exposure to a moderate degree of hypoxia for 30 minutes leads to degeneration of symmetrical synapses belonging to the GABA aspinous large stellate cells (Sloper *et al.* 1980). This evidence raises the possibility that seizures in children or adolescents, that have suffered asphyxia or cerebral hypoxia in the perinatal period, may be a consequence of a selective loss of GABAergic inhibitory neurons.

Pyridoxine phosphate is required as cofactor for the synthesis of GABA by GAD and impaired GABA synthesis is almost certainly responsible for the seizures observed in infants suffering from a dietary deficiency of pyridoxine, or from the inborn metabolic disorder, pyridox-ine dependency, in which the requirement for pyridoxine is increased (Coursin 1964).

Measurement of cerebrospinal fluid GABA concentration has provided some support for GABA deficiency as an aetiological factor. As shown in Table 17.1 several studies have reported lowered levels of CSF GABA in chronic epilepsy and in febrile convulsions even though most patients were on anticonvulsant medication.

Table 17.1. Lumbar CSF GABA content in patients with epilepsy

Controls			Patients				
pmol/ml	n	Age (years)	pmol/ml	n	Age (years)	Seizure type (n)	Reference
239 ± 76	19	42 ± 15	162 ± 71	8	45 ± 14	Generalised, TC (3) Complex partial (3) Simple partial (2)	Manyam et al. (1980)
239 ± 21	20	32 ± 3	139 ± 12	21	29 ± 2	Generalised, TC (5) Complex partial (8) Simple partial (8)	Wood et al. (1979)
210	16	4.6	134	23	1.6	Febrile convulsions	Löscher et al. (1981)
174	41	5.7	121 (untreated)	15	2.9	Infantile spasms (9) Partial (11)	Löscher & Siemes (1985)
			161 (treated)	17	5.9	Myoclonic (4) Generalised TC (4) Miscellaneous (3)	

Seizure activity is induced by all drugs that impair the synthesis or postsynaptic action of GABA (Meldrum 1975, 1979). These seizures are focal if the drug is applied to the cortex or hippocampus, or generalised if the drug is given systemically.

The synthesis of GABA is impaired by a wide range of drugs that inhibit GAD (see Chapter 11). At least three distinct mechanisms of inhibition are effective. Thus 3-mercaptopropionic acid and malic and glutaric acid inhibit by substrate competition. Various hydrazides, isoniazid, thiosemicarbazide, methyl-dithiocarbazinate, methoxypyridoxine, and 4-deoxypryridoxine inhibit by cofactor antagonism, impairing the synthesis or coenzymic action of pyridoxal phosphate (Meldrum 1975). Convulsions produced by L-allylglycine are due to irreversible inhibition of GAD by a metabolite, 2-keto-4-pentenoic acid (Orlowski et al 1977).

The postsynaptic inhibitory action of GABA can be blocked by drugs acting at three distinct sites on the GABA receptor/ionophore complex (see also Chapters 11, 12 and 20). Firstly, bicuculline and related compounds produce convulsions by competing with GABA for its recognition site. Secondly, picrotoxinin, the so-called cage convulsants (tetramethylenedisulphotetramine, p-chlorophenylsilatrane and various bicyclophosphate esters) and some convulsant barbiturates bind to a 'picrotoxinin binding site' which appears to be closely related to the chloride ionophore (Olsen 1982) and prevents the increase in chloride conductance that is the physiological effect of the combination of GABA with its recognition site. Thirdly 'inverse agonists', such as the convulsant β-carbolines, act on the benzodiazepine receptor but decrease rather than enhance the effect of GABA (Meldrum & Braestrup 1985).

When given systemically all three types of GABA antagonist produce generalised seizures with relatively short latencies. The site of initiation of the seizures is not definitively established. The concentration of bicuculline or picrotoxin required to initiate focal cortical seizures in the motor area appears to be higher than that attained following systemic injections. However, a region in the deep prepyriform cortex is exceptionally sensitive to the convulsant action of bicuculline (Piredda & Gale 1986).

Pharmacological enhancement of GABA-mediated inhibition

It is not generally practicable to enhance the action of GABA by administering either it or its precursor, glutamate, systemically. It may however be possible to achieve an anticonvulsant effect by administering GABA entrapped in liposomes (Loeb *et al.* 1986). Table 17.2 lists seven possible pharmacological mechanisms for enhancing GABA-mediated inhibition. Among drugs used clinically the most powerful anticonvulsant effects that can be attributed to enhanced GABA-mediated inhibition are those of the benzodiazepines in primary generalised epilepsies.

Table 17.2. Pharmacological mechanisms leading to enhancement of GABA-mediated inhibition

GABA agonists, e.g. muscimol, THIP
GABA prodrugs, e.g. Cetyl-GABA, progabide, dihydropyridine, GABA-benzylester
Facilitation of GABA release
Inhibition of GABA-transaminase, e.g. γ-vinyl GABA, ethanolamine-O-sulphate
Allosteric enhancement of the affinity of the GABA recognition site, e.g. benzodiazepines, β-carbolines
Action on chloride ionophore to facilitate or prolong its opening, e.g. barbiturates
Inhibition of reuptake of GABA into neurons or glia, e.g. nipecotic acid, THPO

Enhancement of the effect of GABA through an action on the chloride ionophore has been demonstrated for barbiturates, but its precise relation to the clinical effectiveness of barbiturates is less clear.

GABA agonists

By definition a GABA agonist acts at the GABA recognition site of a GABA receptor complex to reproduce the physiological effect of GABA. The most potent agonist at the $GABA_A$ receptor is the fungal toxin, muscimol. Recently several GABA analogues have been synthesised which are highly 'selective' for this recognition site (see Fig. 17.1).

Two of these selective $GABA_A$ agonists, muscimol and THIP, are anticonvulsant when tested in various rodent models of epilepsy, including seizures induced by pentylenetetrazol or by GABA antagonists in mice or by sound in genetically susceptible mice. Isoguvacine and homotaurine are ineffective when given systemically, apparently because of limited entry to the brain (Meldrum 1981).

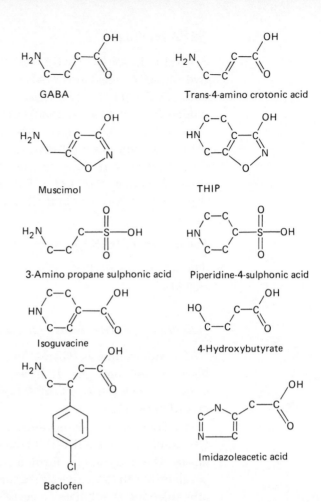

Fig. 17.1. Molecular formulae of GABA agonists.

The potent GABA$_A$ agonists are not, however, useful anticonvulsants. Muscimol and THIP when evaluated in a primate model (photosensitive epilepsy in the baboon, *Papio papio*) do not block photically-induced myoclonus. Indeed they produce rhythmic spike and wave discharges in the EEG and occasional diffuse myoclonus (Pedley *et al.* 1979; Meldrum & Horton 1980). Similar paroxysmal EEG appearances and diffuse myoclonus are seen in patients (with schizophrenia or Huntington's chorea) who have been given muscimol experimentally. Possibly, the diffuse activation of postsynaptic GABA$_A$ receptors, renders inoperative the normal antiepileptic action of the GABA system, which depends on the activation of postsynaptic receptors with a specific timing and spatial relationship to ongoing activity.

The GABA$_B$ agonist L-baclofen when tested in photosensitive baboons depresses photically-induced myoclonic responses, but also induces rhythmic spike and wave discharges (Meldrum & Horton 1974; Meldrum 1981).

GABA prodrugs

Several lipid soluble GABA derivatives that enter the brain and can be hydrolysed to yield free GABA have been tested in animal models as anticonvulsants. Among these cetyl-GABA is active in some rodent models (Frey & Loscher 1980) but it is not proven that hydrolytic release of GABA into the synaptic cleft is responsible for this activity. A brain delivery system for a GABA-benzyl ester has been devised employing a dihydropyridine-pyridinium salt that upon oxidation is trapped in the brain (Anderson *et al.* 1987). This appears to produce behavioural effects dependent on intracerebral release of GABA.

Facilitation of GABA release

There is relatively little data concerning drugs with a specific action of this kind.

Inhibition of GABA-transaminase activity

GABA-transaminase (GABA-T) is a mitochondrial enzyme found in both neurons and glia. It is not directly involved in the inactivation of synaptically released GABA (see Inhibition of GABA reuptake below and Chapter 11).

Several compounds have been described that are 'irreversible' catalytic inhibitors of GABA-T. These are analogues of GABA that are acted on by the enzyme to form a reactive intermediate that combines covalently with the active site of the enzyme (Metcalf 1979). They include ethanolamine-O-sulphate, γ-acetylenic GABA and γ-vinyl GABA and gabaculine. These compounds produce a massive and sustained increase in brain GABA content (4–10 fold increase over 4–48 hours). Anticonvulsant effects can be demonstrated in a wide variety of rodent models of epilepsy with a time course comparable to the increase in brain GABA content. In baboons with photosensitive epilepsy a similarly sustained antiepileptic effect is seen after γ-vinyl GABA or γ-acetylenic GABA (Meldrum & Horton 1978). γ-vinyl GABA has a useful therapeutic action in patients with 'drug resistant' epilepsy (Rimmer & Richens 1986).

These observations demonstrate that inhibition of GABA-T can lead to an anticonvulsant effect. This is presumably because there is a secondary increase in the quantity of GABA released synaptically or a secondary impairment of GABA reuptake. A selective enhancement of synaptosomal GABA content has been demonstrated, transiently after γ-acetylenic GABA, but in a sustained fashion after γ-vinyl GABA.

Allosteric enhancement of the affinity of the GABA recognition site

(See section on anticonvulsant drugs p. 326–8.)

Action on chloride ionophore

As above.

Inhibition of GABA reuptake

Synaptically released GABA is inactivated in the mammalian nervous system by reuptake into neurons and glia. There are high and low-affinity sodium dependent uptake systems. GABA is a highly flexible molecule and the distance between the two charged groups in the GABA zwitterion is less when it interacts with the high affinity GABA carrier than when it acts at the GABA postsynaptic recognition site. Thus there are GABA analogues which act selectively on reuptake (Krogsgaard-Larsen 1980). These include cis-3-aminocyclohexane carboxylic acid, nipecotic acid and guvacine. Most of these compounds do not cross the blood–brain barrier because of their high ionised/un-ionised ratio. However, when applied iontophoretically in the mammalian CNS they can be shown to enhance the inhibition produced by the iontophoretic application of GABA and they also enhance physiological inhibition due to GABA.

The anticonvulsant action of inhibitors of GABA uptake has been tested against sound-induced seizures in susceptible (DBA/2) mice using intracerebroventricular injection (Meldrum *et al.* 1982). Protection is seen after nipecotic and cis-4-hydroxynipecotic acid and THPO, the latter being also effective following intraperitoneal injection. Two compounds that inhibit neuronal uptake but are inactive against GABA uptake into astrocytes (L-2, 4-diaminobutyric acid and ACHC) both induce spontaneous myoclonus and seizures, possibly because they are transported into GABA nerve terminals and displace the neurotransmitters and thus reduce its release. Esters of nipecotic acid, guvacine or cis-4-hydroxynipecotic acid can be used as prodrugs, yielding the active agents following intracerebral hydrolysis (Meldrum *et al.* 1982).

The evidence that a failure in GABA function is responsible for any major syndromes of epilepsy in man remains weak. Nevertheless there is overwhelming evidence that impairment of GABA-mediated inhibition leads to seizures and that enhancement of physiological inhibition due to GABA has a potent anticonvulsant effect in many models of epilepsy. From the therapeutic point of view it is clear that enhancement of inhibitory processes that are spatio-temporally selective in relation to ongoing neuronal activity, whilst preserving the functional integrity of feedback mechanisms, is probably best achieved by the mechanisms attributed to the benzodiazepines and to the barbiturates. GABA agonists or direct GABA mimetics are unlikely to achieve this.

Taurine

Taurine depresses neuronal firing when applied iontophoretically and this inhibition in the cortex and in the lateral geniculate is blocked by strychnine and bicuculline (Curtis & Johnston 1974). The physiological role of taurine in the brain remains to be defined.

Several claims relating to taurine in epilepsy remain controversial. A report that taurine content was reduced in human focal epileptogenic tissue was not subsequently confirmed (Perry *et al.* 1975). The concentration of taurine in plasma was also said to be elevated in adult patients with primary generalised seizures, secondarily generalised seizures or partial complex seizures. However, plasma taurine concentration is low in children with 3/sec spike-wave epilepsy, and in their first degree relatives (Van Gelder *et al.* 1980). A study of plasma and urinary taurine concentration in a mixed population of 41 epileptic subjects reports elevated plasma taurine and an increase in the proportion of low excretors of taurine in the group with epilepsy (Goodman *et al.* 1980). Both these studies offer interpretations in terms of genetically determined abnormalities of amino acid transport mechanisms, that are seen as part of the polygenic background favouring the development of epilepsy.

Intracerebroventricular taurine appears to raise electrical seizure threshold in rats with audiogenic seizures, but not in normal rats (Laird & Huxtable 1978) and a therapeutic effect has been claimed for systemic taurine both for experimental and spontaneous epilepsy in cats and for focal epilepsy in man. However, any therapeutic action of taurine in man appears to occur only in a proportion of patients with partial epilepsy and to be most marked in the first month of treatment (Takahashi & Nakane 1978).

Excitatory amino acids

The intracortical or intracerebroventricular injection of glutamate or aspartate or other excitatory amino acids leads to focal or generalised seizure activity. Particularly potent as a focal convulsant is kainic acid, a toxin derived from seaweed. Systemic administration of these excitant amino acids can also induce seizures, which in the case of kainic acid predominantly involve the limbic system.

Glutamate and aspartate

Reductions in the concentration of glutamate and aspartate have been reported in animal and human epileptogenic foci although this is not a consistent observation in man. Glutamate release into cortical superfusates occurs with increased epileptic discharges. Such observations could be interpreted as consequences of enhanced activity.

The recent description of potent and specific antagonists of excitatory amino acids (see Fig. 13.2) has permitted the investigation of their anticonvulsant properties. When administered intracerebroventricularly in DBA/2 mice, antagonists of excitation due to NMDA (e.g. γ-glutamylglycine, 2-amino-5-phosphonopentanoic acid and 2-amino-7-phosphono-heptanoic acid) block sound-induced seizures (Croucher *et al.* 1982). These NMDA antagonists are also active against sound-induced, and chemically-induced, seizures in rats or photically-induced seizures in baboons following systemic administration (Meldrum *et al.* 1983).

Cysteic, homocysteic acid

There is a paucity of data concerning the sulphur amino acids. Homocysteine given systemically is a convulsant, but its mechanism of action is uncertain; homocysteine is a pyridoxal phosphate antagonist and thus can impair GABA synthesis. However, seizures induced by homocysteine are exacerbated by pyridoxal phosphate or pyridoxamine and alleviated by hydrazine (Hurd *et al.* 1981). In children with homocystinuria, cystathionine synthetase activity is reduced and homocysteine accumulates in the brain, and may be responsible for the seizures sometimes observed in this condition.

Acetylcholine

ACh has a modulatory role through its muscarinic receptors. ACh enhances the excitatory action of neurotransmitters that increase sodium or calcium conductance (see Chapter 6). Nevertheless, an antiepileptic effect of low doses of anticholinesterases (such as eserine) has been reported (Williams & Russell 1941), which may be the pharmacological counterpart of the physiological suppression of spike and wave discharges by enhanced alertness.

The major evidence linking central cholinergic transmission with epilepsy is the induction of seizures by cholinergic agonists or by inhibitors of cholinesterase. Thus the direct application of cholinergic agonists (such as carbachol) to the cerebral cortex induces focal spikes or seizures. Acetylcholinesterase inhibitors produce similar effects focally but also produce generalised seizures when given systemically, e.g. eserine (in high doses), or the irreversible organophosphate inhibitors, such as di-isopropylfluorophosphate. Seizures induced by cholinergic agonists or by reversible or irreversible inhibitors of cholinesterase can be terminated or prevented by prior administration of atropine or scopolamine.

Antimuscarinic drugs do not possess significant anticonvulsant properties in any spontaneous syndrome of epilepsy in man but large oral doses of choline, in a small open study in patients with partial epilepsy, were associated with an increased frequency of seizures. These were, however, shortened and followed by more rapid recovery. Anticholinergics do not have significant anticonvulsant actions in the standard animal models of epilepsy. Thus overactivity within a central (muscarinic) cholinergic system is unlikely to be responsible for the major syndromes of epilepsy in man.

Neuropeptides

More than 20 peptides have been shown to be present in the central nervous system, usually with a regionally selective distribution, but little evidence is available concerning their role in epilepsy. Nevertheless both convulsant and anticonvulsant actions have been claimed for morphine and related compounds, and similar phenomena have now been described in experiments utilising the 'opiate' peptides (enkephalins and endorphins).

Opiates and antagonists

The acute administration of high doses of morphine, heroin or related opioids can induce seizures in man and animals, as can the withdrawal of opiates or the administration of the antagonist naloxone, in habituated subjects (see Meldrum & Menini 1981). Study of seizure thresholds in rodent models of epilepsy shows that opioids acting preferentially on the mu receptor (such as morphine and etorphine) raise seizure threshold and this effect is antagonised by low doses of naloxone (Cowan *et al.* 1979).

Endogenous opiate peptides

Methionine-enkephalin, leucine-enkephalin and β-endorphin occur in separate neuronal systems and probably fulfil separate functions. Given systemically these three compounds are inactive on seizure thresholds because of rapid breakdown and limited access to the brain. Given systemically FK 33-824, a stable synthetic analogue of methionine-enkephalin that enters the brain, raises seizure threshold in a manner similar to morphine. In rodents intracerebroventricular injection of methionine-enkephalin, leucine-enkephalin or β-endorphin induces transient electrographic seizure discharges, sometimes with a limbic origin. However, similar convulsant effects have not been found after intracerebroventricular or focal limbic injections of opiate peptides in primates (see Meldrum & Menini 1981).

Overactivity or supersensitivity within enkephalinergic systems has been postulated as an aetiological factor in epilepsy, but there is no direct evidence for it. Naloxone is not anti-epileptic in man at the relatively low dose-levels so far tested.

Monoamines

The diverse physiological roles of the monoamines in the brain ensure that major disturbances in these systems will have secondary effects on epileptogenesis although there is little evidence for a primary role of any monoaminergic system in epileptic phenomena in man, with the possible exception of serotonin in post-hypoxia myoclonus. All generalisations relating to monoamines and epilepsy are, however, subject to exceptions. What is true of one syndrome or test system is commonly not true of others.

Depletion of cerebral monoamines by compounds that interfere with storage mechanisms (reserpine, tetrabenazine, etc.) facilitates seizures in several rodent test systems, including electroshock and pentylenetetrazol seizures. Audiogenic seizures in DBA/2 mice are enhanced by reserpine and this effect is transiently reversed by the amine precursors L-DOPA or 5-HTP. The effects of inhibitors of tyrosine hydroxylase, tryptophan hydroxylase, or dopamine β-hydroxylase are relatively weak and sometimes discordant between models, but broadly seizure thresholds are lowered by impairing monoamine synthesis. Important exceptions are:

1 barbiturate withdrawal convulsions (which are diminished or prevented by giving α-methyl-p-tyrosine to inhibit tyrosine hydroxylase)

2 absence seizures in tottering mice (which are prevented by 6-hydroxy dopamine destruction of noradrenergic fibres).

Dopamine, NA and 5-HT agonists have protective effects in specific syndromes of epilepsy, mostly those in which sensory precipitation can be demonstrated ('reflex epilepsy'). Antagonists are sometimes protective, sometimes weakly proconvulsant. Interpretation of these pharmacological observations is complicated by the probable role of 'autoreceptors' and other types or presynaptic monoaminergic mechanism (see Vizi 1979).

Several anticonvulsants, including barbiturates, benzodiazepines, and sodium valproate decrease the turnover of monoamines (Bonnycastle et al. 1957). This effect is not essential to their anticonvulsant action but appears to be secondary to enhanced GABAergic activity. In several rodent test systems the anticonvulsant action of phenytoin, acetazolamide and some other anticonvulsants is reduced if monoamine synthesis or storage is impaired.

Many authors have studied the concentration in the cerebrospinal fluid of metabolites of monoamines, in the hope of detecting some abnormality of monoaminergic metabolism or activity that might be:

1 a predisposing factor to epilepsy

2 a consequence of epilepsy

3 a result of anti-epileptic therapy.

Such studies show that there are no changes in MOPEG, the major metabolite of noradrenaline. The acid metabolites of serotonin and dopamine, i.e. 5-HIAA and HVA are either normal, low-normal or significantly reduced, in untreated or subtherapeutically treated epileptic patients. A more dramatic relative reduction in 5-HIAA or HVA concentration is seen when children with generalised tonic-clonic seizures are compared with controls after probenecid is given to block the outward transport of the acid metabolites. This evidence is in favour of a reduced turnover of serotonin and dopamine in these children with grand mal seizures. In children with frequent infantile spasms or those studied shortly after admission for febrile convulsions or status epilepticus HVA is elevated substantially in CSF, whereas 5-HIAA and MOPEG are not different from controls. This indicates an increase in dopaminergic activity secondary to seizure discharges.

Dopamine

The role of DA in the control of movement is probably part of the explanation for the powerful influence of dopamine agonists on reflex epilepsy and on models where somatosensory afferents play a critical role in the development of seizures and their almost total lack of effect in other models, particularly chemically-induced seizures.

Thus the DA agonist apomorphine completely blocks photically-induced myoclonus in photosensitive baboons (Anlezark et al. 1981) and prevents photically-induced spike and wave discharges in susceptible patients (Quesney et al. 1980). The site of this protective action is not known but is certainly central, as the effect is not blocked by domperidone, a dopamine receptor antagonist that does not cross the BBB (Anlezark et al. 1981). It is not known whether dopamine agonists are effective in other forms of reflex epilepsy in man, but L-DOPA has a protective effect in some cases of action myoclonus (Lhermitte et al. 1972).

Apomorphine and other dopamine agonists are effective against audiogenic seizures in DBA/2 mice (Anlezark et al. 1981). Focal spikes induced by cobalt in the rat neocortex are blocked by dopamine agonists given systemically or focally into the striatum. Such spike discharges appear to be under a cortico-striatal influence that is modified by the dopaminergic system. In contrast seizures induced by pentylenetetrazol in rodents or by allylglycine in baboons are exacerbated, not alleviated, by the administration of apomorphine or other dopamine agonists (Anlezark & Meldrum 1978; Soroko & McKenzie 1970).

Dopamine antagonists acting centrally, such as the neuroleptic phenothiazines and butyrophenones, are weakly proconvulsant. In baboons with photosensitive epilepsy haloperidol enhances the number of spikes and waves on the EEG (Meldrum et al. 1975). With chemically-induced convulsions chlorpromazine is protective. In about 1% of psychiatric patients with no history of epilepsy, phenothiazines precipitate seizures.

Noradrenaline

Studies of NA on cerebellar Purkinje cells show it enhances both excitatory and inhibitory inputs (Moises & Woodward 1980) although there appears to be a preferential enhancement of the inhibitory effects of GABA, mediated by β-adrenoceptors. A similar neuromodulatory role has been demonstrated for NA in the hippocampus (Segal & Bloom 1976). In cortical slices low concentrations of adrenaline facilitate the stimulated release of excitatory amino acids whilst high concentrations depress neurotransmission (Collins *et al.* 1984). Depletion of cerebral catecholamines by reserpine or tetrabenazine or by 6-OH DA facilitates seizures in a wide variety of animal models including electroshock and chemically-induced seizures and audiogenic seizures in rats and mice. However, such effects are weak or absent in primate models of epilepsy (see Altshuler *et al.* 1976) or in man.

The use of drugs which mimic or block the synaptic actions of noradrenaline has given somewhat divergent results in animal models of epilepsy. In reflex epilepsy anticonvulsant effects are produced by NA and by α_2 agonists. Thus adrenaline (100 μg) or NA (250 μg) given intracerebroventricularly, block photically-induced myoclonus in baboons (Altshuler *et al.* 1976). In DBA/2 mice protection against audiogenic seizures follows the administration of α_2 agonist drugs, such as clonidine or oxymetazoline (Horton *et al.* 1980). This effect is reversed by α_2 antagonist drugs such as yohimbine and piperoxan. A similar protective effect of clonidine, with reversal by yohimbine, is seen in air-blast induced seizures in susceptible gerbils (Löscher & Czuczwar 1987). Anticonvulsant effects of α_2 agonist drugs also occur in pentylenetetrazol seizures (Papanicolaou *et al.* 1982; Löscher & Czuczwar 1987). Intracerebroventricular injection of α_1 antagonists, such as prazosin and phentolamine, induces epileptic activity (Horton *et al.* 1980).

A contrasting effect has been demonstrated for focal cortical or hippocampal seizure discharges. Focal cortical epileptiform activity induced by penicillin is suppressed by locus coeruleus stimulation in the rat. This effect is blocked by prazosin (and enhanced by yohimbine), suggesting that it depends on NA acting at an α_1 adrenoceptor (Neumann 1986).

Both proconvulsant and anticonvulsant effects of β-adrenoceptor antagonists have been reported. Propranolol raises the threshold for electrically or chemically induced seizures in rodents and protects against audiogenic seizures in mice. However rather high doses are required and the phenomenon does not show stereo-specificity (Anlezark *et al.* 1979), thus it is probably due to the membrane stabilising effect of propranolol rather than a specific action on β-adrenoceptors. An exacerbation of chemically-induced seizures by ($\pm$) propranolol has also been reported. This is consistent with the enhancement of GABA inhibitory phenomena by NA acting at β-adrenoceptors, but other mechanisms remain possible. Major effects on seizure incidence of α- and β-adrenoceptor antagonists have not been described in man.

Many abnormalities of noradrenergic systems have been reported in the genetic and acquired forms of epilepsy. In the tottering mouse (a recessive syndrome due to the tg gene and manifest as ataxia, myoclonus and cortical spike wave discharges accompanied by behavioural episodes resembling absence attacks) there is an overgrowth of the locus coeruleus ascending adrenergic system that is closely linked to the seizure tendency (preventing its development in the neonatal period blocks seizure development) (Noebels 1984). The number of α_1 adrenoceptor binding sites (measured with [^{3}H] prazosin) is slightly lower in the whole brain of DBA/2 mice compared with a non-seizure susceptible strain (Jazrawi & Horton 1986). Similarly in genetically-epilepsy prone rats there is reduced number of α_1 adrenoceptor binding sites in the frontal cortex (compared with normal Sprague-Dawley rats; Nicoletti *et al.* 1986). In human cortical foci removed surgically an increase in tyrosine hydroxylase activity and a decrease in the density of α_1-adrenoceptors has been described (Sherwin *et al.* 1986). In this case the decrease in the α_1 adrenoceptors would appear to be secondary to enhanced NA release. Noradrenaline concentrations decrease markedly, apparently due to enhanced release, during drug-induced seizure activity in rats (Calderini *et al.* 1978; Vezzani & Schwarcz 1985). This might lead to a down-regulation of α_1 adrenoceptors as a consequence of seizure activity. However, in the best-studied animal model of acquired epilepsy, amygdala-kindled epilepsy in the rat, there are no changes in NA turnover and concentration (Okazaki *et al.* 1986) but there is a sustained down-regulation of β-adrenoceptor binding sites (McIntyre & Roberts 1983; Stanford & Jeffreys 1985).

5-HT

In the light of the evidence for at least two major types of 5-HT receptor (with different distributions and different actions) it is not surprising that the use of 5-HT precursors and agonists gives rise to both convulsant and anticonvulsant effects according to the dose and experimental model studied. In man their most significant effect is protection against action myoclonus.

5-HT; myoclonic syndromes and reflex epilepsy in animals and man

Several myoclonic syndromes (head jerks and whole body myoclonus) have been described in guinea pigs, rats and mice following the administration of rather high doses of 5-HT precursors or agonists. Similar syndromes are evoked by tryptophan following pretreatment with a monoamine oxidase inhibitor, or by 5-methoxy-N,N, dimethyltryptamine. All these myoclonic syndromes are readily blocked by cyproheptadine or metergoline, and less effectively by methysergide or mianserin. These syndromes would appear to be due to action of 5-HT, or its agonists, at postsynaptic 'excitatory' sites ('5-HT$_2$ receptors'), either in the cortex or in the brainstem.

The principal myoclonic syndrome responding to serotoninergic therapies is 'intention' or 'action' myoclonus occurring as a sequel to brain hypoxia or head injury. A marked therapeutic effect is seen for 6–8 hours after the intravenous infusion of 5-HTP 2–5 mg/kg (Lhermitte *et al.* 1972; Chadwick *et al.* 1977) in a proportion of patients. Responsive patients have electrophysiological evidence for a brainstem origin of their myo-clonus, and also show low CSF 5-HIAA content. It is possible that this form of action myoclonus is a result of inadequate function within a serotoninergic system. Long-term therapy with oral 5-HTP is only moderately effective, partly because of limitations imposed by gastro-intestinal side-effects. Some patients with essential myoclonus or myo-clonus of intention type, but with other aetiologies, also show a response to L-5-HTP.

In baboons with photosensitive epilepsy, L-5-HTP has a powerful protective action against photically-induced myoclonus (at doses of 15–30 mg/kg) (Wada *et al.* 1972). Various agonists including LSD 25, psilocybin and dimethyltryptamine also effectively block photically-induced myo-clonus in baboons and audiogenic seizures in DBA/2 mice. These protective effects in reflex epilepsy are probably partially at the level of afferent transmission.

Spontaneous spike and wave discharges in photosensitive baboons are reduced by LSD 25, but enhanced by 5-HTP and by psilocybin, suggesting a different action of these agonists at the cortical level.

Adenosine

Adenosine is released from neurons during seizure activity and shows an anticonvulsant action in some *in vitro* and *in vivo* models of epilepsy. Of the two principal receptor subtypes described for adenosine, A_1 receptors induce inhibition of adenylate cyclase whilst A_2 receptors activate it. Alkylxanthines such as caffeine and theophylline act as antagonists at both receptor sub-types. Functional studies suggest that A_2 receptors occur postsynaptically and inhibit cell firing and A_1 receptors presynapti-cally to decrease neurotransmitter release. There is probably a third receptor sub-type, A_3, related to calcium entry into nerve terminals (Ribeiro & Sebastião 1986) In hippocampal slices the depression of synaptic transmission induced by adenosine appears to be mediated by the A_1 receptors (Lee *et al.* 1983). There is autoradiographic evidence for the location of adenosine receptors on axon terminals of excitatory neurons (Goodman *et al.* 1983). The release of glutamate from dentate slices is enhanced by 2-chloroadenosine (Dolphin & Archer 1983).

The anticonvulsive action of adenosine and its analogues has been studied in hippocampal slices exposed to penicillin or bicuculline. Adenosine or L-N6 isopropyladenosine (L-PIA) potently suppress epilep-tiform discharges indicating an effect on A_1 receptors (Lee *et al.* 1984). Experiments using antidromic stimulation have provided evidence that a postsynaptic dendritic site is involved. *In vivo* an anticonvulsant action of adenosine and of A_1 agonists has been shown against pentylenetetrazol seizures in rats and mice (Dunwiddie & Worth 1982; Murray *et al.* 1985). Theophylline antagonises this effect and exerts a proconvulsant action on its own. Limbic seizures induced by pilocarpine are facilitated by aminophylline and blocked by 2-chloro-adenosine (Turski *et al.* 1985). Sound-induced seizures in DBA/2 mice are also blocked by 2-chloro-adenosine or by NECA, and this effect is abolished by pretreatment with methylxanthines or by preventing the hypothermia induced by the adenosine analogues (Bowker & Chapman 1986). The process of kindling induced by amygdala stimulation is accelerated by systemic administration of the adenosine antagonist aminophylline and slowed by papaverine which blocks adenosine reuptake. Kindled seizures are suppressed by adenosine agonists (Dragunow & Goddard 1984).

Several anticonvulsant drugs (notably carbamazepine, barbiturates and benzodiazepines) have been shown to interact with the adenosine system *in vitro*. Actions both on adenosine binding and on adenosine uptake have been reported (Skerritt *et al.* 1983; Weir *et al.* 1984). Chronic carbamazepine administration to rats leads to an increase in adenosine receptor number (Marangos *et al.* 1985), suggesting an antagonist action. Barbiturates appear to act as selective antagonists of the A_1 receptor as they antagonise the inhibitory effect of PIA on adenylate cyclase (Lohse *et al.* 1985).

Anticonvulsant drugs and neurotransmitters

An ideal account of the mechanism of action of anticonvulsant drugs would start from a description of actions at the molecular level and proceed to explain how the consequent changes in neuronal properties prevented or terminated abnormal patterns of firing.

About 10 chemical classes of anticonvulsant drugs are in clinical use, and a vastly greater number of chemical structures possess anticonvulsant activity in animal models. Many active compounds have certain features of molecular structure in common (Fig. 17.2). The eight principal structure groups are:

1 barbiturates (phenobarbitone and primidone),
2 hydantoins (diphenylhydantoin, ethytoin),
3 dibenzazepines (carbamazepines),
4 oxazolidinediones (trimethadione),
5 succinimides (ethosuximide),
6 benzodiazepines (diazepam, clonazepam),
7 sulphonamides (acetazolamide, sulthiame),
8 short chain fatty acids (sodium valproate).

Animal models indicate at least two modes of anticonvulsant drug action. Thus rank order of potency for protection against maximal electroshock seizures is completely different from that for elevation of the threshold to pentylenetetrazol seizures (Krall *et al.* 1978). This corresponds to the clinical differentiation between drugs effective against partial seizures (hydantoin, carbamazepine) and drugs effective against the absences of petit mal (succinimides, tridiones). Some drugs (valproate, benzodiazepines) have a broad spectrum of activity being effective against primary

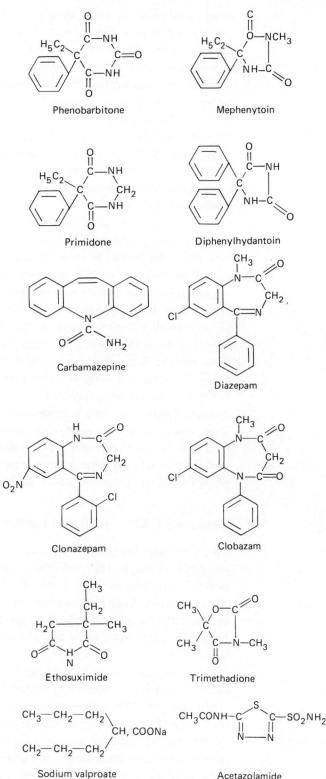

Fig. 17.2. Structural formulae of the principal anti-convulsant drugs.

generalised seizures (including petit mal) and against partial seizures (including complex partial seizures or temporal lobe epilepsy). Thus, we are dealing with at least two major types of action, which may be shown in different proportions by different drugs.

Anticonvulsant drugs produce a variety of effects on cerebral function beyond suppression of seizures. Some of these effects are shown strongly by particular types of drug (e.g. anxiolysis and muscle hypotonia by benzodiazepines, sedation and anaesthesia by barbiturates). However, signs of cerebellar toxicity (nystagmus, ataxia, dysarthria) occur as an acute toxic side-effect in the majority of anticonvulsant drugs, suggesting a close relationship between mechanism of anticonvulsant activity and of cerebellar toxicity.

On the basis of the neuronal pathophysiology described, possible mechanisms of action of anticonvulsant drugs include enhancement of inhibitory feedback mechanisms, stabilisation of resting membrane potentials, or other membrane changes to prevent paroxysmal depolarising responses, changes in synaptic properties to limit sustained activity, or to reduce the upper limit of activity in excitatory pathways. There is physiological evidence to support all these possibilities. The most general hypothesis and the most substantial body of evidence concerns enhancement of GABA-mediated inhibition. Phenomena relating to this mechanism have been clearly demonstrated for benzodiazepines, valproate, barbiturates, and phenylhydantoin. There is weaker evidence that barbiturates, hydantoins and valproate diminish excitatory synaptic action. Experiments of several kinds show effects of hydantoins, carbamazepines (and also benzodiazepines, and barbiturates), on membrane properties, including effects on ionic pumping mechanisms, and membrane protein phosphorylation systems. These topics are reviewed in detail below.

Enhanced GABA-mediated inhibition

Direct evidence for this mechanism comes from two types of experiments, recording of single unit activity *in vivo* or intracellular recording from isolated preparations *in vitro*. *In vivo* experiments allow accurate comparison between anticonvulsant doses and those modifying single unit activity, but often fail to establish the exact site of action of the drug. *In vitro* experiments allow the accurate analysis of postsynaptic membrane effects.

In *in vivo* studies, enhanced inhibitory effects after either stimulation of an intrinsic, presumed GABAergic, pathway or the iontophoretic application of GABA have been reported after benzodiazepine administration for the hippocampus and for the neocortex. Presynaptic inhibition in the spinal cord is also enhanced by benzodiazepines. Similarly, barbiturates have been shown to enhance both GABA-mediated postsynaptic inhibition in the hippocampus and presynaptic inhibition in the spinal cord. Enhancement of inhibition due to exogenous GABA has been reported after valproate in the neocortex or brainstem, although enhancement of inhibition due to GABAergic pathways has not been demonstrated.

In vitro studies have mostly employed cultured spinal neurons (MacDonald & Barker 1979; MacDonald 1983). Barbiturates augment inhibition due to exogenous GABA. The anticonvulsant phenobarbital prolongs the opening of chloride channels by GABA, whereas the anaesthetic/sedative barbiturate pentobarbital directly increases chloride conductance. Valproic acid also augments GABA-induced inhibition in cultured neurons.

Benzodiazepine binding and the GABA-receptor complex

Isotopically labelled benzodiazepines show high-affinity binding to brain membrane preparations that is not competitive with other known neurotransmitters (see Chapter 20). This binding is enhanced in the presence of GABA or certain GABA agonists, such as muscimol and homotaurine and decreased by bicuculline and by some GABA agonists (e.g. THIP). These findings led to the postulation of a GABA/benzodiazepine receptor complex controlling a Cl^- ionophore. Such a complex has now been purified and its primary structure determined (Stephenson & Barnard 1986; Scholfield et al. 1987). Actions at the GABA/benzodiazepine receptor correlate with specific anticonvulsant properties of benzodiazepines. The rank order for the relative potency of a wide range of benzodiazepines to displace isotopically labelled diazepam from membrane binding sites corresponds closely to their relative potency against pentylenetetrazol seizures but not their potency against maximal electroshock seizures (Möhler & Okada 1977). Benzodiazepine antagonists that compete for the specific binding sites (such as imidazodiazepines or β-carbolines) also block the anticonvulsant action of benzodiazepines against pentylenetetrazol (Hunkeler et al. 1981; Meldrum & Braestrup 1985).

Picrotoxinin binding and the chloride ionophore

A wide variety of both convulsant and anticonvulsant drugs compete with dihydropicrotoxinin for binding. Among convulsants the so-called 'cage-convulsants' (e.g. bicyclophosphates and tetramethylene disulphotetramine) are particularly potent but certain convulsant barbiturates and benzodiazepines are also active. Generally the potency of barbiturates at displacing labelled dihydropicrotoxinin correlates better with their hypnotic/anaesthetic activity than with their anticonvulsant potency.

The dihydropicrotoxinin binding site co-purifies with the GABA-benzodiazepine receptor. Thus the binding experiments support the electrophysiological evidence that part of the anticonvulsant action of barbiturates, hydantoins and branched chain fatty acids relates to enhancement of inhibitory transmission through action at a site very closely related to the chloride ionophore (MacDonald 1983).

Anticonvulsant drugs and the further metabolism of GABA

The principal pathway for the further metabolism of GABA in both neurons and glia is by transamination and oxidation to yield succinate, thus completing the GABA shunt on the tricarboxylic acid cycle. GABA-T promotes the formation of succinic semialdehyde from GABA, with the simultaneous conversion of 2-oxoglutarate to glutamate. Succinic semialdehyde dehydrogenase (succinate semialdehyde: $NADP^+$ oxido-reductase) requires oxidised NAD as cofactor and, like GABA-T, is a mitochondrial enzyme. There is also in brain an aldehyde reductase which is NADPH dependent and converts succinic semialdehyde to γ-hydroxy-butyrate (alcohol: NADP oxido-reductase). *In vitro*, using either brain homogenates or enzyme preparations of various degrees of purity, inhibition of all three enzymes has been reported in the presence of anticonvulsant drugs.

Inhibition of either GABA-T or of succinic semialdehyde dehydrogenase has been suggested as the mechanism of anticonvulsant action of valproate (see Chapman *et al.* 1982b). In rodents high doses of valproate acutely increase brain GABA content (Simler *et al.* 1973) although anticonvulsant effects can be seen in the absence of such increases (Anlezark *et al.* 1976). However, it has not been shown that the synaptic release of GABA is enhanced following valproate. The alternative explanation that synaptic GABA concentration rises, because of reduced GABA release following a postsynaptic action of valproate is supported by tracer studies of GABA synthesis rates (Chapman *et al.* 1982a). Similar arguments apply to the less substantial evidence for changes in brain GABA concentration after barbiturates and hydantoins.

Altered excitatory transmission

The most extensive studies on impairment of excitatory transmission concern the barbiturates (especially the anaesthetic barbiturates).

In brain slices the stimulated release of a wide range of neurotrans-mitters is impaired by pentobarbitone (Waller & Richter 1980). The reduced release of transmitter is probably due to impaired Ca^{2+} entry into presynaptic terminals (Goldring & Blaustein 1980). There is also evidence for decreased postsynaptic responsiveness to endogenous transmitters or to acetylcholine or glutamate in the presence of barbiturates.

Evidence relating to actions of other anticonvulsant drugs on excit-atory transmission principally concerns the benzodiazepines. Antagon-ism by benzodiazepines of the excitatory action of dicarboxylic acids has been demonstrated in the frog spinal cord and the rat cerebral cortex.

Membrane and ionic effects

Membrane effects, especially those concerning ionic movements have been most extensively studied with diphenylhydantoin. Observations have been made on whole brain *in vivo* and on isolated preparations including squid giant axons and amphibian skin or bladder.

In whole brain and in isolated axons hydantoin decreases the rise in intracellular sodium concentration that normally occurs during stimulation or activity. This is due to a decreased sodium inward current during activation. Hydantoin reduces calcium fluxes in axons and synaptosomes. In anticonvulsant doses it reduces post-tetanic potentiation and post-tetanic hyperpolarisation (in the spinal cord or peripheral nervous system) (Esplin 1957). Centrally, using hippocampal afferent stimulation, both depression and enhancement of post-tetanic potentiation is found according to the site, and to the dose of hydantoin (Matthews & Connor 1976).

Using dissociated cultures of mouse spinal cord neurons, MacDonald and Barker (1979) and MacDonald *et al.* (1985) have studied the effect of anticonvulsant drugs on membrane excitability and ionic conductances using an intracellular current pulse to induce repetitive firing. This effect is suppressed by concentrations of phenytoin (0.2–1.0 μg/ml) equivalent to those found in the cerebrospinal fluid of patients receiving therapeutic doses. A similar effect is produced by 'therapeutic' concentrations of carbamazepine or valproate and is probably due to a use-dependent block of the sodium conductance channels. The recovery of the channel from inactivation is slowed so that the proportion in the inactive state progressively increases. This effect is also produced by high concentrations of diazepam and it appears to correlate with anticonvulsant activity as assessed in the maximal electroshock test.

In brain membrane or synaptosomal preparations phosphorylation of some proteins is regulated by a Ca^{2+} calmodulin protein kinase system which is inhibited by anticonvulsant concentrations of diphenylhydantoin, carbamazepine or bendzodiazepines. In fact studies with a range of benzodiazepine show that their inhibitory potency correlates with their potency against electroshock seizures, and not against pentylenetetrazol seizures (DeLorenzo *et al.* 1981; DeLorenzo 1986). Thus the anticonvulsant action of hydantoins, carbamazepine, and benzodiazepines in the electroshock test may be related to an action on a calcium-dependent protein kinase in synaptosomal membranes. This could diminish synaptic efficacy and thus reduce the spread of seizure activity.

Summary

The term 'epilepsy' refers to a wide variety of recurrent symptoms or clinical signs, which have a common pathophysiology — the excessively synchronous or sustained discharge, of a group of neurons. At the cellular level this is seen as a 'paroxysmal depolarising shift' in resting membrane potential, associated with a burst of spike discharges. It is not yet possible to say what disorders of synaptic function are associated with the principal syndromes of epilepsy in man. A selective loss of impairment of inhibitory mechanisms (particularly those mediated by GABA) in the neocortex or hippocampus is possibly a contributory factor, but has not yet been definitively established. Biochemical or pharmacological manipulation of the GABAergic inhibitory system, or of amino acid-induced excitation, has powerful effects in animal models of epilepsy. Manipulation of monoaminergic systems modifies the signs of reflex epilepsy in animals and man.

Anticonvulsant drugs have at least two principal mechanisms of action. One is enhancement of GABAergic inhibition through action on postsynaptic membrane components functionally related to the GABA recognition site or to the chloride ionophore. The other mechanism concerns cationic movements and membrane protein phosphorylation in pre-and postsynaptic membranes.

References and further reading

Altshuler HL, Killam EK & Killam KF (1976) Biogenic amines and the photomyoclonic syndrome in the baboon, Papio papio. *J. Pharmacol. Exp. Ther.* **196**, 156–66.

Anderson WR, Simpkins JW, Woodard PA, Winwood D, Stern WC & Bodor N (1987) Anxiolytic activity of a brain delivery system for GABA. *Psychopharmacology* **92**, 157–63.

Anlezark G & Meldrum BS (1978) Blockade of photically-induced epilepsy by dopamine agonist ergot alkaloids. *Psychopharmacology* **57**, 57–62.

Anlezark G, Horton RW, Meldrum BS & Sawaya MCB (1976) Anticonvulsant action of ethanolamine-0-sulphate and di-n-propylacetate and the metabolism of γ-aminobutyric acid (GABA) in mice with audiogenic seizures. *Biochem., Pharmacol.* **25**, 413–17.

Anlezark GM, Horton RW & Meldrum BS (1979) The anticonvulsant activity of the (−) and (+) enantiomers of propranolol. *J. Pharm. Pharmacol.* **31**, 482–3.

Anlezark G, Marrosu F & Meldrum B (1981) Dopamine agonists in reflex epilepsy. In: Morselli PL, Lloyd KG, Löscher W, Meldrum B & Reynolds EH (eds) *Neurotransmitters, Seizures and Epilepsy.* Raven Press, New York. pp. 251–62.

Bonnycastle DD, Giarman NJ & Paasonen MK (1957) Anticonvulsant compounds and 5-hydroxytryptamine in rat brain. *Br. J. Pharmacol.* **12**, 228–31.

Bowker HM & Chapman AG (1986) Adenosine analogues : the temperature-dependence of the anticonvulsant effect and inhibition of 3H-D-aspartate release. *Biochem. Pharmacol.* **35**, 2949–53.

Calderini G, Carlsson A & Nordström C-H (1978) Monoamine metabolism during bicuculline-induced epileptic seizures in the rat. *Brain Res.* **157**, 295–302.

Chadwick D, Jenner P & Reynolds EH (1977) Serotonin metabolism in human epilepsy: the influence of anticonvulsant drugs. *Ann. Neurol.* **1**, 218–24.

Chapman AG, Riley K, Evans MC & Meldrum BS (1982a) Acute effects of sodium valproate and γ-vinyl GABA on regional amino acid metabolism in the rat brain. *Neurochem. Res.* **7**, 1089–105.

Chapman A, Keane PE, Meldrum BS, Simiand J & Vernieres JC (1982b) Mechanism of anticonvulsant action of valproate. *Prog. Neurobiol.* **19**, 315–59.

Collins GGS, Probett GA, Anson J & McLaughlin NB (1984) Excitatory and inhibitory effects of noradrenaline on synaptic transmission in the rat olfactory cortex slice. *Brain Res.* **294**, 211–23.

Commission on Terminology of the International League against Epilepsy (1981) Proposal for revised clinical and electroencephalographic classification of epileptic seizures. *Epilepsia* **22**, 489–501.

Coursin DB (1964) Vitamin B_6 metabolism in infants and children. *Vit. Horm. N.Y.* **22**, 755–83.

Cowan A, Geller EG & Adler MW (1979) Classification of opioids on the basis of change in seizure threshold in rats. *Science* **206**, 465–7.

Croucher MJ, Collins JF & Meldrum BS (1982) Anticonvulsant action of excitatory amino acid antagonists. *Science* **216**, 899–901.

Curtis DR & Johnston GAT (1974) Amino acid transmitters in the mammalian nervous system. *Ergeb. Physiol. Biol. Chem. Exp. Pharmakol.* **69**, 97–188.

DeLorenzo RJ (1986) A molecular approach to the calcium signal in brain: relationship to synaptic modulation and seizure discharge. In: Delgado-Escuita AV, Ward AA, Woodbury DM & Porter RJ (eds) *Advances in Neurology 44, Basic Mechanisms of the Epilepsies*. Raven Press, New York. pp. 435–64.

DeLorenzo RJ, Burdette S & Holderness J (1981) Benzodiazepines inhibition of the calcium-calmodulin protein kinase system in brain membrane. *Science* **213**, 546–9.

Dolphin AC & Archer ER (1983) An adenosine agonist inhibits and a cyclic AMP analogue enhances the release of glutamate but not GABA from slices of rat dentate gyrus. *Neurosci. Lett.* **43**, 49–54.

Dragunow M & Goddard GV (1984) Adenosine modulation of amygdala kindling. *Exp. Neurol.* **84**, 654–65.

Dunwiddie TV & Worth T (1982) Sedative and anticonvulsant effects of adenosine analogs in mouse and rat. *J. Pharmacol. Exp. Therap.* **220**, 70–6.

Edmonds HL, Hegreberg GA, Van Gelder NM, Sylvester DM, Clemmons RM & Chatburn CG (1979) Spontaneous convulsions in beagle dogs. *Fed. Proc.* **38**, 2424–8.

Esplin D (1957) Effect of diphenylhydantoin on synaptic transmission in the cat spinal cord and stellate ganglion. *J. Pharmacol. Exp. Ther.* **120**, 301–23.

Frey H-H & Löscher W (1980) Cetyl GABA: effect on convulsant thresholds in mice and acute toxicity. *Neuropharmacology* **19**, 217–20.

Goddard GV, McIntyre DC & Leech CK (1969) A permanent change in brain function resulting from daily electrical stimulation. *Neurology* **25**, 295–30.

Goldring JM & Blaustein MP (1980) Barbiturates: physiological effects II. In: Glaser GH, Penry JK & Woodbury DM (eds) *Antiepileptic Drugs: Mechanisms of Action*. Raven Press, New York. pp. 523–31.

Goodman HO, Connolly BM, McLean W & Resnick M (1980) Taurine transport in epilepsy. *Clin. Chem.* **26**, 414–19.

Goodman RR, Kuhar MJ, Hester L, Snyder SH (1983) Adenosine receptors: autoradiographic evidence for their location on axon terminals of excitatory neurons. *Science* **220**, 967–9.

Horton R, Anlezark G & Meldrum B (1980) Noradrenergic influences on sound induced seizures. *J. Pharmacol. Exp. Ther.* **214**, 437–42.

Hunkeler W, Möhler H, Pieri L, Polc P, Bonetti EP, Cumin R, Schaffner R & Haefely W (1981) Selective antagonists of benzodiazepines. *Nature* (London) **290**, 514–16.

Hurd RW, Hammond EJ & Wilder BJ (1981) Homocysteine induced convulsions: enhancement by vitamin B_6 and inhibition by hydrazine. *Brain Res.* **209**, 250–4.

Jazrawi SP & Horton RW (1986) Brain adrenoceptor binding sites in mice susceptible (DBA/2J) and resistant (C57 b1/6) to audiogenic seizures. *J. Neurochem.* **47**, 173–7.

Krall RL, Penry JK, White BG, Kupferberg HJ & Swinyard EA (1978) Antiepileptic drug development: II. Anticonvulsant drug screening. *Epilepsia* **19**, 409–28.

Krogsgaard-Larsen P (1980) Inhibitors of the GABA uptake systems. *Mol. & Cell. Biochem.* **31**, 105–21.

Laird HE & Huxtable RJ (1978) Taurine and audiogenic epilepsy. In: Barbeau A & Huxtable RJ (eds) *Taurine and Neurological Disorders*. Raven Press, New York. 339–57.

Lee KS, Schubert P, Reddington M & Kreutzberg GW (1983) Adenosine receptor density and the depression of evoked neuronal activity in the rat hippocampus in vitro. *Neurosci. Lett.* **37**, 81–5.

Lee KS, Schubert P & Heinemann U (1984) The anticonvulsive action of adenosine: a postsynaptic, dendritic action by a possible endogenous anticonvulsant. *Brain Res.* **321**, 160–4.

Lhermitte F, Marteau R & Degos CF (1972) Analyse pharmacologique d'un nouveau cas de myoclonies d'intention et d'action post-anoiques. *Rev. Neurol.* **126**, 107–14.

Loeb C, Besio G, Mainardi P, Scotto P, Benassi E & Bo GP (1986) Liposome-entrapped - aminobutyric acid inhibits isoniazid-induced epileptogenic activity in rats. *Epilepsia* **27**, 98–102.

Lohse MJ, Klotz KN, Jakobs KH & Schwabe U (1985) Barbiturates are selective antagonists at A_1 adenosine receptors. *Neurochem. Res.* **45**, 1761–70.

Löscher W, Rating D & Siemes H (1981) GABA in cerebrospinal fluid of children with febrile convulsions. *Epilepsia* **22**, 697–702.

Löscher W & Siemes H (1985) Cerebrospinal fluid γ-aminobutyric acid levels in children with different types of epilepsy: effect of anticonvulsant treatment. *Epilepsia*. **26**, 314–19.

Löscher W & Czuczwar SJ (1987) Comparison of drugs with different selectivity for central α_1- and α_2-adrenoceptors in animal models of epilepsy. *Epilepsy Research* **1**, 165–72.

MacDonald RL & Barker JL (1979) Enhancement of GABA-mediated postsynaptic inhibition in cultured mammalian spinal cord neurons: a common mode of anticonvulsant action. *Brain Res.* **167**, 323–36.

MacDonald RL (1983) Mechanisms of anticonvulsant drug action. In: Pedley TA & Meldrum BS (eds) *Recent Advances in Epilepsy I*. Churchill Livingstone, Edinburgh. pp. 1–23.

MacDonald RL, McLean MJ & Skerritt JH (1985) Anticonvulsant drug mechanisms of action. *Fred. Proc.* **44**, 2634–9.

Manyam NVB, Katz L, Hare TA, Gerber JC & Grossman MH (1980) Levels of γ-aminobutyric acid in cerebrospinal fluid in various neurologic disorders. *Arch. Neurol.* (Chicago) **37**, 352–5.

Marangos PJ, Weiss SRB, Montgomery P, Patel J, Narang PK, Cappabianca AM & Post RM (1985) Chronic carbamazepine treatment increases brain adenosine receptors. *Epilepsia* **26**, 493–8.

Markand ON, Garg BP & Brandt IK (1982) Non-ketotic hyperglycinemia: electroencephalographic and evoked potential abnormalities. *Neurology* **32**, 151–6.

Matthews WD & Connor JD (1976) Effects of diphenylhydantoin and diazepam on hippocampal evoked responses. *Neuropharmacology* **15**, 181–6.

McIntyre DC & Roberts DCS (1983) Long-term reduction in beta-adrenergic receptor binding after amygdala kindling. *Exp. Neurol.* **61**, 582–91.

McIntyre DC & Racine RJ (1986) Kindling mechanisms: Current progress on an experimental epilepsy model. *Prog. Neurobiol.* **27**, 1–12.

Meldrum BS (1975) Epilepsy and GABA-mediated inhibition. *Int. Rev. Neurobiol.* **17**, 1–36.

Meldrum B (1979) Convulsant drugs, anticonvulsants and GABA-mediated neuronal inhibition. In: Krogsgaard-Larsen P, Scheel-Kruger J & Kofod H (eds) *GABA-Neurotransmitters*. Munksgaard, Copenhagen. pp. 395–405.

Meldrum B (1980) Photically-induced epilepsy in the baboon, *Papio papio*. In: Rose FC (ed) *Animal Models of Neurological Disease*. Pitman, Tunbridge Wells. pp. 202–16.

Meldrum B (1981) GABA-agonists as antiepileptic agents. In: Costa E, di Chiara G & Cessa GL (eds) *GABA and Benzodiazepine Receptors* Raven Press, New York. pp. 207–17.

Meldrum BS & Horton RW (1974) Neuronal inhibition mediated by GABA, and pattern of convulsions in photosensitive baboons with epilepsy (Papio papio). In: Harris P & Mawdsley C (eds) *The Natural History and Management of Epilepsy*. Churchill Livingstone, Edinburgh. pp. 55–64.

Meldrum B & Horton R (1978) Blockade of epileptic responses in the photosensitive baboon, *Papio papio*, by two irreversible inhibitors of GABA-transaminase, γ-acetylenic GABA (4-amino-hex-5-ynoic acid) and γ-vinyl GABA (4-amino-hex-5-enoic acid). *Psychopharmacology* **59**, 47–50.

Meldrum B & Horton R (1980) Effects of the bicyclic GABA agonist, THIP, on myoclonic and seizure responses in mice and baboons with reflex epilepsy. *Eur. J. Pharmacol.* **61**, 231–7.

Meldrum BS & Menini CH (1981) Effect of morphine, enkephalins, β-endorphin and related compounds on seizure thresholds. In: Morselli PL, Lloyd KG, Loscher W, Meldrum B & Reynolds EH *Neurotransmitters, Seizures and Epilepsy*. Raven Press, New York. pp. 185–94.

Meldrum BS, Anlezark G, Balzano E, Horton RW & Trimble M (1975) Photically induced epilepsy in *Papio papio* as a model for drug studies. In: Meldrum BS & Marsden CD (eds) *Advances in Neurology* Vol. 10. Raven Press, New York. pp. 119-28.

Meldrum BS, Croucher MJ & Krogsgaard-Larsen P (1982) GABA-uptake inhibitors as anticonvulsant agents. In: Okada Y & Roberts E (eds) *Problems in GABA Research.* Excerpta Medica, Amsterdam. pp. 182-91.

Meldrum BS, Croucher MJ, Badman G & Collins JF (1983) Antiepileptic action of excitatory amino acid antagonists in the photosensitive baboon, *Papio papio. Neuroscience Lett.* **39**, 101-4.

Meldrum BS & Braestrup C (1984) GABA and the anticonvulsant action of benzodiazepines and related drugs. In: Bowery N (ed), *Actions and Interactions of GABA and Benzodiazepines.* Raven Press, New York. pp. 133-53.

Meldrum BS & Corsellis JAN (1984) Epilepsy. In: Blackwood W & Corsellis JAN (eds) *Greenfield's Neuropathology,* 4th ed. pp. 921-50. Arnold, London.

Metcalf BW (1979) Inhibitors of GABA metabolism. *Biochem. Pharmacol.* **23**, 1705-12.

Miles R & Wong RKS (1987) Inhibitory control of local excitatory circuits in the guinea-pig hippocampus. *J. Physiol.* **388**, 611-29.

Mody I & Heinemann U (1987) NMDA receptors of dentate gyrus granule cells participate in synaptic transmission following kindling. *Nature* **326**, 701-4.

Möhler H & Okada T (1977) Benzodiazepine receptor: demonstration in the central nervous system. *Science* **198**, 849-51.

Moises HC & Woodward DJ (1980) Potentiation of GABA inhibitory action in cerebellum by locus coeruleus stimulation. *Brain Res.* **182**, 327-44.

Murray TF, Sylvester D, Schultz CS & Szot P (1985) Purinergic modulation of the seizure threshold for pentylenetetrazol in the rat. *Neuropharmacology* **24**, 761-6.

Neumann RS (1986) Suppression of penicillin-induced focal epileptiform activity by locus coeruleus stimulation: Mediation by an α_1-adrenoceptor. *Epilepsia* **27**, 359-66.

Nicoletti F, Barbaccia ML, Iadarola MJ, Pozzi O & Laird HE (1986) Abnormality of α_1-adrenergic receptors in the frontal cortex of epileptic rats. *J. Neurochem.* **46**, 270-3.

Noebels JL (1984) A single gene error of noradrenergic axon growth synchronizes central neurones. *Nature* **310**, 409-11.

Noebels JL & Sidman RL (1979) Inherited epilepsy: Spike-wave and focal motor seizures in the mutant mouse tottering. *Science* **204**, 1334-6.

Okazaki MM, Warsh JJ & Burnham WM (1986) Unchanged norepinephrine turnover and concentrations in amygdala-kindled rat brain regions 2 months postseizure. *Exp. Neurol.* **94**, 81-90.

Olsen RW (1982) Drug interactions at the GABA receptor ionophore complex. *Ann. Rev. Pharmacol. Toxicol.* **22**, 245-77.

Orlowski M, Reingold DF & Stanley ME (1977) D- and L-stereoisomers of allylglycine: convulsive action and inhibition of brain L-glutamate decarboxylase. *J. Neurochem.* **28**, 349-53.

Palayoor ST, Seyfried TN & Bernard DJ (1986) Calcium ATPase activities in synaptic plasma membranes of seizure-prone mice. *J. Neurochem.* **46**, 1370-75.

Papanicolaou J, Summers RJ, Vajda FJE & Louis WJ (1982) Anticonvulsant effects of clonidine mediated through central α_2 adrenoceptors. *Europ. J. Pharmacol.* **77**, 163-6.

Pedley TA, Zuckermann EC & Glaser GH (1969) Epileptogenic effects of localized ventricular perfusion of ouabain on dorsal hippocampus. *Exp. Neurol.* **25**, 207-19.

Pedley TA, Horton RW & Meldrum BS (1979) Electroencephalographic and behavioural effects of a GABA agonist (Muscimol) on photosensitive epilepsy in the baboon, Papio papio. *Epilepsia* **20**, 409-16.

Perry TL, Hansen S, Kennedy J, Wada JA & Thompson GB (1975) Amino acids in human epileptogenic foci. *Arch. Neruol.* (Chicago) **32**, 752-4.

Peterson SL (1986) Glycine potentiates the anticonvulsant action of diazepam and phenobarbital in kindled amygdaloid seizures of rats. *Neuropharmacology* **25**, 1359-63.

Piredda S & Gale K (1985) A crucial epileptogenic site in the deep preperiform cortex. *Nature* **317**, 623-5.

Prince DA (1968) The depolarization shift in epileptic neurons. *Exp. Neurol.* **21**, 467-85.

Quesney LF, Andermann F, Lai S & Prelevic S (1980) Transient abolition of generalised photosensitive epileptic discharge in man by apomorphine, a dopamine receptor agonist. *Neurology* **30**, 1169-74.

Ribak CE, Harris AB, Vaughn JE & Roberts E (1979) Inhibitory, GABAergic nerve
terminals decrease at sites of focal epilepsy. *Science* **205**, 211–14.

Ribeiro JHA & Sebastião AM (1986) Adenosine receptors and calcium: basis for proposing a
third (A3) adenosine receptor. *Progr. Neurobiol.* **26**, 179–209.

Rimmer EM & Richens A (1984) Double blind study of γ-vinyl GABA in patients with
refractory epilepsy. *Lancet* **i**, 189–90.

Rosenblatt DE, Lauter CJ, Baird HR & Trans EG (1977) ATPase in animal models of
epilepsy. *J. Mol. Med.* **2**, 137–44.

Schofield PR, Darlison MG, Fujita N, Burt DR, Stephenson FA, Rodriguez H, Rhee LM,
Rhamachondran J, Reale V, Glencorse TA, Seeburg PH & Barnard EA (1987) Sequence
and functional expression of the GABA$_A$ receptor shows a ligand-gated receptor superfamily. *Nature* **328**, 221–7.

Schwartzkroin PA & Wyler AR (1980) Mechanisms underlying epileptiform burst discharge.
Ann. Neurol. **7**, 95–107.

Segal M & Bloom FE (1976) The actions of norepinephrine in the rat hippocampus IV. The
effects of locus coeruleus stimulation on evoked hippocampal unit activity. *Brain Res.*
107, 513–25.

Seiler N & Sarhan S (1984) Synergistic anticonvulsant effects of GABA-T inhibitors and
glycine. *Naunyn-Schmiedebergs Arch. Pharmac.* **326**, 49–57.

Seyfried TN & Glaser GH (1985) A review of mouse mutants as genetic models of epilepsy.
Epilepsia **26**, 143–50.

Sherwin A, Robitaille Y, Quesney L, Reader T, Olivier A, Briere R, Andermann E,
Andermann F, Feindel W, Leblanc R, Matthew E, Ochs R, Villemure J & Gloor P (1986)
Noradrenergic abnormalities in human cortical seizure foci. In: Engel Jr J. (ed)
*Fundamental Mechanisms of Human Brain function: Opportunities for Direct Investi-
gations in Association with the Surgical Treatment of Epilepsy*. Raven Press, New
York.

Simler S, Ciesielski L, Maitre M, Randrianarisoa H & Mandel P (1973) Effect of sodium n-
dipropylacetate on audiogenic seizures and brain γ-aminobutyric acid level. *Biochem.
Pharmacol.* **22**, 1701–8.

Skerritt JH, Davies LP & Johnston GAR (1983) Interactions of the anticonvulsant
carbamazepine with adenosine receptors. 1. Neurochemical studies. *Epilepsia* **24**,
634–42.

Sloper JJ, Johnson P & Powell TPS (1980) Selective degeneration of inter-neurons in the
motor cortex of infant monkeys following controlled hypoxia: a possible cause of
epilepsy. *Brain Res.* **198**, 204–9.

Soroko FE & McKenzie GM (1970) The effects of apomorphine and dexamphetamine on
metrazol-induced convulsions in the rat and mouse. *Pharmacologist* **12**, 253–5.

Stanford SC & Jefferys JGR (1985) Down-regulation of α_2 and β-adrenoceptor binding sites
in rat cortex caused by amygdalar kindling. *Exp. Neurol.* **90**, 108–17.

Stephenson FA & Barnard EA (1986) Purification and characterization of the brain
GABA/benzodiazepine receptor. In: Olsen RW & Venter JC (ed.) *Benzodiazepine/
GABA Receptors and Chloride Channels*. A.R. Liss, New York.

Takahashi R & Nakane Y (1978) Clinical trial of taurine in epilepsy. In: Barbeau A &
Huxtable RJ (eds) *Taurine and Neurological Disorders*. Raven Press, New York. pp.
375–85.

Turski WA, Cavalheiro EA, Ikonomidou C, Mello LM, Bortolotto ZA & Turski L (1985)
Effects of aminophylline and 2-chloroadenosine on seizures produced by pilocarpine in
rats: morphological and electroencephalographic correlates. *Brain Res.* **361**, 309–23.

Van Gelder NM, Janjua NA, Metrakos K, MacGibbon B & Metrakos JD (1980) Plasma amino acids in 3/sec spike/wave epilepsy. *Neurochem. Res.* **5**, 659–70.

Vezzani A & Schwarcz R (1985) A noradrenergic component of quinolinic acid-induced
seizures. *Exp. Neurol.* **90**, 254–8.

Vizi ES (1979) Presynaptic modulation of neurochemical transmission. *Progr. Neurobiol.*
12, 181–90.

Wada JA, Balzano E, Meldrum BS & Naquet R (1972) Behavioural and electrographic
effects of L-5-hydroxytryptophan and D, L parachloro-phenylalanine on epileptic
Senegalese baboon (Papio papio). *Electroencephalogr. Clin. Neurophysiol.* **33**, 520–6.

Waller MB & Richter JA (1980) Effects of pentobarbital and Ca^{++} on the resting and K^+-stimulated release of several endogenous neurotransmitters from rat midbrain slices. *Biochem. Pharmacol.* **29**, 2189-98.

Weir RL, Padgett W, Daly JW & Anderson SM (1984) Interaction of anticonvulsant drugs with adenosine receptors in the central nervous system. *Epilepsia* **25**, 492-8.

Williams D & Russell WR (1941) Action of eserine and prostigmine on epileptic cerebral discharges. *Lancet* **i**, 476-9.

Wood JH, Hare TA, Glaeser BS, Ballenger JC & Post RM (1979) Low cerebrospinal fluid γ-aminobutyric acid content in seizure patients. *Neurology* **29**, 1203-8.

18   Schizophrenia

F. OWEN AND A.J. CROSS

Schizophrenia is a general term given to a group of mental disorders which have several clinical features in common. The most prominent features of schizophrenia are:

1 auditory hallucinations.
2 delusions, often of a paranoid nature.
3 passivity feelings.
4 blunting or incongruity of affect.
5 disorganisation of logical thought.

Not all of these symptoms need be present for the diagnosis to be made. The onset of schizophrenia can take place at any age but is most common in the 15–35 years age group.

Evidence for a genetic basis of schizophrenia

The evidence for the operation of genetic factors in the aetiology of schizophrenia is strong, although the extent of their operation is controversial. There are some differences in the diagnosis of schizophrenia from place to place and from time to time which may have contributed to this controversy. The incidence of schizophrenia varies a little around 1% in those countries (mainly Western Europe) where it has been studied. This fairly constant incidence has, in itself, been put forward as being indicative of a genetic basis for schizophrenia. However, the investigations have been carried out in societies that have much in common and it could be argued that non-genetic factors which might produce schizophrenia may be present in equal intensities in these societies. The strongest evidence in favour of the involvement of genetic factors in the aetiology of schizophrenia has emerged from studies on twins. From the geneticist's point of view the interest in twins arises from the fact that identical or monozygotic twins have identical genotypes, whereas fraternal or dizygotic twins have genotypes that differ as much as for siblings. It is now generally accepted that the concordance for schizophrenia in monozygotic twins is at least 50% and that the concordance is at least four times as high in monozygotic twins compared with dizygotic twins. Other highly suggestive evidence for the genetic transmission of schizophrenia has come from studies of the incidence of schizophrenia in the biological and adoptive parents of schizophrenics who had been adopted early in life. It has been clearly demonstrated that the incidence of schizophrenia is significantly higher in biological parents compared with adoptive parents. Although the genetic evidence is strong, it does not exclude environmental influences in the generation of schizophrenia. An interesting anecdote is that of the Gerrain quadruplets. These monozygotic quadruplets each developed schizophrenia, yet the course and outcome of the illness was different in each case. One recovered almost completely, another achieved some degree of adjustment, the remaining two are still hospitalized, one with fluctuating severity of illness and the other with a more serious deteriorating form of the disease.

There is no simple Mendelian mode of inheritance of schizophrenia. Both polygenic and single gene (with incomplete penetrance) hypotheses have been proposed and the subject is still a matter of debate. Overall the genetic evidence is sufficiently compelling to suggest that a neurochemical approach might prove fruitful in identifying some factors contributing to the precipitation of schizophrenia. The genetics of schizophrenia has been comprehensively reviewed by Rosenthal and Kety (1968).

Biochemical hypotheses of schizophrenia

The biochemical hypotheses that have generated the most interest over the past 30 years or so are listed in Table 18.1

Table 18.1. Biochemical hypotheses of schizophrenia

Hypothesis	Reference
(a) Transmethylation aberration	Osmond & Smythies (1952)
(b) 5-HT abnormalities	Woolley & Shaw (1954)
(c) Noradrenergic deficits	Stein & Wise (1971)
(d) Reduced monoamine oxidase activity	Murphy & Wyatt (1972)
(e) Excessive central dopaminergic function	Randrup & Munkvad (1972)

Transmethylation

The possibility that schizophrenia is induced by an endogenous toxin coursing through the brain has, for many years, inspired attempts to show an effect of plasma or urine fractions from schizophrenics on biological test systems or to demonstrate the presence of abnormal metabolites in these body fluids. The possibility that abnormal methylation reactions took place in schizophrenics was suggested by Osmond *et al.* (1952). These workers pointed out that 3, 4-dimethoxy-phenylethylamine (DMPE) was a potent producer of catatonic-like states in animals. Since dopamine is 0-methylated to 3-methoxytyramine under the action of catechol-0-methyltransferase (COMT) it seemed possible that under some pathological conditions 3-methoxytyramine could be further 0-methylated to form DMPE. There followed a number of reports purporting to have identified

DMPE after paper chromatography of urinary extracts from at least 50% of schizophrenics but never or very rarely in controls. DMPE was indicated by a 'pink spot' on paper chromatograms. However, later studies either failed to detect a 'pink spot' in urine from schizophrenics or detected it in urine from non-schizophrenic controls. Moreover the 'pink spot' hypothesis became much less attractive when it was shown that doses of up to 1 gram of DMPE were without effect on mentally normal volunteers. This is no longer an active area of research and the early positive findings can probably be explained on the basis of diet or drug treatment. A similar theory was also proposed based on the production of endogenous hallucinogenic compounds from indoleamines. The N-methylated indoleamines, in particular NN-dimethyltryptamine (DMT), have been the subject of considerable research. The enzymes necessary to produce DMT from dietary tryptophan are present in man and it seems clear that DMT is produced but in very low concentrations. An early report that DMT occurred more frequently in the blood of schizophrenics was not confirmed by a later study.

The transmethylation hypothesis persisted for several years largely because of the consistent finding that large doses of the amino acid methionine caused a marked exacerbation in the condition of many schizophrenics. The effects of various amino acids were tested, sometimes in conjunction with monoamine oxidase inhibitors, but only methionine caused any obvious effects. It seemed, therefore, that the effect of methionine administration lent strong support to the transmethylation hypothesis since this amino acid can act as a methyl donor in the body after conversion to its active form S-adenosyl-methionine. This also is no longer a popular area of biochemical research in schizophrenia.

Serotonergic (5-HT) theories

The serotonergic hypotheses, involving either a deficit or excess of 5-HT, were proposed by Wooley and Shaw (1954), who had been studying serotonergic compounds for use as antihypertensive drugs. They observed that many drugs which resembled 5-HT in chemical structure, e.g. harmine, bufotenin, yohimbine and lysergic acid diethylamide (LSD), caused mental disturbances in man. In addition each of these compounds affected the behaviour of experimental animals in a manner indicative of some change of mental function. Because some of these compounds had 5-HT as well as anti 5-HT like properties, Wooley and Shaw were unable to predict whether schizophrenia was the result of a deficit or an excess of 5-HT and post-mortem studies have failed to provide any evidence for either alternative. 5-Hydroxyindole acetic acid (5-HIAA), the major end product of 5-HT metabolism in the brain, is unchanged in brains of schizophrenics indicating no change in 5-HT turnover in the illness.

Noradrenergic deficits

Stein and Wise (1971) proposed that the lack of goal directed behaviour apparent in many schizophrenics was the result of a degeneration of central noradrenergic neurons. Subsequently they reported a decrease in post-mortem brain samples from schizophrenics of the activity of dopamine-β-hydroxylase which catalyses the hydroxylation of dopamine to NA and is a marker for noradrenergic neurons. However, two later reports failed to confirm this deficit in dopamine-β-hydroxylase activity and additional investigations into the brain concentration of NA and its metabolites provided no evidence for a loss of noradrenergic neurons in schizophrenia.

Monoamine oxidase activity

Since the initial report by Murphy and Wyatt (1972) of a significant decrease in platelet monoamine oxidase (MAO) activity in chronic schizophrenia there has been considerable interest in the suggestion that low platelet MAO activity might be a genetic marker for vulnerability to the disease. This hypothesis was particularly attractive since there were previous undisputed reports of the exacerbation of symptoms after administration of monoamine oxidase inhibitors to schizophrenic patients. There then followed a number of reports on platelet MAO activity in schizophrenia with several groups confirming the initial finding of decreased enzyme activity and others unable to demonstrate any difference between controls and schizophrenics. In addition, studies on post-mortem brain tissue failed to find any deficit in MAO activity in several brain regions from schizophrenic patients. Monoamine oxidase, particularly the platelet enzyme, is still being actively researched although its relevance to schizophrenia remains obscure.

The dopamine hypothesis

The dopamine hypothesis of schizophrenia arose from two separate lines of evidence. Firstly it has been established that amphetamines and other DA releasing drugs can induce, in mentally normal individuals, a state closely resembling paranoid schizophrenia and that they can exacerbate the symptoms of an existing psychosis. Secondly, neuroleptic drugs, that are effective in the treatment of schizophrenia, belong to several different chemical classes but have in common the ability to block the DA receptor either in terms of inhibiting the dopamine induced stimulation of adenylate cyclase or in their ability to displace the high affinity binding of ligands to the receptor binding site (see Chapter 8). From these two lines of evidence the dopamine hypothesis was formulated, i.e. that schizophrenia is associated with excessive dopaminergic function in the central nervous system.

Clinical evaluation of the dopamine hypothesis

The observation that certain neuroleptics of the thioxanthene class existed in isomeric forms with one isomer very much more potent than the other in blocking DA receptors *in vitro* provided the basis for a clinical evaluation of the dopamine hypothesis. A drug of particular interest was flupenthixol (Fig. 18.1) since both the α (or cis-) and the β (or trans-) isomers are usually included in the oral preparation of the drug, which is effective in the treatment of schizophrenia, but the DA receptor blocking potency of the drug resides almost exclusively in the α-isomer. The α-isomer is potent both at inhibiting DA sensitive adenylate cyclase activity and in displacing the high affinity binding of [^{3}H]-haloperidol to the DA receptor itself. In a double-blind controlled trial the clinical efficacies of α- and β-flupenthixol were compared with placebo in 45 acutely ill schizophrenics. Patients were rated by standardised clinical interview at weekly intervals. The results are presented in Fig. 18.2. With this rating scale the lower the rating the greater the improvement in the schizophrenic symptoms. The study revealed that α-flupenthixol was significantly better than either β-flupenthixol or placebo in ameliorating the positive symptoms of schizophrenia — positive symptoms being defined as hallucinations, delusions and thought disorder. These findings are consistent with the view that the sole therapeutic effect of neuroleptic drugs is derived from their DA receptor blocking activity. It should be pointed out that α-flupenthixol is also more potent than β-flupenthixol at blocking 5-HT receptors although it seems unlikely that the antipsychotic activity of α-flupenthixol is attributable to its 5-HT receptor blocking potency since it is well established that the correlation between 5-HT

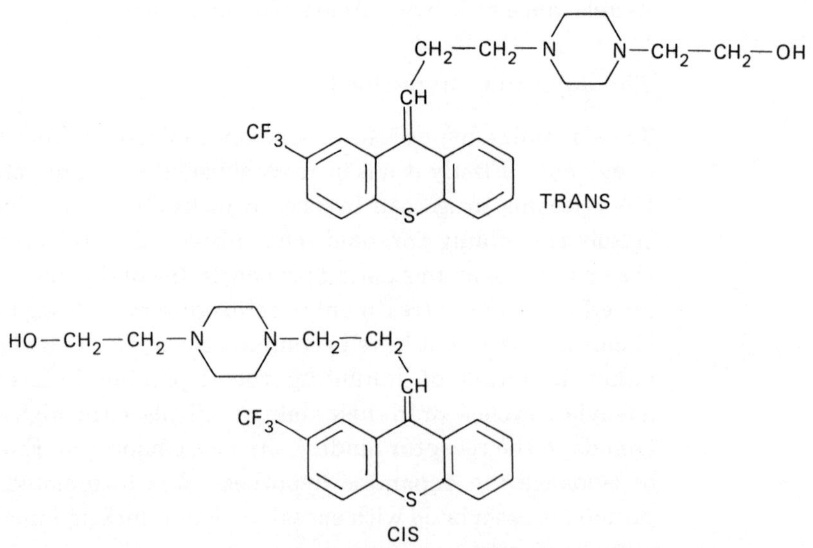

Fig. 18.1. Chemical structure of the isomers of flupenthixol.

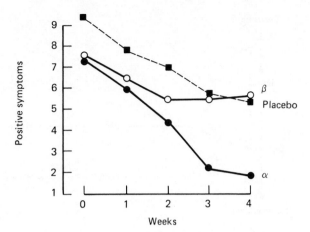

Fig. 18.2. Effects of α-flupenthixol, β-flupenthixol or placebo on the positive symptoms of schizophrenia.

receptor blocking potency (assessed by ligand binding techniques) and antipsychotic activity is poor.

Biochemical evaluation of the dopamine hypothesis

Indices of central DA metabolism in schizophrenia have been assessed by measuring the concentration of its metabolites in cerebrospinal fluid (CSF), by tests of DA mediated endocrine function and by direct studies on post-mortem brain tissue from schizophrenic patients. Dopamine synthesis and metabolism is outlined in Fig. 18.3 (see also Chapter 7). Briefly the amino acid tyrosine is hydroxylated to form dihydroxyphenyl-alanine (DOPA) under the action of tyrosine hydroxylase (TH), which is the important rate-limiting enzyme in the synthesis of catecholamines and DOPA is then decarboxylated to form DA. This is inactivated under the influence of monoamine oxidase (MAO) to form dihydroxyphenyl acetic acid (DOPAC) which is then further metabolised to form the major end product homovanillic acid (HVA) by 0-methylation, catalysed by catechol-O-methyl transferase (COMT). Dopamine can also be 0-methylated to form 3-methyoxytyramine (3MT) which can then be deaminated by MAO to form HVA. It could be envisaged that the suspected increase in dopaminergic function in schizophrenics could be brought about by excess DA concentrations in the synapse produced either by an increase in TH activity or as a result of deficits in MAO or COMT activities. In the former case increased levels of metabolites such as HVA might be expected and in the latter case possibly decreased levels. An evaluation of the likelihood of these possibilities based on results of (a) CSF studies, (b) studies of plasma prolactin levels and (c) post-mortem studies are discussed below.

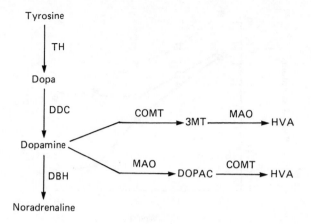

Fig. 18.3. Dopamine metabolism in the central nervous system. (See text for abbreviations.)

CSF studies

CSF assessment of HVA has been used as an index of central DA turnover. The technique used depends on the phenomenon that propenecid blocks the egress of acidic metabolites, such as HVA, from the CSF. The rise in HVA concentration in the CSF in a given time may therefore be taken as an index of the rate the metabolite is leaving the brain and therefore an index of the rate of DA turnover. The strategy had previously been tested in Parkinson's disease and in the amphetamine psychosis. Parkinson's disease is associated with degeneration of nigro-striatal and mesolimbic DA pathways and as expected the decrease in DA turnover was detected by decreased HVA concentrations compared with controls. Also an increase in HVA accumulation has been detected by the probenecid technique in the amphetamine psychosis. It seemed likely therefore that if schizophrenia is associated with increased DA turnover in the brain, it ought to be readily demonstrable by assessing HVA in the CSF using the probenecid technique. However, a number of studies have failed to produce any evidence of increased HVA production and hence DA turnover in schizophrenia using this technique. It has to be concluded therefore, that a general increase in DA turnover does not occur in the brains of schizophrenics or that if an increase in turnover does exist it must occur in a relatively discrete brain region such that the increased HVA production is obscured in the amount produced by dopamine neurons as a whole.

Neuroendocrine studies

There is good evidence from histochemical studies that monoamines control aspects of pituitary function. In particular there is strong evidence to suggest that the tuberoinfundibular dopamine system modulates prolactin release. Thus if there were a general increase in DA release in schizophrenics then plasma prolactin levels should be decreased compared with controls. Certainly it has been well established that the adminstration of neuroleptic drugs results in a significant increase in plasma prolactin levels in man. However, studies on schizophrenics have yielded no evidence that there is a decrease in plasma prolactin associated with the illness. These results indicate that if there is an increase in dopaminergic function in the brains of schizophrenics. It does not include the tuberoinfundibular dopamine system.

Post-mortem neurochemical studies

A direct approach to assessing dopaminegic mechanisms in schizophrenia has been made by studying post-mortem brain tissue. The impetus for such studies came from the successful demonstration of the neurochemical dysfunctions in Parkinson's disease and Huntington's chorea. The results of the major studies on (i) DA and its metabolites and (ii) enzymes responsible for synthesising and inactivating DA in relation to schizophrenia are summarised below.

Dopamine and its metabolites

The largest study of DA and its metabolites in the brains of schizophrenics was a collaborative investigation between the Division of Psychiatry at the Clinical Research Centre, Harrow and the MRC Neurochemical Pharmacology Unit at Cambridge, England. In this study the concentration of DA and HVA were determined in samples of caudate and nucleus accumbens from 44 control subjects and 46 schizophrenics. The results are presented in Table 18.2. Dopamine concentrations were significantly increased in caudate samples in the CRC series and in the nucleus accumbens samples in the Cambridge series. Homovanillic acid concentrations were significantly decreased in the caudate in the CRC series and significantly increased in the putamen in the Cambridge series. Dopamine turnover is often expressed as the HVA/DA ratio and the calculation of this ratio for the results of the above study are presented in Table 18.3. The only significant difference between the groups was a decrease in DA turnover in the caudate samples from schizophrenics in the CRC series of brains. It has been established that the large difference in DA turnover between the two series of brains in the nucleus accumbens was because the CRC series of brains were dissected according to a more restricted concept of the extent of this nucleus in the brain. The discrepancies in the details of the findings between the two groups may reflect the post-mortem instability of the metabolites, particularly DA which is known to be relatively unstable post-mortem. Nevertheless the results provided no evidence to suggest an increase in DA turnover in brains of schizophrenics.

Bacoupolos *et al.* (1979) reported significant increases in HVA in temporal, frontal and orbital frontal cortices but not in putamen or

Table 18.2. Dopamine and HVA concentrations in post-mortem brain samples from controls and schizophrenics

	CRC results, Controls (*n* = 19)	Schizophrenics (*n* = 18)
Caudate		
Dopamine	1.6 ± 0.3	2.5 ± 0.3*
HVA	5.4 ± 0.3	3.8 ± 0.5**
Putamen		
Dopamine	2.0 ± 0.4	2.2 ± 0.3
HVA	4.7 ± 0.5	5.9 ± 0.6
Nucleus Accumbens		
Dopamine	0.9 ± 0.3	0.7 ± 0.1
HVA	4.7 ± 0.5	5.5 ± 0.5
	Cambridge results, Controls (*n* = 25)	Schizophrenics (*n* = 28)
Caudate		
Dopamine	1.7 ± 0.2	2.0 ± 0.2
HVA	4.3 ± 0.4	5.6 ± 0.8
Putamen		
Dopamine	2.4 ± 0.2	2.5 ± 0.3
HVA	7.4 ± 0.6	10.3 ± 0.9**
Nucleus Accumbens		
Dopamine	1.4 ± 0.1	2.0 ± 0.1***
HVA	4.4 ± 0.4	4.9 ± 0.6

Values are means ± SE μ/g tissue; *$P < 0.05$; **$P < 0.02$; ***$P < 0.01$.

Table 18.3. Dopamine turnover (as HVA/DA)

	CRC		Cambridge	
	Controls	Schizophrenia	Controls	Schizophrenia
Caudate	4.7 ± 0.7	1.9 ± 0.4*	2.9 ± 0.4	3.0 ± 0.5
Putamen	4.0 ± 0.9	3.8 ± 0.7	3.7 ± 0.4	4.5 ± 0.5
Nucleus accumbens	11.1 ± 2.1	11.9 ± 2.2	3.1 ± 0.5	3.0 ± 0.5

*$P < 0.001$, values as means ± SE

nucleus accumbens of neuroleptic treated schizophrenics compared with controls. However, in a small number of patients not receiving neuroleptics the increase in HVA in cortical areas was not observed. Thus this study, too, provided no evidence for increased DA turnover in brains of schizophrenics.

A study of post-mortem tissue by Reynolds (1983) has implicated an increase in DA concentrations in the amygdala specifically in the left cerebral hemisphere of schizophrenics (Table 18.4). This finding seems particularly interesting, since there is some evidence to suggest that

Table 18.4. Catecholamine concentrations in bilaterally dissected post-mortem brain tissue

	Left		Right	
Amygdala				
Dopamine				
Schizophrenics	96.1*	(79.3−116.4)	55.7*	(46.0−67.5)
Controls	57.3	(46.7−70.4)	50.8	(41.4−62.4)
Noradrenaline				
Schizophrenics	58.7	(49.9−69.0)	61.5	(52.3−72.4)
Controls	54.2	(45.5−64.4)	63.2	(53.1−75.1)
Caudate nucleus				
Dopamine				
Schizophrenics	2185	(1889−2527)	2612	(2258−3021)
Controls	2572	(2202−3005)	2121	(1815−2478)

Assays were carried out on samples from 16 schizophrenics and 14 controls; values are geometric means with 95% confidence limits in brackets; *$P < 0.001$, all other left or right differences are not significant.

schizophrenia is associated with a dysfunction in the left temporal lobe, e.g. an association between a schizophrenia-like psychosis and temporal lobe epilepsy has been frequently observed. This promising finding requires replication and in particular the measurement of HVA concentrations in the same samples to determine whether this increase in DA in the left amygdala of schizophrenics represents an increase in DA turnover.

Enzymes related to dopamine metabolism

The activities of the enzymes involved in the metabolism of DA have been assessed in post-mortem brain tissue from controls and schizophrenics and the results are consistent with the findings for DA metabolites. Thus there is general agreement that the activities of tyrosine hydroxylase, dopa decarboxylase, monoamine oxidase and catechol-O-methyltransferase in brain samples from schizophrenics are similar to those in samples from controls.

Glutamate decarboxylase and choline acetyltransferase

Apart from enzymes involved directly in the metabolism of dopamine, glutamate decarboxylase (GAD) and choline acetyltransferase (ChAT) have also attracted considerable attention. Glutamate decarboxylase catalyses the formation of GABA from glutamic acid and is a marker for GABAergic neurons. Choline acetyltransferase catalyses the production of ACh from choline and acetyl Co-A and is a marker enzyme for cholinergic neurons. Both GABA and acetylcholine containing neurons have been reported to interact with dopaminergic mechanisms and hence changes in these two systems have also been implicated in the aetiology of schizophrenia.

Glutamate decarboxylase activity has been reported to be normal in schizophrenic brains and also to be significantly decreased. However, it subsequently became clear that in the latter study a preponderance of schizophrenics compared with controls had died with bronchopneumonia and the terminal hypoxia had an adverse effect on post-mortem GAD activity. It is now generally agreed that GAD activity is unchanged in brains of schizophrenics.

Choline acetyl transferase has been reported to be normal, decreased and increased in schizophrenic brains. However, there are several factors which affect the activity of the enzyme post-mortem which are probably sufficient to explain these discrepant findings. Choline acetyltransferase activity has been shown to be increased by neuroleptic medication and to decrease with age in some brain regions. As is the case for GAD it is now generally agreed that ChAT activity is unchanged in brains of schizophrenics.

Ligand binding studies in schizophrenia

It seems clear that DA turnover is unchanged in schizophrenia. Also at least two neurotransmitter systems that interact with DA, i.e. ACh and GABA are also unchanged. Although these findings lend no support to the DA hypothesis of schizophrenia, it had been suggested prior to the enzyme and metabolite studies that the suspected aberration in dopaminergic transmission may be located at the postsynaptic DA receptor. With the advent of ligand binding technique suitable for studying the DA receptor it became possible to evaluate this suggestion. In addition the binding of ligands to several other putative neurotransmitter receptors have been investigated in brains from schizophrenics.

Dopamine D_2 receptors

Not surprisingly the majority of ligand binding studies in schizophrenia have been concerned with assessing DA receptors. Initial studies used [^{3}H]-spiperone or [^{3}H]-haloperidol as ligand and it was soon established that these ligands were binding to D_2 and not D_1 receptors. The results of one such study using [^{3}H]-spiperone as ligand are shown in Fig. 18.4. There was a significant increase in [^{3}H]-spiperone binding in the schizophrenic group in all three brain regions investigated. In this study [^{3}H]-spiperone was at 0.8 nM in the binding procedure, therefore in order to determine whether the increased binding in schizophrenic brains was due to an increase in the number of receptors or increased affinity of the receptor for [^{3}H]-spiperone a Scatchard analysis was carried out on saturation data in samples of caudate nucleus and the result is shown in Fig. 18.5. There was a greater than 100% increase in the number of D_2 re-

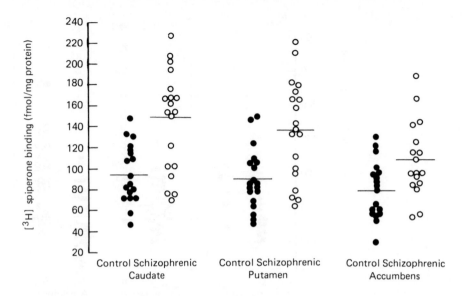

Fig. 18.4. Tritiated spiperone binding in brain samples from controls and schizophrenics.

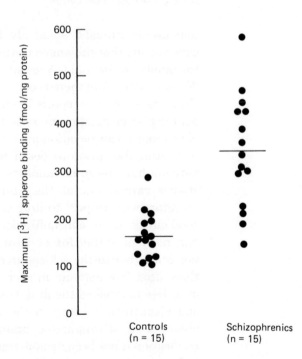

Fig. 18.5. Maximum [³H]-spiperone binding in samples of caudate nucleus from controls and schizophrenics.

ceptors in samples from schizophrenics. It seemed, therefore, that the dopamine hypothesis of schizophrenia could be sustained on the basis that the suspected dopaminergic overactivity was mediated through an increase in DA receptors rather than increased DA turnover and there is now general agreement that D_2 receptors are increased in number in brains of schizophrenics. However, what is not in agreement is how this

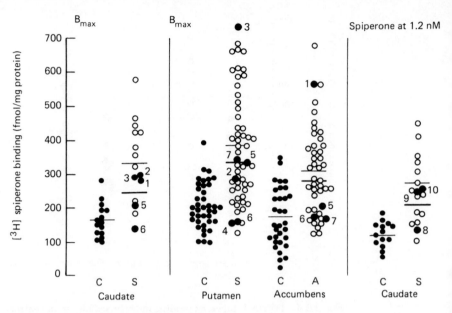

Fig. 18.6. Summary of studies on dopamine D_2 receptors in schizophrenia carried out at the Clinical Research Centre.

increase is brought about. It has been well established in animal experiments that prolonged neuroleptic treatment leads to an increase in the number of striatal DA receptors although usually only to the extent of 25–50%. Therefore there is considerable controversy over whether or not the increase in D_2 receptors in schizophrenic brains is solely the result of neuroleptic medication or related to the disease process. Some studies have reported an elevation in D_2 receptor numbers in schizophrenics who were drug-free prior to death whilst others have reported that such patients have receptor numbers similar to controls. A summary of the studies carried out at the Clinical Research Centre, Harrow on D_2 receptors with respect to drug treatment is presented in Fig. 18.6. The solid circles in the schizophrenic groups represent those 10 patients who had been drug-free for at least one year prior to death. The heavy horizontal bar in the schizophrenic group represents the mean value of these drug-free patients in each case. In every study the mean for the drug-free (as well as the drug-treated) patient was significantly elevated above controls. To support the view that the increase in D_2 receptors observed in schizophrenic brains was not solely due to neuroleptic medication it has been demonstrated that there is no significant elevation in D_2 receptors in patients dying with Huntington's chorea or Alzheimer's disease who had received neuroleptic treatment before death compared with similar patients who had not received these drugs (Fig. 18.7 and 18.8). Although, in general, some of these patients received doses of neuroleptics lower than those received by schizophrenics, some had received comparable doses for several years.

By contrast Mackay *et al.* (1980) reported that the density of D_2

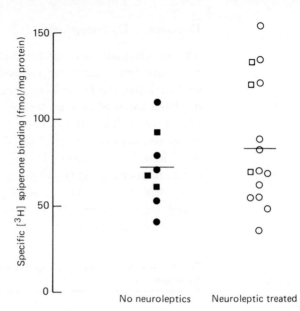

Fig. 18.7. Tritiated spiperone binding in drug-treated and drug-free patients with Huntington's chorea.

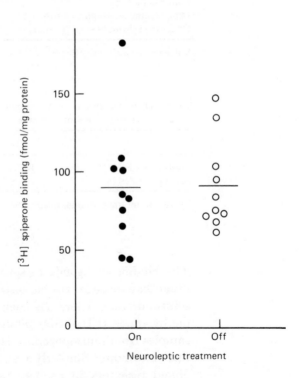

Fig. 18.8. Tritiated spiperone binding in brain samples from drug-treated and drug-free patients with Alzheimer's disease.

receptors was significantly increased in a psychotic group compared with controls in the caudate nucleus and the nucleus accumbens but that this increase was limited to those patients who had been receiving neuroleptics up until death. The controversy over neuroleptic treatment and the state of the D_2 receptor in schizophrenia remains unresolved.

Dopamine D_1 receptors

Tritiated flupenthixol was originally proposed as a selective ligand for D_1 receptors, but it was later realised that [^{3}H]-flupenthixol bound equally well to dopamine D_1 and D_2 receptors. The binding of [^{3}H]-flupenthixol has been assessed in drug-treated, drug-free schizophrenics and controls (Table 18.5). Tritiated flupenthixol binding was significantly increased compared with controls in both drug-treated and drug-free schizophrenics. When the binding of [^{3}H]-flupenthixol was resolved into its D_1 and D_2 components by using the highly selective D_2 antagonist, domperidone, to define the D_2 component in samples from drug-free schizophrenics, it was found that only the D_2 component was significantly elevated above controls (Table 18.6).

Table 18.5. Maximum [^{3}H]-flupenthixol binding in caudate nucleus of controls and schizophrenics

	B_{max} (fmol/mg protein)
Controls ($n = 8$)	370 ± 44
Drug-treated schizophrenics ($n = 7$)	637 ± 80**
Drug-free schizophrenics ($n = 8$)	566 ± 46*

Values as mean $\pm$ SE; *$P < 0.02$; **$P < 0.01$.

Table 18.6. D_1 and D_2 components [^{3}H]-flupenthixol binding in caudate nucleus of controls and drug-free schizophrenics

	D_1	D_2
Controls ($n = 9$)	104 ± 16	57 ± 9
Schizophrenics ($n = 6$)	133 ± 11	109 ± 16*

Values as fmol/mg protein; mean $\pm$ SE. *$P < 0.02$ vs controls.

The binding of ligands to several putative neurotransmitter receptors other than those for DA has also been studied in post-mortem brains from schizophrenics. There has been a report of decreased [^{3}H]-lysergic acid diethylamide ([^{3}H]-LSD) binding to 5-HT receptors in frontal cortex samples from schizophrenics. However, a later study was unable to confirm this finding. Similarly a report of decreased [^{3}H]-naloxone binding to opioid receptors in caudate nucleus of schizophrenics could not be replicated in a subsequent study. Other receptors or binding sites, which have been found to be unchanged in brains of schizophrenics include GABA, benzodiazepine, muscarinic and α- and -β-adrenoreceptors.

Thus of the neurotransmitter receptors assessed in schizophrenic brains, there is some agreement that only the D_2 receptor is increased in number but not general agreement on whether or not this is due to the effects of neuroleptic medication or part of the disease process. Ligand binding studies in post-mortem brains of schizophrenics have been reviewed (Owen *et al.* 1983).

In vivo studies

Recently considerable advances have been made in the development of ligands for the assessment of neurotransmitter receptor in living human subjects. With respect to schizophrenia, [77Br]-bromospiperone ([77Br]-BrSp) has been of particular interest (Fig. 18.9). Since it is a ligand for the D_2 receptor, bromospiperone (BrSp) is a potent displacer of [3H]-spiperone binding *in vitro* and increases plasma prolactin levels in the rat. After tail vein injection of [77Br]-BrSp the distribution of radioactivity in the brain is consistent with the known distribution of DA receptors, i.e. high in the striatum which is rich in DA receptors and low in the cerebellum which is devoid of DA receptors. Moreover the relatively high levels of [77Br]-BrSp in rat striatum after tail vein injection can be sterospecifically displaced by the isomers of flupenthixol. In addition it has been reported that in the rat, after chronic haloperidol administration, striatal DA receptor supersensitivity can be demonstrated both by increased [3H]-spiperone binding *in vitro* and by increased striatal [77Br]-BrSp content. There can be little doubt that [77Br]-BrSp is a ligand for D_2 receptors. (77Bromine is a γ-emitting source with a half-life of 56 hours and hence is suitable for clinical studies. [77Br]-BrSp has been administered to a small number of human volunteers. After intravenous injection of the ligand, good reconstructed images have been obtained after a 1-hour data acquisition period using a computer assisted gamma camera. Such a system generates axial, coronal or sagittal images of the radioactivity in the brain and it is possible from these images to quantify the ligand bound to the receptor. A computer reconstructed axial section is illustrated in Fig. 18.10, which demonstrates, clearly, the increased concentration of [77Br]-BrSp in the striatum. Since the striatum is rich in DA receptors and the cerebellum essentially devoid of DA receptors the striatum: cerebellum ratio of [77Br]-BrSp can be used an an index of the number of DA receptors in the striatum. This technique has been applied

Fig. 18.9. Chemical structure of [77Br]-bromospiperone.

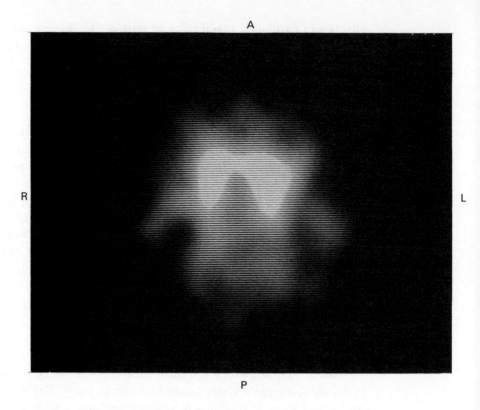

Fig. 18.10. Axial section depicting [^{77}Br]-bromospiperone distribution in the brain of a human volunteer. A, anterior. P, posterior. R, right. L, left.

to a small number of drug-free schizophrenics and controls and the result is illustrated in Fig. 18.11. There was a small but significant increase in striatum: cerebellum ratios of [^{77}Br]-BrSp in the schizophrenics compared with controls. Clearly more work is required to confirm and extend these initial results.

Concluding remarks

It should always be borne in mind that schizophrenic illnesses are heterogeneous and their pathology may also be heterogeneous. Biochemical studies on post-mortem brains have been carried out on relatively small numbers and the possibility that the particular psychoses of certain sub-groups of schizophrenics may be associated with the different biochemical hypotheses discussed above cannot be ruled out. On the basis of CSF and post-mortem studies, it seems clear that a primary overactivity of DA neurons is not present in the brains of schizophrenics, although the lateralisation of the amine in this condition requires further investigation. If in some cases it does turn out that increased D_2 receptors are indeed re-

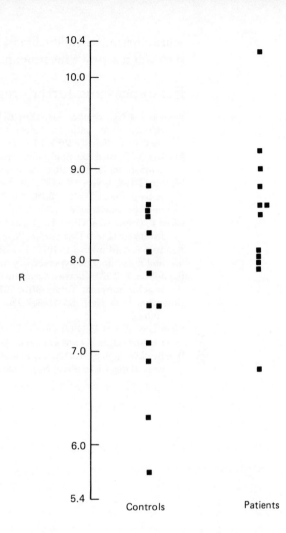

Fig. 18.11. Striatum: cerebellum ratios (R) of [^{77}Br]-bromospiperone in controls and schizophrenics.

lated to some forms of schizophrenia, it would still leave some questions unanswered. Firstly DA receptor blockade is complete within hours of initiation of neuroleptic medication and yet the attenuation of schizophrenic symptoms often takes two to three weeks. Also, if the illness in some cases is related to increased D_2 receptors, it is surprising that discontinuation of neuroleptic medication does not lead to an exacerbation of symptoms more frequently that is the case. Nevertheless it would seem that whatever the underlying defect in schizophrenia, the effects can be slowly amieliorated by neuroleptic blockade of DA receptors. Clearly, at best, increased D_2 receptors could only form part of the biological basis for schizophrenia.

Research in schizophrenia may soon benefit from advances in molecular genetics so that it may be possible to map the precise genetic defects and then in turn to establish the expression of these particular genes. Such an approach is well underway in the simple autosomal dominant condition of Huntington's chorea. The likely diversity of schizophrenia will undoubtedly present problems but it is to be hoped that they will not prove insurmountable.

References and further reading

Bacoupolos NC, Spokes EG, Bird ED & Roth RH (1979) Antipsychotic drug action in schizophrenic patients: Effect on cortical dopamine metabolism after long term treatment. *Science* **205**, 1405–7.

Mackay AVP, Bird ED, Spokes EG, Rossor M & Iversen LL (1980) Dopamine receptors and schizophrenia: drug effect or illness. *Lancet* **ii** 915–6.

Murphy DL & Wyatt RJ (1972) Reduced MAO activity in blood platelets from schizophrenic patients, *Nature* **238**, 225–6.

Osmond H & Smythies JR (1952). Schizophrenia: a new approach. *J. Ment. Sci.* **98**, 309–15.

Owen F, Cross AJ & Crow TJ (1983) Ligand binding studies in brain of schizophrenics. In: Strange PG (ed) *Cell Surface Receptors*. Ellis Horwood, Chichester.

Randrup A & Munkvad 1 (1972) Evidence indicating an association between schizophrenia and dopaminergic hyperactivity in the brain. *Orthomol. Psychiat.* **1**, 2–7.

Reynolds GP (1983) Increased concentrations and lateral asymmetry of amygdala dopamine in schizophrenia. *Nature* **305**, 527–9.

Rosenthal D & Kety SS (1968) *The Transmission of Schizophrenia*. Pergamon Press, Oxford.

Stein L & Wise CD (1971) Possible etiology of schizophrenia: progressive damage to the noradrenergic reward system by 6-hydroxydopamine. *Science* **171**, 1032–6.

Woolley DW & Shaw E (1954) A biochemical and pharmacological suggestion about certain mental disorders. *Proc. Nat. Acad Sci.* **40**, 228–31.

19 Depression

J.M ELLIOTT AND J.D. STEPHENSON

To the layman, depression is a commonly recognised emotion experienced by many people in response to adverse circumstances. In the clinical sense, however, depression can be a debilitating condition associated with distinct physical symptoms, withdrawal from normal social behaviour and, in about 15% of severe depressives, suicide. If left untreated, the depression will normally remit of its own accord only to return again after a varying interval (months or years). The introduction of antidepressant drugs has led to reduced suffering for both patients and their families and quicker recovery than would otherwise occur. Unfortunately, as will be seen, the drugs are not always effective and there is a need for better and more rapidly acting compounds.

Depression, together with mania, is termed an affective disorder since the major change apparent in such people is that of mood or 'affect'. A number of clinical features are associated with depression, some of which appear innocuous in themselves but together compose a well-recognised condition. These include:

1 depressed mood, which in milder cases may be a transient, recurring phenomenon, but in more severe cases is persistent and unresponsive to normal stimuli.

2 negative self-concept (self-deprecation), observed as a severe lack of self-confidence and self-worth.

3 changes in motor activity, which may become apparent as either retardation (lack of motivation, poverty of movement) or agitation (hyperactivity, persistent repetition of tasks).

4 physiological symptoms, the most common of which include early morning wakening, loss of appetite, loss of libido and general tiredness.

Mania in many ways is the opposite of depression and is characterised by heightening of mood (apparent as elation or even euphoria), irritability or hostility, poor insight into the consequences of sudden irrational decisions and in the most severe form, delusions and hallucinations. Some patients experience depression interspersed with episodes of mania, so-called manic-depressives. Indeed, the natural progression of depressive illness often begins with several minor episodes of depression, developing over a number of years into more serious and frequent depressive phases then eventually into regular and rapid fluctuations between depression and mania.

As in many areas of medicine, classification of depression into distinct categories would be useful in the attempt to identify the aetiology and predictive outcome of treatment. Although not totally exclusive, a number of broad distinctions have been drawn. Depression interspersed with periods of mania is termed 'bipolar' whilst that seen in the absence of manic symptoms is termed 'unipolar'. Bipolar depression displays a stronger hereditary trait than unipolar depression, hence not only do the children of bipolar depressed patients have a higher than average incidence of depression but this is also more likely to be of the bipolar than unipolar type. Depression with physical symptoms (insomnia, anorexia, retardation and altered diurnal rhythms) and no apparent cause is described as 'endogenous' and is generally more severe than 'reactive' depression, which may be precipitated by external events and is frequently associated with anxiety. Often the endogenous types of depression responds better to drug treatment than the reactive type, although this may reflect the inability of drugs to treat the primary defect in the latter case. However, the distinction between endogenous and reactive depression is still a matter of debate among psychiatrists.

A number of systems for classifying depression have been introduced and in order to estimate the severity of the illness various rating scales have been devised. That most widely used is the Hamilton Depression Rating Scale. This scale assesses the patient on 17 items which encompass the most common symptoms of all types of depression, the cumulative score reflecting the intensity of the illness. The important elements of any such rating scale are that they should be sensitive to changes in the intensity of the illness and demonstrate a high degree of inter-rater reliability, hence eliminating the subjective elements of diagnosis which may vary considerably between investigators.

Origins of the monoamine deficiency hypotheses of depression

The monoamines, noradrenaline (NA) and 5-hydroxytryptamine (5-HT) have been closely identified with the affective disorders since the 1960s as a result of observations that reserpine caused depression in a small proportion of patients prescribed the drug as an antihypertensive. When administered to rodents, reserpine produced a syndrome which included profound sedation, reduced locomotion, ptosis and hypothermia, effects considered analogous to the somatic changes accompanying the affective state produced in man. It was observed that these effects of reserpine could be prevented by prior treatment of the animals with the then novel antidepressants, iproniazid and imipramine. This antagonism formed the basis of early screening tests for antidepressant activity.

Reserpine was known to prevent the intraneuronal storage of the monoamines allowing them to leak into the cytoplasm where they were metabolised by mitochondrial monoamine oxidase (MAO). This interference with vesicular storage resulted in a gradual depletion of monoamines from the brain. However, in animals pretreated with iproniazid, a monoamine oxidase inhibitor, administration of reserpine caused monoamines, rather than their deaminated metabolites, to 'leak' from the neurons with the result that excitation occurred instead of sedation. Imipramine also prevented the sedative effects of reserpine and it was later shown to produce this effect by inhibiting the neuronal reuptake of NA thereby potentiating the effects of any NA released. This effect of imipramine was first described in the sympathetic nervous system but it is now known to exert a similar action in the CNS where it also inhibits the uptake of 5-HT.

Therefore by the mid-1960s, the association had been made between drugs which altered the affective state in man and central NA and 5-HT concentrations in animals. This association contributed to the formulation of the monoamine theories of affective disorder. Thus the catecholamine hypothesis of Schildkraut (1965) postulated that ' ... some, if not all, depressions are associated with an absolute or relative deficiency of catecholamines, particularly NA at functionally important receptor sites in the brain. Elation conversely may be associated with an excess of such amines ... ' Other, mostly European, authors proposed instead that indoleamines rather than NA were deficient in depression (Coppen 1967). Because the tricylic antidepressants (TCAs) and monoamine oxidase inhibitors (MAOIs) affected uptake and metabolism of both 5-HT and NA and because reserpine interfered with the intraneuronal storage of both monoamines, it was not possible to determine whether NA or 5-HT was more relevant. It was also suggested that there may be some patients with a selective deficiency of NA, while other patients, displaying essentially the same symptoms, may have a 5-HT deficiency.

Acute pharmacology of tricyclic antidepressants

Imipramine was the first of a series of tricyclic antidepressants to be used clinically. It is structurally related to chlorpromazine but when tested in patients suffering from a variety of mental disorders it was found to be devoid of antipsychotic activity but instead to be an effective antidepressant. Comparison of the structure of the two molecules shows the two phenyl rings of imipramine to be at an angle to each other, wheareas in the chlorpromazine molecule, the two phenyl rings are aligned in the same plane as the third ring (Fig. 19.1). It is to this difference that the shift from antipsychotic to anti-depressant activity has been attributed.

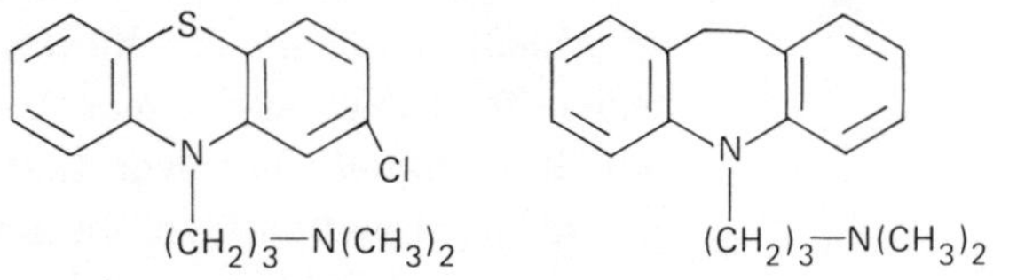

$(CH_2)_3$—$N(CH_3)_2$

Chlorpromazine

$(CH_2)_3$—$N(CH_3)_2$

Imipramine

Fig. 19.1. Structural analogy between imipramine and chlorpromazine.

In 1959, Sigg reported that imipramine increases the pressor responses of the cardiovascular system and contractile responses of the cat nictitating membrane to injected NA and this was shown (Hertting et al. 1961) to be due to inhibition of the uptake of infused NA into peripheral tissues thereby increasing its availability at postsynaptic receptor sites. A similar action on neuronal uptake of NA within the CNS was later demonstrated. Unexpected, was the finding that large doses of amitriptyline could reverse the pressor responses to adrenaline, which is not taken up like NA, because of its chlorpromazine-like α-adrenoceptor blocking activity. Therefore the final effect of certain tricyclic antidepressants is the resultant of these two opposing actions as can be demonstrated in cats after chronic denervation of one nictitating membrane. In such animals amitriptyline, which is a more potent α-adrenoceptor blocking agent than imipramine, will potentiate responses of the innervated membrane to injections of NA but dose dependently reduce responses of the super-sensitive denervated membrane.

Typically the α_1-adrenoceptor blocking properties of those tricyclic antidepressants which are tertiary amines are greater than those which are secondary amines. Although the tricyclics are considerably less potent than selective antagonists such as prazosin, α_1-adrenoceptor blockade will be achieved in clinical practice because therapeutic doses of the antidepressants are much greater.

Tricyclic antidepressants also inhibit the uptake of [^{3}H]5-HT into brain slices. Ross and Renyi (1969) observed that imipramine and amitriptyline were more potent inhibitors of 5-HT uptake than their respective metabolites, desipramine and nortriptyline. These metabolites are secondary amines formed by oxidative N-demethylation of the parent compounds. More extensive structure activity relationships of the tricyclic antidepressants have demonstrated that the tertiary amines are generally more potent inhibitors of 5-HT uptake than the corresponding secondary amines (Fig. 19.2) but they do not exhibit selectivity for 5-HT (Fig. 19.3). In contrast, the secondary amines show far greater selectivity towards inhibition of NA uptake than 5-HT uptake. The tricyclic antidepressants also display antagonistic activity at 5-HT$_2$ receptors but this aspect of their actions is less easily studied.

Given the pedigree of imipramine as phenothiazine-like it is not surprising that it also possesses antihistaminic and cholinolytic properties. Of the tricyclics, amitriptyline is the most potent antagonist at muscarinic cholinoceptors. It has about one-tenth the potency of atropine but because therapeutic doses of the antidepressants are relatively large, significant blockade is achieved in vivo. This is evidenced by atropine-like side-effects such as dry mouth, urinary retention, impairment of memory etc. It is unlikely, however, that muscarinic receptor blockade contributes to antidepressant activity because the more potent, selective cholinolytics which are available are not known to possess antidepressant activity and some newer non-tricyclic antidepressants such as bupropion, nomifensine, viloxazine and trazodone are practically devoid of such activity.

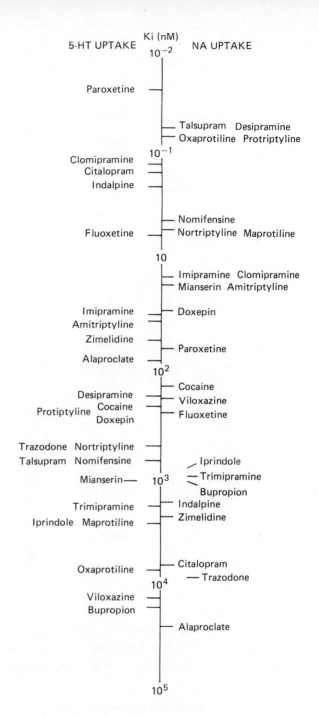

Fig. 19.2. Potency of some antidepressants to block noradrenaline (10 nM) and 5-HT (10 nM) uptake into synaptosomes prepared from occipital and temporal cortex of rat brain (noradrenaline) and whole brain, excluding brainstem and cerebellum (5-HT). The data was obtained from Hytell (1982).

Several tricyclic antidepressants, particularly the tertiary amines, are more potent H_1-receptor antagonists than established antihistamines such as diphenhydramine and mepyramine. The equilibrium dissociation constant (K_B) for mepyramine on the guinea pig ileum is 1000 pM compared with 56 pM and 84 pM for doxepine and amitriptyline

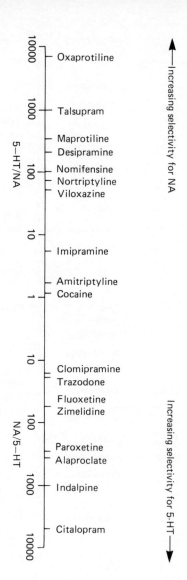

Fig. 19.3. *In vitro* selectivity of some antidepressants for NA and 5-HT uptake mechanisms. The data was obtained from Hytell (1982).

respectively (Figge *et al.* 1979). It is likely that the sedation produced by certain antidepressants, e.g. doxepin and amitriptyline is primarily due to central H_1 receptor antagonism.

Clinical aspects

Following the proposal of the monoamine hypothesis, attempts were made to identify deficits in the activity of monoamine transmitters in depressed patients by measurement of the concentration of these transmitters and their metabolites in various body fluids. The major metabolic products of the monoamine neurotransmitters are outlined in Fig. 19.4 (see also Figs 7.3 and 8.2).

Fig. 19.4. Metabolic products of the action of monoamine oxidase (MAO) and/or catechol-O-methyltransferase (COMT) on NA, DA and 5-HT.

Noradrenaline	MAO/COMT	MOPEG (3-methoxy,4-hydroxyphenylethylglycol)
	MAO	DOPEG (3,4 dihydroxyphenylethylglycol)
	COMT	Normetanephrine
	MAO/COMT	VMA (vanillylmandelic acid)
Dopamine	MAO/COMT	HVA (homovanillic acid)
	MAO	DOPAC (3,4, dihydroxyphenylacetic acid)
5-Hydroxytryptamine	MAO	5-HIAA (5-hydroxyindole acetic acid)

5-Hydroxytryptamine

Initial studies of cerebrospinal fluid (CSF) samples suggested that the concentrations of 5-HT and 5-HIAA were lower in depressed patients than in euthymic control subjects (Ashcroft *et al.* 1966). However, subsequent investigations have been unable to confirm this as a consistent finding (see Green & Costain 1979). One possible interpretation of such confusing data is that these indoleamines may show a bimodal distribution among depressed patients, with low concentrations being particularly associated with suicidal tendencies (Ashberg *et al.* 1976). However, such studies are no longer common since the lumbar puncture method of obtaining samples of CSF exposes patients to unnecessary risks. Furthermore, there is considerable debate as to the origin of the indoleamines within lumbar CSF, since there are known to be active 5-HT neurons within the spinal cord. Indeed a study of CSF samples taken simultaneously from both the lumbar spinal cord and from the brain ventricles showed poor correlation in terms of indoleamine content (Curzon *et al.* 1980). It seems likely, therefore, that the concentration of indoleamines in lumbar CSF could reflect 5-HT activity in the spinal cord and the low values reported in some studies may simply reflect the reduced motor activity frequently associated with depression rather than a primary biochemical defect within the brain.

Studies of urinary samples is not applicable in the case of 5-HT since the content of indoleamines originating from the brain is small by comparison with that synthesised and released by entero-chromaffin cells within the gut.

The studies outlined above have attempted to assess 5-HT activity in depressed patients by *ex vivo* measurement of indoleamines. An alternative approach is the direct measurement of brain indoleamines in postmortem tissue. Again, initial results suggested a significant decrease in brain 5-HT content, particularly in the raphe nuclei where the serotonergic cell bodies are located (Lloyd *et al.* 1974) but subsequent studies have not confirmed this apparent deficit (Beskow *et al.* 1976). However, postmortem studies introduce a number of problems not encountered in *ex vivo* analysis (Cooper *et al.* 1985). Principally it is frequently the case that little is known of the psychiatric history or drug treatment regimen of the patient shortly before death, particularly in the case of suicide victims. Indeed the assumption that suicide victims are necessarily depressed is controversial. Also the subjects used as the control group should be clearly matched to the test group particularly in terms of the agonal state of the patient at the time of death. Finally the monoamine neurotransmitters are quite labile molecules, therefore minimal post-mortem delay is essential for accurate determination.

Catecholamines

Metabolism of NA by MAO and/or COMT leads to a number of metabolites (Fig. 19.4, see also Fig. 7.3) of which MOPEG (3-methoxy, 4-hydroxy-phenylglycol) is probably the major product from within the central nervous system. Brain post-mortem levels of both NA and DA are generally agreed to be unchanged in depressed patients. Measurement of CSF catecholamines and metabolites have produced conflicting results, some reporting a decrease which others have been unable to confirm (see Green & Costain 1979).

Measurement of urinary MOPEG produced inconsistent reports of decreased levels in depressed patients until the patients were subdivided into unipolar and bipolar type, when it became apparent that low levels of MOPEG were observed in bipolar depressives during the depression phase and were increased during the manic phase (Schildkraut 1978). It is therefore questionable whether these changes in NA activity are related to the mood of the patient or to the level of activity associated with the particular mood.

Metabolic enzymes

In addition to measurement of the monoamines and their metabolites, studies have also been made of the activity of associated metabolic enzymes, specifically monoamine oxidase (MAO), catechol-O-methyl transferase (COMT) and dopamine beta-hydroxylase (DBH). Since routine assay of brain enzyme activity was clearly impossible the approach adopted was to investigate enzyme activity in peripheral tissues. In the case of a genetic abnormality, which may result in a change in the activity of an enzyme, it would be anticipated that such a change should be apparent at peripheral as well as central sites. Hence the peripheral tissue could then act as a trait marker for depression. Unfortunately, no such trait marker has been succesfully identified.

No significant differences were observed in the activity of DBH, as located in plasma or CSF, or COMT, located in erythrocytes, between depressed patients and controls. Analysis of MAO from platelets initially suggested increased activity in depressed patients, but further study refuted this finding, demonstrating instead a close familial association of enzyme activity which was independent of any affective disorder.

It is clear from the above that clinical findings lend little support to the proposed deficit in neuronal monoamines as the primary biochemical lesion responsible for depression.

Problems with the monoamine theory

The main arguments which have been advanced against the monoamine deficiency hypotheses are as follows:

1 Measurements of monoamine metabolites in depressed patients and of post-mortem monoamine concentrations in the brains of suicide victims have not unequivocally identified a monoamine deficit.

2 Some newly introduced antidepressant drugs, the so-called 'second generation' or 'atypical' antidepressants such as iprindole and mianserin, fail to inhibit monoamine uptake into neurons while some long-established monoamine uptake inhibitors, notably cocaine and amphetamine, are devoid of antidepressant activity.

3 Whereas blockade of monoamine reuptake by tricyclic anti-depressants is of rapid onset, the therapeutic response in depressed patients is delayed by up to three weeks despite daily medication. This cannot be entirely explained by the clinical practice of prescribing antidepressants at low doses initially and then gradually increasing the dose (to minimise side-effects) because after electroconvusive shock therapy (ECT) maximal clinical benefit, while more rapid, is still not achieved until after 6–8 shocks administered 2–3 days apart.

None of these objections alone is sufficiently sound for rejecting the hypothesis that antidepressant action is due to an increase in monoamine concentration at postsynaptic receptor sites but together they provide a powerful argument for its re-examination and suggest that antidepressants act in a more complex manner than that envisaged by the monoamine deficiency hypotheses of depression. Current research is therefore very much focused on studying the long-term changes in monoamine systems produced by daily administration of antidepressants to experimental animals, usually rats. So far this research has concentrated on determining changes in receptor populations after repeated antidepressant administration but behavioural and electrophysiological studies have been valuable in attributing functional relevance to the observed receptor changes particularly in those instances when these have been inconsistent.

Atypical antidepressants

The original group of antidepressant drugs were either monoamine uptake inhibitors, tricyclic in structure and derived from the imipramine molecule, or were non-selective MAO inhibitors and included hydrazines, hydrazides and sympathomimetic amines. The chemical structures of some of these compounds are shown in Figs. 19.5 and 19.6.

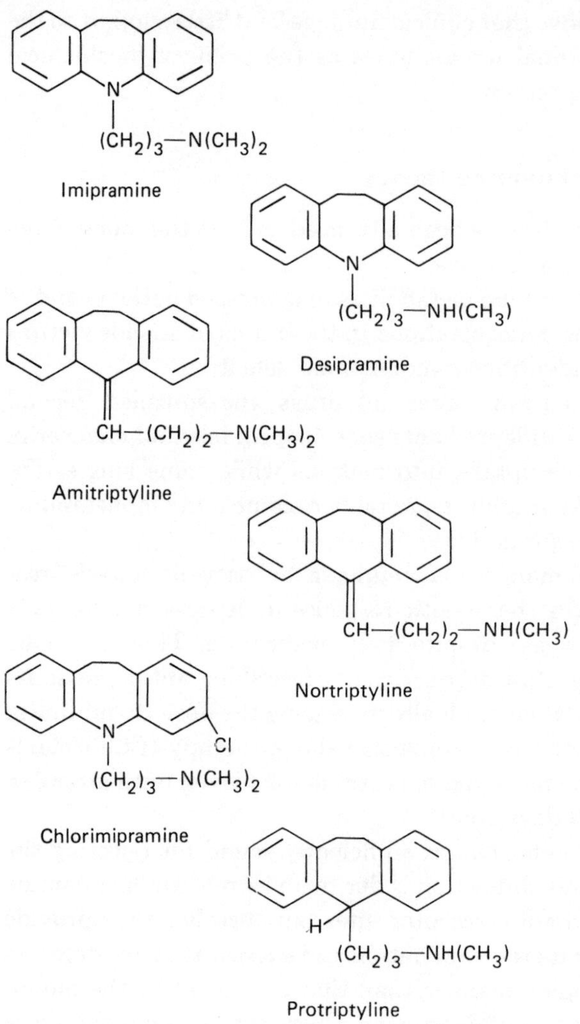
N
$(CH_2)_3$—$N(CH_3)_2$
Imipramine
N
$(CH_2)_3$—$NH(CH_3)$
Desipramine
CH—$(CH_2)_2$—$N(CH_3)_2$
Amitriptyline
CH—$(CH_2)_2$—$NH(CH_3)$
Nortriptyline
N
Cl
$(CH_2)_3$—$N(CH_3)_2$
Chlorimipramine
H
$(CH_2)_3$—$NH(CH_3)$
Protriptyline

Fig. 19.5. Chemical formulae of some tricyclic antidepressants. Tertiary amines are shown to the left and secondary amine to the right.

Unfortunately, tricyclic antidepressants are beneficial in only approximately three-quarters of depressed patients within a 3–4 week treatment period (compared with a 30–40% placebo response) and the use of MAO inhibitors, which are no more effective than the tricyclics, is severely restricted by the occurrence of severe, sometimes fatal, hypertensive crises in patients after ingestion of foodstuffs containing various amines such as tyramine, histamine and phenethylamine. Another disadvantage of tricyclic antidepressants is that they are highly toxic in overdosage. This is a particularly undesirable feature of drugs which are given to a patient population who are most at risk from self-poisoning. In fact, tricyclic antidepressants are the commonest cause of drug-induced life-threatening CNS depression and are responsible for about 350 deaths per year in England and Wales alone. ECT remains the most effective and rapid treatment for severe endogenous depression but its use is now restricted to 'drug-resistant depressives' and to those patients for whom a

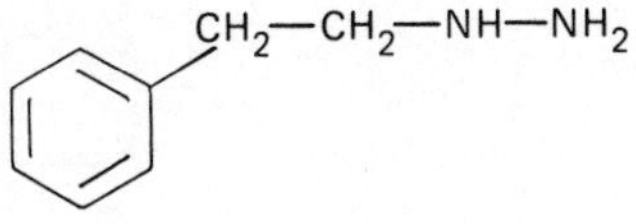

Phenelzine

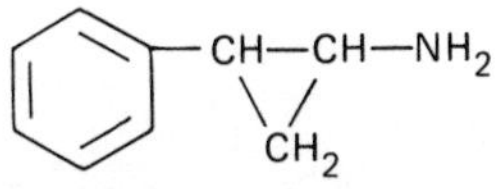

Tranylcypromine

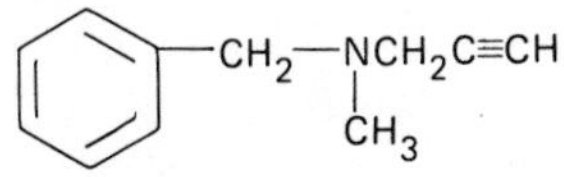

Pargyline

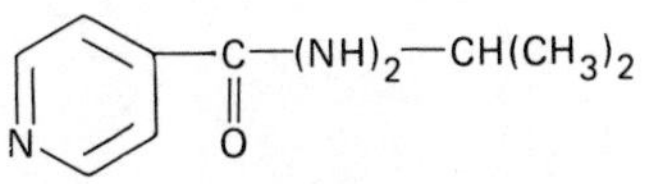

Fig. 19.6. Chemical formulae of some monamine oxidase inhibitors.

Iproniazid

delay of at least 3 weeks before occurrence of a therapeutic effect would be unacceptable because of the risk of death from suicide, inanition etc. Therefore, in an attempt to obtain safer, more effective and more rapidly acting drugs a number of putative antidepressants have been introduced with widely differing chemical structures and pharmacological actions. These are known as 'second generation' or 'atypical' antidepressants. Some notes on the more important of these are given below and their chemical formulae are shown in Fig. 19.7.

Iprindole

Iprindole differs from imipramine only in the configuration of the ring system. It has negligible effects on monamine uptake mechanisms and does not affect NA turnover. It was the first of the 'atypical' antidepressants introduced into clinical practice and it became the standard 'atypical' antidepressant for studies in which antidepressants were administered chronically to animals although Zis and Goodwin (1979) concluded that its superiority over placebo in clinical trials had not been proven.

Mianserin

Mianserin is a tetracyclic which was first synthesised as a 5-HT antagonist; it is also a potent antihistamine. Its potential as an

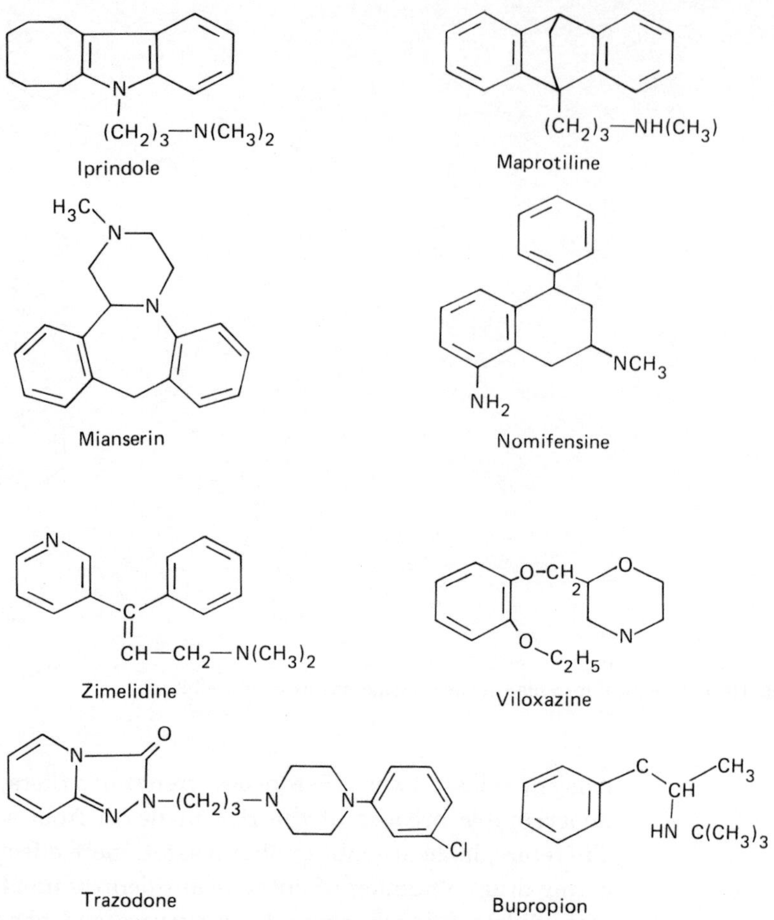

Fig. 19.7. Chemical formulae of some atypical antidepressants.

antidepressant was suspected from its effects on the computerised EEG in volunteers. *In vitro*, mianserin selectively inhibits NA uptake but this action is absent *in vivo*. Given acutely to animals, mianserin increases NA turnover by blockade of presynaptic α_2 receptors but it appears that this effect is lost with repeated administration over several days. Although it appears to be less effective than the tricyclic antidepressants it is relatively free of side-effects — apart from a temporary sedative effect, which can be attributed to its antihistaminic activity, and weight gain.

Bupropion

This is a chloropropiophenone which has negligible effects on 5-HT and NA reuptake, only weakly inhibits DA uptake but reverses tetrabenazine-induced sedation and potentiates the effects of L-DOPA. It is without effect on monoamine oxidase and has no anticholinergic or antihista-minic effects. Bupropion has few side-effects making it suitable for use in geriatric patients and in patients with cardiovascular problems.

Maprotiline

Maprotiline is a bridged tricyclic which otherwise resembles the conventional tricyclics. Maprotiline inhibits NA uptake selectively with very little effect on 5-HT uptake and only moderate anticholinergic effects. Its antidepressant activity is similar to that of the standard tricyclic antidepressants, the most important side-effect being induction of seizures. The hydroxy derivative of maprotiline, oxaprotiline, also possesses antidepressant activity and is the most selective and potent NA uptake inhibitor available for clinical usage. It is of particular value for research purposes because there are two enantiomers, the uptake blocking properties residing in the (+)-enantiomer.

Nomifensine

Nomifensine is a tetrahydroisoquinoline. It is alone among the antidepressants in being a potent inhibitor of DA as well as NA reuptake. Its structure remotely resembles that of the β-phenethylamines and it has excitant properties which have been attributed to possible DA release and inhibition of its reuptake. Clinically, exacerbation of both manic and psychotic symptoms have been noted but the drug has recently been withdrawn from usage because of unwanted side-effects.

Trazodone

Trazodone is a triazolopyridine derivative. It is inactive in the standard screening tests for antidepressant activity. It does not antagonise tetrabenazine or reserpine induced sedation, it has virtually no effect on catecholaminergic mechanisms and it does not inhibit MAO. Trazodone is an antagonist at 5-HT receptors and in high concentrations it inhibits 5-HT reuptake.

Viloxazine

Viloxazine is an oxazine derivative of propranolol. It is a moderately potent but selective inhibitor of NA uptake with only minimal effects on 5-HT and DA uptake. It has little antihistaminic and cholinolytic activity and therefore is free from the sedative side-effects of the tricyclic antidepressants and is less cardiotoxic than the tricyclics.

Zimelidine

Zimelidine is a bicyclic compound and a potent selective inhibitor of 5-HT uptake without significant effects on cholinergic, histaminergic and catecholaminergic systems. However, the in vivo metabolite, norzimelidine is less selective and weakly inhibits NA reuptake. It is the best documented of the selective 5-HT uptake inhibitor type of antidepressant but hypersensitivity reactions in some patients caused its withdrawal in 1983.

Adaptive changes following chronic antidepressant administration

Administered acutely, monoamine uptake inhibitors and monoamine oxidase inhibitors reduce turnover of brain 5-HT and NA, the magnitude of the reduction correlating with the amount of uptake blockade or enzyme inhibition. One mechanism by which this might be achieved is illustrated by the reduction in the spontaneous firing rate of neurons of the locus coeruleus following acute administration of an inhibitor of NA uptake or of monoamine oxidase (Scuvee-Moreau & Dresse 1979). This effect, which would lead to a reduction in NA release from terminals of the locus coeruleus and hence a reduction in transmitter turnover, is due to activation of soma-dendritic α_2-adrenoceptors on locus coeruleus neurons. Recurrent inhibitory collaterals arising from the locus coeruleus are thought to release NA onto these α_2-adrenoceptors thereby reducing the neuronal activity. It has also been shown that inhibitors of 5-HT uptake reduce the firing rate of 5-HT neurons in the dorsal raphe nuclei, presumably by an analogous mechanism. Following daily administration of various antidepressants for periods of from 5 days to 3 weeks this relation between uptake inhibition and monoamine turnover was found to hold no longer with authors reporting increases, decreases or no change in turnover. Since the drugs continue to inhibit either MAO or monoamine uptake when administered chronically, adaptive changes must have occurred.

Segal *et al.* (1974) were the first to propose that when given chronically antidepressants might produce compensatory changes which would affect neurotransmission in the opposite direction to that produced by acute administration. Reserpine administered daily for 8 days significantly increased tyrosine hydroxylase activity whereas desipramine similarly administered, reduced activity of the enzyme. Thus conditions assumed to reduce central NA activity actually increased synthesising capacity and *vice versa*. It was proposed that these presynaptic adaptive changes were of primary importance in the action of drugs which precipitated or alleviated depression and that depressed patients had catecholamine receptors of 'heightened responsiveness', that is, depression was associated with enhanced catecholaminergic transmission. It had previously been assumed that the acute increase in monoaminergic transmission which resulted from the increased synaptic concentrations of 5-HT and/or NA caused by antidepressant administration persisted with continued administration of the antidepressants.

Effects of antidepressants on beta-adrenoceptors

A major breakthrough in the search for a common mechanism of antidepressant action was the finding of Vetulani & Sulser (1975) that the once daily administration of desipramine to rats for at least 3 weeks diminished the response of the NA sensitive adenylate cyclase system, in slices of the limbic forebrain, to applied NA. This observation was followed by the findings of Banerjee et al. (1977) and Sarai et al. (1978) that daily repeated administration of desipramine also reduced the binding of radioligands to β-adrenoceptors in rat forebrain due to a reduction in the number of binding sites (Bmax) rather than an altered affinity (K_D). These two events — reduction in the number of β-adrenoceptors and subsensitivity of the NA-sensitive adenylate cyclase — were presumed to be functionally linked although there is evidence that in the rat the stimulation of cyclic AMP production by NA is not mediated entirely by β-adrenoceptors (Mobley & Sulser 1979). These results established a temporal relationship between changes in sensitivity of β-adrenergic mechanisms and the therapeutic response to antidepressants and led Vetulani and Sulser (1975) to propose that the adaptive changes in receptor sensitivity were fundamental to the clinical antidepressant effect.

Receptor binding studies

[^{3}H]-Dihydroalprenolol and [^{125}I]-iodohydroxybenzylpindolol are the radioligands most commonly used for determining β-adrenoceptor numbers. Both compounds are antagonists and neither distinguishes between the β_1- and β_2- subtypes of the receptor. With the exception of the cerebellum where β_2-adrenoceptors predominate, 55–65% of β-adrenoceptors in the rat brain are of the β_1- subtype. These have a much higher affinity for NA than the β_2-adrenoceptors suggesting they are likely to be primarily involved in neuronal function (Minneman et al. 1979). The β-adrenoceptor down-regulation observed after chronic administration of desipramine is restricted to the β_1-subtype.

The ability of chronically administered desipramine to down-regulate β-adrenoceptors in the brains of rats by 30–40% has been confirmed in many studies and the finding has been extended to include other tricyclic antidepressants, e.g. imipramine, amitriptyline, chlorimipramine etc. (see reviews by Sugrue 1983 and Charney et al. 1981). Beta-adrenoceptor down-regulation also occurs in the rat forebrain after repeated administration of MAO inhibitors such as pargyline, tranylcypromine and the selective MAO A inhibitor, clorgyline, and also by repeated electroconvulsive shocks. However, there may be species differences because desipramine does not down-regulate β-adrenoceptors in the guinea pig forebrain.

It is presumed that the down-regulation of rat brain β-adrenoceptors is caused by maintained high concentrations of NA in the synaptic cleft because destruction of presynaptic NA terminals with 6-hydroxydopamine prevented desipramine from reducing receptor numbers (Schweitzer *et al.* 1979). There are regional differences in the rate of down-regulation. Cortical β-adrenoceptors are lost more rapidly than those in the hippocampus while in the striatum, the receptor numbers do not change. Factors which may be responsible for these regional variations in the rate and degree of down-regulation include the density of the noradrenergic innervation within the region, the local turnover rates of NA and the relative importance of uptake, diffusion and metabolism to the termination of the action of NA at the postsynaptic site.

The picture becomes less clear, however, when the effects of the atypical antidepressants are considered. In the paper in which Banerjee *et al.* (1977) first showed desipramine to cause β-adrenoceptor down-regulation upon repeated administration it was also reported that iprindole caused down-regulation. Iprindole only weakly inhibits NA uptake and does not enhance responses to injected NA. The fact that it caused down-regulation of β-adrenoceptors was fundamental to Banerjee *et al.* (1977) proposing β-adrenoceptor down-regulation as a common mechanism of antidepressant action. Results for mianserin are equivocal with down-regulation being reported in only one out of several publications and this author, Clements-Jewry (1978), commented on the smallness of the effect (an 18% reduction in the number of receptors). Bupropion, an antidepressant without acute effects on noradrenergic mechanisms, has been claimed to both reduce (Gandolfi *et al.* 1983) and not to affect (Ferris & Beaman 1983) cortical β-adrenoceptors after chronic administration to rats. Other drugs for which antidepressant activity has been claimed and which do not lead to a reduction in receptor numbers include the highly selective 5-HT uptake inhibitors, fluoxetine and citalopram, and the selective NA uptake inhibitor, nisoxetine (Mishra *et al.* 1979).

If the therapeutic effect of antidepressants is due to β-adrenoceptor down-regulation, there should be clinical benefit from hastening the process. In patients it would be impractical to give massive doses of antidepressants because of unpleasant and dangerous side-effects. An alternative approach would be to administer an α_2-adrenoceptor antagonist, such as idazoxan or yohimbine together with an established antidepressant. The rationale for this approach is that inhibition of the presynaptic control of NA release would increase the synaptic concentration of NA above that caused by inhibition of its uptake alone which could in any case increase α_2-adrenoceptor activity and decrease release. Several groups have reported that in rats a combination of yohimbine or phenoxybenzamine with desipramine produces down-regulation of cortical β-adrenoceptors within 1–4 days but whether this would result in a more rapid clinical response is not yet known; yohimbine does not appear to be of value as an adjunct to tricyclic antidepressants in the treatment of drug-resistant patients.

Adenylate cyclase studies

Stimulation of β-adrenoceptors increases adenylate cyclase activity and the production of second messenger cyclic AMP. Since this may generate the postsynaptic response to receptor stimulation any alteration in its activity would manifest itself as a change in the sensitivity of the NA mechanism. In 1976, Vetulani *et al.* reported that daily injections of either desipramine or the atypical antidepressant iprindole to rats for 4 weeks or daily electroconvulsive shocks for 4 days reduced the sensitivity of the noradrenaline-sensitive cyclic AMP generating system in slices prepared from limbic forebrains. The ability to induce subsensitivity of the adenylate cyclase system is shared by many antidepressant drugs but not by other types of psychoactive drugs such as the anxiolytic benzodiazepines, neuroleptics and antihistamines. Of particular interest was the finding that some antidepressants which did not reduce β-adrenoceptor numbers nevertheless reduced the adenylate cyclase response, e.g. mianserin, zimelidine, nisoxetine, etc. However, there are still antidepressants which do not reduce the adenylate cyclase response, e.g. the selective 5-HT uptake inhibitors, fluoxetine and citalopram.

The mechanisms whereby subsensitivity of the adenylate cyclase system can occur without a reduction in β-adrenoceptor numbers are not fully understood. It is now well established that stimulation of adenylate cyclase by catecholamines involves at least three physically separable components: the hormone receptor, the catalytic adenylate cyclase enzyme and a guanyl nucleotide regulatory subunit which enables coupling of the receptor to the enzyme. Exposure of various cell types (glioma, lymphoma, frog erythrocytes etc.) to isoprenaline *in vitro* has shown that the process of catecholamine-induced desensitisation occurs in at least two stages. The first stage is rapid in onset, reversible and involves modification of receptor-adenylate cyclase coupling with consequent loss of hormone responsiveness but no change in receptor numbers. The second stage occurs after more prolonged incubation for several hours and is identified by receptor loss which is not reversible except by synthesis of new receptors (Su *et al.* 1979; Wessels *et al.* 1978). Whether a similar uncoupling of the receptor-adenylate cyclase complex is responsible for those instances of antidepressant-induced subsensitivity of the adenylate cyclase system in the absence of changes in receptor numbers is not known. When cortical slices from desipramine-treated rats were incubated with isoprenaline, β-adrenoceptor binding sites were further reduced. This effect of isoprenaline was reversible and was proportionally similar to that obtained in control animals (Dibner & Molinoff 1979). The results demonstrate that the reduction in β-adrenoceptor numbers obtained in rats after chronic treatment with desipramine, and to other drugs which increase NA availability, is not maximal. It remains to be determined whether the acute isoprenaline-induced and chronic desipramine-induced receptor decreases are different processes or sequential stages of one process.

Beta-adrenoceptor numbers in rat brain have so far only been measured with antagonist ligands such as [³H]-dihydroalprenolol which do not discriminate between high and low agonist affinity forms of the receptor. Activation of adenylate cyclase is believed to be associated with the high affinity agonist state of the receptor. Studies of isoprenaline-induced desensitisation of β-adrenoceptors on frog erythrocytes using the agonist ligand, [³H]-hydroxybenylisoprenaline (which preferentially binds to the high affinity state), show a much closer correlation between β-adrenoceptor binding and loss of adenylate cyclase sensitivity. Unfortunately there are no reports of the use of this ligand on brain tissue.

Functional studies

Electrophysiological

This inhibitory effect of β-adrenoceptor activation on cerebellar and cortical cell firing rate (see Chapter 9) has been widely used to assign functional significance to the reductions in β-adrenoceptor numbers. Olpe and Schellenberg (1980) demonstrated a statistically significant reduction in the inhibitory effect of iontophoretically applied NA to cingulate cortical cells after rats had received daily injections of an antidepressant. The antidepressants tested (desipramine, clomipramine, maprotiline and tranylcypromine) were all effective and the onset of the effect paralleled that of β-adrenoceptor down-regulation. In a different type of experiment, Huang et al. (1980) showed that the spontaneous firing rates of rat hippocampal pyramidal cells were increased after 3 weeks of daily injections of desipramine. This effect was attributed to reduced neuronal activity in the locus coeruleus with consequent loss of inhibitory input to the hippocampal cells because when the locus coeruleus was stimulated electrically its' ability to inhibit the hippocampal cells was unaffected (Huang 1979). It is unfortunate that these authors did not measure β-adrenoceptor binding in the hippocampus because down-regulation of these receptors is known to be of slower onset in this structure than in the cortex but iontophoretic studies have not demonstrated a change in the responsiveness of hippocampal pyramidal cells to NA in rats which received chronic administration of various antidepressants.

Woodward and his colleagues (Woodward et al. 1979; Yeh & Woodward 1983) have shown how β-adrenoceptor modulation of the activity of other transmitter systems may itself be modified by antidepressant treatment. They showed that iontophoretic application of NA to cerebellar Purkinje cells reduced their firing rate but did not affect the response of the cells to activation of their conventional inputs (i.e. excitatory amino acid inputs from mossy and climbing fibres and inhibitory GABAergic inputs from basket cells). Chronic administration of desipramine reduced the sensitivity of the Purkinje cells to NA and diminished the ability of NA to enhance the inhibitory responses to GABA; sensitivity of the cells to GABA alone was unaffected by desipramine.

Pineal gland

The pineal gland receives a noradrenergic innervation from postganglionic sympathetic fibres whose cell bodies lie in the superior cervical ganglion. Stimulation of the nervous supply causes melatonin (N-acetyl-5-methoxytryptamine) to be synthesised and released, an effect mediated by β_1-adrenoceptor activation and cyclic AMP production. This production of melatonin displays a diurnal rhythm being maximal during the dark. In rats, the night-time rise in melatonin was reduced by chronic treatment with desipramine and imipramine, an effect associated with reduced pineal β-adrenoceptors (Heydorn *et al.* 1982; Friedman *et al.* 1984), which demonstrates that NA uptake inhibition is unable to offset the consequences of the reduced receptor numbers. Maprotiline and amitriptyline given to rats daily for periods of at least 10 days reduced the increase in pineal melatonin content in response to incubation with isoprenaline *in vitro* but the atypical antidepressants, mianserin and iprindole and the selective 5-HT uptake inhibitor, fluoxetine were without effect (Cowen *et al.* 1983). The lack of effect of iprindole could be because a minimum of 4 weeks daily treatment is required for it to effect down-regulation of β-adrenoceptors (Friedman *et al.* 1984).

Effects of antidepressants on alpha$_2$-adrenoceptors

Interest in the effects of antidepressants on α_2-adrenoceptors stemmed from the observation that mianserin was an antagonist at these receptors. Blockade of presynaptic α_2-adrenoceptors by mianserin would be expected to increase release of NA into the synapse and hence increase noradrenergic neurotransmission. Presynaptic α_2-adrenoceptors located on the cell bodies and dendrites (soma-dendritic receptors) modulate the firing frequency of the neurons whereas those located in the terminal region attenuate NA release. Many α_2-adrenoceptors, however, appear to be located postsynaptically (see Chapter 7).

Receptor binding studies

Alpha$_2$-adrenoceptors have been labelled using both agonist ([³H]-clonidine) and antagonist ([³H]-yohimbine, [³H]-rauwolscine) radioligands. The number of binding sites identified by agonist radioligands is substantially less (about 50%) than that for antagonist ligands, since only those α_2-adrenoceptors linked to the inhibitory guanine nucleotide binding protein (Gi) are labelled by agonists at high affinity. Debate continues as to which is the better ligand for assessment of functional α_2-adrenoceptors. At first inspection, it would seem that the agonist sites represent those most intimately associated with adenylate cyclase, the major second messenger of this receptor. However, the association between receptor and nucleotide binding protein is a labile one, highly sensitive to changes in the concentration of guanine nucleotides and both divalent and monovalent cations. Hence minor changes in these factors within the tissue may have major effects on the apparent receptor density as estimated by agonist radioligands. Furthermore, the current concept of the receptor-adenylate cyclase system envisages free association between the component proteins (receptors, nucleotide binding protein and adenylate cyclase) within the membrane in which all the receptors may have a functional role. In such a case, an estimate of the total α_2-adrenoceptor population, as indicated by antagonist radioligands, may serve as a better guide to potential receptor function.

In view of the above, it is not surprising that estimations of the effects of chronic antidepressant treatments on α_2-adrenoceptor populations have produced conflicting results. Sugrue (1982) found chronic administration of the monoamine oxidase inhibitor, pargyline to reduce [^{3}H]-clonidine binding whereas repeated administration of several other antidepressants which included desipramine, imipramine, amitriptyline, mianserin and electroconvulsive shocks, were without effect in the rat. In contrast, decreased [^{3}H]-clonidine binding was reported in the rat cortex after imipramine (Campbell & McKernan 1982), in the rat limbic system after amitriptyline (Smith et al. 1981) and in several brain regions following electroconvulsive shock (Stanford & Nutt 1982).

Functional studies

Noradrenaline turnover

At low doses clonidine preferentially stimulates α_2-adrenoceptors thereby reducing NA release and hence NA turnover. Turnover was estimated by Sugrue (1981) from the brain concentration of MOPEG. Out of five antidepressants given to rats twice daily for 14 days, only desipramine attenuated the response to clonidine. It was concluded that production of presynaptic α_2-adrenoceptor subsensitivity was not a common action of antidepressants.

Behavioural

In rats and mice low doses of clonidine produce a behavioural syndrome consisting of sedation, reduced locomotor activity and hypothermia. These effects are attenuated by chronic administration of antidepressant drugs suggesting the development of α_2-adrenoceptor subsensitivity by antidepressant treatment. However, single doses of desipramine have also been reported to slightly reduce the sedation and reduction in motor activity produced by clonidine. This is of interest because Pelayo et al. (1980) have shown that desipramine directly antagonises the actions of clonidine at presynaptic α_2-adrenoceptors but not the actions of α-methylnoradrenaline at the same receptors.

Electrophysiological

Local iontophoretic application of NA or clonidine or systemic administration of clonidine slows the spontaneous firing rate of neurons in the locus coeruleus whereas administration of yohimbine has the opposite effect. The fact that yohimbine alone increases the neuronal firing rate is evidence that the nucleus is under tonic inhibitory noradrenergic control, presumably from recurrent collaterals arising from the locus coeruleus neurons themselves. Acute administration of desipramine mimics the effect of locally applied NA presumably by increasing the synaptic concentration as a result of amine uptake inhibition. The response to desipramine is markedly attenuated in animals which have been given repeated daily injections of the antidepressant; the response to clonidine is also similarly attenuated. However, this ability of desipramine (and of imipramine) to render presynaptic α_2-adrenoceptors subsensitive is not shared by clomipramine demonstrating that it is not a common property even of tricyclic antidepressants.

Effects of antidepressants on alpha$_1$-adrenoceptors

Receptor binding studies

Chronic antidepressant treatment has failed to show any consistent changes on α_1-adrenoceptor binding of rat brain homogenates. This is surprising in view of the fact that many antidepressants are α_1 antagonists, particularly doxepin, trimipramine, amitriptyline and mianserin, and might therefore have been expected to increase the number of α_1-adrenoceptor binding sites. The general lack of effect could be attributed to problems resulting from the use of an antagonist ligand, usually [^{3}H]-WB 4101, whose selectivity has been questioned.

Functional studies

Behavioural

These have been limited by the poor penetration of available α_1-adrenoceptor agonists into the brain. Large doses of clonidine produce increased locomotor activity in rats, an effect blocked by α_1-adrenoceptor antagonists, unaffected by reserpine pretreatment and mimicked by intraventricular injection of phenylephrine, an α_1-adrenoceptor agonist. Maj and his co-workers (Maj *et al.* 1979) have shown that chronic, but not acute administration of mianserin or a tricyclic antidepressant enhanced the stimulant effects of clonidine; clonidine-induced aggression in mice was also potentiated by chronic administration of various antidepressants. The recent introduction of selective α_1-adrenoceptor agonists .such as St 785, an imidazolidine which readily penetrates to the brain, will facilitate the direct confirmation of this enhanced α_1-adrenoceptor sensitivity by various antidepressants.

Electrophysiological

The dorsal lateral geniculate nucleus in the thalamus receives an excitatory input from the locus coeruleus and iontophoretic application of NA also increases the firing rate of its neurons, an effect blocked by α_1-adrenoceptor antagonists. The excitatory responses to NA were enhanced after repeated daily administration of desipramine, imipramine, clomipramine, amitriptyline and iprindole (Menkes & Aghajanian 1981). This enchancement could not be attributed solely to inhibition of NA uptake because iprindole only weakly inhibits this process and responses to the iontophoretic application of phenylephrine, which is a poor substrate for uptake, were also potentiated. Neurons of the rat facial motor nucleus are quiescent in anaesthetised animals unless excited by afferent inputs or local application of glutamate. Simultaneous iontophoresis of NA augments this activity through α_1-adrenoceptors, and this was enhanced in rats pretreated with one of several antidepressants for 14–20 days (Menkes *et al.* 1980). The antidepressants which were active in this respect were desipramine, imipramine, amitriptyline and iprindole; the selective 5-HT uptake inhibitor, fluoxetine was without effect.

Thus despite any consistent effect of repeated administration of antidepressants on α_1-adrenoceptor binding, behavioural and electrophysiological experiments indicate that responses mediated by these receptors are enhanced.

Effects of antidepressants on 5-HT receptors

Antidepressants display a wide spectrum of acute effects on serotonergic mechanisms ranging from drugs such as citalopram, a potent and selective 5-HT uptake inhibitor devoid of affinity for the 5-HT receptor, to mianserin which is a potent 5-HT antagonist without 5-HT uptake blocking properties. The majority of the tricyclic antidepressants, particularly the tertiary amines, inhibit 5-HT reuptake but also behave as classical 5-HT antagonists in certain test systems. Attempts to obtain a consistent picture of antidepressant action on central serotonergic mechanisms have been aided by descriptions of 5-HT receptor subtypes e.g. 5-HT_{1A}, 5-HT_2, 5-HT_3 although the classification remains far from established (see Chapter 8 below).

Receptor binding studies

5-HT_2-receptors

A range of antidepressants down-regulate the number of 5-HT_2 receptors in rat cortex after repeated daily administration for at least 3–4 weeks.

They include tricyclic antidepressants such as imipramine, desipramine and amitriptyline, atypical antidepressants like iprindole, mianserin and trazodone and several MAO inhibitors (pargyline, tranylcypromine etc). The down-regulation observed after the 5-HT_2 antagonist mianserin is of interest not only because chronic administration of an antagonist usually leads to an increase in receptor numbers but also because the effect, albeit slightly smaller, is also seen 48 hours after a single injection of mianserin (Blackshear & Sanders-Bush 1982). Also puzzling is the finding that highly selective 5-HT uptake inhibitors such as citalopram and fluoxetine do not decrease cortical 5-HT_2 receptor numbers after their repeated administration to rats. Perhaps the degree of postsynaptic receptor stimulation by these drugs is limited by presynaptic control whereas tricyclic antidepressants antagonise the presynaptic autoreceptors.

Onset of 5-HT_2-receptor down-regulation has been achieved within 3 hours by administering a 5-HT uptake inhibitor together with a monoamine oxidase inhibitor, presumably by virtue of their different actions on serotonergic mechanisms (Koshikawa *et al.* 1985) and within 4 days by administering phenoxybenzamine with trazodone (Taylor *et al.* 1981). The mechanism for this last interaction is uncertain but Green and Nutt (1983) have suggested it may be due to induced β-adrenoceptor downregulation hastening the onset of a similar effect on 5-HT_2-receptor numbers.

The relevance of 5-HT_2 receptor down-regulation to the therapeutic action of tricyclic antidepressants, already in doubt because of the acute blocking effect of mianserin at these receptors and the lack of effect of the selective 5-HT uptake inhibitors on these receptor populations, is made more doubtful by the observation that repeated electroconvulsive shocks increase the density of [^{3}H]-spiperone binding.

5-HT_1 receptors

Effects of chronic antidepressant administration on 5-HT_1 receptor numbers in rat brain are conflicting. Down-regulation of 5-HT_1 receptors in rat forebrain has been most consistently obtained after chronic administration of non-selective MAO inhibitors and after the selective MAO-A inhibitor, clorgyline. The selective MAO-B inhibitor, selegeline was without effect. Desipramine has been reported to down-regulate the number of 5-HT_1 binding sites but in the majority of studies it has been found to be without effect as have other tricyclic antidepressants, selective 5-HT uptake inhibitors and electroconvulsive shocks.

Functional studies

Behavioural

Interpretation of the effects of tricyclic antidepressant administration on behaviours evoked by 5-HT agonists is complicated by their antagonistic activity at these receptors. For example, head twitches (i.e. 5-HT_2 mediated effect) evoked in mice by 5-methoxydimethyl-tryptamine (5-MeODMT) were equally attenuated irrespective of whether the 5-HT agonist was given 1 hour after a single injection of either imipramine or amitriptyline or 1 hour after the last of 28 daily injections. However, when the interval between injection of the antidepressant and of 5-MeODMT was increased to 48 hours, head twitches were significantly more frequent in the mice which had received repeated antidepressant injections. This ability to antagonise 5-MeODMT-evoked head twitches was not shared by desipramine and iprindole, two antidepressants devoid of 5-HT receptor blocking activity (Friedman *et al.* 1983). The gradual emergence of an enhanced 5-HT response over 48 hours after ceasing antidepressant administration is consistent with the direct antagonistic effects of amitriptyline and imipramine being responsible for the initial attenuation of the effects of 5-MeODMT but it must be remembered that clinically, the therapeutic response is obtained during continued antidepressant therapy. Enhanced responses to 5-HT receptor agonists have also been obtained after repeated electroconvulsive shocks. In contrast to these results, the ability of zimelidine, a selective 5-HT uptake inhibitor, to enhance prolactin and growth hormone secretion in rats was lost after its chronic administration and the number of head twitches evoked in mice by 5-HTP and 5-MeODMT given 24 hours after the last injection of zimelidine was also reduced.

Electrophysiological

Aghajanian (1981) identified three types of 5-HT receptor, S_1, S_2, S_3 on the basis of unit responses to 5-HT agonists and antagonists. This classification differs from the accepted $5\text{-HT}_1/5\text{-HT}_2/5\text{-HT}_3$ scheme derived from radioligand binding and behavioural studies. S_1 receptors were characterised on neurons of the facial motor nucleus and their activation facilitated the depolarising action of excitatory amino acids (like 5-HT_2 receptors). Sensitivity of these receptors to iontophoretic application of 5-HT was enhanced after chronic administration of several tricyclic antidepressants but not after the selective 5-HT uptake inhibitor, fluoxetine. That this enhancement was not simply due to amine uptake inhibition was also shown by the finding of enhanced responses to 5-MeODMT which is not taken up into presynaptic terminals (Menkes *et al.* 1980).

Stimulation of S_2 receptors caused a decrease in the firing rate of the raphé nuclei and the receptors were therefore presumed to be presynaptic autoreceptors (like 5-HT_{1A} receptors). There is a good correlation between the 5-HT uptake blocking activities of tricyclic antidepressants and their abilities to reduce the firing rate of the raphé nuclei upon acute administration. However, after repeated daily administration of antidepressants the firing rate returns to normal and it has been shown that this is due to S_2 receptor subsensitivity (de Montigny & Blier 1984).

The third receptor S_3, is associated with inhibition of non-5-HT neurons in the ventral lateral geniculate nucleus and dorsal hippocampus of the rat. Sensitivity of these receptors to 5-HT was enhanced by chronic administration of various tricyclic antidepressants, by mianserin and by repeated electroconvulsive shocks. Several selective 5-HT uptake inhibitors (fluoxetine, zimelidine, citalopram, etc.) did not alter S_3 receptor sensitivity (de Montigny *et al.* 1984 for references).

Effects of antidepressants at GABA receptors

Recently, several types of antidepressant (amitriptyline, desipramine, citalopram, pargyline and viloxazine) have been shown to increase the density of $GABA_B$ receptor binding sites in rat frontal cortex after chronic administration (Pilc & Lloyd 1984). It is too soon to evaluate the significance of these findings, particularly since there is a report of $GABA_B$ receptors in the whole cortex being unaffected by chronic administration of desipramine and zimelidine to rats (Cross & Horton 1986), but it is of interest because the effect is exhibited by widely different antidepressants. The description of $GABA_B$ receptors on noradrenergic nerve terminals may provide a link between these findings and those on noradrenergic mechanisms.

Antidepressant binding sites

High affinity binding sites for [^{3}H]-imipramine have been described in both rat and human brain and in human platelets. Surprisingly, such binding is displaced with high affinity by a range of tricyclic antidepressants which inhibit 5-HT reuptake but less readily by the selective 5-HT uptake inhibitors such as paroxetine. Because the ability of tricyclic antidepressants to displace [^{3}H]-imipramine binding is closely correlated with their ability to inhibit 5-HT uptake, it is presumed that the imipramine binding site is intimately associated with the 5-HT uptake mechanism. High affinity binding sites to [^{3}H]-desipramine have also been described and appear to be associated with the uptake mechanism for NA. As is to be expected from their presynaptic location, the densities of the [^{3}H]-imipramine and [^{3}H]-desipramine binding sites in rat brain are decreased by selective lesions of serotonergic and noradrenergic pathways respectively.

The majority of studies report [^{3}H]-imipramine binding to be decreased in platelets from untreated depressives as compared with platelets from a matched population of normal subjects. The studies performed during antidepressant treatment and following recovery from depression are not so consistent in their findings probably because of a residual antidepressant effect. Nevertheless the results from euthymic patients in which a long interval was allowed to elapse between cessation of antidepressant treatment and the receptor assay, indicate a normalisation of [^{3}H]-imipramine binding sites. This suggests that lowered [^{3}H]-imipramine binding may be a state-dependent, rather than a trait-dependent marker.

Lithium

Cade (1970) describes how, in an attempt to determine the factor responsible for the greater toxicity in guinea pigs of intraperitoneal injections of urine from manic patients than of urine from normals, depressives and schizophrenics, he noted that uric acid potentiated the toxicity of urea. A practical difficulty in studying this phenomenon was the comparative insolubility of uric acid and therefore he used the most soluble urate, lithium urate. Unexpectedly, lithium urate exerted a protective effect against urea and when given alone to guinea pigs it diminished their responsiveness to external stimuli. Because lithium salts had been widely used for the treatment of gout (lithium urate) and as an hypnotic (lithium bromide) there were no ethical considerations to prevent their immediate use in manic patients. Lithium carbonate and citrate were found to be effective and although this is now widely recognised, there was a delay of several years between the first report of the anti-manic properties of lithium by Cade in 1949 and general clinical acceptance. This was due largely to concern about the toxicity of lithium as identified in earlier studies, a factor which is still important today but which is controlled by monitoring the plasma lithium concentration of patients during treatment.

The biochemical mechanisms underlying the anti-manic effect of lithium are not yet understood. Like antidepressants, there is a delay of 2 to 3 weeks between starting treatment and any clinical improvement. Consequently the biochemical studies of lithium in animals have concentrated on the effects of chronic, rather than acute, treatment. Since mania represents the opposite end of the affect scale to depression, the monoamine hypotheses proposed that mania should be associated with elevated monoamine activity and hence lithium might be expected to reduce the effectiveness of monoamine systems. Indeed early studies showed that lithium given to rats for 2 days increased the turnover and intraneuronal metabolism of NA and to a lesser extent 5-HT. However, treatment for longer periods (2 to 4 weeks) resulted in a normalisation of monoamine turnover.

Contrary to expectation, recent results suggest that lithium causes similar, rather than opposite, changes to those obtained following classical antidepressant treatment. Hence in the rat, chronic lithium treatment decreased the number of β-adrenoceptors and increased the number of α_1-adrenoceptors, as identified by radioligand binding studies, although in some cases these changes did not reach statistical significance. No effect was observed on DA receptors. More important was the ability of lithium to attenuate the receptor response to administration of a second drug. In particular, lithium abolished the supersensitivity response of both β- and α_1-adrenoceptors after treatment of rats with 6-hydroxydopamine and of DA receptors following chronic haloperidol. These effects were reinforced by parallel changes in post-receptor events, such as NA-stimulated adenylate cyclase activity in the former case and apomorphine-induced behavioural changes in the latter.

Independent of its anti-manic effects, lithium is widely used by biochemists studying the phosphatidylinositol second messenger system where it potently inhibits inositol-1-phosphatase, the enzyme which dephosphorylates inositol-1-phosphate to yield inositol. This second messenger system is closely associated with the α_1-adrenoceptor and 5-HT$_2$ receptor, among others. It is possible therefore, that lithium treatment may lower the brain free inositol concentration so that it becomes rate-limiting. Under these circumstances, activity of the inositol-polyphosphate second messenger systems of the brain would be reduced. However, supporting evidence from animal studies of such an effect is not yet available.

The mechanism of lithium's therapeutic action is therefore at present unclear. It must in part be attributed to its ability to mimic to varying degrees, other important cellular cations such as Na^+, K^+, Mg^{2+}, and Ca^{2+}. Given alone, it reduces the responsiveness of many biological systems, e.g. cation transport mechanisms such as Na/K-ATPase. Drug interaction studies consistently demonstrate the ability of lithium to attenuate responses to other drugs. It is possible that the simultaneous attenuation of many diverse biochemical reactions within the brain may represent the true therapeutic mechanism of action of lithium. Such a mechanism would then be evident at the cellular level as a moderation of numerous drug or time-induced biochemical effects and at the clinical level as a damping of the extreme swings in mood between mania and depression (see Knapp 1983). In such an event, it would be futile to search for a specific neurotransmitter system as the key to the biochemical mechanism of action of lithium.

Clinical markers for depression and antidepressant drug action

The development of reliable biochemical markers for depression in man is a major goal. Even with the use of diagnostic criteria and rating scales, at present the assessment of depression relies on the clinical acumen of the psychiatrist. The existence of dependable biochemical tests for depression would aid the psychiatrist in his diagnosis and may also lead to an understanding of the biochemical changes which induce the condition or may bring about its resolution.

The biochemical changes studied in animals, as discussed above, cannot be easily applied to extant human tissue, especially the brain. However, investigations in man do obviate the problem of species differences and the results of biochemical tests in man can be related to the state of the patients' illness, so permitting the identification of state-dependent markers which are not feasible in animal models. Also, the biochemical consequences of antidepressant drugs can be compared with the therapeutic effectiveness of the drugs in man. This may be particularly important if, as indicated by some studies (Braddock *et al.* 1986), the effects of such drugs are different in depressed patients compared with euthymic controls. By contrast the biochemical effect of antidepressants in animals are generally investigated in naive 'non-depressed' animals.

As the analysis of monoamine neurotransmitters and their metabolites in various body fluids has not revealed any consistent defect associated with depression, recent studies have concentrated more on their receptors. One notable exception to this approach however, is the dexamethasone suppression test.

Human receptor studies

As outlined above, the use of radioligand binding and second messenger studies in animal models has identified a number of receptor changes consequent upon chronic antidepressant treatment. Attempts to carry out similar studies in man are limited by the ethical constraints of obtaining tissue, therefore most such work has concentrated on circulating cells which can be easily obtained from blood samples.

The lymphocyte possesses a functional β_2-adrenoceptor positively linked to adenylate cyclase. Mann *et al.* (1985) reported that the activity of isoprenaline-stimulated adenylate cyclase in these cells was reduced in endogenous depressed patients compared with healthy controls without any change in β-adrenoceptor number. However, when the patients were divided into psychomotor agitated and retarded groups only the agitated patients had significantly reduced receptor function, suggesting that the decrease in enzyme activity corresponded more closely with activity level than depression. Circulating catecholamines, glucocorticoids, sex hormones and drugs have been shown to affect lymphocyte β-adrenoceptor numbers. Wright *et al.* (1984) attempted to eliminate these influences by virally transforming lymphocytes into lymphoblastoid cells which could then be passaged for several generations. Utilising this approach, they demonstrated substantially decreased numbers of β-adrenoceptors in lymphoblastoid cell-lines derived from 4 out of 6 manic-depressive patients compared with only 1 out of 18 cell-lines derived from familial euthymic controls. This is particularly interesting in view of the hereditary nature of manic depression and may indicate a genetic susceptibility in affected patients associated with a defect in the β-adrenoceptor.

However, more recent studies have not found β-adrenoceptor numbers of lymphocytes from depressives to be different from those from euthymic controls.

These findings are difficult to correlate with the animal data, which indicated that antidepressant drug treatment itself induced a decrease in β-adrenoceptor function. The difference may be due to the tissues studied or to the fact that in rat brain, the β-adrenoceptor is predominantly of the β_1-type whereas on the lymphocyte it is β_2. Some recent post-mortem brain studies support the hypothesis that β-adrenoceptor numbers are increased in suicidal depressive subjects although other studies report a difference in receptor number compared to control subjects. Indeed the relevance of β-adrenoceptor changes in man to antidepressant treatment has been seriously questioned (Willner 1984).

The platelet demonstrates several of the characteristics of the serotonergic nerve terminal in respect of a specific, high-affinity, sodium-dependent uptake mechanism for 5-HT, vesicular storage of 5-HT and exocytotic release following stimulation (Pletscher 1978). Identification of a specific binding site for [^{3}H]-imipramine on platelets associated with the 5-HT uptake system was followed by reports of a decreased number of such sites in depressed patients compared with euthymic controls (Briley et al. 1980). This difference has been confirmed by a number of independent groups although some negative studies have also been reported (Elliott 1984). This decrease in binding appears to be normalised following treatment and clinical remission of the depression, although the binding change is delayed by some weeks or months following successful treatment. A similar decrease in [^{3}H]-imipramine binding has been reported in post-mortem brain studies of depressed patients although this has also been challenged (Stanley et al. 1982; Owen et al. 1986). Clearly some form of communication must occur between the brain as the 'source' of the depression and the platelet. The most likely candidate is a circulating factor such as a hormone or an agent which at present remains undetected. One suggested possibility is an endogenous imipramine-like compound.

The platelet also exhibits an α_2-adrenoceptor which closely resembles that characterised in human brain tissue (Cheung et al. 1982). Labelling of this receptor by selective α_2-adrenoceptor antagonists demonstrates no significant difference in receptor number between depressive and euthymic subjects (Elliott 1984). Using the partial agonist ligand [^{3}H]-clonidine, however, several groups have reported increased numbers of high-affinity receptors in depressed patients which are normalised following treatment with antidepressants (Garcia-Sevilla et al. 1981; Siever et al. 1984). The complications introduced by the ability of [^{3}H]-clonidine to bind to two sites makes accurate determination of the binding capacities at each site rather difficult. Further studies will be needed to determine whether these investigations reflect a true difference in the binding characteristics of agonist and antagonist ligands in depressed patients.

Neuroendocrine challenge tests

In addition to *ex vivo* receptor studies described above, attempts to measure *in vivo* receptor function have been based on the principle that stimulation of specific central neurotransmitter receptors regulates the release of specific hormones. Assay of the circulating concentration of one such hormone may then act as an indirect measure of central receptor function. The release of several hormones from the anterior pituitary is regulated by nuclei within the hypothalamus whose activity in turn is modified by the action of classical neurotransmitters. Hence growth hormone release can be stimulated by clonidine (acting at α_2-adrenoceptors), apomorphine (DA receptors) or tryptophan (5-HT precursor acting via 5-HT receptors). Assay of the change in hormone level in response to a fixed dose of a suitable challenge drug in depressed compared with euthymic subjects can then be used as an indirect assessment of the sensitivity of that particular receptor.

Using such a protocol, Heninger *et al.* (1984) reported that the increase in plasma prolactin following tryptophan infusion was significantly lower in depressed patients than euthymic controls. Following chronic treatment with antidepressants this response to tryptophan was increased in both depressed and euthymic subjects (Charney *et al.* 1984). This suggests that 5-HT sensitivity within the hypothalamus is reduced in depression and enhanced by chronic treatment with antidepressant drugs.

Similarly, clonidine stimulation of growth hormone release is reported to be weaker in depressed patients than in euthymic controls (Checkley *et al.* 1981), suggesting that depression may also be associated with reduced sensitivity of central α_2-adrenoceptors.

Extrapolation of such results should be tempered by the possibility that hypothalamic changes may not be related to a primary biochemical lesion in depression. In fact, because the release of some pituitary hormones is regulated by a series of hypothalamic interneurons, a deficit in any one interneuronal link will result in a diminished response to all receptors upstream of that deficit. Nevertheless, it is of particular interest that the recent clinical studies reinforce the original monoamine hypotheses that the functional activity of the monoamines appears to be diminished in depression.

Dexamethasone suppression test

Cortisol, which is the predominant corticosteroid in man, shows a clear circadian rhythm with peak plasma concentrations occurring during late morning and the nadir at around midnight (Fig. 19.8). The release of cortisol from the adrenal cortex is regulated by a well characterised negative feedback control mechanism directed by nuclei within the hypothalamus which are sensitive to circulating corticosteroids. Conse-

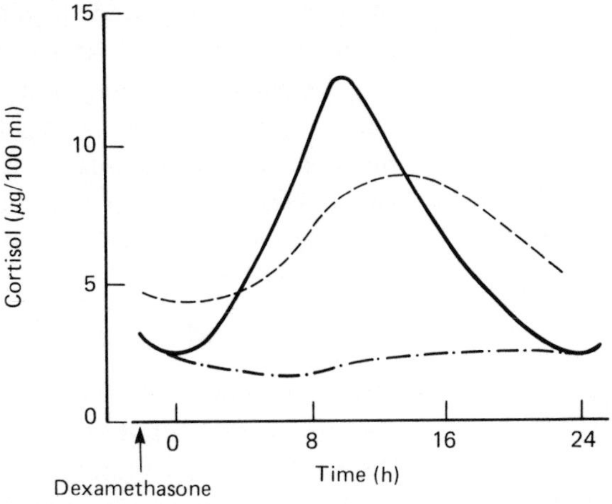

Fig. 19.8. The diurnal rhythm in plasma cortisol secretion in a control subject (solid line) may be suppressed by dexamethasone, 1 mg given orally (— · — · —). The dashed line indicates persistence of cortisol secretion after dexamethasone in a DST positive (non-suppressor) depressed patient (-----).

quently, administration of an exogenous corticosteroid, such as dexamethasone, will inhibit cortisol release from the adrenal by feedback within the hypothalamus. If the dexamethasone is administered in sufficient dose at a time when plasma cortisol is near its minimum (i.e. late evening) then the feedback mechanism will cancel the natural surge in cortisol release that normally occurs after midnight. Hence plasma cortisol concentrations will be much lower than normal when measured later next morning.

In depressed patients, particularly of the endogenous type, there is frequently a hypersecretion of cortisol throughout the day but this effect is not specific for depression. What is found in a substantial proportion of depressives however, is that dexamethasone fails to inhibit the morning rise in plasma cortisol. This effect was refined and characterised by Carroll (1982) as the dexamethasone suppression test (DST). Routinely 1 mg dexamethasone is administered orally to subjects at approximately 22.00 hours and a blood sample taken at 08.00 hours the next morning. If the plasma cortisol is less than 5 μg/100 ml then it is concluded that the natural rise has been successfully suppressed and the subject rates as negative on the DST. In contrast, the subject is said to be DST positive if the plasma cortisol exceeds 5 μg/100 ml.

Initial studies by Carroll (1982) claimed high sensitivity and selectivity for the DST in identifying depressed patients, with approximately 50% depressed patients being DST positive but only 2% of euthymic controls. However, these figures have been questioned by other studies which have reported a less clear distinction between depressed and non-depressed subjects (Hirschfeld *et al.* 1983; Green & Kane 1983).

Although the DST clearly cannot act as a diagnostic test for depression, there does appear to be a significantly higher incidence of DST positives among depressed patients than euthymic subjects. However, the assumption that any one test will be valid for distinguishing all forms of depression may itself be untenable. Given our present understanding of the biochemical mechanisms of the brain, the collectivisation of depression as a single psychopathology may eventually prove as naive as the attempts of physicians two hundred years ago to treat chest-pain in a homogeneous manner. The power of the DST may in fact reside in its ability to characterise a subset of depressed patients for whom a specific biochemical test is available. It remains to be demonstrated however, that this marker is consistent for a particular condition or patient group and that some unifying defect underlies this abnormal response.

Overview and discussion

Dissatisfaction with the original monoamine deficiency hypotheses of depression prompted both clinicians and basic scientists to investigate the chronic rather than the acute effects of antidepressant treatments in their respective experimental models. This approach was initiated by Sulser and his colleagues in an attempt to find a common action for an established tricyclic antidepressant, desipramine and a then novel antidepressant, iprindole, which did not appear to affect monoaminergic mechanisms upon acute administration to rats. Investigation of the chronic effects of antidepressant administration has been of immense value and has produced what is currently the most consistent hypothesis of antidepressant drug action, namely that this is attributable to subsensitivity of central β-adrenoceptor function. It then follows that depression may be due to an enhanced responsiveness of these noradrenergic systems, a hypothesis which is diametrically opposed to the original catecholamine hypothesis of depression. The new hypothesis immediately raises the question, why are lipophilic β-adrenoceptor blocking agents such as propranolol and metoprolol, which readily cross the blood brain barrier, not effective antidepressants? In fact, it is β-adrenoceptor agonists such as salbutamol and clenbuterol which are currently being tested as potential antidepressants.

The hypothesis that antidepressant action is attributable to β-adrenoceptor down-regulation derives from experiments carried out in normal healthy rats for extrapolation to depressed man. There is already evidence of species differences among laboratory animals in the ease with which β-adrenoceptors down-regulate and therefore differences must also be expected to occur between rats and man. Further, there is no known locus for the therapeutic action of antidepressants. In rats, regional variations in receptor distributions have dictated which areas of the brain have been used for biochemical and electrophysiological investigations while in man, neuroendocrine challenge tests provide the only direct access to central receptors and the neurotransmitter control of hormone secretion from the pituitary is recognised as being particularly complex. Other clinical studies have utilised the secretion of melatonin by the pineal gland, a β-adrenoceptor mediated response, and measurements of monoamine metabolites and of receptors on circlating platelets and lymphocytes.

A declared aim of many chronic animal studies has been to search for a common action of antidepressants at the receptor level. This represents an oversimplification. First, it assumes that depression itself is either a homogeneous condition or that it is a heterogenous disorder but responsive to a common treatment. Although some psychiatrists envisage all forms of depression as lying on a continuum, there are strong therapeutic reasons for attempting to identify subtypes within the reactive/endogenous, neurotic/psychotic or unipolar/bipolar divisions of the affective disorders. Benefits would include the possibility of better diagnosis by the use of different genetic and neurochemical markers and the tailoring of drug therapy to the particular subtype. Second, why should all antidepressants act by a common mechanism? — not all antihypertensives do. However, the other extreme that each antidepressants acts by a different mechanism is equally untenable.

It is also simplistic to consider changes in only one transmitter system and to ignore interactions between transmitter systems. For example, enhancement of the locomotor responses of mice to both selective DA and 5-HT receptor agonists (apomorphine and quipazine respectively) by repeated electroconvulsive shocks were prevented by previous lesions of just the ascending noradrenergic pathways with 6-hydroxydopamine. The reduction in β-adrenoceptor numbers produced by chronic administration of desipramine to rats was shown to be dependent on serotonergic mechanisms and could be prevented by previous lesioning of 5-HT pathways with 5,7-dihydroxytryptamine (Green & Deakin 1980).

How therefore, do antidepressants act? Do they increase noradrenergic neurotransmission as might be expected from NA uptake inhibition, α_2-adrenoceptor subsensitivity and increased α_1-adrenoceptor responsiveness or do they attenuate noradrenergic transmission by virtue of reduced β-adrenoceptor numbers?

There are of course complex interactions among central putative neurotransmitter and neuromodulatory systems and examples of how a change in the function of one can effect changes in another have been given. Unfortunately, there is no specific behavioural model of central β-adrenoceptor function but the elegant electrophysiological experiments of Woodward and his colleagues (p. 372) demonstrate how β-adrenoceptor activation can alter neuronal responsiveness to other transmitters. In their studies, desipramine-induced β-adrenoceptor down-regulation diminished the ability of NA to enhance inhibitory responses of cerebellar Purkinje cells to GABA. In contrast in another example described above, the responsiveness of rats to 5-HT and DA agonists was enhanced by electroshock-induced subsensitivity of central β-adrenoceptors.

The up-regulation of $GABA_B$ receptors, if it can be confirmed, may also prove to be of considerable importance. It has been shown that local GABAergic neurons may control the functioning of many neuronal circuits. One of the best studied examples is of the cat's lateral geniculate nucleus in which it has been postulated that GABAergic interneurons gate (i.e. control) the flow of visual information from the retina into geniculate X-cells (Koch 1985). The ubiquitous nature of the GABA receptors suggests that such control mechanisms are commonplace in the CNS and that alterations in GABAergic function could be involved in both the behavioural disturbances associated with the affective disorders and in their alleviation by antidepressants.

The concept that a neuron releases only one transmitter has been shown to be no longer valid by the demonstration of the coexistence of classical amine transmitters with neuropeptides in the same neuron, e.g. 5-HT with substance P. It is too soon to assess the relevance of this to antidepressant drug action but it is expected to be of considerable importance although some peptides, e.g. TRH and ACTH, are already suspected of possessing antidepressant activity. Chronic administration of desipramine to rats has been shown to reduce cortical opiate receptor binding as well as enhance cortical neuron responsiveness.

In the absence of satisfactory animal models of depression, description of a novel drug as an antidepressant must await clinical verification. This is not easy. Depression is an episodic, recurrent illness with periods of spontaneous remission, the cyclical nature of the illness contributing to the high placebo response usually observed during the course of a clinical trial (Fig. 19.9). Other contributing factors are the psychotherapeutic effects of the increased attention given to the patient from the medical and nursing staff and both their, and the patient's, expectations and hope for improvement. For these, and other reasons, double-blind placebo-controlled trials are essential to establish the efficacy of new antidepressants. Inevitably however, the very ill and those patients considered to be a high suicide risk tend to be systematically excluded from these trials

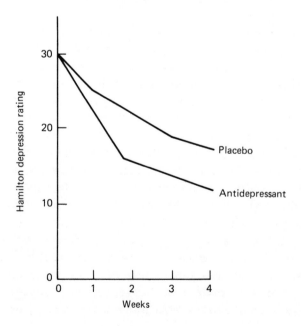

Fig. 19.9. Characteristic time courses of clinical improvement to placebo and to an effective antidepressant in depressed patients.

and therefore those participating may not be representative of all patient groups. It is also important that the number of patients participating in clinical trials, particularly if an established antidepressant is to be compared against a new drug, is sufficiently large to avoid a Type 2 error (i.e. a false negative). Unfortunately, this is often not the case and the evaluation of new antidepressants takes many years to complete. For instance, publications on iprindole first appeared in 1965. Fourteen years later in 1979, Zis and Goodwin claimed that its superiority over placebo had not been established and this is probably still true in 1986. Yet this drug has been used as a standard atypical antidepressant in many chronic animal studies and indeed was partly responsible for the questioning of the original catecholamine hypothesis of depression. Evidence is now accumulating which suggests that some of the atypical antidepressants (e.g. mianserin and citalopram) may be less effective than the tricyclic antidepressants and that to obtain the best antidepressant effect it may be necessary to inhibit the uptake of both NA and 5-HT.

It is therefore clear that we are far from understanding how antidepressants work. The situation is more complex than a few years ago when the monoamine deficiency hypothesis of depression appeared to adequately explain their mechanism of action. It is important to realise however, that despite flaws in the arguments which gave rise to the monoamine hypothesis, many of the clinical observations remain valid. As the elaborate and varied therapeutic mechanisms of the antidepressant drugs are gradually elucidated we would not be surprised if the enhancement of monoamine function was found to constitute a crucial preliminary step in the action of at least some antidepressants.

Acknowledgement

The authors thank Dr SA Checkley for helpful comments on the manuscript.

References and further reading

References marked with an asterisk are recommended for further reading and contain extensive reference lists.

Aghajanian GK (1981) The modulatory role of serotonin at multiple receptors in brain. In: Jacobs BL & Gelperin A (eds) *Serotonin, Neurotransmission, and Behaviour*. MIT Press, Cambridge. pp. 156–85.

Asberg M, Traskman L & Thoren P (1976) 5-HIAA in the cerebrospinal fluid — A biochemical suicide predictor. *Arch gen. Psychiat.* 33, 1193–7.

Ashcroft GW, Crawford TBB, Eccleston D, Sharman DF, McDougal EJ, Stanton JS & Binns JK (1966) 5-Hydroxyindole compounds in the cerebrospinal fluid of patients with psychiatric or neurological diseases. *Lancet* ii, 1059–2.

Banerjee SP, Kung LS, Riggi SJ & Chanda SK (1977) Development of beta-adrenergic receptor subsensitivity by antidepressants. *Nature* (Lond.) 268, 455–6.

Beskow J, Gottfries CG, Roos B-E & Winblad B (1976) Determination of monoamines and monoamine metabolites in the human brain: post mortem studies in group of suicides and in a control group. *Acta Psychiat. Scand.* **53**, 7–20.

Blackshear MA & Sanders-Bush E (1982) Serotonin receptor sensitivity after acute and chronic treatment with mianserin. *J. Pharmacol. Exp. Ther.* **221**, 303–8.

Braddock L, Cowen PJ, Elliott JM, Fraser S & Stump K (1986) Binding of yohimbine and imipramine to platelets in depressive illness. *Biol. Psychiat.* (in press).

Briley M, Langer SZ, Raisman R, Sechter D & Zarifian E (1980) Tritiated imipramine binding sites are decreased in platelets of untreated depressed patients. *Science* **209**, 303–5.

Cade JFJ (1980) The story of lithium. In: Ayd FJ & Blackwell B (eds), *Discoveries in Biological Psychiatry.* J B Lippincott, Philadelphia. pp. 218–29.

Campbell IC & McKernan RM (1982) Central and peripheral changes in alpha-receptors in the rat after chronic tricyclic antidepressants. *Br. J. Pharmac.* **75**, 100P.

Carroll BJ (1982) The dexamethasone suppression test for melancholia. *Br. J. Psychiat.* **140**, 292–304.

Charney DS, Heninger GR & Sternberg DE (1984) Serotonin function and mechanism of action of antidepressant treatment: effect of amitriptyline and desipramine. *Arch. Gen. Psychiat.* **41**, 359–64.

*Charney DS, Menkes DB & Heninger GR (1981) Receptor sensitivity and the mechanism of action of antidepressant treatment. *Arch. Gen. Psychiat.* **38**, 1160–80.

Checkley SA, Slade AP & Shur E (1981) Growth hormone and other responses to clonidine in patients with endogenous depression. *Br. J. Psychiat.* **138**, 51–5.

Cheung Y-D, Barnett DB & Nahorski SR (1982) ^{3}H-Rauwolscine and ^{3}H-yohimbine binding to rat cerebral and human platelet membranes — possible heterogeneity of alpha-2 receptors. *Eur. J. Pharmac.* **84**, 79–85.

Clements-Jewry S (1978) The development of cortical beta-adrenoceptor subsensitivity in the rat by chronic treatment with trazodone, doxepin and mianserin. *Neuropharmacology* **17**, 779–81.

*Cooper SJ, Owen F, Chambers DR, Crow TJ, Johnson J & Poulter M (1985) Post-mortem neurochemical findings in suicide and depression: a study of the serotonergic system and imipramine binding in suicide victims. In: Deakin JFW (ed.) *The Biology of Depression.* Gaskell, Oxford. pp. 53–70.

Coppen A (1967) The biochemistry of affective disorders. *Br. J. Psychiat.* **113**, 1237–64.

Cowen PJ, Fraser S, Grahame-Smith DG, Green AR & Stanford C (1983) The effect of chronic antidepressant administration on alpha-adrenoceptor function of the rat pineal. *Br. J. Pharmac.* **78**, 89–96.

Cross JA & Horton RW (1986) Cortical GABA$_B$ is unaltered following chronic oral administration of desmethylimipramine and zimelidine in the rat. *Br. J. Pharmac.* **89**, 521P.

Curzon G, Kantamanini BD, van Boxel P, Gillman PK Bartlett JR & Bridges PK (1980) Substances related to 5-hydroxytryptamine in plasma and in lumbar and ventricular fluids of psychiatric patients. *Acta Psychiat. Scand.* **61**, (Supp. 280), 3–20.

de Montigny C & Blier P (1984) Effects of antidepressant treatments on 5-HT neurotransmission: electrophysiological and clinical studies. *Adv. Biochem. Psychopharmacol.* **39**, 223–39.

Dibner MD & Molinoff PB (1979) Agonist-induced changes in beta adrenergic receptor density and receptor-mediated responsiveness in slices of rat cerebral cortex. *J. Pharmacol. Exp. Ther.* **210**, 433–9.

*Elliott JM (1984) Platelet receptor binding studies in affective disorders. *J. Affect. Disord.* **6**, 219–39.

Ferris RM & Beaman OJ (1983) Bupropion: a new antidepressant drug, the mechanism of action of which is not associated with down-regulation of postsynaptic beta-adrenergic, seotonergic (5-HT$_2$), alpha$_2$-adrenergic, imipramine and dopaminergic receptors in brain. *Neuropharmacology* **22**, 1257–67.

Figge J, Leonard P & Richelson E (1979) Tricyclic antidepressants; potent blockade of histamine H$_1$ receptors of guinea pig ileum. *Eur. J. Pharmacol.* **58**, 479–83.

Friedman E, Cooper TB & Dallob A (1983) Effects of chronic antidepressant treatment on serotonin receptor activity in mice. *Eur. J. Pharmacol.* **89**, 69–76.

Friedman E, Yocca FD & Cooper TB (1984) Antidepressant drugs with varying pharmacological profiles alter rat pineal beta adrenergic-mediated function. *J. Pharmacol. Exp. Ther.* **228**, 545–50.

Gandolfi 0, Barbaccia ML, Chuang DM & Costa E (1983) Daily bupropion injections for 3 weeks attenuates the NE-stimulation of adenylate cyclase and the number of beta-adrenergic recognition sites in rat frontal cortex. *Neuropharmacology* **22**, 927–9.

Garcia-Sevilla JA, Zis AP, Hollingsworth PJ, Greden JF & Smith CB (1981) Platelet alpha$_2$-adrenergic receptors in major depressive disorder — binding of tritiated clonidine. *Arch. Gen. Psychiat.* **38**, 1327–33.

*Green AR & Costain DW (1979) The biochemistry of depression. In: Paykel E S & Coppen A (eds) *Psychopharmacology of Affective Disorders* Oxford University Press, Oxford. pp. 14–37.

Green AR & Deakin JFW (1980) Brain noradrenaline depletion prevents ECS-induced enhancement of serotonin- and dopamine-mediated behaviour. *Nature* **285**, 232–3.

*Green AR & Nutt DJ (1983) Antidepressants. In: Grahame-Smith DG & Cowen PJ (eds), *Psychopharmacology 1. Part 1 Preclinical Psychopharmacology.* Excerpta Medica, Amsterdam. pp 1–37.

Heninger GR, Charney DS & Sternberg DE (1984) Serotonergic function in depresssion: prolactin response to intravenous trytophan in depressed patients and healthy subjects. *Arch. Gen. Psychiat.* **41**, 398–402.

Hertting G, Axelrod J & Whitby LG (1961) Effects of drugs on the uptake and metabolism of [^{3}H]-norepinephrine. *J. Pharmac. Exp. Ther.* **134**, 146–53.

Heydorn WE, Brunswick DJ & Frazer A (1982) Effect of treatment of rats with antidepressants on melatonin concentrations in the pineal gland and serum. *J. Pharmacol. Exp. Ther.* **222**, 534–43.

Hirschfeld RMA, Koslow SH & Kupfer DJ (1983) The clinical utility of the dexamethasone suppression test in psychiatry. *J. Am. Med. Assoc.* **250**, 2171–4.

Huang YH (1979) Chronic desipramine treatment increases activity of noradrenergic postsynaptic cells. *Life Sci.* **25**, 709–16.

Huang YH, Maas JW & Hu GH (1980) The time course of noradrenergic pre- and postsynaptic activity during chronic desipramine treatment. *Eur. J. Pharmacol.* **68**, 41–47.

Hyttel J (1982) Citalopram — pharmacological profile of a specific serotonin uptake inhibitor with antidepressant activity. *Prog. Neuro-Psychopharmacol. Bio. Psychiat.* **6**, 277–95.

*Knapp S (1983) Lithium. In: Grahame-Smith DG & Cowen PJ (eds) *Psychopharmachology 1. Part 1. Preclinical Psychopharmacology.* Excerpta Medica, Amsterdam. pp. 71–106.

Koch C (1985) Understanding the intrinsic circuitry of the cat's lateral geniculate nucleus: electrical properties of the spine-triad arrangement. *Proc. Roy. Soc.* **B. 225**, 365–90.

Lloyd KG, Farley IJ, Deck JHN & Hornykiewicz O (1974) Serotonin and 5-hydroxyindoleacetic acid in discrete areas of the brain stem of suicide victims and control patients. *Adv. Biochem. Psychopharmac.* **11**, 387–97.

Mann JJ, Brown RP, Halper JP, Sweeney JA, Kocsis JH, Stokes PE & Bilezikian JP (1985) Reduced sensitivity of lymphocyte beta-adrenergic receptors in patients with endogenous depression and psychomotor agitation. *New Eng. J. Med.* **313**, 715–20.

Maj J, Mogilnicka E & Klimek V (1979) The effect of repeated administration of antidepressant drugs on the responsiveness of rats to catecholamine agonists. *J. Neural Transm.* **44**, 221–35.

Menkes DB & Aghajanian GK (1981) Alpha$_1$-adrenoceptor-mediated responses in the lateral geniculate nucleus are enhanced by chronic antidepressant treatment. *Eur. J. Pharmacol.* **74**, 27–35.

Menkes DB, Aghajanian GK & McCall RB (1980) Chronic antidepressant treatment enhances alpha-adrenergic and serotonergic responses in the facial nucleus. *Life Sci.* **27**, 45–55.

Minneman KP, Dibner MD, Wolfe BB & Molinoff PB (1979) Beta$_1$- and beta$_2$-adrenergic receptors in rat cerebral cortex are independently regulated. *Science* **204**, 866–8.

Mishra R, Janowsky A & Sulser F (1979) Subsensitivity of the norepinephrine receptor-coupled adenylate cyclase system in brain: effects of nisoxetine versus fluoxetine. *Eur. J. Pharmacol.* **60**, 379–82.

Mobley PL & Sulser F (1979) Norepinephrine stimulated cyclic AMP accumulation in rat limbic forebrain slices: partial mediation by a subpopulation of receptor with neither alpha or beta characteristics. *Eur. J. Pharmacol.* **60**, 221-7.

Olpe HR & Schellenberg A (1980) Reduced sensitivity of neurones to noradrenaline after chronic treatment with antidepressant drugs. *Eur. J. Pharmacol.* **63**, 7-13.

Owen F, Chambers DR, Cooper SJ Crow TJ, Johnson JA, Lofthouse R & Poulter M (1986) Serotonergic mechanisms in brains of suicide victims. *Brain Res.* **362**, 185-8.

Pelayo F, Dubocovich ML & Langer SZ (1980) Inhibition of neuronal uptake reduces the presynaptic effects of clonidine but not of alpha-methylnoradrenaline on the stimulation-evoked release of ^{3}H-noradrenaline from rat occipital cortex slices. *Eur. J. Pharmacol.* **64**, 143-55.

Pilc A & Lloyd KG (1984) Chronic antidepressants and GABA B receptors. A GABA hypothesis of antidepressant drug action. *Life Sci.* **35**, 2149-54.

Pletscher A (1978) Platelets as models for monoaminergic neurons. In: Youdim MBH, Lovenberg W, Sharman DF & Lagnado JR (eds) *Essays in Neurochemistry and Neuropharmacology.* Vol. 3. John Wiley, Chichester.

Ross SB & Renyi AL (1969) Inhibition of the uptake of tritiated 5-HT in brain tissue. *Eur. J. Pharmacol.* **4**, 270-7.

Sarai K, Frazer A, Brunswick D & Mendels J (1978) Desmethylimipramine-induced decrease in beta-adrenergic receptor binding in rat cerebral cortex. *Biochem. Pharmacol.* **27**, 2179-81.

Schildkraut JJ (1965) The catecholamine hypothesis of affective disorders: a review of supporting evidence. *Am. J. Psychiat.* **122**, 509-22.

Schildkraut JJ (1978) Current status of the catecholamine hypothesis of affective disorders. In: Lipton MA, DiMascio A & KF Killam (eds) *Psychopharmacology: A Generation of Progress.* Raven Press, New York. pp. 1223-34.

Schweitzer JW, Schwartz R & Friedhoff AJ (1979) Intact presynaptic terminals required for beta-adrenergic receptor regulation by desipramine. *J. Neurochem.* **33**, 377-9.

Scuvee-Moreau JJ & Dresse AE (1979) Effect of various antidepressant drugs on the spontaneous firing rate of locus coeruleus and dorsal raphe neurons of the rat. *Eur. J. Pharmacol.* **57**, 219-25.

Segal DS, Kuczenski R & Mandell AJ (1974) Theoretical implications of drug-induced adaptive regulation for a biogenic amine hypothesis of depression. *Biol. Psychiat.* **9**, 147-59.

Sigg EB (1959) Pharmacological studies with Tofranil. *Can. Psychiat. Assoc. J.* **4** (Suppl.), S75-S85.

Smith CB, Garcia-Seville JA & Hollingsworth PJ (1981) Alpha$_2$-adrenoceptors in rat brain are decreased after long-term tricyclic antidepressant drug treatment. *Brain Res.* **210**, 413-18.

Stanford C & Nutt DJ (1982) Comparison of the effects of repeated electroconvulsive shock on alpha$_2$ and beta-adrenoceptors in different regions of rat brain. *Neuroscience* **7**, 1753-7.

Stanley M, Virgilio J & Gershon S (1982) Tritiated imipramine binding sites are decreased in the frontal cortex of suicides. *Science* **216**, 1337-9.

Su Y-F, Harden TK & Perkins JP (1979) Isoproterenol induced desensitization of adenylate cyclase in human astrocytoma cells. *J. Biol. Chem.* **254**, 38-41.

Sugrue MF (1981) Effects of acutely and chronically administered antidepressants on the clonidine-induced decrease in rat brain 3-methoxy-4-hydroxyphenylethylene glycol sulphate content. *Life Sci.* **28**, 377-84.

*Sugrue MF (1983) Chronic antidepressant therapy and associated changes in central monoaminergic receptor functioning. *Pharmac. Ther.* **21**, 1-33.

Taylor DP Allen LE, Ashworth EM, Becker JA, Hyslop DK & Riblet LA (1981) Treatment with trazodone plus phenoxybenzamine accelerates development of decreased type 2 serotonin binding in rat cortex. *Neuropharmacology* **20**, 513-16.

Vetulani J & Sulser F (1975) Action of various antidepressant treatment reduces reactivity of noradrenergic cyclic AMP generating system in limbic forebrain. *Nature* **257**, 495-6.

Vetulani J, Stawarz RJ, Dingell JV & Sulser F (1976) A possible mechanism of action of antidepressant treatments. Reduction in the sensitivity of the noradrenergic cyclic AMP generating system in the rat limbic forebrain. *Naunyn-Schmiedebergs' Arch. Pharmacol.* **293**, 109-14.

Wessels MR, Mullikin D & Lefkowitz RJ (1978) Differences between agonist and antagonist binding following beta-adrenergic receptor desensitization. *J. Biol. Chem.* **253**, 3371-3.

Willner P (1984) The ability of antidepressant drugs to desensitize beta-adrenoceptors is inversely correlated with their clinical potency. *J. Affect. Dis.* **7**, 53-8.

*Woodward DJ, Moises HC, Waterhouse BD, Hoffer BJ & Freedman R (1979) Modulatory actions of norepinephrine in the central nervous system. *Fed. Proc.* **38**, 2109-16.

Wright AF, Crichton DN, Loudon JB, Morten JEN & Steel CM (1984) Beta-adrenoceptor binding defects in cell lines from families with manic-depressive disorder. *Ann. Hum. Genet.* **48**, 20-214.

Yeh HH & Woodward DJ (1983) Alterations in beta adrenergic physiological response characteristics after long-term treatment with desmethylimipramine: Interaction between norepinephrine and gamma-amino butyric acid in rat cerebellum. *J. Pharmacol. Exp. Ther.* **226**, 126-34.

Zis AP & Goodwin FK (1979) Novel antidepressants and the biogenic amine hypothesis of depression. The case for iprindole and mianserin. *Arch. Gen. Psychiat.* **36**, 1097-107.

20   Anxiety

SANDRA V. VELLUCCI

Few members of a demanding modern society can exist for long before experiencing anxiety. It is an emotive state, felt at some time by all normal individuals. Although different authors have ascribed different meanings to the term 'anxiety', and in many cases have used it interchangeably with the terms 'fear' or 'stress', it is generally accepted that anxiety is an unpleasant state accompanied by apprehension, worry, fear, nervousness, tenseness and sometimes conflict. Arousal is usually heightened and this period of greater awareness is tiring both mentally and physically. Often associated with these psychological changes is an increase in sympathetic autonomic nervous system activity which leads to raised blood pressure and heart rate, disturbed respiration, increased skeletal muscle tone, dryness of the throat and mouth and gastrointestinal disturbances. This increased sympathetic discharge gears the individual for a possible increase in energy output. Thus the role of 'normal' or physiological anxiety is to focus attention on a current or future event and subsequently increase the ability of the individual to cope with it.

Anxiety is frequently an anticipatory response caused by the prior knowledge of an impending aversive event which may be inevitable. Once it is realised that no form of response will prevent its occurrence a state of helplessness may be generated. Physiological anxiety is usually short-lived, often with a rapid onset and an abrupt cessation as the aversive event passes. It is only when anxiety becomes excessive or pathological and affects the ability of the individual to lead a normal life that it is considered to be a problem. Approximately 2–4% of the population suffer from pathological anxiety and often no removable causative factor can be identified, thus making it necessary to treat the symptoms clinically with so-called sedative or tranquillising drugs. Generally a sedative drug is one which gives rise to feelings of drowsiness, sluggishness and apathy, effects which are generally ascribed to drugs of the barbiturate group. On the other hand a tranquillising drug is one which produces calmness and serenity and reduces agitation, ideally without giving rise to mental or physical impairment. Drugs of this type are called 'minor' tranquillisers, since they can affect anxiety states but are devoid of significant activity in the 'major' psychoses (e.g. mania and schizophrenia), for which it is necessary to use the 'major' tranquillisers or neuroleptics (see Chapter 18).

Examples of compounds that can exert anxiolytic effects are ethanol, meprobamate, barbiturates and benzodiazepine derivatives. Theoretically the terms 'sedative' and 'anxiolytic' are distinct but in practice this distinction is not clear-cut, as benzodiazepines and barbiturates, for example, can produce both effects depending on the dose administered.

Anxiolytic drugs — historical background

In the past, drugs such as mephenesin, meprobamate and the barbiturates were used in the treatment of anxiety and anxiety states. However, since the introduction of the benzodiazepines, the former compounds are now rarely used in this context and they will only be considered briefly. Meprobamate, a propanediol derivative, was originally synthesised in 1951 and developed as a longer-acting successor to the centrally-acting muscle relaxant, mephenesin. It was used extensively in the treatment of anxiety before the introduction of the benzodiazepines because unlike the barbiturates, which in clinically effective doses can give rise to motor and intellectual impairment, it has a more 'specific' anxiolytic action. In normal therapeutic doses it does not cause significant behavioural impairment and appears to have no effect in non-anxious subjects, unlike the barbiturates which produce effects in both types of subject. Meprobamate was also considered to be a much safer drug than the barbiturates. Little data is available concerning the precise way in which mephenesin and meprobamate act at the neuronal level.

Barbiturates

It is generally accepted that the barbiturates are anxiolytic in subhypnotic doses and that this property is merely a weak reflection of their CNS depressant effects.

Pentobarbitone and closely related substituted barbiturates have been shown to enhance the action of GABA. In high concentrations pentobarbitone appears to have a GABA-mimetic action which can be reversed by picrotoxin. The sedative barbiturates have also been shown to enhance the affinity of benzodiazepine receptors for benzodiazepines. Data from numerous studies including electrophysiological investigations, support the existence of a macromolecular complex in which GABA, benzodiazepine and barbiturate binding sites are coupled to a chloride ionophore (see later). The barbiturate binding site is, however, distinct from the benzodiazepine binding site and it is thought that barbiturates act at the dihydropicrotoxinin binding site (i.e. at a site closely associated with the chloride ionophore) to enhance chloride ion flux (see Olsen 1986). Thus, as both the barbiturates and the benzodiazepines can augment GABA function, albeit by different mechanisms, it is not surprising that these two classes of compounds have several pharmacological properties in common. The barbiturates are now little used in the treatment of anxiety states due to their abuse potential and low therapeutic index.

Benzodiazepines

In 1957, animal studies carried out with the benzodiazepine derivative Ro5-0690 (chlordiazepoxide) indicated that the compound had hypnotic, sedative and anticonvulsant effects, similar to those of meprobamate, in mice and cats. The drug was almost discarded after initial trials, since it was administered in too high a dose to a small group of geriatric patients, producing sedation, severe ataxia and slurring of speech. Re-tested in a group of younger psychoneurotic patients it soon became apparent that chlordiazepoxide was clinically effective in alleviating tension and anxiety. Moreover it filled the need for a drug having a potency mid-way between that of meprobamate and the major tranquillisers (e.g. the phenothiazine derivative, chlorpromazine), and appeared suitable for regular use in non-hospitalised patients. Chlordiazepoxide (Librium) was introduced into clinical practice in 1960 and followed three years later by diazepam (Valium). Thousands of benzodiazepine derivatives have since been synthesised and screened pharmacologically and about 20 of these are currently marketed in the UK and representative structures are shown in Fig. 20.1.

Although this chapter deals mainly with the anxiolytic properties of the benzodiazepines, it must be remembered that these drugs are also used for premedication in anaesthesia, in the treatment of muscle spasms, as anticonvulsants, as hypnotics and in the treatment of alcohol withdrawal. Benzodiazepines have a high therapeutic index and are thus comparatively safe in overdose; 20 times the hypnotic dose of a barbiturate can result in coma and death, whereas it is almost impossible to commit suicide with benzodiazepines taken alone. Benzodiazepines have comparatively few immediately undesirable side-effects, thus making them suitable for use in non-hospitalised patients. They generally have less abuse potential than the barbiturates, do not cause marked induction of hepatic microsomal enzymes, and so do not accelerate their own metabolism or that of other drugs which may be taken concomitantly. Thus the benzodiazepines have superseded the barbiturates as anxiolytic and hypnotic agents and have emerged as the major class of drugs prescribed clinically for the treatment of anxiety states. The clinical importance of benzodiazepines has been emphasised by reports such as that of Lader (1978), stating that in a given year, about 9% of adult males and 19% of adult females received a prescription for either a tranquilliser or a hypnotic, and about 1.5% of the adult population had taken these drugs continuously for at least one year (see Lader & Petursson 1983). Chronic usage of these drugs was reported to be widespread, with a large proportion (up to 60%) of all 'repeat' prescriptions being for drugs of this type. Although in the short-term benzodiazepines have proved to be beneficial in the treatment of anxiety and related disorders their long-term use is questionable as it has been demonstrated that they give rise to

1, 4 Benzodiazepine derivatives

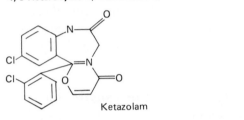

Chlordiazepoxide   Diazepam   Oxazepam

4, 5-Heterocyclo-1, 4-Benzodiazepine

Ketazolam

1, 5-Benzodiazepine   **Imidazodiazepine**   **Triazolobenzodiazepine**

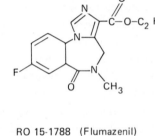

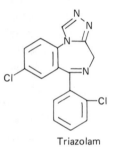

Clobazam   RO 15-1788   (Flumazenil)   Triazolam

Fig. 20.1. The chemical structures of some benzodiazepine derivatives.

tolerance and dependence (Cook & Sepinwall 1975; Vellucci & File 1979). The occurrence of withdrawal symptoms (e.g. seizures) after abrupt cessation of treatment with moderate to high doses of benzodiazepines has also been reported in man (see Greenblatt & Shader 1978). Thus it is not surprising that concern exists about the abuse potential of these compounds.

Despite the high incidence of anxiety in modern society, insight into the biology of this condition has not been easy to obtain. Extensive investigations have been carried out into the neurological and biochemical mechanisms underlying anxiety, but its aetiology is still poorly understood as is the precise way in which drugs such as the benzodiazepines exert their anxiolytic effects.

Animal models of anxiety

In the absence of fully characterised biological indices, anxiety is measured clinically as unpleasant effects reported verbally by patients and because of the subjective nature of this condition, suitable animal models have been difficult to design. Nevertheless, even if such models are not exact replicas of human anxiety they are essential for investigations into the biochemistry of anxiety and the mechanism of action of anxiolytic drugs. Firstly, they must be sensitive in a dose-dependent manner to clinically effective anxiolytics. Secondly the relative potency of different anxiolytic agents should be similar to that found in man and finally animal models should distinguish the effects of anxiolytic from non-anxiolytic drugs. Some of the more commonly used animal models of anxiety will now be described (see also Treit 1985).

Models based on the effects of anxiolytics on unconditioned reactions

1 The active social interaction test (File & Hyde 1978) exploits the social behaviour of pairs of male rats and the way in which this alters under different test conditions. When a pair of male rats is placed in a test chamber in which neither animal has established territory, social interaction will not be dominated by aggressive encounters, and is mostly of an investigative nature. The time spent in active social interaction is greatest when the pairs of rats are tested under a low level of illumination in a test chamber with which they are familiar and decreases if the light level is increased, or if the chamber is unfamiliar and uncertainty maximised (i.e. active social interaction is reduced under conditions that would lead to an increase in 'anxiety'. Drugs with a sedative effect decrease active social interaction in all test conditions but also decrease locomotor activity. On the other hand, anxiolytic activity is revealed by the fact that the decrease in active social interaction that normally occurs as the test conditions are altered is prevented. This test is also sensitive to anxiogenic activity. Anxiogenic substances decrease the time spent in active social interaction in the low light familiar condition, where control scores are highest, but unlike sedative compounds do not decrease locomotor activity. The pattern of results obtained with benzodiazepines in this test is similar to that found clinically. For example, in acute doses chlordiazepoxide (5 mg/kg, i.p.) has a marked sedative effect in the rat, whereas the same dose administered chronically produces a significant anxiolytic effect without causing sedation.

2 Anxiolytic agents tend to increase the locomotor activity of rodents placed in an unfamiliar environment and Crawley and Goodwin (1980) have developed a test based on this observation that also makes use of the natural tendency of rodents to avoid a brightly lit arena. In this test mice are placed on the brightly-lit side of a 2-compartment chamber and the number of transitions between the light and dark sides of the chamber and the locomotor activity are recorded. Anxiolytic drugs produce a dose-dependent increase in light-dark crossings and locomotor activity, whereas non-anxiolytic agents do not. On the other hand anxiogenic compounds decrease the number of transitions between the light and dark sides without decreasing the overall level of locomotor activity.

3 A more recently developed model is the elevated plus maze test. When animals are placed in a plus-shaped maze elevated above the ground with two opposing arms having enclosed sides and the other two being open, it is found that control animals spend only a very small proportion of time in the open arms. The percentage of entries into the open arms of the maze provides a measure of fear-induced inhibition of exploratory activity and is found to be increased by anxiolytic drugs and reduced by anxiogenic compounds (Pellow *et al.* 1985).

Models based on the effects of anxiolytics in traditional learning paradigms

The Geller–Seifter conflict test (Geller & Seifter 1960) and variations thereof have been shown to be reasonable predictors of anxiolytic drug action. In this type of test the rate of occurrence of an easily measured re-sponse (e.g. lever pressing for food reward) is suppressed by punishment (e.g. a mildly aversive electric shock). The ability of a drug to disinhibit, i.e. to increase, the rate of punished behaviour in the presence of the electric shock, defines its anti-anxiety activity. Thus for this particular test, hungry rats are trained to press a lever for a food reward which is usually delivered on a variable interval schedule. When the rate of lever pressing becomes stable a signal is presented to the animal (e.g. a light or sound) during which time the schedule is altered, so that each single lever press is rewarded by food (i.e. the schedule changes from one of variable interval to one of continuous reinforcement). Once the animals have been trained a punishment, usually in the form of a mildly aversive electric shock applied to the feet via the cage floor, is introduced during the continous reinforcement periods. Thus during this time, when the animal presses the lever it will not only receive a food pellet, but also an electric shock. This is assumed to create a state of emotional conflict within the animal, hence the name of the test. If the level of the shock is very carefully adjusted so as to produce a stable but low rate of responding, an anxiolytic drug will restore the rate of responding towards normal. An excellent correlation between anticonflict effect and clinical potency of anxiolytics can be obtained. Benzodiazepines and other anxiolytic com-pounds (e.g. meprobamate, low doses of ethanol and barbiturates) all produce an increase in the rate of punished responding. Unpunished responding is not generally affected by these drugs unless sedative doses are used. The close relationship between anticonflict and clinical activity can be further demonstrated with chronic benzodiazepine treatment. For example the anticonflict effect of oxazepam has been shown to increase, and its depressant effect on unpunished responding to decrease with this treatment (Margules & Stein 1968). Although the conflict procedure appears to fulfil the major criteria for a valid behavioural test of anxiolytic agents the conflict period usually suppresses responding to very low rates, so that additional suppression is difficult to obtain, thus hindering the concomitant detection of anxiogenic drugs.

More recently a drug discrimination procedure has been described which can detect potential anxiolytic or anxiogenic activity (Lal & Shearman 1982). A rat is placed in a test chamber containing two levers and trained to press one lever for food reward when treated with an anxiogenic drug, such as a low dose of pentylenetetrazole (PTZ) and the second lever when treated with the drug vehicle or any non-anxiogenic drug. The animal's perception of the drug's action provides a cue (the so-called interoceptive discriminable stimulus, IDS) for the selection of the appropriate lever. Other drugs may subsequently be tested to see whether they will produce the same response as the test drug or whether the animal selects the vehicle-appropriate lever instead. Thus an animal will learn to discriminate the state of 'anxiety' induced by an anxiogenic drug, revealing this learning by pressing the appropriate lever. Anxiolytics have been shown to antagonise these stimuli in a dose-dependent manner with rank orders of potency similar to those reported clinically.

Neurotransmitters in anxiety

The normally transient and ill-defined nature of anxiety in man has made it difficult to evaluate in terms of neurotransmitter malfunction. Similarly, in animals the state of 'anxiety' produced in some of the tests described earlier is usually an acute effect and therefore unlikely to be reflected by significant, easily measurable changes in central neurotransmitter turnover. Thus most of the data relating to the neurochemical basis of anxiety has been obtained in animals by either (1) looking at changes in brain neurotransmitter function which may be evoked by treatment, particularly chronic treatment, with benzodiazepines and other anxiolytic or anxiogenic compounds, and (2) investigating possible modifications of behaviour produced in these tests after procedures such as lesion placement or treatment with drugs that have known effects on CNS neurotransmitter function.

Noradrenaline (NA) and dopamine (DA)

Significant decreases in the turnover of NA and DA in the rat cerebral cortex and corpus striatum respectively, have been reported to occur following benzodiazepine treatment. Benzodiazepines have also been found to block stress-induced increases in DA turnover but there is no other evidence to link DA with anxiety. Phenothiazine derivatives, such as chlorpromazine, reduce noradrenergic (and dopaminergic) function but do not prevent the suppression of punished behaviour in the conflict test; neither do α-and β-adrenergic antagonists. Thus antianxiety activity does not appear to involve noradrenergic blockade. Indeed intracerebroventricular (i.c.v.) injection of NA was found to increase the antipunishment activity of systemically administered benzodiazepines (Stein *et al.* 1973), lending further support to the idea that anticonflict action does not depend solely on a reduction in noradrenergic activity. At the same time NA i.c.v. antagonised the depressant effect of the benzodiazepine derivative, oxazepam on non-punished behaviour, suggesting that the depressant (sedative) action of these drugs may be mediated by a reduction in noradrenergic function. This was further supported by the finding that the decreased NA turnover and sedative effects evoked by a single injection of oxazepam in the rat rapidly undergo tolerance and are no longer observed after chronic treatment whereas the anxiolytic effects are still evident. Thus it appears that the decrease in noradrenergic function that is observed during the initial stages of benzodiazepine treatment is associated with the depressant or sedative effects of this class of compounds and not with their anxiolytic effects.

More recently evidence has emerged which indicates that clonidine (a partial agonist at α_2-adrenoceptors) attenuates opiate withdrawal symptoms and reduces pathological anxiety, fear or panic. Since these psychopharmacological effects appear to be associated with behaviours mediated by the (noradrenergic) locus coeruleus, the activity of which is inhibited by clonidine, it has been suggested that locus coeruleus pathways may play a role in the mediation of some types of anxiety (Charney & Redmond 1983). In the monkey, electrical stimulation of this region or the administration of the α_2-adrenoceptor antagonist, piperoxan, produced an increase in the frequency of parameters associated with fear or anxiety, whereas locus coeruleus lesions or clonidine-treatment have the opposite effect. Clonidine also has anticonflict effects in the rat although it was ineffective in a model of anxiety based on novelty-induced inhibition of food intake. However, as the possibility now exists that altered noradrenergic function may underlie certain forms of anxiety such as that seen in patients suffering from panic attacks and anxiety with depression, this requires further investigation.

5-HT

Several pharmacological studies have suggested that a reduction in the function of 5-HT pathways in the brain results in an anxiolytic effect and that the anxiolytic effects of the benzodiazepines are mediated by a reduction in central 5-HT neurotransmission (see File & Vellucci 1978; Saner & Pletscher 1979; Collinge *et al.* 1983). Reducing 5-HT function with parachloro-phenylalanine or α-propyl-dopacetamide (inhibitors of tryptophan hydroxylase) or with non-specific 5-HT antagonists such as methysergide, cinanserin, cyproheptadine or bromolysergic acid, generally produces anxiolytic effects in various animal models (see Cook & Sepinwall 1975; Stein *et al.* 1973). Some authors, however, have failed to show this, or an ability of 5-HT agonists to modify the anticonflict effects of chlordiazepoxide (see e.g. Blakely & Parker 1973; Shepherd *et al.* 1982) or to exert anxiogenic effects (see Gardner 1986). Some of the discrepancies that have arisen may be due to the different animal models of anxiety used, and to the numerous differences in experimental procedures that have been employed to alter central 5-HT neurotransmission. For example, reduced 5-HT function has been produced by electrolytic or neurotoxic lesions, by synthesis inhibition, or by relatively non-specific 5-HT receptor antagonists. Conversely, enhanced 5-HT function has been produced by 5-HT uptake inhibitors, 5-HTP, 5-HT itself or by non-specific 5-HT receptor agonists (e.g. quipazine, N,N-dimethyltryptamine). Some of the procedures employed (e.g. lesions) have affected localised areas of the CNS, whereas others (e.g. systemic administration of *p*CPA), have affected the entire brain. Furthermore it is well-known that different agonists or antagonists vary in potency and binding site specificity (for example cyproheptadine has also been shown to interact with GABA-linked chloride ionophores with a similar potency to pentobarbitone (Squires *et al.* 1983)). Nevertheless benzodiazepines have been shown to inhibit the firing of 5-HT neurons in the midbrain raphe nuclei (Laurent *et al.* 1983) and a link between these 5-HT projections and the possible neuroanatomical and neurochemical substrates of anxiety has been proposed.

The link between 5-HT pathways and the control of anxiety has been further strengthened by the characterisation of, and development of, specific ligands for different 5-HT receptors in the CNS. Their use in various animal models of anxiety show that a reduction of 5-HT neurotransmission can evoke anxiolytic effects in animals whereas enhancement of 5-HT evokes an anxiogenic response (see Chopin & Briley 1987).

GABA

Although a great deal of evidence has accumulated from extensive physiological and biochemical studies which indicate that benzodiazepines act specifically by augmenting GABA function, at least as far as their anticonvulsant and muscle relaxant effects are concerned, it has not been easy to demonstrate a clear association between changes in GABA function and anxiolytic activity. Studies have shown that the GABA-mimetic, muscimol, administered peripherally possesses some anti-conflict activity, although the effect was not found to be dose-related or associated with the potentiation of benzodiazepine activity (Sepinwall & Cook 1980). This could, however, be explained by the fact that muscimol is rapidly metabolised, with only a small proportion of a systemically

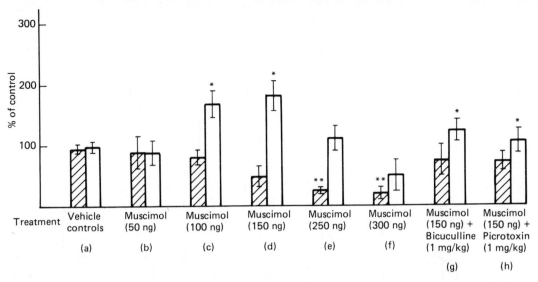

Fig. 20.2. Modification of the effect of muscimol (150 ng i.c.v., 15 min. before testing) on unpunished (shaded columns) and punished (open columns) responding by bicuculline and picrotoxin (1 mg/kg, i.p.) administered at the same time as and 5 min after muscimol, respectively. The effect of various doses of muscimol injected i.c.v. 15 min before testing is also shown (b–f). The ordinate shows the response rate as a percentage of the corresponding untreated control response, where the latter is 100%. Drug treatments are indicated on the abscissa. Each value represents the mean (±SEM) obtained from 10 rats using a conflict paradigm. Significantly different from corresponding control groups: *$P < 0.05$; **$P < 0.001$. (From Vellucci & Webster 1984b.)

administered dose entering the CNS. When administered i.c.v., muscimol can indeed produce a dose-related anticonflict effect which can be abolished by the GABA antagonists bicuculline and picrotoxin (see Fig. 20.2). Muscimol has also been shown to potentiate the anticonflict effects of low doses of diazepam. Conversely, the pharmacological effects of benzodiazepines can be inhibited by GABA antagonists or GABA synthesis inhibitors (see Zakusov *et al.* 1977; Vellucci & Webster 1984b).

If increased GABA function does play a role in reducing anxiety then one might expect that GABA-transaminase inhibitors, such as amino-oxyacetic acid (AOAA) would also possess anxiolytic properties, but there is no evidence to support this. However, the increased brain GABA concentrations produced by AOAA appear to be associated primarily with non-nerve terminal components (e.g. neuronal perikarya and glial cells) and thus do not give a true reflection of functionally available GABA in the CNS. Further support for an involvement of GABAergic mechanisms in anxiety comes from the observation that the anticonvulsant drug sodium valproate has potent anticonflict effects which appear to be related to its activity at the picrotoxinin binding site where it is believed to act by prolonging the life-time of GABA-receptor regulated chloride ionophores (Ticku & Davis 1981). Sodium valproate produces a dose-related anticonflict effect which is comparable with that of chlordiazepoxide or diazepam and can be blocked by picrotoxin but not bicuculline (see Fig. 20.3).

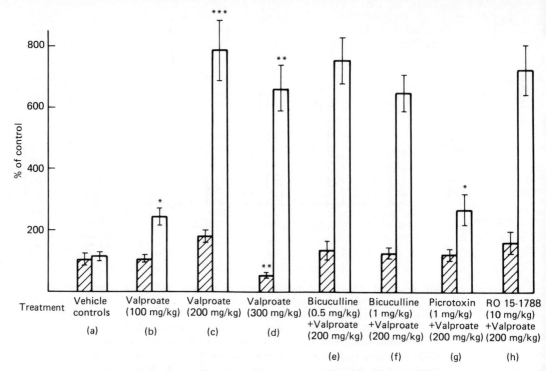

Fig. 20.3. Modification of the effects of sodium valproate (200 mg/kg, i.p. 5 min before testing) on unpunished (shaded columns) and punished (open columns) responding by bicuculline (0.5 and 1.0 mg/kg, i.p.), picrotoxin (1.0 mg/kg, i.p.) and RO15-1788 (10 mg/kg, i.p.) administered 10, 5 and 10 min. before valproate, respectively. The effects of various doses of valproate administered 5 min before testing are also shown (b–d). The ordinate shows the response rate as a percentage of the corresponding untreated control response, where the latter is 100%. Drug treatments are indicated on the abscissa. Each value represents the mean (±SEM) obtained from 10 rats using a conflict paradigm. Significantly different from corresponding control groups: *$P < 0.05$; **$P < 0.005$; *** $P < 0.001$. (From Vellucci & Webster 1984.)

Possible sites of action of the benzodiazepines and related anxiolytic compounds

Raphe nuclei

Evidence exists to indicate that ascending 5-HT projections from the midbrain raphe nuclei may be involved in the mediation of behavioural suppression that occurs in certain animal models such as the conflict test (see Thiebot *et al.* 1982; Soubrie *et al.* 1981). It is well-established that the midbrain raphe nuclei (including the dorsal raphe nucleus, DRN) give rise to the 5-HT innervation of limbic structures. In addition to 5-HT receptors, DRN neurons also possess receptors for GABA and glycine and recently evidence has been put forward to indicate the possible co-existence of 5-HT and GABA in neurons at this site (Nanopoulos *et al.* 1982). It is therefore conceivable that any modification of the GABA input to the raphe nuclei could subsequently affect the 5-HT system. Indeed it has been demonstrated that electrolytic lesions of the habenular nuclei can block the ability of GABA agonists to reduce 5-HTP accumulation in nerve terminals and cell bodies (i.e. in the raphe nuclei) and that chlordiazepoxide applied to the DRN reduced 5-HT release in terminal areas of 5-HT axons (Soubrie *et al.* 1983), an effect that could be prevented by intra-raphe 5,7-dihydroxytryptamine (5,7-DHT) pretreatment (Soubrie *et al.* 1981; Thiebot *et al.* 1980; Thiebot *et al.* 1982). A similar blockade of the effects of GABA-mimetics was noted after ibotenate-induced lesions of the habenula but not after electrolytic lesions of the stria medullaris (which conveys most of the afferents to the habenula). Therefore GABAergic inhibition of ascending 5-HT neurons exerted at the medial and dorsal raphe nuclei (see Fig. 9.1) is likely to depend on ongoing activity in habenulo-raphe pathways, and GABA may exert its inhibitory control over these 5-HT neurons by decreasing a facilitatory influence on these cells exerted by the habenula. Additionally, acute systemic injection of GABA-mimetic substances can reduce 5-HTP accumulation in 5-HT nerve terminal regions (e.g. prefrontal cortex, olfactory tubercule, septum, corpus striatum and spinal cord) as well as in corresponding cell-body regions (raphe dorsalis, medianus, pontis and magnus). Decreases in 5-HT synthesis induced by intra-raphe muscimol infusions have been shown to be restricted to the corresponding projection areas. These effects could be antagonised by bicuculline which was, however, ineffective in the absence of a GABA-mimetic. The above data therefore suggest that GABA exerts an inhibitory (non-tonic) control over central 5-HT neurons located in the raphe nuclei (Nishikawa & Scatton 1985).

These findings, coupled with the observations that GABA and chlordiazepoxide injected directly into the DRN exert anticonflict effects (Thiebot & Soubrie 1983; Thiebot *et al.* 1980) and that picrotoxin injected into the DRN increases cerebral cortical 5-HT turnover and can reverse the depressant effects of diazepam on 5-HT turnover (Collinge *et al.* 1983), provide further support for the idea that the change in 5-HT turnover and the behavioural effects observed after benzodiazepine treatment are indirect and are secondary to the interaction of benzodiazepines with GABA neurotransmission in this system. The postulated relevance of the 5-HT projections from the DRN in anxiety is further emphasised by the observation that animals with 5,7-DHT lesions of the DRN exhibit a behavioural profile in the active social interaction test which is similar to that seen in animals treated with anxiolytic drugs (Collins *et al.* 1979). In addition lesions of 5-HT pathways at the level of the ventral tegmentum (with 5, 7-DHT) have been shown to have the following effects, firstly to cause a release of response suppression which was acquired before lesioning, with the size of the response being similar to that noted following the systemic administration of benzodiazepines. Secondly such lesions prevent acquisition of response suppression noted in a punishment paradigm (Iversen 1983).

Recently Hobbs *et al.* (1984) have shown that microinjection of benzodiazepine receptor ligands such as β-carboline-3-carboxylic acid methyl ester (β-CCM; see later) into the DRN of the rat produced an anxiogenic profile which could be specifically blocked by the benzodiazepine receptor antagonist RO15–1788.

Amygdala

The ventral 5-HT pathway projecting from the raphe nuclei innervates several diencephalic and telencephalic structures. The amygdala is of particular interest in this context as it receives a rich 5-HT innervation from the raphe and contains glutamic acid decarboxylase (GAD) the GABA synthesising enzyme. Benzodiazepine receptors have been shown to be concentrated in the cortical and basolateral amygdaloid nuclei (Niehoff & Kuhar 1983). Lesions at this site in rats have been shown to impair responses to fear-inducing novelty and benzodiazepine injections at this site have been reported to have anxiolytic effects (Thomas & Iversen 1985; Petersen & Scheel-Kruger 1982) that could be reversed by bicuculline.

Nevertheless, although it can be seen that lowered 5-HT neuronal activity induced by a variety of manipulations in the midbrain raphe nuclei and the amygdala mimics the effects of systemically administered benzodiazepines, the precise way in which this occurs remains to be established. The issue is further complicated by the demonstration that punished response rates can be increased further by benzodiazepine treatment in raphe-lesioned or pCPA-treated rats (see Thiebot et al. 1982, 1984; Hodges & Green 1984), suggesting that additional pathways may also be involved. For example it has been shown that overactivity of noradrenergic systems in the brain may underlie certain forms of anxiety and hence it has been proposed that the locus coeruleus may be an additional important site at which benzodiazepines act. There is, however, some controversy concerning the nature of the interaction between the benzodiazepine receptor/GABA receptor/chloride ionophore complex in the locus coeruleus. Although this region contains GABA receptors and nerve terminals as well as benzodiazepine receptors, and both GABA and flunitrazepam can inhibit locus coeruleus impulse flow, benzodiazepines do not potentiate GABA-induced inhibitions at this site and conversely benzodiazepine-induced inhibitions cannot be potentiated by GABA. This apparent anomaly requires further investigation.

How do benzodiazepines augment GABA function?

It is now necessary to consider how the benzodiazepines may augment GABA function at the neuronal level. Schmidt et al. (1967), were the first to report the potentiation, by diazepam, of presynaptic inhibition in the cat spinal cord. However, the importance of these findings as far as the mechanism of action of benzodiazepines was concerned, was not recognised for several years because at that time the existence of presynaptic inhibition had not been fully established. When the role of GABA as an inhibitory transmitter was eventually confirmed, Polc *et al.* (1974) re-investigated the effects of diazepam in the cat spinal cord. Diazepam and other pharmacologically active benzodiazepines were found to increase the amplitude and duration of the dorsal root potential (synaptically-induced depolarisation of primary afferent endings) and to enhance presynaptic inhibition of monosynaptic excitation of spinal motoneurons. These effects were prevented by bicuculline. If endogenous GABA is then depleted by the GAD inhibitor thiosemicarbazide, presynaptic inhibition is abolished and can no longer be restored or evoked by benzodiazepines, indicating that they do not possess intrinsic GABA-mimetic activity (Polc & Haefely 1977). Of course this does not mean that the benzodiazepines modulate all GABA-mediated neurotransmission, but they enhance GABA mediated post- and presynaptic inhibition in the cuneate nucleus without affecting the synaptic excitation of cuneothalamic relay cells and these effects were blocked by GABA antagonists and by depleting endogenous GABA. Benzodiazepines also enhance GABA-mediated recurrent inhibition on hippocampal and cerebral cortical pyramidal cells as well as its inhibition of cultured hypothalamic neurons. Similar effects were also observed in the nigrostriatal GABA pathway. Thus data from electrophysiological studies have established that the action of benzodiazepines depends on the existence of a functional GABA system and since benzodiazepines fail to affect re-uptake, release or turnover of GABA, attention was focused on the GABA receptor as a possible site of action of these drugs. There is, however, no evidence to indicate that benzodiazepines are GABA receptor agonists. As benzodiazepines specifically augment the function of GABA but not that of other neurotransmitters, yet do not act on GABA receptors or increase synaptic concentrations of GABA it was, therefore, suggested that they could exert this effect by acting at a specific site or sites adjacent to the GABA receptor, i.e. on their own receptors.

Benzodiazepine receptors

The use of radiolabelled benzodiazepines led to the discovery of saturable, stereospecific binding sites on neuronal elements in the mammalian CNS with a high affinity for benzodiazepines and the excellent correlation obtained between the affinity of various benzodiazepines for these binding sites and their pharmacological potencies in man and animals provided strong evidence that they represent the pharmacological sites of action of these drugs (Braestrup & Squires 1978). Scatchard analysis of equilibrium binding (see Chapter 4) in several buffer systems initially indicated the existence of a single homogeneous class of binding sites, although more recent experiments have suggested the existence of two or more distinct neuronal binding sites (Squires *et al.* 1979). In addition to the neuronal binding sites which have affinity for benzodiazepines at nanomolar concentrations, a 'micromolar' receptor has also been reported to exist in the brain which is analogous to the benzodiazepine binding sites found peripherally, e.g. in the kidney. This classification has been based on the respective binding affinities of these sites for 1,4-benzodiazepine derivatives. For example clonazepam is a potent displacer of $[^3H]$-diazepam binding at 'nanomolar' receptors but is virtually inactive at displacing $[^3H]$-diazepam from 'micromolar' receptors. On the other hand the benzodiazepine derivative R05-4864 (which differs from diazepam by a single chloride substituent in the 4' position of the 'C' (benzene) ring), inhibits the binding of diazepam to 'micromolar' receptors. These, as yet unexplained, differences in binding characteristerics may therefore be used to distinguish between 'nanomolar' and 'micromolar' binding sites and to provide a quantitative measure of the proportion of each type of site present in a given brain region (assuming ligand specificity). 'Nanomolar' binding sites are believed to be analogous to the high affinity binding sites for benzodiazepines that mediate the anxiolytic, anticonvulsant, hypnotic, sedative and muscle relaxant properties of these compounds. R05-4864 does however, have pharmacological actions (e.g. convulsant effects) that may be mediated by an effect at the picrotoxin site (Pellow & File 1984).

The binding of nanomolar concentrations of benzodiazepines to brain membrane preparations is enhanced in the presence of GABA agonists and a reciprocal effect of benzodiazepines on GABA binding can also be shown, thus suggesting that a functional relationship exists between the GABA receptor and the benzodiazepine receptor. The two are however distinct entities, as neither GABA nor bicuculline displace benzodiazepines from their receptors and vice versa.

Benzodiazepines bind to their receptors and augment the effects of GABA via an allosteric interaction with a GABA receptor which has the characteristics of the $GABA_A$ receptor (see Chapter 12), the resultant effect being an increase in the number of chloride channel openings induced by a given GABA concentration (Barker & Owen 1986). In the absence of GABA, benzodiazepines have no effect on chloride ion flux. Although nanomolar benzodiazepine receptors are associated with receptors of the $GABA_A$ type, not all $GABA_A$ receptors are associated with benzodiazepine receptors, and indeed the regional distribution of these two receptor classes, although similar, is not exactly parallel. It is considered that a macromolecular complex exists consisting of a GABA binding site linked to a chloride ionophore and a benzodiazepine binding site. Specific sites associated with the chloride ionophore to which barbiturates and substances such as picrotoxin can bind are also present within this complex. Recently the receptor complex has been purified with these binding sites intact. Its subunit structure has been shown to be $\alpha_2\beta_2$, with the α-subunit containing the benzodiazepine binding site and the β-subunit the GABA binding site (Sigel & Barnard 1984).

Benzodiazepine receptor ligands. Agonists, antagonists and inverse agonists

Small amounts of β-carboline-3-carboxylic acid ethyl ester (β-CCE) were isolated from human urine and mammalian brain extracts by Braestrup et al. (1980). This compound has a very high affinity for brain benzodiazepine receptors with an IC_{50} value against [³H]-diazepam binding in rat forebrain membranes of 4–7 nM compared with 5 nM for clonazepam, the most potent 1,4-benzodiazepine derivative in general clinical use. β-CCE also has high specificity for benzodiazepine receptors and does not displace GABA, dopamine, noradrenaline, acetylcholine or opiates from their binding sites in the brain. It has some affinity for 5-HT receptors but this is more than 100 times less than that for benzodiazepine receptors. The fact that β-CCE has effects on 5-HT receptors is not surprising in view of the structural similarity between β-carbolines and the harmala alkaloids. Although β-CCE is actually an artefact of the extraction procedure used by Braestrup et al. (1980) and is not considered to be an endogenous substance it has proved to be a useful research tool with which to investigate benzodiazepine receptor mechanisms.

The pharmacological effects of β-CCE are opposite to those of the clinically useful benzodiazepines. In suitable doses it antagonises the anticonvulsant effects of benzodiazepines when given either peripherally or centrally, potentiates the effects of PTZ, lowers the seizure threshold to bicuculline and overcomes the locomotor inhibitory effects of flurazepam in rodents (Oakley & Jones 1980; Tenen & Hirsch 1980; Nutt et al. 1982), and produces convulsions in monkeys. It also reverses the anxiolytic effects of benzodiazepines in the Geller-Seifter conflict test (Vellucci & Webster 1982) and exhibits anxiogenic activity (File et al. 1982). There are other β-carboline derivatives which bind to benzodiazepine receptors (e.g. β-carboline carboxylic acid methyl ester (β-CCM), which like β-CCE, is proconvulsant and methyl 6,7-dimethoxy-4-ethyl-β-carboline (DMCM) which is a potent convulsant and like β-CCE and β-CCM is anxiogenic at non-convulsant doses. In contrast, 6-benzyloxy-4-methoxy methyl-β-carboline-3-carboxylic acid ethyl ester (ZK 93423) and its 5-benzyloxy homologue (ZK 91296) are anticonvulsants and have been classified as full agonist and partial agonist, respectively. The structures of various β-carboline derivatives are shown in Fig. 20.4.

Apart from the β-carbolines several imidazodiazepine derivatives, e.g. RO15-1788 (flumazenil, ethyl-8-fluoro-5,6-dihydro-5-methyl-6-oxo-4H-imidazo [1,5-a][1,4] benzodiazepine-3-carboxylate) have been found to specifically inhibit [³H]-diazepam binding to brain synaptosomal fractions and to specifically antagonise the behavioural, electrophysiological and biochemical effects of clinically useful benzodiazepines in a variety of experimental paradigms (Hunkeler et al. 1981). Although numerous investigators have confirmed these observations it has also been reported, however, that RO15-1788 has intrinsic pharmacological effects. High

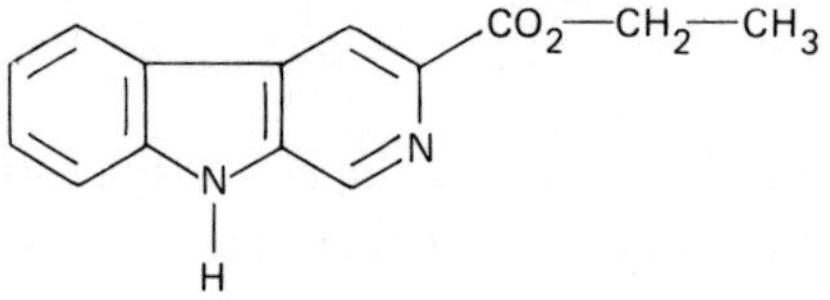

βCCE

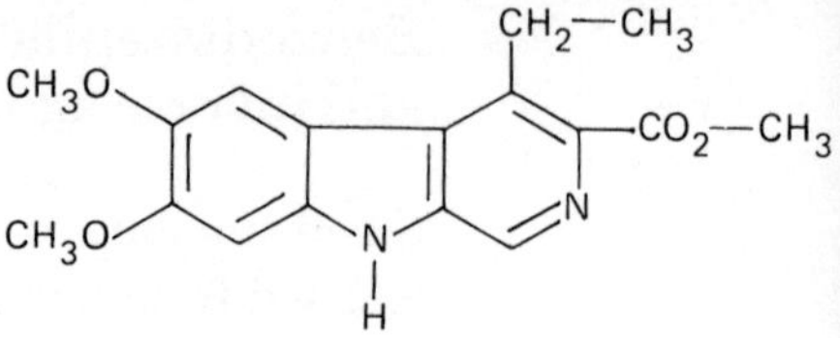

DMCM

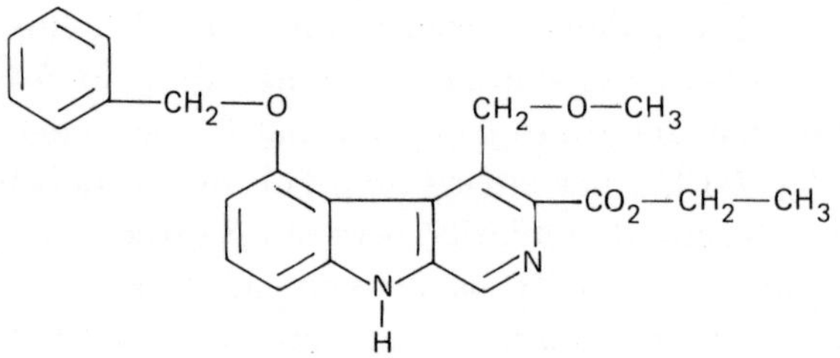

ZK 91 296

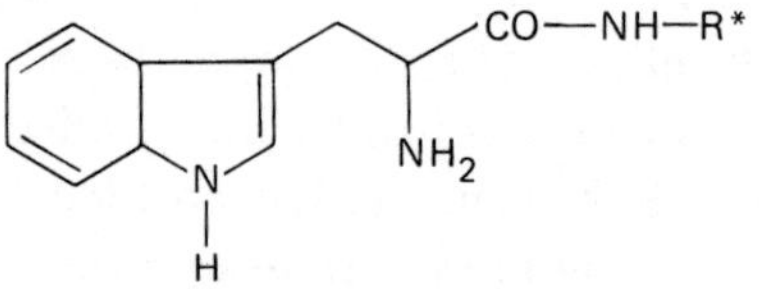

(* e.g. glycine residue)

Typtophan-containing peptide

Fig. 20.4. The chemical structures of some β-carboline derivatives.

doses of the compound have been shown to have anticonvulsant effects (Nutt *et al.* 1982; Vellucci & Webster 1983), and studies in animal paradigms of anxiety have indicated an anxiogenic profile (File *et al.* 1982). Thus although the classification of R015-1788 as a benzodiazepine antagonist is not in question, as it is able to antagonise the effects of other compounds that act at benzodiazepine receptors, it can no longer be classified as a true antagonist in view of the fact that it possesses intrinsic activity. Another putative benzodiazepine antagonist is the β-carboline derivative ZK 93426, but this too has been shown to have intrinsic activity.

On the basis of their pharmacological activity benzodiazepine receptor ligands have therefore been divided into the following groups:

1 'Agonists' — these have the characteristic therapeutic effects of the benzodiazepines (i.e. anticonvulsant, sedative, muscle relaxant, anxiolytic and hypnotic effects). Examples are diazepam and chlordiazepoxide.

2 'Inverse Agonists' — these have effects opposite to those of the 'agonists' and thus have convulsant and anxiogenic properties. An example is the β-carboline derivative DMCM.

3 'Competitive' or 'Neutral Antagonists' — these should have no intrinsic activity but should inhibit the pharmacological actions of 'agonists' and 'inverse agonists'. To date no true 'neutral antagonist' of benzodiazepine receptors has been reported to exist.

4 Finally there are 'partial agonists' (e.g. RO17-1812 and ZK 91296) and 'partial inverse agonists' (e.g. ZK 90866, FG 7142 and CGS 8216, the latter being a pyrazoloquinolinone derivative) which also act at benzodiazepine receptors.

Thus agents acting at benzodiazepine receptors form a continuum of compounds ranging from agents with potent agonist effects to agents which are full inverse agonists (see Table 20.1 for examples). The benzodiazepine receptor represents a unique example of a receptor for which ligands exist that can apparently produce opposite effects. The ligands can also be described as having either positive efficacy (benzodiazepine-like) or negative efficacy (having effects opposite to those of the benzodiazepines) whereas true competitive receptor antagonists will have no efficacy. The use of the term 'inverse agonist' may be criticised on the grounds that it lacks a sound theoretical basis. However, it does aptly reflect the complex pharmacology of benzodiazepine receptors and their ligands and raises the question of how benzodiazepine receptor occupancy is translated into different pharmacological responses.

Table 20.1. Actions of some benzodiazepine receptor ligands

	Actions	Substances
Agonists	Anxiolytic	Benzodiazepines
		Triazolopyridazines
	Anticonvulsant	CGS 9896
		ZK 91296
Antagonists		RO 15-1788
		RO 15-1788
	Anxiogenic	CGS 8216
		FG 7142
		βCCE
Inverse agonists	Convulsant	βCCM
		DMCM

The mechanism by which drugs evoke a conformational change in a receptor may be explained by assuming that the drug binds to different conformations of the receptor with different affinities. In simple terms a receptor may exist in two conformational states, namely a 'ground' state and an 'active' state which are in equilibrium, with the degree of receptor activation being dependent on the number of receptors that are present in the active conformation. An agonist may be considered to bind selectively to the active state of the receptor, an antagonist has equal affinity for both states or higher affinity for the inactive state, whereas a partial agonist will possess some selectivity for the active state but will not have as high an affinity for it as a full agonist. This concept has been applied to the benzodiazepine receptor/GABA receptor/chloride ionophore complex (Ehlert 1986). Thus in this complex the ground and active conformations may be considered to represent closed and open states of the chloride channel, respectively. GABA will bind selectively to the open state of the receptor-chloride channel complex, causing it to remain open thus enhancing chloride flux. Benzodiazepine agonists (e.g. diazepam and chlordiazepoxide) which are also considered to bind selectively to the open state of the receptor-channel complex will therefore enhance GABA binding and indeed evidence from binding studies has confirmed this. However the selectivity of benzodiazepine agonists for the open state of the receptor-chloride channel complex is not as great as that of GABA and thus benzodiazepines are unable to enhance chloride flux in the absence of GABA. The convulsant effects of DMCM may be interpreted on the basis that it binds selectively to the closed state of the receptor complex and allosterically inhibits the binding of GABA and indeed it has been demonstrated that inverse agonists like DMCM can reduce the affinity of GABA for its receptors and vice versa. A substance with equal affinity for the ground and active states should have no observable effect of its own, irrespective of whether GABA is present but should, however, antagonise the effects of other ligands which are either benzodiazepine receptor agonists or inverse agonists. So far a true benzodiazepine receptor antagonist lacking any intrinsic activity has not been found.

Dissociation of pharmacological effects: different benzodiazepine receptors

In clinical practice although a given benzodiazepine derivative is used preferentially for the treatment of a given condition (e.g. chlordiazepoxide as an anxiolytic, diazepam as a muscle relaxant, clonazepam as an antiepileptic and flurazepam and nitrazepam as hypnotics), most 1,4-benzodiazepine derivatives are able to produce all of these effects and with most of them there exists very little separation between anxiolytic and sedative properties.

Recently the 1,5-benzodiazepine derivative, clobazam (Fig. 20.1) has shown a good separation between anxiolytic doses and those producing sedation. In view of the obvious advantages of separating these properties attempts have been made to find new compounds which exhibit anxiolytic properties but which lack the sedative and ataxic effects that are manifested by most of the classical 1,4-benzodiazepine derivatives. One class of compounds that has a wide separation between anxiolytic/ anticonvulsant and sedative doses are the triazolopyridazine derivatives (e.g. CL 218, 872). These readily cross the blood–brain barrier and selectively inhibit [³H]-diazepam and [³H]-flunitrazepam binding with a potency range similar to that of the benzodiazepines themselves. Structurally triazolopyridazines are similar to the purines (Fig. 20.5). Unfortunately CL 218, 872 cannot be used clinically as it has been reported to have hepatotoxic effects in animals.

The wide range of compounds that are known to bind to benzodiazepine receptors and the difference in their range of activities has led to the suggestion that these receptors consist of a heterogeneous population. It has been demonstrated that triazolopyridazine derivatives, unlike the 1,4-benzodiazepine derivatives, inhibit the binding of [³H]-diazepam to CNS membrane preparations with shallow dose-response curves, yielding Hill coefficients of less than one (0.6–0.7) (Squires *et al.* 1979). Also incompatible with the presence of a single class of neuronal benzodiazepine receptors with non-interacting sites was the observation that β-CCE exhibited regional selectivity for benzodiazepine receptors. Its affinity for cerebellar receptors is high ($K_i = 1$ nM), whereas its potency in the hippocampus is 4–7 times less. Data from studies of various brain regions in which [³H]-flunitrazepam was displaced by β-CCE have indicated the existence of two apparently distinct subclasses of 'nanomolar' benzodiazepine receptor (termed Bz_1 and Bz_2 receptors). Further support for this came from data obtained with CL 218, 872. Analysis of the ability of this compound to inhibit the binding of [³H]-benzodiazepine derivatives to rat cerebral cortical membranes yielded curvilinear Scatchard plots, which could be resolved into two components. Thus β-CCE and some triazolopyridazine derivatives have a greater affinity for Bz_1 receptors, whereas most of the classical 1,4-benzodiazepine derivatives that are used clinically have equipotent effects at both types of receptor. Subsequent biochemical studies have shown that the cerebellum contains mainly receptors of the Bz_1 type (90% of the total) whereas 75% of cerebral cortical and 50–60% of hippocampal receptors are of this type. Significant proportions of Bz_1 receptors are also found in the amygdala and medial thalamus. Most other brain regions contain roughly equal proportions of both receptor types, but high concentrations of Bz_2 receptors have been reported to exist in the putamen, superficial layers of the superior colliculus and ventromedial hypothalamus.

The finding that [³H]-flunitrazepam becomes irreversibly (covalently) bound to its receptors when the membrane preparation is incubated in the presence of ultraviolet light has enabled the receptor-protein complex to be extracted, purified and its molecular weight determined (Sieghart & Karobath 1980). Two major protein fractions of molecular weight 55 000 and 51 000 daltons, P_{55} and P_{51}, respectively have been isolated. The P_{51} component comprised approximately 50% of the total radioactive protein in the hippocampus, 70% of that in the cerebral cortex and 90% of that in the cerebellum. This seemed to correspond very well with the distribution of the Bz_1 receptor, whereas the P_{55} fraction corresponds with the distribution of Bz_2 receptors. Thus on the basis of biochemical and pharmacological studies the possibility arises that different benzodiazepine receptor subclasses may be linked to specific pharmacological and physiological effects. If this is so, then the anxiolytic and anticonvulsant properties of these drugs may be mediated by Bz_1 receptors, whereas the sedative and hypnotic actions may be mediated by Bz_2 receptors. This obviously has important applications in the design of new drugs. Although Bz_1 and Bz_2 receptors appear to show a distinct and consistent regional distribution in the CNS and differ in ontogeny, with Bz_2 receptors predominating in the rat brain at birth and in the immediate post-natal period thus suggesting a true heterogeneity, it has not been possible to differentiate between the two receptor sub-types with monoclonal antibodies.

Endogenous ligands for the benzodiazepine receptor

As specific binding sites for benzodiazepines exist in the CNS one might address the question as to whether or not there exists a specific endogenous ligand (or ligands) for these receptors and if so what is the nature of this ligand and what is its precise physiological or pathological function. Needless to say, considerable efforts have been directed towards attempting to isolate and characterise such a ligand, which might be expected to play a fundamental role in the aetiology of anxiety. Although it is quite possible that an interaction may occur between benzodiazepine receptors and GABA receptors without invoking the existence of an endogenous ligand, or modulator, several endogenously-occurring substances have been proposed for this role in addition to the β-carbolines, considered previously.

Peptides

GABA modulin

This is a basic protein of molecular weight 17 000 daltons, located in postsynaptic membranes and is believed to non-competitively inhibit the binding of GABA to specific high affinity sodium-independent recognition sites via an allosteric mechanism (Guidotti et al. 1982; Vaccarino et al. 1985). GABA modulin has been shown to be a substrate for a Ca^{2+} and cyclic AMP-dependent protein kinase which catalyses the incorporation of 4 mol of phosphate/mol of protein. This changes the biological activity of GABA modulin, thus abolishing its inhibitory action on GABA binding. It has been suggested that as there are high concentrations of GABA in the brain, the high affinity GABA binding sites may be fully saturated with their physiological ligand (i.e. GABA) and thus lack the capacity to respond to variations in synaptic GABA concentrations. Therefore it is possible that GABA modulin could modulate GABAergic function at the synaptic level by altering the proportion of high affinity

GABA recognition sites located postsynaptically, and indeed dephosphorylated GABA modulin is known to selectively reduce the B_{max} of these high affinity binding sites. Benzodiazepine receptors and GABA modulin have different characteristics thus eliminating the possibility that they are the same entity. Nevertheless it has been proposed that the benzodiazepines interact with GABA modulin in some way such that when benzodiazepines bind to their receptors they displace GABA modulin, thus preventing it from exerting an inhibitory effect on GABA binding. The observations relating to the possible existence of GABA modulin have, however, not been confirmed by other workers.

Diazepam binding inhibitor (DBI)

It has been suggested that the brain also contains an endogenous ligand, or endacoid, that can reduce the binding of benzodiazepines to rat brain membrane preparations (Guidotti et al. 1983). This substance has been named diazepam binding inhibitor (DBI) and is a polypeptide of molecular weight 11 000 daltons. The active component of DBI is thought to be an 18 amino acid sequence (an octadecaneuropeptide, ODN; Guidotti et al. 1986; Gray et al. 1986) which is very similar in structure and distribution to another polypeptide, endozapine (Shoyab et al. 1986). DBI and ODN have been found to displace benzodiazepines and β-carbolines from synaptosomes and from cerebral cortical neurons and astrocytes in primary cell cultures (Bender & Herz 1986). Guidotti et al. (1986) studied the pharmacological profile of DBI using various techniques and reported that the peptide competitively inhibited the binding of benzodiazepines or β-carbolines to rat cerebellar granule cells in primary culture, reduced GABA-mediated chloride channel opening in spinal cord neurons as determined using the patch-clamp technique and had a proconflict effect in the rat which could be prevented by pre-treatment with RO15-1788.

Tryptophan containing peptides

If the proposed endogenous ligand for benzodiazepine receptors is a small peptide then it is possible that the receptors may be able to recognise some of its constituent amino acids. When all the naturally-occurring amino acids were tested for inhibition of [^{3}H]-flunitrazepam binding to rat brain membranes (Squires et al. 1979), L-tryptophan was found to be the strongest inhibitor (ED_{50} = 5 mM). Several dipeptides were also reported to be active, with L-tryptophyl glycine being the most potent (IC_{50} = 80 μM), making it about ten times more potent than postulated ligands such as inosine or hypoxanthine. (see Fig. 20.5). It is interesting to note that the Trp-Gly sequence is found in amino acid residues 52–58 of β-lipotrophin (Trp-Gly-Ser-Pro-Pro-Lys-Asp). This sequence also contains two other amino acids which displace [^{3}H]-flunitrazepam, i.e. proline and aspartate, and is part of a near-repeat of a sequence found in

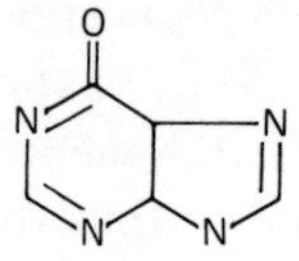

Hypoxanthine

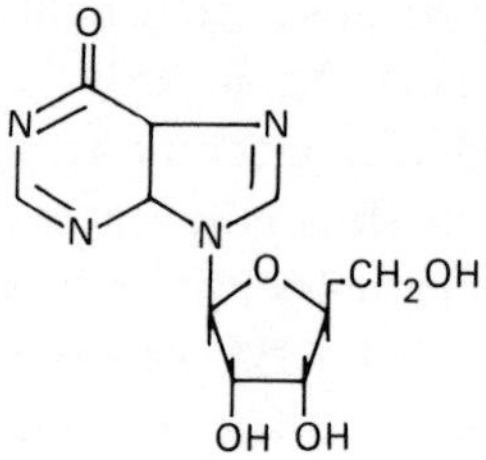

Inosine

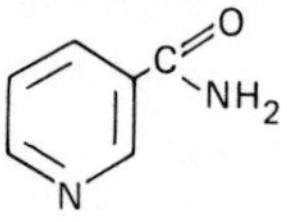

Nicotinamide

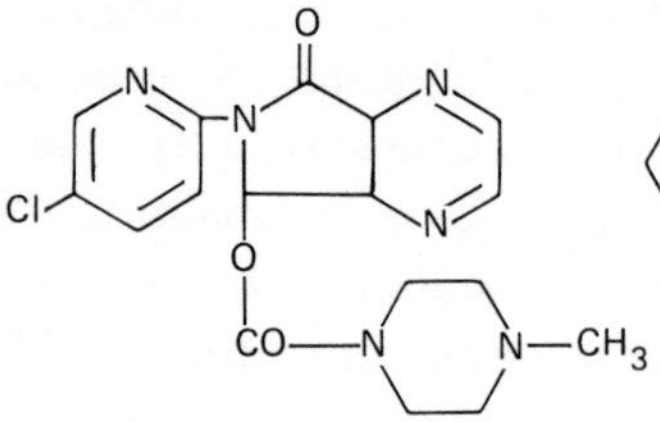

Zopiclone

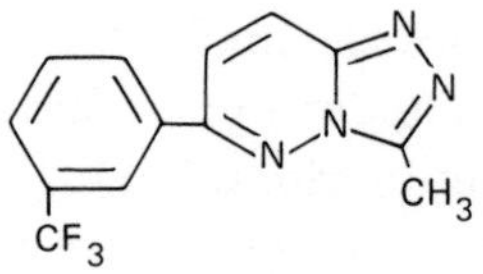

CL-218872

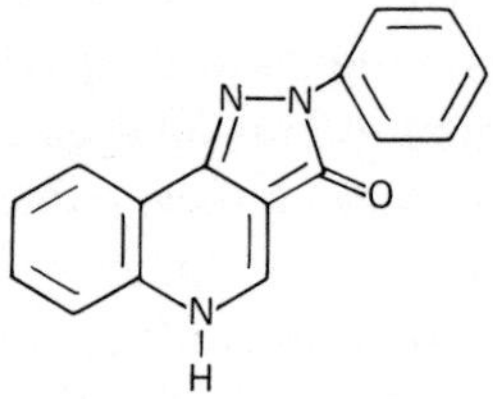

CGS-8216

Fig. 20.5. Some benzodiazepine receptor ligands.

corticotrophin (ACTH) which also occurs in a large precursor protein of molecular weight 30 000 daltons.

It is known from biochemical studies that if tryptophan-containing peptides are subjected to the same chemical procedures as those employed in the original extraction of β-CCE (i.e. heating the extract in acid ethanol at 80°C for 20 hours), then β-CCE itself is formed. Thus β-CCE may be an extraction artefact originating specifically from tryptophyl peptides that occur naturally in the CNS and, indeed a striking structural similarity between tryptophyl-glycine and β-CCE has been noted (Vellucci & Webster 1981; see Fig. 20.4). It is therefore possible that a tryptophan-containing peptide or closely related structure may prove to be an endogenous benzodiazepine receptor ligand and there is evidence that low concentrations of tryptophyl-glycine injected i.c.v. in mice have anticonvulsant properties and can potentiate the effects of diazepam (Vellucci &

Webster 1981). Tryptophan-containing peptides have been shown to exist in various brain regions (Edvinsson *et al.* 1973) but their precise function remains to be elucidated.

Inosine and hypoxanthine

Extracts from brain tissue have yielded low molecular weight, thermostable, non-lipid, non-protein compounds which competitively inhibit benzodiazepine receptor ligand binding to brain membrane fragments but have little or no affinity for peripheral benzodiazepine binding sites. These substances were subsequently identified as inosine and hypoxanthine but like other purines they are such low-affinity inhibitors of diazepam binding, with IC_{50} values ranging from 300 μm, for 2-deoxyguanosine to 2 mM for adenosine (inosine = 0.9 mM, hypoxanthine = 0.7 mM), that it seems to preclude them from being physiological modulators of benzodiazepine receptors. However, studies have revealed that only a comparatively small fraction (10–20%) of the total benzodiazepine receptor population needs be occupied to produce a pharmacological effect (see Marangos *et al.* 1979). Thus if IC_{10} or IC_{20} values for purinergic inhibition of diazepam binding are relevant physiologically, then the micromolar concentrations that exist *in vivo* (20–60 μM) could be sufficient to occupy the percentage of receptors required to produce a pharmacological effect, especially since it has been shown that the brain concentrations of inosine and hypoxanthine increase following electrical or chemical depolarisation of brain tissue.

Whilst binding studies alone cannot reliably establish whether putative endogenous ligands are agonists or antagonists, *in vivo* studies with purine derivatives indicate that they have some pharmacological properties in common with the benzodiazepines (e.g. i.c.v. inosine and 2′deoxyinosine increase seizure latency following PTZ and protect mice from convulsions induced by 3-mercaptopropionic acid). The concentrations of inosine achieved in the brain in these experiments are sufficient to inhibit the binding of [³H]-diazepam to its receptors. However, the possibility that inosine is an agonist at benzodiazepine receptors was only partially confirmed by electrophysiological studies on spinal cord neurons in primary cultures that contain benzodiazepine receptors and it is now considered unlikely to act as an endogenous ligand.

Adenosine

Adenosine, a selective agonist for purinergic P_1 receptors, has been shown to have sedative, anticonvulsant and anxiolytic effects with a potency similar to that of inosine and hypoxanthine. Benzodiazepines are able to inhibit adenosine uptake in the CNS, an effect which is not reversed by benzodiazepine 'antagonists' such as RO15-1788. Indeed, it has been demonstrated that RO15-1788 has similar effects on adenosine uptake to benzodiazepine agonists (Morgan *et al.* 1983). It is possible therefore that the intrinsic benzodiazepine-like effects of compounds such as RO15-1788 could be mediated by adenosine. It is interesting to note that doses of RO15-1788 that have no effect on convulsions induced by low doses of PTZ are able to effectively antagonise convulsions induced by the methylxanthine derivative, caffeine (Vellucci & Webster 1984a), which is believed to cause convulsions by antagonising adenosine.

Nicotinamide

This naturally-occurring substance has only low affinity for the benzodiazepine binding site *in vitro* (IC_{50} = 3.9 mM) but like the benzodiazepines, increases brain 5-HT concentrations and has hypnotic, anticonvulsant, muscle-relaxant, antiaggressive and anticonflict effects. If nicotinamide is to exert a physiological effect, then its efficacy would need to be high in view of the low concentrations present in the brain (0.1 μmol/g rat whole brain) and its low affinity for benzodiazepine receptors. Electrophysiological experiments have shown that the potency of nicotinamide is equivalent to that of the highly potent benzodiazepines (Mohler *et al.* 1979). If nicotinamide does exert benzodiazepine-like actions in the CNS, this may shed light on some mental disorders that accompany nicotinamide deficiency states. However, present evidence casts doubt on the role of this compound as an endogenous benzodiazepine receptor ligand.

A putative endogenous benzodiazepine

De Blas & Sangameswaran (1986) produced hybridoma cell lines secreting monoclonal antibodies to benzodiazepines by immunising mice with a conjugate of benzodiazepine-bovine serum albumin. These antibodies had a high affinity for diazepam, flunitrazepam and RO5-4864 (K_D values in the nanomolar range). One class of these monoclonal antibodies has subsequently been used to demonstrate the existence of endogenous benzodiazepine-like molecules in the brain. These molecules appeared to be of neuronal origin and exhibited a regional distribution. The substance was subsequently purified by immunoaffinity chromatography and shown to have benzodiazepine agonist activity, to be of low molecular weight and to be resistant to proteases. The substance was capable of displacing agonists, inverse agonists and antagonists from nanomolar (central-type) benzodiazepine receptors but not from micromolar (peripheral-type) receptors. Chemically the substance, which has been detected in bovine and human brain, has a structure similar to that of N-desmethyl diazepam, the major metabolite of diazepam. The binding of the substance to benzodiazepine receptors was increased by GABA. However, at present, its precise origin has not been established and the possibility that it originated from dietary components, e.g. fungi (in which the ability to synthesise benzodiazepines has been demonstrated) cannot be discounted.

Non-benzodiazepine anxiolytic compounds

The search for anxiolytic drugs that are devoid of sedative and ataxic properties has led to the development of several putative anxiolytics that are structurally unrelated to benzodiazepines and do not exert their pharmacological effects via an action at benzodiazepine receptors. Examples of such compounds are buspirone, ipsapirone and ritanserin. These compounds have been shown to influence 5-HT systems and have thus helped to provide further evidence for the possible involvement of 5-HT pathways in the neurobiology of anxiety.

Buspirone

The effects of buspirone in animal models of anxiety are somewhat inconsistent although clinically the drug is reported to be active as an anxiolytic, devoid of the sedative, anticonvulsant and muscle-relaxant

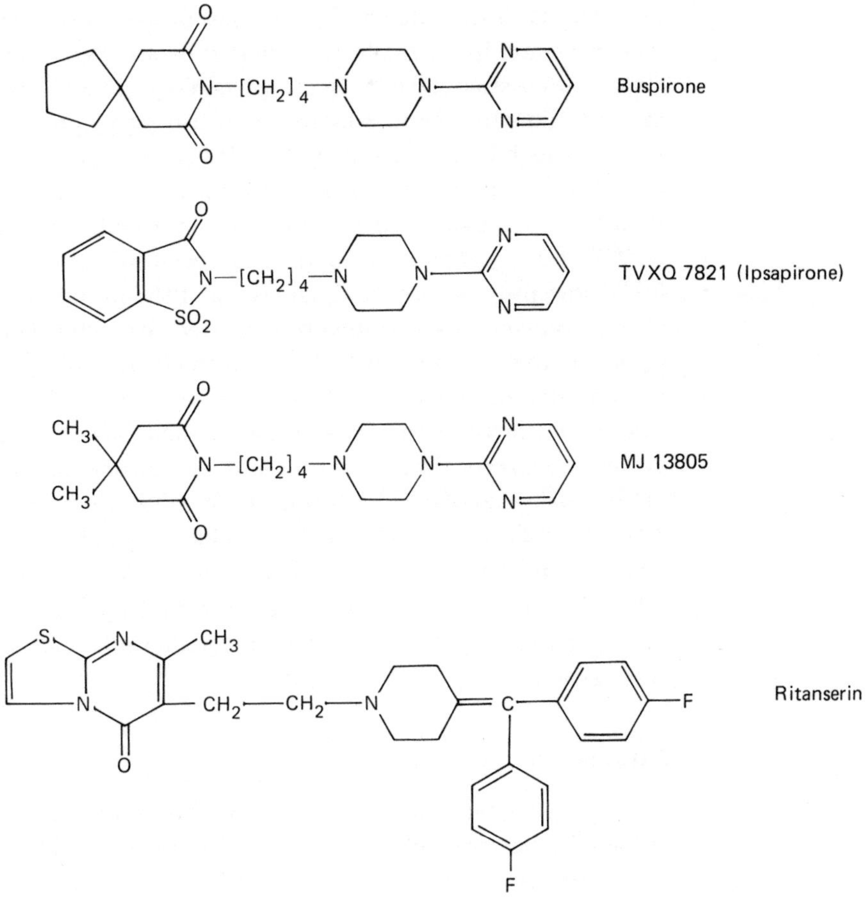

Fig. 20.6. Structures of some putative anxiolytic compounds that do not interact directly with benzodiazepine receptors.

properties which the 1,4-benzodiazepine derivatives possess (Goldberg & Finnerty 1979; Rickels *et al.* 1982). Chemically buspirone is unlike the benzodiazepines and does not interact with either benzodiazepine or GABA binding sites but there is now evidence to indicate that buspirone and its dimethyl analogue (MJ 13805; see Fig. 20.6), can specifically affect 5-HT-mediated processes in the CNS (Glaser & Traber 1983; Hall *et al.* 1985; Van Der Maelen & Wilderman 1984). More specifically buspirone is believed to act on 5-HT1$_A$ receptors (Gozlan *et al.* 1983) which may play an important role in the action of anxiolytics (see Traber & Glaser 1987).

Ipsapirone (TVXQ 7821)

This compound bears a structural resemblance to buspirone and is also selective for 5-HT$_{1A}$ binding sites in the CNS (e.g. in calf hippocampal membrane preparations) and is probably an agonist or partial agonist at these sites (Dompert *et al.* 1985; Traber *et al.* 1984). Ipsapirone also exhibits anxiolytic effects in animals but does not have sedative, ataxic or anticonvulsant effects. The proposal that the anxiolytic effects of buspirone and ipsapirone are mediated by an effect on 5-HT$_{1A}$ sites (see Chapter 9) is supported by electrophysiological and behavioural data. For example, buspirone and 8-hydroxy-2-(di-n-propylamino) tetralin (8-OH-DPAT, which binds selectively to 5-HT$_{1A}$ sites) produce dose-dependent reductions in spike height in hippocampal slice preparations and in a drug discrimination model, both buspirone and ipsapirone generalise to 8-OH-DPAT. Such generalisation did not occur if agonists for 5-HT$_{1B}$ or 5-HT$_2$ receptors were tested. Of course if the proposed anxiolytic effects of buspirone and ipsapirone are mediated through 5-HT$_{1A}$ sites it might be of use, in helping us to understand the neurobiology of anxiety, to determine the exact anatomical location(s) of these sites and to establish whether buspirone and ipsapirone act as agonists or antagonists. Current evidence suggests that buspirone and ipsapirone activate autoreceptors on the cell bodies of 5-HT neurons in the midbrain raphe nuclei, again like 8-OH-DPAT. Thus they would be able to inhibit the firing of 5-HT neurons and so decrease 5-HT function, although the result of their effects in the various parts of the brain that receive afferent projections from the raphe nuclei (e.g. in the amygdala septo-hippocampal region) is less certain.

Ritanserin

Data from ligand binding studies and the observation that it is able to antagonise but not generalise to the LSD discriminable stimulus have led to the conclusion that ritanserin is a highly selective, high affinity, slowly-dissociating antagonist at 5-HT$_2$ receptors with no partial agonist properties (Leysen *et al.* 1985). Clinical trials suggest that ritanserin has anxiolytic activity which is qualitatively different from that of the benzodiazepines (Ceulemans *et al.* 1984), although data from animal models is less conclusive (Gardner 1986; Colpeart *et al.* 1985).

Drug-induced anxiety in man

Some of the compounds that are reported to have an anxiogenic effect in animal models of anxiety also have an anxiogenic effect when administered to healthy human volunteers. Thus PTZ has been reported to induce anxiety in man when administered in sub-convulsant doses (Rodin 1958). Other drugs that are known to interact with the GABA receptor-benzodiazepine receptor-chloride ionophore complex (e.g. picrotoxin) can also induce anxiety. A congener of β-CCE which is metabolically more stable, namely N-methyl-β-carboline-3-carboxamide (FG7142), has been administered to healthy volunteers and was found to induce severe anxiety with the subjects reporting inner tension, restlessness, and a feeling of impending doom. These symptoms were accompanied by an increase in heart rate, blood pressure and plasma cortisol concentration (Dorow *et al.* 1983). Centrally acting α_2-adrenoreceptor antagonists such as piperoxan and yohimbine have been shown to have anxiogenic effects in patients and healthy subjects. For example Charney *et al.* (1983) demonstrated an increase in anxiety following 30 mg yohimbine, which could be antagonised by clonidine or diazepam, accompanied by autonomic symptoms and an increase in plasma MHPG concentrations which could be antagonised by clonidine but not diazepam.

High doses of caffeine can produce anxiety symptoms. The discontinuation of opiates, some antidepressants, clonidine and benzodiazepines themselves may sometimes be accompanied by sleep disturbances, irritability, dysphoria and anxiety, with overt seizures occurring in the more severe cases (see also Dorow 1985).

Benzodiazepines as hypnotics

Although the electrophysiological changes that characterise the different stages of the sleep-waking cycle have been extensively studied, our knowledge of the precise neuroanatomical pathways and neurotransmitter systems involved in the production of sleep and the maintenance of the sleep-waking cycle is far from complete. Consequently it is not surprising that the way in which hypnotic drugs act to produce their pharmacological effect has not been fully elucidated. In this section the neuropharmacology of sleep will be discussed only very briefly and an attempt will be made to suggest possible mechanisms whereby the benzodiazepines might exert their hypnotic effects.

Evidence obtained from studies in the cat indicates that 5-HT may be involved in sleep-regulating mechanisms. The adminstration of *p*CPA in doses that induce an 80–90% decrease in cerebral 5-HT synthesis produces insomnia (Pujol *et al.* 1971). On the other hand the adminstration of 5-HTP to *p*CPA-treated animals, in doses that restore brain 5-HT to 60% of normal levels temporarily restores normal sleep patterns. Jouvet (1972), put forward the idea that the 5-HT-containing perikarya of the raphe system play a prominent role in sleep induction, since thé destruction of this system is followed by insomnia, the degree of which is found to be proportional to the extent of the raphe lesions, and thus to the decrease in 5-HT synthesis and release. However, when the animals are monitored over a longer period of time their sleep pattern tends to return towards normal (Morgane & Stern 1974). Similarly, Adrien *et al.* (1977) lesioned the raphe dorsalis and centralis in new-born rats, but even though the 5-HT concentration was decreased to 5–10% of normal when the animals were studied at 3 weeks, their sleep pattern was not significantly different from that of the corresponding controls.

The noradrenaline-containing neurons of the rostral part of the locus coeruleus ascending in the dorsal noradrenergic pathway, are involved in the maintenance of tonic cortical arousal, as are ascending cholinergic pathways. The inhibitory effects of GABA on acetylcholine systems might also be important since cholinergic pathways appear to influence rapid eye movement (REM) sleep, changing it to slow wave sleep (see e.g. Masserano & King 1982). This will not be discussed here, however. According to the monoamine theory of sleep, it is believed that there are reciprocal interactions between 5-HT and noradrenergic systems. Thus destruction of the rostral portion of the raphe, which leads to insomnia, is followed by an increase in the activity of the noradrenergic neurons in the dorsal noradrenergic bundle, while destruction of the latter is followed by an increase in activity in the rostral raphe system and by hypersomnia. Thus it has been suggested that non-REM sleep is initiated by the synaptic release of 5-HT originating in the rostral raphe nuclei in the brainstem. REM sleep, on the other hand, is believed to be initiated by the release of 5-HT from neurons originating in the caudal raphe nuclei, whereas wakefulness and cortical arousal depend on the noradrenergic neurons of the anterior locus coeruleus. Obviously it is difficult to reconcile directly the evidence that a decrease in the activity of the raphe system produces insomnia with the idea that the benzodiazepines, which are used as hypnotics, may produce some of their pharmacological effects (e.g. anxiolytic effects) by decreasing the activity of the same system. However, the precise role of 5-HT in the regulation of consciousness is by no means unequivocal and indeed there is evidence that fails to support the theory that 5-HT plays a role in the production of non-REM sleep. Thus it has been demonstrated that electrical stimulation of raphe neurons or the administration of 5-HT precursors, fails to increase total sleep time and may even cause arousal. The release of 5-HT from the DRN is decreased during slow wave sleep and REM sleep, when compared with wakefulness and it has been reported that the raphe magnus and median raphe units exhibit reduced discharge in slow-wave sleep when compared with wakefulness. This evidence is not inconsistent with the idea that benzodiazepines may be exerting their hypnotic effect by reducing 5-HT turnover in the raphe nuclei.

In practice it is highly likely that the raphe system is not the only important site at which the benzodiazepines act to exert this effect. Indeed there is evidence that these drugs can influence the pathway that descends from the limbic forebrain to the noradrenergic cells in the locus coeruleus (Haefely *et al.* 1975), with the net effect that the overall activity of this noradrenergic pathway, which is essential for the maintenance of wakefulness and cortical arousal, is reduced, thus promoting sleep.

Evidence indicates that Bz_2 receptors may be involved in mediating the sedative/hypnotic actions of these drugs and that benzodiazepine-receptor mediated effects may be essential in the physiological control of sleep. Studies using membranes prepared from various regions of hamster brain following 50 minutes of non-REM sleep or a comparable period of wakefulness, suggest the presence of an endogenous inhibitor of benzodiazepine binding in the 3000 g supernatant prepared from the brains of awake animals, which is absent in sleeping animals. The relevance of this observation and whether or not this proposed inhibitor of benzodiazepine binding bears any relationship to the putative endogenous sleep-enhancing substance, delta sleep-inducing peptide (DSIP, Monnier *et al.* 1977) has not been established.

It is well-known that an important cause of insomnia is anxiety and indeed sleep-disturbance is a regular component of anxiety states, depression and psychotic disorders and in individuals undergoing emotional or psychological trauma. Short-acting benzodiazepines (e.g. temazepam) have been useful in promoting sleep in patients who normally have difficulty in falling asleep and it is possible that the anxiolytic action of these drugs contributes to this effect. However, as benzodiazepines in adequate doses are able to promote sleep even in normal (non-anxious) individuals or animals, the anxiolytic effect is by no means the only way whereby these drugs promote sleep.

References and further reading

Adrien J, Bourgoin S & Hamon M (1977) Midbrain lesion in the newborn rat. 1. Neurophysiological aspects of sleep. *Brain Res.* **127**, 99–100.

Barker JL & Owen DG (1986) Electrophysiological pharmacology of GABA and diazepam in cultured CNS neurons. In: Olsen RW & Venter JC (eds) *Benzodiazepine/GABA Receptors and Chloride Channels: Structural and Functional Properties.* Alan Liss: New York. pp. 135–65.

Bender AS & Hertz L (1986) Octadecaneuropeptide (ODN; 'anxiety peptide') displaces diazepam more potently from astrocytic than from neuronal binding sites. *Eur. J. Pharmac.* **132**, 335–6.

Blakely TT & Parker LF (1973) The effects of parachlorophenylalaine on experimentally induced anticonflict behaviour. *Pharmco. Biochem. Behav.* **1**, 609–13.

Braestrup C, Nielsen RF & Olsen CE (1980) Urinary and brain β-carboline-3-carboxylates as potent inhibitors of brain benzodiazepine receptors. *Proc. Natl. Acad. Sci. USA* **77**, 2288–92.

Braestrup C & Squires RF (1978) Brain specific benzodiazepine receptors. *Br. J. Psych.* **133**, 249–60.

Ceulemans D, Hoppenbrouwers ML Gelders Y & Reyntjens A (1984) Serotonin blockade or benzodiazepines. What kind of anxiolysis? *Proc. 14th CINP Congress, Florence, Abster. P727.*

Charney DS, Heninger GR & Redmond DE (1983) Yohimbine induced anxiety and increased noradrenergic function in humans: effects of diazepam and clonidine. *Life Sciences* **33**, 19-29.

Charney DS & Redmond DE (1983) Neurological mechanisms in human anxiety. Evidence supporting central noradrenergic hyperactivity. *Neuropharmacology* **22**, 1531-6.

Chopin P & Briley M (1987) Animal models of anxiety: the effect of compounds that modify 5-HT neurotransmission. *Trends Pharm. Sci.* **8**, 383-8.

Collinge J, Pycock CJ & Taberner PV (1983) Studies on the interaction between cerebral 5-hydroxytryptamine and γ-aminobutyric acid in the mode of action of diazepam in the rat. *Br. J. Pharmac.* **79**, 637-43.

Collins GGS, File SE, Hyde JRG & Macleod N (1979) The effects of 5,7-dihydroxytryptamine lesions of the median and of the dorsal raphe nuclei on social interaction in the rat. *Br. J. Pharmac.* **66**, 114P.

Colpeart FC, Meert TF, Niemegeers CJE & Janssen PJE (1985) Behavioural and 5HT antagonist effects of ritanserin: A pure and selective antagonist of LSD discrimination in rat. *Psychopharmacology* **86**, 45-54.

Cook L & Sepinwall J (1975) Behavioural analysis of the effects and mechansim of action of benzodiazepines. In: Costa E & Greengard P (eds) *Mechanism of Action of Benzodiazepines.* Raven Press, New York. pp. 1-28.

Costa E. Guidotti A & Toffano G (1978) Molecular mechanisms mediating the action of diazepam on GABA receptors. *Br. J. Psych.* **133**, 239-48.

Crawley J & Goodwin FK (1980) Preliminary report of a simple behavioural model for the anxiolytic effects of benzodiazepines. *Pharmacol., Biochem. & Behav.* **13**, 167-70.

De Blas A & Sangameswaran L (1986) Current topics. 1. Demonstration and purification of an endogenous benzodiazepine from the mammalian brain with a monoclonal antibody to benzodiazepines. *Life Sci.* **39**, 1927-36.

Dompert WU, Glaser T & Traber J (1985) TVXQ 7821: Identification of 5HT$_1$ binding sites as a target for a novel putative anxiolytic. *NS Arch. Pharmacol.* **328**, 467-70.

Dorow R (1985) Anxiety and its generation by pharmacological means. In: Iversen SD (ed.) *Psychopharmacology, Recent Advances and Future Prospects.* Oxford University Press, Oxford. pp. 100-12.

Dorow R , Horowski R, Paschelke G, Amin M & Braestrup (1983) Severe anxiety induced by FG7142, a β-carboline ligand for benzodiazepine receptors. *Lancet* **i**, 98-9.

Edvinsson L, Hakanson R, Ronnberg A-L & Sundler F (1973) Tryptophyl polypeptides in rat brain. *J. Neurochem.* **20**, 897-99.

Ehlert FJ (1986) 'Inverse agonist', cooperativity and drug action at benzodiazepine receptors. *Trends Pharmacol. Sci.* Jan. 28-32.

File SE & Hyde JRG (1978) Can social interaction be used to measure anxiety? *Br. J. Pharmac.* **62**, 19-24.

File SE, Lister RG & Nutt DJ (1982) The anxiogenic action of benzodiazepine antagonists. *Neuropharmacology* **21**, 1033-7.

File SE & Vellucci SV (1978) Studies on the role of ACTH and of 5HT in anxiety, using an animal model. *J.Pharm. Pharmac.* **30**, 105-10.

Gallager DW (1978) Benzodiazepines: potentiation of a GABA inhibitory response in the dorsal raphe nucleus. *Europ. J. Pharmac.* **49**, 133-43.

Gardner CR (1986) Recent developments in 5HT-related pharmacology of animal models of anxiety. *Pharmacol, Biochem. Behav.* **24**, 1479-85.

Geller I & Seifter J (1960) The effects of meprobamate, barbiturates, d-amphetamine and promazine on experimentally-induced conflict in the rat. *Psychopharmacologia* **1**, 482-92.

Glaser T & Traber J (1983) Buspirone, action on serotonin receptors in calf hippocampus. *Europ. J. Pharmac.* **88**, 137-8.

Goldberg HL & Finnerty RJ (1979) The comparative efficacy of buspirone and diazepam in the treatment of anxiety. *Am. J. Psych.* **136**, 1184-7.

Gozlan H, El Mestikawy SE, Pichat L, Glowinski J & Hamon M (1983) Identification of pre-synaptic serotonin autoreceptors using a new ligand, [^{3}H]-PAT. *Nature* **305**, 140-2.

Gray PN, Glaister D, Seeburg PH, Guidotti A & Costa E (1986) Cloning and expression of cDNA for human diazepam binding inhibitor, a natural ligand of an allosteric regulatory site of the γ-aminobutyric acid type A receptor. *Proc. Natl. Acad. Sci.* **83**, 7547.

Greenblatt DJ & Shader RI (1978) *Benzodiazepines in Clinical Practice.* Raven Press, New York.

Guidotti A, Ferrero P, Fujimoto M, Santi RM & Costa E (1986) Studies of endogenous ligands (endocoids) for the benzodiazepine/β-carboline binding site. In: Biggio G & Costa E (eds) *GABAergic Transmission and Anxiety. Advances in Biochemical Psychopharmacology* **41**, p. 137. Raven Press, New York.

Guidotti A, Konkel DR, Ebstein B, Corda MG, Wise BC, Krutzsch H, Meek JL & Costa E (1982) Characterization and purification to homogeneity of a rat brain protein (GABA-modulin). *Proc. Natl. Acad. Sci. USA.* **79**, 6084-8.

Hall MD, El Mestikawy S, Emerit MB, Pichat L, Hamon M & Gozlan H (1985) [³H] 8-hydroxy-2-(di-n-propylamino) tetralin binding to pre-and postsynaptic 5-hydroxy-tryptamine sites in various regions of the rat brain. *J. Neurochem.* **44**, 1685-96.

Hobbs A, Paterson IA & Roberts MHT (1984) The effects on social interaction of microinjection of R015-1788 into the nucleus raphe dorsalis of the rat. *Br. J. Pharmac.* **82**, 241P.

Hodges H & Green S (1984) Evidence for the involvement of brain GABA and serotonin systems in the anticonflict effects of chlordiazepoxide in rats. *Behav. Neural Biol.* **40**, 127-54.

Hunkeler W, Mohler H, Pieri L, Polc P, Bonetti EP, Cumin R, Schaffner R & Haefely W (1981) Selective antagonists of benzodiazepines. *Nature* **290**, 514-16.

Iversen SD (1983) Where in the brain do benzodiazepines act? In: Trimble MJ (ed.) *Benzodiazepines Divided.* John Wiley, Chichester. pp. 167-83.

Jouvet M (1972) The role of monamines and acetylcholine-containing neurons in the regulation of the sleep-waking cycle. *Ergeb. Physiol. Biol. Chem. exp. Pharmacol.* **64**, 166-307.

Lader M (1978) Benzodiazepines- the opium of the masses? *Neuroscience* **3**, 159-65.

Lader M & Petursson H (1983) Long-term effects of benzodiazepines. *Neuropharmacology* **22**, 527-33.

Lal H & Shearman GT (1982) Attenuation of chemically-induced anxiogenic stimuli as a novel method for evaluating anxiolytic drugs: a comparison of clobazam with other benzodiazepines. *Drug Dev. Res Suppl.* **1**, 127-34.

Laurent J-P, Margold M, Humbel V & Haefely W (1983) Reduction by two benzodiazepines and pentobarbitone of the multi-unit activity in substantia nigra, hippocampus, nucleus locus coeruleus and dorsal raphe nucleus of 'encephale isole' rats. *Neuropharmacology* **22**, 501-12.

Leysen JE, Gommeren W, Van Gompel P, Wijnants J, Janssen PFM & Laduron PM (1985) Receptor binding properties in vitro of ritanserin, a very potent and long-acting serotonin-S₂ antagonist. *Mol. Pharmacol.* **27**, 600-11.

Liljequist S & Engel JA (1984) Reversal of the anticonflict action of valproate by various GABA and benzodiazepine antagonists. *Life Sci.* **34**, 2525-33.

Marangos PH, Paul SM, Goodwin FK, Syapin P & Skolnick P (1979) Purinergic inhibitor of diazepam binding to rat brain *in vitro*. *Life Sci.* **24**, 851-8.

Margules L & Stein L (1968) Increase of 'antianxiety' activity and tolerance to behavioural depression during chronic administration of oxazepam. *Psychopharmacologia* **13**, 74-80.

Masserano JM & King C (1982) Effects on sleep of acetylcholine perfusion of the locus coeruleus of cats. *Neuropharmacology* **21**, 1163-7.

Mohler H, Polc P, Cumin R, Pieri L & Kettler R (1979) Nicotinamide is a brain constituent with benzodiazepine-like actions. *Nature* **278**, 563-5.

Monnier M, Dudler L, Gaechter R, Maier PF, Tobler HJ & Schoenenberger GA (1977) The delta-sleep-inducing peptide (DSIP). Comparative properties of the original and synthetic nonapeptide. *Experientia* **33**, 548-52.

Morgan D, Lloyd HGE & Stone TW (1983) Inhibition of adenosine accumulation by a CNS benzodiazepine antagonist (R015-1788) and a peripheral benzodiazepine receptor ligand (RO05-4864). *Neurosci. Lett.* **41**, 183-8.

425   ANXIETY

Morgane PJ & Stern WC (1974) Chemical anatomy of brain circuits in relation to sleep and wakefulness. *Adv. Sleep Res.* **1**, 1–31.

Nanopoulos D, Belin MF, Maitre M, Vincendon G & Pujol JF (1982) Immunocytochemical evidence for the existence of GABAergic neurones in the nucleus raphe dorsalis. Possible existence of neurones containing serotonin and GABA. *Brain Res.* **232**, 375–89.

Niehoff DL & Kuhar MJ (1983) Benzodiazepine receptors: localization in rat amygdala. *J. Neurosci.* **3**, 2091–7.

Nielsen M & Braestrup C (1980) Ethyl-β-carboline-3-carboxylate shows differential benzodiazepine receptor interaction. *Nature* **286**, 606–7.

Nishikawa T & Scatton B (1985) Inhibitory influence of GABA on central serotonergic transmission. Involvement of the habenulo-raphe pathways in the GABAergic inhibition of ascending cerebral serotonergic neurones. *Brain Res.* **331**, 81–90 (also 91–103).

Nutt DJ, Cowen PJ & Little HJ (1982) Unusual interactions of benzodiazepine receptor antagonists. *Nature* **295**, 436–8.

Oakley NR & Jones BJ (1980) The pro-convulsant and diazepam-reversing effects of ethyl-β-carboline-3-carboxylate. *Europ. J. Pharmac.* **68**, 381–2.

Olsen RW, Yang J, King RG, Dilber A, Stauber GB & Ransom RW (1986) Barbiturate and benzodiazepine modulation of GABA receptor binding and function. *Life Sci.* **39**, 1969–76.

Pellow S, Chopin P, File SE & Briley M (1985) Validation of open: closed arm entries in an elevated plus-maze as a measure of anxiety in the rat. *J. Neuroscience Methods* **14**, 149–67.

Pellow S & File SE (1984) Behavioural effects of R05-4864 a ligand for peripheral-type benzodiazepine binding sites. *Life Sci* **35**, 229–40.

Petersen EN & Scheel-Kruger J (1982) The GABAergic anticonflict effect of intra-amygdaloid benzodiazepines demonstrated by a new water lick conflict paradigm. In: Spiegelstein MY & Levy A (eds) *Behavioural Models and the Analysis of Drug Action. Proc. 27th OHOLO Conference.* pp. 467–73. Elsevier, Amsterdam.

Pieri L & Biry P (1985) Isoniazid-induced convulsions in rats: effects of R015-1788 and β-CCE. *Europ. J. Pharmac.* **112**, 355–62.

Polc P & Haefely W (1977) Effects of systemic muscimol and GABA in the spinal cord and superior cervical ganglion in the cat. *Experientia* **33**, 809.

Polc P, Mohler H & Haefely W (1974) The effect of diazepam on spinal cord activities; possible sites and mechanisms of action. *N.S. Arch. Pharmacol.* **284**, 319–37.

Pujol JF, Buguet A, Froment JL, Jones B & Jouvet M (1971) The central metabolism of serotonin in the cat during insomnia: a neurophysiological and biochemical study after p-chlorophenylalanine or destruction of the raphe system. *Brain Res.* **29**, 195–212.

Rickels K, Weisman K, Norstad N, Singer M, Stoltz D, Brown A & Danton J (1982) Buspirone and diazepam in anxiety. A combined study. *J. Clin. Psychiat.* **43**, (52), 81–6.

Rodin E (1958) Metrazol tolerance in a 'normal' volunteer population. *EEG Clin. Neurophysiol.* **10**, 433–6.

Saner A & Pletscher A (1979) Effect of diazepam on cerebral 5-hydroxytryptamine synthesis. *Europ. J. Pharmac.* **55**, 315–8.

Shephard RA, Buxton DA & Broadhurst PL (1982) Drug interactions do not support the reduction in serotonin turnover as the mechanism of action of benzodiazepines. *Neuropharmacology* **21**, 1027–32.

Shoyab M, Gentry LE Marquardt H & Todaro GJ (1986) Isolation and characterisation of a putative endogenous benzodiazepineoid (endozepine) from bovine and human brain. *J. Biol. Chem.* **261**, 1196.

Sepinwall J & Cook L (1980) Mechanism of action of the benzodiazepines: behavioural aspect. *Fed. Proc.* **39**, 3024–31.

Sieghart M & Karobath M (1980) Molecular heterogeneity of benzodiazepine receptors. *Nature* 286–7.

Sigel E & Barnard RA (1984) A γ-aminobutyric acid/benzodiazepine receptor complex from bovine cerebral cortex. *J. Biol. Chem.* **259**, 7219–23.

Soubrie P, Blas C, Feron A & Glowinski J (1983) Chlordiazepoxide reduces *in vivo* serotonin release in the basal ganglia of encephale isole but not anaesthetized cats. Evidence for a dorsal raphe site of action. *J. Pharmac. Exp. Ther.* **226**, 526–32.

Soubrie P, Thiebot MH, Jobert A & Hamon M (1981) Serotoninergic control of punished behaviour. Effects of intra-raphe microinjections of chlordiazepoxide, GABA and 5HT on behavioural suppression in rats. *J. Physiol.* (Paris) **77**, 449.

Squires RF, Benson DI, Braestrup C, Coupet J, Klepner CA, Myers V & Beer B (1979) Some properties of brain specific benzodiazepine receptors: new evidence for multiple receptors. *Pharmacol. Biochem. Behav.* **10**, 825–30.

Squires RF, Casida JE, Richardson M & Saederup E (1983) [^{35}S]-t-butyl bicyclophosphorothionate binds with high affinity to brain-specific sites coupled to γ-aminobutyric acid-A and ion recognition sites. *Mol. Pharmacol.* **23**, 326.

Squires RF, Saederup E, Crawley JN, Skolnick P & Paul SM (1984) Convulsant potencies of tetrazoles are highly correlated with actions on GABA/benzodiazepine/picrotoxin receptor complexes in brain. *Life Sci.* **35**, 1439–44.

Stein L, Wise CD & Berger BD (1973) Antianxiety action of benzodiazepines: decrease in activity of serotonin neurones in the punishment system. In: Garattini S Mussini E & Randall LO (eds) *The Benzodiazepines*, Raven Press, New York. pp. 299–326.

Tenen SS & Hirsch JD (1980) β-carboline-3-carboxylic acid ethyl ester antagonizes diazepam activity. *Nature* **288**, 609–10.

Thiebot MH, Hamon M & Soubrie P (1982) Attenuation of induced anxiety in rats by chlordiazepoxide. Role of the raphe dorsalis benzodiazepine binding sites and serotonergic neurones. *Neuroscience* **7**, 2287–94.

Thiebot MH, Jobert A & Soubrie P (1980) Chlordiazepoxide and GABA injected into raphe dorsalis release the conditioned behavioural suppression induced in rats by a conflict procedure without nociceptive component. *Neuropharmacology* **19**, 633–41.

Thiebot MH, Soubrie P & Hamon M (1984) Evidence against the involvement of serotonergic neurones in the antipunishment activity of diazepam in the rat. *Psychopharmacology* **82**, 355–9.

Thomas SR & Iversen SD (1985) Correlation of [^{3}H]-diazepam binding density with anxiolytic locus in the amygdaloid complex of the rat. *Brain Res.* **342**, 85–90.

Ticku MK & Davis WC (1981) Effect of valproic acid on [^{3}H]-diazepam and [^{3}H]-dihydropicrotoxinin binding sites at the benzodiazepine-GABA receptor-ionophore complex. *Brain Res.* **223**, 218–22.

Traber J, Davies MA, Dompert WU, Glaser T, Schuurman T & Seidel PR (1984) Brain serotonin receptors as a target for the putative anxioltic TVXQ 7821. *Brain Res. Bull.* **12**, 741–4.

Traber J & Glaser T (1987) 5-HT$_{1A}$ receptor-related anxiolytics. *Trends Pharmacol. Sci.*, **8**, 432–7.

Treit D (1985) Animal models for the study of anti-anxiety agents: A review. *Neurosci. Biobehav. Rev.* **9**, 203–22.

Vaccarino F, Tronconi BMC, Panula P, Guidotti A & Costa E (1985) GABA-modulin: A synaptosomal basic protein that differs from small myelin basic protein of rat brain. *J. Neurochem.* **44**, 278–90.

Van der Maelen CP & Wilderman RC (1984) Iontophoretic and systemic administration of the nonbenzodiazepine anxiolytic drug buspirone causes inhibition of serotonergic dorsal raphe neurons in rat. *Fed. Proc.* **43**, 947.

Vellucci SV & File SE (1979) Chlordiazepoxide loses its anxiolytic action with long term treatment. *Psychopharmacology* **62**, 61–5.

Vellucci SV & Webster RA (1981) Modification of diazepam's antileptazol activity by endogenous tryptophan-like compounds. *Europ. J. Pharmac.* **76**, 255–9.

Vellucci SV & Webster RA (1982) Antagonism of the anticonflict effects of chlordiazepoxide by β-carboline-carboxylic acid ethyl ester, RO15-1788 and ACTH$_{(4-10)}$. *Psychopharmacology* **78**, 256–60.

Vellucci SV & Webster RA (1983) Is RO15-1788 a partial agonist at benzodiazepine receptors? *Europ. J. Pharmacol.* **90**, 263–8.

Vellucci SV & Webster RA (1984)a Antagonism of caffeine-induced seizures in mice by RO15-1788. *Europ. J. Pharmacol.* **97**, 289–93.

Vellucci SV & Webster RA (1984)b The role of GABA in the anticonflict action of sodium valproate and chlordiazepoxide. *Pharmacol. Biochem. Behav.* **21**, 845–51.

Zakusov VV, Ostrovskaya RU, Kozhechkin SN, Markovich VV, Molodavkin GN & Voronina TA (1977). Further evidence for GABAergic mechanisms in the action of benzodiazepines. *Arch. Int. Pharmacodyn.* **229**, 313–26.

21   Alzheimer's disease

CHRISTINE M. SMITH

Interest in Alzheimer's disease, a degenerative disease of the brain, has increased greatly in the last ten years. Demographic trends of increasing numbers of older people in developed countries have focused attention on this condition which is associated with progressive and irreversible dementia, and is particularly prevalent in the elderly. Biochemical findings of a cholinergic deficiency in the brains of patients with this disease have provided much of the impetus for increased interest and research effort.

Dementia is a syndrome of global impairment of mental function. It has been estimated that the prevalence of dementia may be as high as 10% in people over 65 years, rising to 20% in those aged over 80. There are many causes of dementia and these include other degenerative diseases of the brain, e.g. Parkinson's disease, vascular disorder and, less commonly, toxic or metabolic conditions (Table 21.1).

Table 21.1. Examples of causes of dementia

Alzheimer's disease*
Vascular disease (= 'Multi-infarct' dementia)
Mixed Alzheimer's disease and 'multi-infarct' dementia
Parkinson's disease*
Hypothyroidism
Alcoholic dementia

*Degenerative diseases of the brain.

Alzheimer's disease alone or in combination with vascular disease is a common cause of dementia. In institutionalised patients with severe dementia, post-mortem studies have suggested that about 50% had Alzheimer's disease, approximately 20% had multi-infarct disease, and 15–20% had a combination of the two conditions. In clinical studies of patients admitted to neurological or psychiatric units for evaluation of mental function, Alzheimer's disease or an unrecognised cause of dementia, was diagnosed by exclusion of other conditions causing dementia, in 24–57% of the patients in the individual studies. These studies have used selected samples and do not give a reliable indication of the prevalence of Alzheimer's disease as a cause of dementia in the community. However, both types of investigation do indicate that Alzheimer's disease is an important cause of the severer forms of dementia which are referred for hospital evaluation and which may require institutional care in the later stages.

Pathology and clinical features

The diagnosis of Alzheimer's disease (AD) can only be made with certainty by microscopic examination of the brain. The disease is named after Alois Alzheimer (1907) who found two characteristic pathological changes, senile plaques and neurofibrillary tangles, in the brain of a middle-aged woman dying demented with memory loss, disorientation and gross deterioration of intellectual function. This patient was only 51 years old, but the clinical and neuropathological similarities between the patient's pre-senile disorder and the more common senile condition were evident to Alzheimer who believed that pre-senile and senile cases were the same disorder. Subsequently neuritic plaques consisting primarily of abnormal axon terminals associated with extracellular amyloid, and neurofibrillary tangles of paired helical filaments within the cell body of neurons have been found in both pre-senile and the more common senile cases. These plaques and tangles are not specific for AD, since they are also found in the brains of boxers known to be 'punch drunk' during life, in some patients with Parkinson's disease, and in some elderly subjects known to have had a normal intellect during life. However, in general, pathological change is less extensive in the brains of these groups compared to Alzheimer patients, where the distribution of pathological change may also be different. In AD the temporal, frontal and parietal association areas of the cortex are particularly affected, but the primary visual, somatosensory and motor areas show little damage. The hippo-campus and amygdala are also severely affected. An additional pathologi-cal change, granulovacuolar degeneration which consists of intracellular vacuoles in hippocampal pyramidal neurons is found more frequently than in normal old age. Although qualitative differences between the Alzheimer's disease presenting in younger and older patients have not been established, there are some pathological and clinical grounds for recognising a more rapidly progressive form of the disease occurring in younger patients.

Alzheimer's disease commonly presents with a relatively isolated disturbance of memory for recent events. Some features of the memory disorder are characteristic. For example, the patient has difficulty remembering peoples names, but little or no difficulty in recognising faces at least in the early stages of the disease. In some patients a language disturbance is also an early manifestation and anaphasia-like syndrome develops. Other, and usually later features include geographical disorien-tation and apraxia so that a patient may not be able to go out alone or dress himself. As the disease progresses there is a global disturbance in all aspects of higher brain function and in the later stages motor disturbance and double incontinence may occur. Despite the high prevalence and devastating nature of this condition, until recently there was very little known about it.

Neurotransmitters in Alzheimer's disease

Cholinergic system

Biochemical studies

The first large scale biochemical studies of the brains of patients with AD were begun in the early 1970s. Using post-mortem tissue from patients and age matched controls Bowen *et al.* (1976) showed a reduction of about 50% in choline acetyltransferase (ChAT) in the frontal cortex of patients with AD which appeared to be correlated with the number of plaques and tangles. This and subsequent studies showed that ChAT activity was not dependent on the agonal state of the patient and was also stable after death. In contrast, glutamate decarboxylase (GAD) levels which were also reduced in the cortex of patients with AD, appeared to be related to the terminal state of the patient, rather than the presence of AD since a slow death can produce substantial losses of GAD activity by a mechanism perhaps involving anoxia. Confirmation of reduced ChAT levels in AD soon followed and Perry *et al.* (1977, 1978) showed that the reduction of ChAT activity was greatest in the hippocampus, an area markedly affected by Alzheimer neuropathology. In addition the reduction in ChAT and also acetylcholinesterase (AChE) activity correlated with the number of senile plaques in the cortex and with the extent of intellectual impairment, using test data obtained within six months of death. Whilst the findings with ChAT suggest that a cholinergic deficit might be important in AD, the observations with AChE are more difficult to interpret since unlike ChAT it is also found in dopaminergic and noradrenergic neurons. However, ChAT activity may not be rate limiting (its theoretical capacity to synthesise ACh is far in excess of the actual rate of ACh synthesis *in vivo*), and therefore ACh synthesis from $[U^{-14}C]$ glucose, together with choline uptake was measured in cortical biopsy samples removed from demented patients for diagnostic purposes by Bowen's group. In samples predominantly from the temporal lobe, synthesis of ACh was markedly reduced only in the demented patients who showed the histological features of AD. Choline uptake and ChAT activity were also significantly reduced. These findings directly demonstrated a cholinergic deficit in AD and confirmed that previous findings of reduced ChAT levels were not due to the terminal condition of the patient or to post-mortem artefact. All these findings taken together indicated a reduction in presynaptic cholinergic activity, but most studies using quinuclidinyl benzilate (QNB) or other muscarinic ligands failed to show changes in muscarinic binding sites. This suggests that postsynaptic cholinergic receptors may be relatively intact in AD, except perhaps in the hippocampus where modest reductions in muscarinic receptors have been reported in some studies. Recent evidence for subclasses of muscarinic receptors has raised questions, however, about the status of muscarinic receptors in AD. Certainly binding studies, with the novel antagonist drug pirenzepine, do not give simple mass action binding curves and are consistent with the presence of several receptor subclasses. Its high affinity site (M_1), which is concentrated in hippocampus, cortex and striatum but not in cerebellum (or heart or ileum), see Chapter 6, is reported to be unaltered in AD but the lower affinity (M_2) sites appear to be reduced.

Cholinergic pathways

The presynaptic cholinergic deficit is not uniform for although reductions in ChAT have been found in all cortical areas examined, maximal reductions are found in temporal cortex and in the hippocampal formation. In contrast, many subcortical areas are not affected, and changes in ChAT have been shown to be confined to about a third of the areas examined. These include the amygdala and two basal forebrain areas, the septal nuclei and substantia innominata. The loss of ChAT in these forebrain areas is of particular interest as these structures are believed to represent the origins of major cholinergic projections to the hippocampus and neocortex (Fibiger 1982). Lesion of particular forebrain areas followed by determination of ChAT levels in possible target areas has been used to map projections which have been further delineated by retrograde transport studies using horseradish peroxidase injected into target areas as well as immunocytochemical techniques to directly demonstrate that cell bodies within the basal forebrain complex are cholinergic. In primates, the cholinergic cell bodies of the basal forebrain have been divided into groupings which include the medial septal nucleus, the vertical limb of the diagonal band, and the nucleus basalis of Meynert. Several other terms including the substantia innominata have been used to describe the nucleus basalis area (see Fig. 6.2). In the rat, lesions in an analogous area result in reductions in ChAT activity of up to 70% which are mainly confined to cerebral cortex, whereas lesions affecting the other cell groups reduce ChAT activity by about 70% in the hippocampal formation. Retrograde tracing studies in primates are consistent with these findings and show that whereas the nucleus basalis neurons mainly terminate in many areas in the cortex and in the amygdala, the medial septal nuclei and cell bodies in the vertical limb of the diagonal band innervate the hippocampus. With knowledge of the organisation of these cholinergic pathways, the basal forebrain nuclei have been examined in post-mortem tissue from patients with AD. Examination of the nucleus basalis has demonstrated a 70% loss of cell bodies and ChAT in this area in younger patients with AD (Coyle *et al.* 1983), which might suggest that any reduction of ChAT in the cortex results from a degeneration of cell bodies in the nucleus basalis. However, in elderly patients with AD the neuronal loss in the nucleus basalis has been found to be only slight despite reduction of ChAT in the cortex and it has been suggested that, at least in these patients, the cortical abnormality may be primary and that the alterations in the nucleus basalis may reflect retrograde changes. Moreover, findings in Parkinsonian patients, particularly those with cognitive impairment or dementia, raise questions about the fundamental importance of changes in the nucleus basalis in relation to dementia in AD. The loss of neurons from the nucleus basalis has been found to be greater in Parkinsonian patients than in elderly AD patients, although dementia is generally more severe in AD. Because of findings like these and observations that other neurotransmitters, particularly cortical somatostatin are reduced in AD, it has been suggested that the dementia of AD relates to primary cortical abnormalities. It is possible that in addition to degeneration of extrinsic cholinergic pathways to the cortex, there is also degeneration of an intrinsic cholinergic system, as lesions of forebrain areas in the rat do not totally abolish ChAT activity in the cortex. Recently immunocytochemical techniques have demonstrated ChAT positive cell bodies in the cortex of the rat. It is important to clarify to what extent any intrinsic cortical cholinergic neurons are affected in patients with AD and whether these neurons show degenerative changes. Detailed histological studies should also be carried out in the medial septal area and the nucleus of the diagonal band in AD because a variety of evidence from animal studies suggests it provides a major cholinergic input to the hippocampus formation. There is also some evidence that the hippocampus contains an intrinsic system of cholinergic neurons, but the distribution and connection of these cells, and whether they are affected in AD is not known.

Studies of both AChE histochemistry and ChAT immunohistochemistry indicate that staining for these enzymes is fairly intact in the large interneurons of the striatum and so it appears that there is some anatomical specificity in the cholinergic deficits in AD, even though its pattern has not yet been fully characterised. Further studies of the cholinergic system in patients with AD and also in animals, particularly primates, should help clarify the pathophysiology of this disease and add to our basic knowledge of the structure and function of the central cholinergic system.

Noradrenaline (NA) and 5-HT

In addition to the cholinergic deficit in AD there is also evidence for damage to an ascending noradrenergic system. Reduced concentrations of NA and also reduced activity of the noradrenergic marker, dopamine-β-hydroxylase have been found in the cerebral cortex. Noradrenergic nerve endings in the cortex arise from cell bodies located in the locus coeruleus within the brainstem (see Fig. 7.1), and there is a loss of cells in this area particularly in younger patients dying with AD. However, the cortical noradrenergic impairment does not seem to be as extensive as the cholinergic deficit and one study has shown reduced levels of ChAT irrespective of whether there was cell loss from the locus coeruleus. However, autopsy and biopsy studies in temporal cortex from patients with AD have indicated that reduced synthesis of ACh is significantly correlated with cognitive impairment whereas autopsy NA levels, although reduced particularly in early onset AD, were not related to disease severity. Levels of the major metabolite of NA, 3-methoxy-4-hydroxy-phenylglycol, were significantly increased in early onset but not late onset AD, suggesting that there is a major compensatory increase in NA turnover in younger patients dying of AD. This may account for the lack of correlation between NA levels and disease severity. Despite the loss of presynaptic NA markers, the number of cortical adrenoceptor binding sites (α and β) appears unchanged and it has been suggested that the alterations in NA neurons may not be closely related to AD. There is also some evidence of an abnormality of the 5-HT system in AD. Reduced levels of both cortical 5-HT and the metabolite 5-hydroxyindoleacetic acid (5-HIAA) have been reported in several studies. Uptake of 5-HT is also reduced in biopsy tissue from temporal cortex. The cortical 5-HT deficit may reflect damage of the ascending pathways from the raphe nucleus which shows dense neurofibrillary tangle formation and cell loss in AD. 5-HT receptors are the only ones which have been found to be consistently reduced in AD, although it is not known whether loss of 5-HT receptors occurs because of down-regulation of receptors or loss of postsynaptic cells carrying these receptors. Using displacement by spiperone to define subclasses of $5\text{-}HT_1$ and $5\text{-}HT_2$ receptors (Table 9.1) it has been found that although both types of receptor are reduced in AD, receptors of the 5-HT_2 type are predominantly affected. However, both changes in 5-HT receptors and also 5-HT concentrations do not appear to be related to disease severity.

Amino acids

In contrast to the findings on brain amine systems, changes in amino acid and peptide neurotransmitters appear to be less extensive. As described previously changes in GAD were attributed to the agonal state of the patient. Subsequently GAD activity has been found to be unchanged in cortical biopsy samples. Normal concentrations of GABA have been found in subcortical areas. Several areas of cortex have been examined and within the cortex significant reductions in GABA levels of about 30% are restricted to the temporal lobe. K^+-evoked release of amino acids has also been carried out by Bowen's group on biopsy tissue which showed markedly reduced ACH synthesis. Release of GABA, aspartate, and glutamate were no different from control values. Although this suggests sparing of cortical glutamergic neurons, findings of increased [³H]-glutamate binding in caudate nucleus may suggest up regulation of glutamate receptors in response to damage of the cortico-striatal glutamergic projection.

Peptides

Five neuropeptides, cholecystokinin (CCK), vasoactive intestinal polypeptide (VIP), somatostatin (SRIF), neurotensin (NT), and substance P (SP) have been measured in several cortical and sub-cortical areas (Ferrier *et al.* 1983). Levels of SRIF, but not those of the other four peptides were reduced in temporal, frontal and parietal cortex, but increased in the substantia innominata in AD. SRIF and also NT levels were reduced in the septum, but apart from this SRIF was the only peptide showing major alteration. It has also been demonstrated that cortical somatostatin-immunoreactive cell bodies in temporal lobe structures (temporal cortex, hippocampus and amygdala) showed neuronal degeneration and that many neurons containing tangles were also somatostatin positive (Roberts *et al.* 1985). Moreover, changes in somatostatin are significantly associated with the severity of dementia at the time of death. This has led to the supposition that cortical somatostatin containing neurons are a primary focus for AD. Until recently somatostatin was the only neuropeptide whose brain levels were known to be reduced in AD. However, the levels of corticotrophin-releasing factor (CRF) have now been found to be lowered in several brain areas of patients with AD. Although CRF levels were found to be reduced by more than 50% in frontal and temporal cortex, larger reductions were found in occipital cortex (80%) and caudate nucleus (70%). CRF receptor binding is increased in these areas and this up-regulation of receptors contrasts with decreased somatostatin receptors in AD. It is not yet known whether CRF neurons are associated with senile plaques and neurofibrillary tangles.

Relationship between cholinergic and other neurotransmitter systems and variation in the pattern of neurotransmitter deficits between different groups of patients

In some cases the changes in somatostatin (SRIF) were associated with the general pattern of neuropathological and ChAT deficits (i.e. cortex, septum, substantia innominata) but not in others (i.e. amygdala and hippocampus). Only in temporal cortex and substantia innominata was there a significant correlation between ChAT activity and SRIF levels. However, whilst the correlation was positive in the temporal cortex so that subjects who had low ChAT activity also had low SRIF levels, in the substantia innominata subjects with the lowest ChAT levels had the highest SRIF levels. The finding of concomitant changes in ChAT and SRIF may relate to severity of disease rather than a direct relationship between them. In animal studies lesions of the nucleus basalis area have been shown to result in a reduction of ChAT activity in the cortex, but to have no effect on SRIF levels. It therefore appears that SRIF is not localised in cholinergic neurons originating in the nucleus basalis area. Thus, whilst the changes found in SRIF levels may appear to be associated with damage to ascending cholinergic pathways from the basal forebrain, the relationship between these systems is not clear. In the case of CRF the loss of peptide is inconsistent with the loss of ChAT, being greatest in occipital cortex and caudate nucleus and not significantly changed in hippocampus, amygdala or substantia innominata.

In other studies of patients with AD reductions in SRIF levels have only been found in the temporal lobe. Similarly, reductions in GABA levels have been observed in several cortical areas, rather than restricted to the temporal lobe as described above. There are other indications that the pattern of neurotransmitter changes in AD varies between groups of patients. Of particular interest is a study by Rosser et al. (1984) where ChAT activity, NA, and GABA levels were measured in post-mortem tissue and the results analysed according to age of death. Patients over 80 had a relatively mild cholinergic deficit, which spared the frontal cortex, and was selective in that the only other neurotransmitter affected was SRIF and this deficit was confined to the temporal lobe, which also exhibited the lowest ChAT activity. In contrast, patients under 80 years had a more severe and generalised cholinergic deficit together with changes in NA, GABA and somatostatin in several brain areas. Although the general severity of dementia appeared to be similar in the two groups of patients, it is possible that the older group died at an earlier stage of the disease. Of course, the different patterns of biochemical deficit may also reflect a different disease process in early and late onset AD. This would agree with other evidence which suggests that both neuropathological changes and clinical features may be more severe in patients with early onset of disease.

In conclusion there are several neurotransmitter changes in AD and the relation between them is not clear. However, this should not lead to therapeutic nihilism since although the dopamine abnormality in Parkinson's disease is a critical one, this disease is also associated with a wide spectrum of other neurotransmitter changes. It may also be relevant that the cholinergic and somatostatin changes which may be more obvious in older AD patients, are significantly associated with the severity of dementia at the time of death. Whilst further studies are needed to clarify the specificity of the cholinergic deficit and the reasons for the vulnerability of cholinergic neurons the cholinergic deficit in AD has appeared of sufficient clinical relevance to encourage attempts to treat this disease by boosting central cholinergic function.

Drug therapy in Alzheimer's disease

Augmenting cholinergic function

Most studies with cholinergic drugs in AD have concentrated on attempts to improve memory in this condition and there are a number of reasons for this. Firstly, the memory defect is usually an early symptom of the disease and it is likely, as in Parkinson's disease that patients will respond better to drug treatment in the early stages of the disease before neuronal degeneration has progressed too far. Also patient compliance with test procedures is feasible in the early stages of the disease and therefore the results are more reliable and easier to interpret. Secondly, and more importantly, there is some theoretical basis to predict that cholinergic drugs might be useful in improving memory deficits. As described earlier the cholinergic deficit in the hippocampus and temporal lobes is particularly marked in AD, and there is neuropsychological evidence to suggest that damage to these areas is associated with memory disorder in man. Also in animals, hippocampal lesions particularly with concomitant amygdala lesions give rise to certain types of memory deficit. It has been known for a long time that anticholinergic drugs like hyoscine impair memory in man, and there is some evidence that cholinergic drugs for example, physostigmine, may improve memory at least in some normal volunteers (Davis *et al.* 1978). Another reason for focusing on memory in drug studies is that some test procedures are available for assessing drug induced changes. Other early behavioural symptoms of AD, e.g. impairment of judgement and logical thought are more difficult to evaluate and in any case a basic memory deficit may contribute to these.

There are three general classes of drugs available that may increase cholinergic transmission and be of potential benefit in AD (see Table 21.2). These are:

1 Drugs like choline which may increase the synthesis and/or release of ACh

2 Anticholinesterases which cross the blood–brain barrier

3 Agonists for cholinergic receptors.

Table 21.2. Some approaches to drug therapy in Alzheimer's disease

Augment cholinergic function	
1 Increase synthesis	Give precursor — choline, phosphatidylcholine (lecithin)
2 Reduce metabolism	Anticholinesterases, physostigmine, tetrahydroaminoacridine (THA)
3 Muscarinic agonists	Arecoline (also nicotinic), oxotremorine
4 Increase release	4-aminopyridine
Augment glucose and oxygen utilisation	
1 Vasodilators	Uncertain role
2 Metabolic stimulants	Co-dergocrine mesylate (ergot alkoloids), piracetam

Choline

Originally it was thought that choline, a precursor of acetylcholine, might act in analogous fashion to levodopa on the dopamine system and make more ACh available in the brain. Therefore in early studies of cholinergic agents in AD, choline in the form of a choline salt or lecithin preparation was administered. Lecithin (phosphatidyl choline) is a natural source of choline which is found in many foodstuffs including eggs and fish. On a normal diet plasma choline levels are usually maintained within narrow limits and quite large amounts of choline need to be administered to increase plasma levels significantly. In one double blind crossover study in which 9 g of choline were administered for two weeks no drug effects were observed on a large battery of memory tests (Smith *et al.* 1978). A variety of other studies of choline given in various doses and for longer periods of time have also failed to provide good evidence for an improvement in memory function. One reason for these negative results may be that ACh synthesis in cholinergic nerve terminals appears to be directly linked to choline uptake via a sodium dependent high affinity transport system which is almost completely saturated under normal conditions. In animal studies, *in vivo* and *in vitro*, increasing the amounts of available choline has not normally been shown to have any effect on turnover or release of ACh. However, choline treatment has been reported to facilitate ACh synthesis under some conditions, so that that depletion of ACh by direct electrical stimulation can be reduced by pretreatment with choline, possibly because under some conditions of increased demand a low-affinity uptake system transports the extra choline needed for ACh synthesis.

Generally it has not been possible to demonstrate an improvement in memory with choline in normal volunteers, although Sitram *et al.* (1978) found that a single 10 g oral dose of choline significantly enhanced serial learning of lists of words, with the degree of improvement produced by the drug being inversely proportional to a subject's performance on placebo. Mohs and Davis (1982) evaluated the effects of choline in subjects who had earlier received physostigmine. They found that choline had no significant effect on average performance, but the subjects who had improved most when given physostigmine tended to show slight improvement after choline. These results suggest that choline may have some weak effects on memory. Choline may also slightly potentiate the beneficial effects of anticholinesterase drugs on memory in AD.

Anticholinesterases

Small improvements in memory on word recall tasks were seen when the anticholinesterase tetrahydroaminoacridine (THA) was given in combination with lecithin to mild to moderately impaired patients with AD but did not occur when either substance was given alone (Kaye *et al.* 1982). In other studies anticholinesterase drugs given alone have improved performance slightly. The drug usually used, physostigmine, has generally been given by intravenous infusion or subcutaneous injection and laboratory-style memory tests have been used. Although small improvements in memory performance have been seen in some studies, these have often been restricted to certain types of memory test and then only to some aspects of performance. On recall tasks where patients are usually asked to remember lists of words, physostigmine appears to be more effective in reducing the number of mistakes or inappropriate responses, rather than the number of words correctly recalled (Smith & Swash 1979). Also in recognition tasks physostigmine appears mainly to reduce the number of false positive responses rather than improve identification of correct or previously shown items (Mohs & Davis 1982).

These findings of apparently selective effects of anticholinesterase drugs are perhaps not surprising. Memory is not a unitary function. Studies both in animals and man suggest that memory is a differentiated process that has various biological substrates. It may be that a multiplicity of neurotransmitter deficits and structural changes in AD mitigates against complete restoration of normal cognitive functioning. On the other hand, it may be naive to think of these rather artificial laboratory tasks as complete measures of cognitive function and indicators of what the drug may achieve in modifying everyday performance. Informed evaluation of these preliminary results and the development of rational screening tests for drugs which may produce benefit in AD must await greater knowledge of cognitive deficits in AD, and of the ways in which cholinergic drugs modify cognitive processes. In the meantime, as there is some evidence to suggest that at least some performance errors are a feature of AD, these preliminary results appear sufficiently interesting to warrant clinical trials of these drugs in AD.

One recent study which was more clinically based suggest that oral administration of physostigmine is associated with clinical improvement in a few patients (Mohs et al. 1985). This study also employed a rating scale which assessed not only memory function but also included measures of language function, apraxia and mood. Further studies will be needed to establish whether significant clinical improvement occurs. One rate limiting step in carrying out clinical trials with physostigmine is that physostigmine only has a short half-time, of about 30 minutes. Indeed in many drug studies unpromising results may have been obtained because there was little or no drug in the body. To achieve sustained plasma levels of physostigmine it will probably need to be administered as some type of sustained release preparation. The recent development of a sensitive high pressure liquid chromatography (HPLC) method, which can measure low levels of physostigmine in plasma, should prove useful in enabling rational physostigmine regimens to be developed (Whelpton & Moore 1985). Both human and animal experiments have shown that intravenously administered physostigmine has a narrow 'therapeutic window' and optimal doses vary from subject to subject. In elderly monkeys reliable improvement of memory has been demonstrated with intravenous physostigmine administration, but the optimal dose varied widely — from 0.005 mg/g to 0.05 mg/g between animals. Also although slight improvements in memory can be demonstrated in normal volunteers, larger doses worsen performance and are associated with nausea, autonomic effects and sometimes depressive symptomatology. If anticholinesterase drugs prove not to be clinically useful their evaluation will at least have contributed to the development of methodology to look at other possible approaches to treatment.

Cholinergic agonists

Both choline and AChE drugs rely on relatively intact presynaptic cholinergic neurons as a basis for their activity. This may be avoided by administering cholinergic agonists acting directly at postsynaptic receptor sites since the majority of studies have shown that these are not reduced in AD compared to age-matched controls. Unfortunately it is by no means certain that these drugs would act in a manner equivalent to ACh released from neurons. One factor to consider is that memory may depend on phasic activity in the brain and therefore 'amplification of the signal' using an AChE drug may be more appropriate than indiscriminate stimulation of receptors. Despite these uncertainties there is a small amount of evidence that this approach might be worth pursuing. Arecoline, an agonist at both nicotinic and muscarinic receptors has been shown to enhance learning in both normal young volunteers and elderly monkeys. Also in a small study an intravenous infusion of arecoline appeared to improve recognition memory in patients with AD. In contrast preliminary studies of orally administered pilocarpine have not yielded positive results in AD. The longer acting muscarinic drug oxotremorine and similar compounds are now undergoing investigation. One limiting factor with some agonists like oxotremorine is that activation of pre-synaptic muscarinic receptors occurs leading to reduced release of endogenous acetylcholine. Drugs acting with some selectivity on postsynaptic receptors are being developed and may be more successful. It is currently thought that muscarinic agonists would be most appropriate as not only do muscarinic receptors greatly outnumber nicotinic receptors in the brain, but the latter are unchanged in AD. Of course administration of muscarinic agonists will be associated with unwanted effects mediated peripherally and centrally, although unwanted effects might be expected to be less than with anticholinesterases which will facilitate transmission at all cholinergic synapses. Nausea, autonomic effects, and depressive and extrapyramidal symptoms are likely and some of these have already been reported in normal volunteer studies. With the recent growth of attempts to subdivide muscarinic receptors (see Chapter 6) it may be expected that more selective muscarinic agonists may be available in the future although studies on receptors in the brain are at an early stage. It appears from ligand binding studies that M_1 and M_2 receptors are present in the brain with the former being most numerous in neocortex hippocampus and striatum, and the latter in mid-brain, cerebellum and hind-brain. Unfortunately, little is known about the types of response mediated by these receptors.

Other means of increasing cholinergic functions

Another approach to the problem is to attempt to increase the release of ACh by the use of drugs like 4-amino-pyridine. This has been used in man in some types of neuromuscular junction disorder and preliminary studies in AD appear encouraging.

In contrast to earlier modest results with cholinergic drugs in AD, very encouraging results have been reported recently in response to orally administered tetrahydroaminoacridine (THA). This is an anticholinesterase drug with a longer biological half-time than physostigmine and although no pharmacokinetic studies have been done, it appears that its duration of action is at least 6 hours. Patients showed marked improvement in tests of orientation and memory and formal assessment of their disease severity was improved. In patients who took the drug for an average of twelve months, there were also striking improvements in everyday behaviour, so that one patient was able to resume work on a part-time basis and another to cope with housework again. Unwanted cholinergic effects such as nausea, diarrhoea and sweating were seen mainly soon after starting treatment and could be controlled either by reducing the dose or by giving the peripherally acting anticholinergic drug, glycopyrrolate. The mechanism of action of THA is unclear at present. Although its actions are usually attributed to its anticholinesterase properties, the pharmacology of THA warrants further investigation. Since it is structurally similar to 4-aminopyridine it may also increase the release of ACh. In addition, THA causes some inhibition of monoamine oxidase in rat liver. It is not known whether THA has effects on brain amine systems, but 4-aminopyridine does increase NA turnover in the brain. Possible effects on brain amine systems are worth considering because mood elevation may be associated with positive behavioural change in AD.

Other possible approaches currently being considered include alternative methods of increasing ACh synthesis, administration of a cholinergic neurotrophic factor and transplantation of cholinergic nervous tissue. The availability of acetylcoenzyme A has been suggested as a rate limiting factor worth exploring in AD. It has been shown that the synthesis of ACh is very sensitive to treatments which interfere with the oxidation of glucose or pyruvate to acetylcoenzyme-A, and further reference will be made to this later on. However, at the moment there is no practical way of increasing the availability of acetylcoenzyme A.

Another suggestion recently put forward is that AD, may result from the lack of a neurotrophic hormone released from target cells of cholinergic afferents. This has been argued because a large reduction in ChAT in the nucleus basalis area and the neocortex has been seen in elderly cases of AD, yet the number of cells in the nucleus basalis was very near normal. Degenerative changes in subcortical nuclei may therefore be secondary to degeneration of cortical cholinergic axons brought about by a deficiency of a trophic factor. It has also been postulated that somatostatin or a somostatin-like peptide could under normal circumstances control the release of such a neuronal trophic factor. It is therefore possible that treatment with a cholinergic neurotrophic factor or suitable peptide, might reduce degeneration of central cholinergic systems in Alzheimer's disease. The effects of cholinergic neurotrophic factors on central neurons are being investigated but animal studies of the effects of somatostatin on memory have been disappointing.

In Parkinson's disease attempts are being made to correct for dopamine deficiency by transplanting fetal brain tissue into the caudate nucleus. Some regeneration of central cholinergic connections has been observed in animals with central neural transplants and transplants from the septal area have been reported to reverse learning deficits in aged rats. It is therefore feasible that in the future this approach may be attempted in AD.

Miscellaneous drugs

It has been shown that patients with AD can respond favourably to antidepressant drugs with a reduction in confused behaviour, presumably because depressive features are exacerbating the organic dementia. However, it is common experience that tricyclic antidepressant therapy often increases confusion in AD patients and it is therefore wise to give one of the less sedative drugs, e.g. imipramine. Also in view of the anticholinergic properties of some of these drugs, and the cholinergic deficit in AD an appropriate choice is one of the newer drugs, not only with less sedative properties, but with minimal anticholinergic actions too.

The point has already been made that in AD the severity of dementia is correlated to the amount of brain tissue damaged. This is consistent with studies of cerebral blood flow and oxygen and glucose utilisation which also correlate with severity of dementia. It was assumed for many years that most types of senile dementia including AD were actually caused by reduced blood supply to the brain. On the basis of this several vasodilator drugs were introduced including cyclandelate which is still in use. However, this approach has recently been largely abandoned as it seems likely that reduced blood flow is secondary to decreased neuronal activity in AD. In addition there has been doubt whether these drugs achieve their aim because being nonselective they have peripheral vasodilator effects and may cause a net reduction in cerebral perfusion. It has also been considered that reduced glucose and oxygen utilisation is secondary to degeneration of brain tissue. However, there has been a recent revival of interest in drugs that may be 'metabolic stimulants'. This is because some of these drugs have yielded positive behavioural effects in animal studies. There is also some indirect evidence that a metabolic defect many underlie the cholinergic deficiency in AD.

Hypoxia has been found to greatly reduce the synthesis of ACh. Even a reduction in oxygen supply of 10% decreases the synthesis of ACh by about 90% but much larger reductions in oxygen supply than this are necessary to reduce ATP levels. It is thought that this preferential reduction in ACh synthesis occurs because glucose and pyruvate are used for ATP production rather than synthesis of acetyl CoA for acetylation of choline to ACh.

In summary it is considered that as both brain carbohydrate metabolism and ACh synthesis are reduced in AD, 'metabolic stimulants' are worth trying. It is important to note that in the past and sometimes now, some of these drugs are actually classified as vasodilators because they increase local blood supply by promoting carbon dioxide formation. Co-dergocrine mesylate, a combination of ergot alkaloids is marketed as Hydergine and is the oldest of these drugs. It is still widely used both in AD and in multi-infarct dementia but there is a lot of uncertainty about it's mode of action and efficacy. There is some evidence in animals that it increases electrical activity of the brain and can promote glucose metabolism under conditions of ischemia. Many controlled clinical trials of this drug have been carried out and positive results obtained in some of these. Interpretation of these results is made difficult by the fact that patients with various types of dementia, not just AD, have usually been included. Also many different types of assessment procedures have been used to evaluate the drug, and actual measures of cognitive performance have not usually been included. One review of controlled clinical trials reported statistically significant improvement in the behaviour of patients with senile dementia of mixed aetiology in a large proportion of trials and by careful analysis of the measures used suggested that any improvement in behaviour may be secondary to an antidepressant effect of Hydergine. However, in some studies there appears to be some evidence of improvement in cognitive function independent of an improvement in mood. There are several other metabolic stimulants also of a fairly long history which are not in routine clinical use at the moment. These include centrophenoxine and nafronyl, but the efficacy of these is uncertain. There is now much more interest in piracetam, which is also usually classified as a metabolic stimulant, although it is also considered to be a so-called 'nootropic drug'. Piracetam is a cyclic derivative of γ-aminobutyric acid but it does not appear to act as an agonist or antagonist with any known transmitter substance. The drug has been shown to increase levels of ATP and this property is currently thought to be responsible for some improvement of learning in animal studies. Bartus *et al.* (1983) have shown that piracetam can improve memory in some elderly monkeys. Despite this, clinical studies, both in AD and multi-infarct dementia have not given clear cut results. However, the findings in animal studies have been sufficiently encouraging to prompt development of piracetam analogs including oxiracetam and pramiracetam and these drugs are being evaluated in AD.

Finally it should be mentioned that there have been speculations that certain peptides, e.g. adrenocorticotrophic hormone (ACTH) and vasopressin, and also opioid antagonists might be usefully employed in AD, but preliminary clinical studies have not been encouraging.

Conclusion

Many drug treatments have been evaluated in Alzheimer's disease and some of these are still in routine use. Despite this, there is no drug of established efficacy to treat cognitive deficits in this condition. However, the prospects for development of such a drug are considerably brighter than they were ten years ago. The recent study of neurotransmitter systems means that a rational approach to treatment is now being pursued and preliminary attempts to boost cholinergic function do appear promising. At the same time it has been recognised that some established psychoactive drugs hitherto used indiscriminantly to treat some of the symptoms of AD, e.g. amitriptyline for depressive symptoms and chlorpromazine for severe behavioural disturbance may exacerbate confusion and are best replaced by drugs of their class or alternative drugs with less anticholinergic properties. The neuropharmacological developments have also directed attention to the necessity for accurate diagnosis of AD during life and the need for better tools in order to assess performance both in the laboratory and when this appears promising, in everyday life. They have also focused attention on the need to identify the nature of the processes causing a fairly selective degeneration of some neurotransmitter pathways rather than others. It is likely that any of the putative pharmacological approaches discussed may only at best have a modest effect in temporarily alleviating symptoms and attempts to find out the cause of the disease should also be rigorously pursued. In some cases, particularly with younger patients, there is a hereditary basis for AD but there must at least be another factor, possibly viral or environmental, that must be present for the disease to develop, especially in older patients. There is no doubt that research into AD will continue to be carried out on every level because the scale of the problem is enormous, both in economic and in human costs.

(*See Addendum, p. 444.*)

References and further reading

Alzheimer A (1907) Uber eine eigenartge Erkrankung der Hirnrinde. *Zentralbl. Nervenheilk* **30**, 177-9.

Bartus RT, Dean RL & Beer B (1983) An evaluation of drugs for improving memory in aged monkeys: implications for clinical trials in humans. *Psychopharmacol. Bull.* **19**, 168-84.

British Medical Bulletin (1986) **42**, No 1.

Bowen DM. Smith CB, White P, & Davison AN (1976) Neurotransmitter-related enzymes and indices of hypoxia in senile dementia and other abiotrophies. *Brain* **99**, 459-96.

Coyle JT, Price DL & De Long MR (1983) Alzheimer's disease: A disorder of cortical cholinergic innervation. *Science* **219**, 1184-9.

Davis KL, Mohs RC, Tinklenberg JR, Pfefferbaum GA, Hollister LE & Kopell BS (1978) Physostigmine: Improvement of long term memory processes in normal humans. *Science* **201**, 272-4.

Ferrier IN, Cross AJ, Johnson JA, Roberts GW, Crow TJ, Corsellis JAN, Lee YC, O'Shaughnessy D, Adrian TE McGregor GP, Baracese-Hamilton AJ, & Bloom SR (1983) Neuropeptides in Alzheimer type dementia. *J. Neurol. Sci.* **62**, 159-70.

Fibiger HC (1982) The organisation of some projections of cholinergic neurons of the mammalian forebrain. *Brain Res. Rev.* **4**, 327-88.

Kaye WH, Sitaram N, Weingartner H, Ebert MH, Smallberg S & Gillin J (1982) Modest facilitation of memory in dementia with combined lecithin and anticholinesterase treatment. *Biol. Psych.* **17**, 275-80.

Mohs RC & Davis KL (1982) A signal detectability analysis of the effect of physostigmine on memory in patients with Alzheimer's disease. *Neurobiol. Aging* **3**, 105-10.

Perry EK, Perry RH, Blessed G & Tomlinson BE (1977) Necropsy evidence of central cholinergic deficits in senile dementia. *Lancet* **i**, 189.

Perry EK, Tomlinson BE, Blessed G Bergmann K, Gibson PH & Perry RH (1978) Correlation of cholinergic abnormalities with senile plaques and mental test scores in senile dementia. *Br. Med. J.* **ii**, 1457-9.

Roberts GW, Crow TJ & Polak JM (1985) Location of neuronal tangles in somatostatin neurones in Alzheimer's disease. *Nature* **314**, 92-4.

Rossor MN (1982) Neurotransmitters and C.N.S. disease – Dementia. *Lancet* **ii**, 1200-04.

Rossor MN, Iversen LL, Reynolds GP, Mountjoy CQ & Roth M (1984) Neurochemical characteristics of early and late onset types of Alzheimer's disease. *Br. Med. J.* **288**, 961-4.

Sitaram N, Weingartner H, & Gillin JC (1978) Human serial learning: Enhancement with arecoline and choline and impairment with scopolamine. *Science* **201**, 274-6.

Smith *et al.* (1978) Choline in Alzheimer's disease. *Lancet* **ii**, 318.

Smith CM & Swash M (1979) Physostigmine in Alzheimer's disease. *Lancet* **i**, 42.

Smith CM (1984) Drugs and human memory. In: Sanger DJ & Blackmore DE (eds), *Aspects of Psychopharmacology*. Methuen, London. pp. 140-74.

Soni N & Kam P (1982) 4-aminopyridine - a review. *Anaesth. Intens. Care* **10**, 120-5.

Summers WK, Majovski LV, Marsh GM *et al.* (1986) Oral tetrahydroaminoacridine in long-term treatment of senile dementia, Alzheimer type. *N. Eng. J. Med.* 315, 1241-5.

Whelpton R & Moore T (1985) Sensitive liquid chromatographic method for physostigmine in biological fluids using dual-electrode electrochemical detection. *J. Chromatography* **341**, 361-71.

Editorial addendum

Amino acids in Alzheimer's disease

One stimulus to the study of ACh function in AD was the knowledge that antimuscarinic drugs impair memory acquisition. Other drugs which cause amnesia are the dissociative anaesthetics such as phencyclidine and ketamine, which are non-competitive antagonists at the excitatory amino acid NMDA receptor (Chapter 13) and the benzodiazepines, which augment the action of GABA at the $GABA_A$ receptor.

NMDA antagonists block learning behaviour in animals and the long term potentiation (LTP) in hippocampal neurons which is thought to be important in the memory process. These properties would not make such drugs obvious candidates for the treatment of AD except that the excitatory amino acid can also be neurotoxic. High concentrations of glutamate may produce biochemical changes like those seen in AD, and NMDA applied to the cortex of rats produces retrograde degeneration of the important cholinergic neurons in the nucleus basalis. Of more relevance is the fact that anoxic destruction of cultured hippocampal or cortical neurons can be prevented by NMDA antagonists as can the neuronal damage that follows forebrain ischaemia after vascular occlusion *in vivo*. Thus it appears that many of the neurons important for memory acquisition and function may be destroyed by the excessive activation — presumably through endogenously released glutamate — of the same NMDA receptors that are normally involved in memory processing. Whilst the case for glutamate and NMDA receptor dysfunction in AD obviously requires further study (see Maragos *et al.* 1987), especially as reductions in NMDA receptors have been reported, it appears that glutamate neurons may also suffer the same degeneration as afflicts others in AD. At present it seems that any value of the NMDA antagonists in protecting against neuronal damage could be offset by their blocking normal memory acquisition.

Since benzodiazepines cause amnesia, their antagonists and more particularly the inverse agonists (Chapter 20), might have the opposite effects. In humans, one benzodiazepine antagonist, the β-carboline derivative ZK 93426, has been reported to show some improvement in the performance of learning and memory tests without invoking anxiety. It also improves acquisition in animal learning tests and counteracts the impairment in acquisition caused by scopolamine, as does the β-carboline inverse agonist DMCM. The role of benzodiazepines and GABA in memory acquisition and in AD is uncertain but diazepam, like muscimol, inhibits ACh release and turnover in rat cortex and there is a high concentration of benzodiazepine binding sites on the cholinergic neurons of the substantia innominata. Thus the cholinergic innervation of the cortex may come under a GABA inhibitory control augmentable by benzodiazepine agonists but reduced by their antagonists or inverse agonists. Any possible value of benzodiazepine antagonists or inverse agonists in AD (see Sarter *et al.* 1988) could, however, be countered by the fact that such patients may need to be sedated by benzodiazepines. Obviously the treatment of AD through manipulating the amino acids presents many problems.

References

Maragos WF, Greenamyre JT, Penny Jr, JB & Young AB (1987) Glutamate dysfunction in Alzheimer's disease: an hypothesis. *Trends Neurosci* **10**, 65–8.
Sarter M, Schneider HH & Stephens DN (1988) Treatment strategies for senile dementia: antagonist β-carbolines. *Trends Neurosci.* **11**, 13–17.

Pain transmission and analgesia

A.H. DICKENSON

Pain is a common but uniquely personal sensation. In addition to the sensory, psychological and indeed emotional responses to the stimulus, autonomic and motor reactions are intermingled with the unpleasant nature of the stimulus. Whether provoked by trauma, surgery, disease, inflammation or other causes, pain represents a major clinical problem. It has become apparent that pain can be subdivided into acute or chronic forms. Acute pain does not outlast the tissue pathology itself and effectively serves as an important survival or warning signal as witnessed by the poor prognosis of those, thankfully rare, suffering from a congenital insensitivity to pain. Chronic pain, on the other hand, outlasts the normal healing period or results from a chronic tissue pathology and can have adverse effects on both the quality and duration of life, due to sympathetic, motor and psychological disturbances (insomnia, anorexia, depression, anxiety etc.) resulting from the continuing pain.

Although the treatment, care and outcome of these two forms of pain differ the treatment in terms of analgesic drugs does not and choice of analgesics relates more to the degree of severity of the pain than its duration.

The two main groups of analgesic drugs are the non-steroidal anti-inflammatory drugs (NSAIDs) and the opiate analgesics such as morphine. The former are only really effective against mild to moderate pain and opiates are used for moderate or severe suffering. The NSAIDs have predominately peripheral effects although some as yet poorly characterised central effects have been described. By contrast, the opiates produce analgesia by central actions although their side-effects arise from both central and peripheral actions.

The past decade has seen an enormous increase in our understanding of how peripheral stimuli are transmitted to, received by and modulated in the central nervous system. In addition to the therapies derived from this knowledge there has been a corresponding increase in our comprehension of the pharmacology of pain and analgesia particularly with regard to the mode of action of opiate compounds. Another intensive field of study has been the attempts to identify the neurotransmitters in the afferent and intrinsic neural circuits involved in transmitting and modulating painful messages.

The pathways of pain, if indeed they exist in a specific sense, are complex and subject to modulatory influences at many stages between the periphery and the higher centres of the CNS. However, there are neural circuits within which afferent fibres and neurons can be characterised as responding to noxious stimuli and hence can be presumed to be involved in pain processes.

Pain receptors, unlike other sensory receptors such as Pacinian corpuscles which respond to skin indentation, have not been identified. It is therefore presumed that nociceptors, pain sensory receptors, must be the free bared nerve endings found profusely in the dermal and epidermal layers. Pain is transmitted from these free endings by an unknown transduction process but the endings connect to the spinal cord, where the first synapses occur, by the Aδ, fine myelinated or C fibres which remain unmyelinated. Since these fibres have little or no myelin, they conduct slowly, Aδ fibres in the range of 4–30 m/sec and C fibres less than 2.5 m/sec. Hence in a large mammal such as man, noxious messages from the feet may take a second to reach the lumbar spinal cord.

These primary afferent fibres, accessible to electrophysiological techniques in man and animals, are responsive to noxious stimuli. Some high threshold thermoreceptive or mechanoreceptive Aδ fibres have been found but many of the C fibres are polymodal responding to intense thermal, mechanical and chemical stimuli and exhibit activity proportional to the intensity of the stimulus. However, there is evidence for sensitisation and desensitisation of the receptor. In addition to the innervation of cutaneous tissue, Aδ and C fibres innervate cardiac muscle and the tooth pulp and analogous fibres (group III and group IV afferents), carry painful information from the skeletal muscle.

The non-steroidal anti-inflammatory drugs (NSAIDs) block the cyclooxygenase which converts arachidonic acid to prostaglandins and so are able to prevent the sensitisation of receptors to alogenic substances — hence their peripheral analgesic effects. Local anaesthetics, either by a direct action on the fibres or on the dorsal root ganglion, can actually block the transmission of the sensory signals.

It is at the next stage in the pathway that opiates can act both at the level of the spinal cord, where the first synapses occur, and higher in the CNS. Opiates can reduce the pain messages at the spinal level either by direct actions within the cord or through controls descending from the brain. These descending controls together with the local controls within the spinal cord produce powerful effects which can alter the intensity, modality, spatial and temporal aspects of the noxious messages. Since it is at the level of the spinal cord that the noxious messages can be greatly altered, before being transmitted onwards and where reflex motor responses to pain are generated, it is obviously important to known how the messages are mediated and modulated in the spinal cord.

The axons of the stimulated cells in the spinal cord pass upwards towards higher centres of the CNS in addition to generating local circuits. The ascending nociceptive pathways travel in the ventrolateral and dorsolateral funiculi of the spinal cord and terminate mainly in the

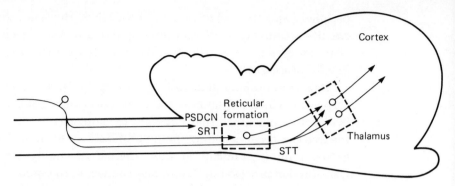

Fig. 22.1. Ascending nociceptive pathways from spinal cord to reticular formation, thalamus and cortex. PSDCN, postsynaptic dorsal column nucleus; SRT, spinoreticular tract; STT, spinothalamic tract.

thalamus and reticular formation over a wide area. Some of the spinoreticular axons then project to the thalamus and further connections arise from this latter area to cortical regions (Fig. 22.1). Although all these sites are potential areas of pain modulation the profound changes at the spinal level influence the high representation of pain at this first stage in the pathway.

In the following sections I will consider the evidence for various substances that have been implicated as neurotransmitters involved in the synaptic transmission of nociceptive inputs either by:

1 their release from primary afferent nerve terminals or,

2 their role in transmission within the dorsal horn or,

3 in mediating descending control over the response to afferent inputs.

Primary afferent neurotransmitter candidates

Peripheral fibres have been divided into several classes on the basis of their pattern of innervation, function and diameter but under non-pathological conditions the fine diameter thinly myelinated Aδ and unmyelinated C fibres carry the majority of painful messages although these fibres may well subserve other functions.

The cell bodies of all peripheral fibres located in the spinal and trigeminal ganglia form both a peripheral and a central process. The large A fibres convey mainly innocuous tactile and proprioceptive information. The peripheral nociceptors which are excited by high intensity mechanical, electrical, thermal and noxious chemical stimuli are probably undifferentiated free endings and their central terminals can now be mapped using sensitive anatomical techniques. The nociceptor population of afferents in these fibre populations are mostly polymodal — particularly in the rat which has been widely used in these studies — and so respond equally well to the various forms of noxious stimuli.

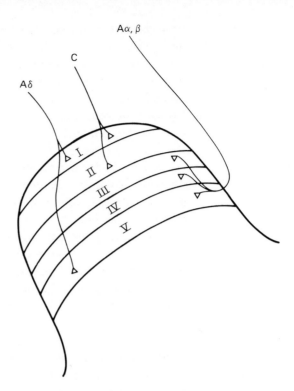

Fig. 22.2. Schematic representation of the termination of different afferent inputs in the various lamina of the dorsal horn of the spinal cord. Note that whilst most nociceptive fibres (C and Aδ) terminate in lamina I and II (apart from some Aδ in lamina V), the non-nociceptive (Aα and β) terminals are mainly found in the deeper lamina III, IV and V.

These fine afferent fibres synapse in the outer or superfical layers of the dorsal horn of the spinal cord, above and in a zone which because of its translucent appearance in unstained sections is known as the substantia gelatinosa. The tactile fibres terminate deeper in the dorsal horn (Fig 22.2). This separation of terminations has been used in conjunction with mapping the location of the various putative primary afferent neurotransmitters using immunocytochemical means and has proved a useful technique in linking mediator with modality. On the basis of this anatomical arrangement, nociceptive neurons in the dorsal horn, some of which are projection cells sending axons into the ascending spinoreticular and spinothalamic tracts, respond either exclusively or with an additional tactile input to noxious stimuli depending on their location.

By default, the transmitter(s) in the primary afferent nociceptive fibres are likely to be either amino acids or peptides. The well demonstrated roles of ACh and NA in other parts of the nervous system are not paralleled in the dorsal horn and 5-HT, DA and GABA, other seemingly likely candidates, are clearly not involved in pain transmission from the periphery to the spinal cord.

The two major amino acids which may have an excitatory role in the primary afferent transmission are L-glutamate and L-aspartate. The techniques used at present cannot separate out the metabolic from the transmitter roles of these compounds nor has their anatomical location been charted. There is, however, evidence for glutamate in synaptosomes, an uptake system in afferent terminals and small ganglion cells and release from large diameter dorsal column fibres. There is an uneven distribution of glutamate in the spinal cord and there are reports of a possible reduction from control levels following peripheral nerve lesions. Dorsal root ganglion cells, grown in culture with spinal cord cells have been used as a model of transmission into the spinal cord. In this system the fast EPSP recorded in the spinal neurons by stimulation of a ganglion cell seems to be produced by glutamate. The evidence for a role of aspartate is scanty and overall neither of these amino acids can as yet be assigned a role in afferent neurotransmission especially with regard to a particular modality.

One is therefore left with peptides and there has been much interest currently in these compounds with special attention paid to substance P. The approaches and conclusions reached provide a good illustration of the modern techniques required and associated pitfalls encountered in the study of transmitter function in defined pathways for relatively novel compounds.

substance P is an eleven amino acid peptide discovered in 1931 by von Euler and Gaddum. After a flurry of intense research over the past few years, it has now been identified in both small cell bodies in the dorsal root ganglion and in central terminals in the superficial dorsal horn. It is released by peripheral noxious stimuli, decreased levels accompany dorsal root section and local application excites nociceptive neurons although often with a long latency and slow offset of response. Interpretation of some of these results is difficult since there are intrinsic and bulbospinal substance P neurons but overall the results indicate some role in afferent transmission in C fibres.

Proof of such a role has been hampered by the lack of specific or suitable substance P antagonists but recent studies suggest that these compounds, which have potential as analgesic agents, may soon become available. Because of the lack of antagonists many studies on substance P have made use of the dramatic effects of capsaicin, the pungent ingredient in the chilli pepper. Capsaicin has a neurotoxic effect on $A\delta$ and C fibres when given to neonatal animals but spares the cell bodies. Applied to man (onto the skin) capsaicin elicits a sensation of burning pain. Hence changes following capsaicin treatment have been studied.

The administration of capsaicin at first releases then depletes the spinal cord of substance P from the primary afferents and the animals so treated have a reduced sensitivity to mechanical and chemical noxious stimuli but not always to thermal stimuli. Acute administration of capsaicin to adult rats depletes substance P without destruction of the peripheral C fibres and again the behavioural responses to noxious stimuli are reduced.

The ensemble of these studies lead to the concept that substance P was a, or the, primary afferent transmitter in pain pathways. Whilst seemingly justified by the available evidence two findings have led to a reappraisal of this role. Firstly it was realised that substance P was not the only peptide influenced by capsaicin and that vasoactive intestinal peptide (VIP), somatostatin (SRIF) and cholecystokinin (CCK), which are all located in primary afferents, like substance P, could be similarly depleted. Hence any or all of these peptides may fulfill the role suggested for substance P by the experiments with capsaicin. Additionally local application of capsaicin to a nerve which depletes substance P does not alter C fibre transmission into the spinal cord but rather would seem to impair the somatotopic map of the outside world since receptive fields of central neurons are shifted. It is hence conceivable that the nociceptive deficits after capsaicin may result from the inability of the animal to locate the stimulus.

Whilst the role of substance P remains debatable, other possible candidates mount up. As stated before, SRIF, VIP and CCK are contained in and released from small afferent fibres and although the latter peptides are clearly excitatory some studies indicate inhibitory effects of somatostatin: whether this is primary afferent inhibition or an effect mediated by interneurons is unclear. Somatostatin is located in small ganglion cells which do not contain substance P whilst CCK coexists with substance P and so the possibility of a separate or simultaneous release of these latter peptides exists. Another peptide, methionyl-tyrosyl-lysine may be an inhibitory primary afferent transmitter in proprioceptive fibres and there are now hints that ATP may be another candidate although the modality of the afferents using ATP is unknown.

The role of VIP and CCK in the spinal cord are unknown although the former seems to be located in visceral afferents and not cutaneous nerves. Both peptides are found in extremely high concentrations in forebrain areas and electrophysiological experiments in these areas have demonstrated powerful excitatory effects of these compounds.

Moving centrally into the spinal cord the existence of substance P, somatostatin, CCK and VIP in intrinsic neurons as well as the afferents has been demonstrated but other opiate and non-opiate peptides and amino acids are present leading to a complex pharmacological and physiological organisation. Thus whilst the precise neurotransmitter(s) involved in the transmission of afferent sensory nociceptive inputs into the cord is uncertain there is much evidence for the peptides and non-peptide substances discussed above in playing some role in afferent transmission. It is now necessary to consider the neurotransmitters involved in the local modification of sensory input within the dorsal horn of the cord.

Dorsal horn neurotransmitter candidates

Table 22.1 lists the ever increasing number of opioids and other peptides as well as amino acids located in the dorsal horn. In addition to substance P and somatostatin, neurotensin has been shown to influence nociceptive

Table 22.1. Neurotransmitter candidates found in the dorsal horn of the spinal cord and thought to be associated mainly with the terminals of primary afferent, dorsal horn neurons or descending axons

Primary afferent fibres	Substance P
	Somatostatin
	Vasoactive intestinal polypeptide (VIP)
	Cholecystokinin (CCK)
	Glutamate
	ATP
Dorsal horn intrinsic neurons	Enkephalin
	Dynorphin
	Substance P
	Somatostatin
	VIP
	CCK
	Bombesin
	Neurotensin
	Glutamate
	Aspartate
	GABA
	Glycine
Descending axons	5-Hydroxytryptamine
	Noradrenaline
	Dopamine
	Enkephalin
	Substance P
	Thyrotrophin releasing factor (TRH)

neurons but there is a lack of information regarding the exact role of these peptide compounds in central sensory processing.

Glutamate and aspartate excite most classes of dorsal horn cells and are hence unlikely to play exclusive roles in nociceptive events, although subdivisions (see Chapter 13) of amino acid receptors may have differential locations.

GABA, in contrast to the excitatory amino acids, can be localised anatomically by mapping the distribution of glutamic acid decarboxylase (GAD), the enzyme involved in the synthesis of GABA from glutamate and this shows it to be concentrated in the superficial dorsal horn where C fibres dominate. It is now clear that GABA receptors are not homogeneous (see Chapter 12) and it is the effects mediated by the GABA$_A$ (bicuculline sensitive) receptor which are implicated in the GABA induced depolarisation of 1a spinal afferents and large A cutaneous fibres, as well as the fine C fibres. However, the GABA$_B$ receptor binding sites, which predominate in the outer dorsal horn are reduced by neonatal capsaicin treatment which destroys fine afferent fibres and so implies a presynaptic location on terminals of those fibres (Aδ and C) associated with nociceptive input. Baclofen, agonist for the GABA$_B$ receptor, is able to reduce the C fibre input to dorsal horn nociceptive neurons and produce behavioural antinociception. There may then be a differential control of large and fine afferent inputs by these two subtypes of GABA receptors.

By far the greatest increase in our knowledge of neurotransmitters in the dorsal horn has concerned the opioid compounds. Despite the widespread use of morphine in the form of opium over many thousands of years and by many civilisations it was only in 1973 that hints as to the mechanisms of its potent effects on the nervous system were realised. In this year a saturable, stereospecific binding of opiates to neuronal tissue was demonstrated and this evidence for an opiate receptor was followed by an intense and successful hunt for the endogenous ligands. These are again peptides of varying sizes and again the list of opioid peptides discovered increases each year. Paradoxically, the discovery of the opiate receptor and the endogenous ligands has improved dramatically our understanding of the action of morphine but the physiological roles of the endogenous opioids remains little understood.

The opioid peptides and indeed all other peptides, substance P, SRIF etc., are produced in the neuronal cell body in the form of a propeptide (precursor or parent), consisting of the neuropeptide and a string of amino acids which signal the transfer of the large peptide from the genetic apparatus and endoplasmic reticulum to the Golgi apparatus. Here the propeptide is formed in granules and then transported by axonal transport to the terminal. En route, or in the terminal, the precursor peptide is enzymatically cleaved to produce the active peptide which is released from the terminal by a calcium dependent process. This synthesis and transport of peptides differs markedly from the precursor uptake and synthesis of other non-peptide transmitters (e.g. acetyl choline) in the terminal and is obviously a slower process. Whereas active reuptake is common for other neurotransmitters, predominating for central noradrenaline, peptides are inactivated only by enzymatic breakdown. The enkephalins are cleaved in three positions and there is much interest in prolonging the actions of peptides by enzyme inhibitors and protected analogs of the peptide. Other than opiate receptors, little is known about peptide receptors (Chapter 14), although substance P receptors have been recognised.

The major differences between non-peptide and peptide neurotransmission have several important implications and these will be discussed at the end of this chapter.

Returning to the opioid peptides it is now clear that a whole family of peptides are produced from these major propeptide precursors (see Table 22.2). Leucine and methionine enkephalin were the first opioid peptides to be found and consist of 5 amino acids with a single different amino acid end sequence. The enkephalins have a widespread distribution, with highest concentrations in the basal ganglia and amygdala but also densely clumped in the brainstem thalamus and substantia gelatinosa. The cell bodies containing endorphins are confined to the pituitary hypothalamic-axis and adrenal medulla and the release of endorphin with

Table 22.2. Structures (amino acid sequence) of the three major opioid propeptide precursors

Proenkephalin	→	Tyr-Gly-Gly-Phe-(Met/Leu)-OH
enkephalin (methionine and leucine)		
Pro-opiocortin	→	Tyr-Gly-Gly-Phe-Met-Thr-Ser-Glu-Lys-Ser-Gln-Thr-Pro-Leu-Val-Thr-Leu-Phe-Lys-Asn-Ala-Ile-Lys-Asn-Ala-Tyr-Lys-Lys-Gly-Glu-OH β-endorphin also ACTH
Prodynorphin	→	Tyr-Gly-Gly-Phe-Leu-Arg-Arg-Ile-Arg-Pro-Lys-Leu-Lys-Trp-Asp-Asn-Gln-OH dynorphin

ACTH and the catecholamines from these areas may relate to a role of endorphin in stress. Exogenously applied endorphin, by a variety of routes, is analgesic in animals and man but only in high doses. Unfortunately despite attempts to correlate CSF levels of endorphin with acupuncture and deep-brain-stimulation produced analgesia and also with analgesic requirements post-operatively the role of endorphins is not yet understood. Dynorphin too, has no defined physiological role as yet.

This cornucopia of opioid peptides is paralleled by subclasses of the opiate receptor which on the basis of binding studies and behavioural techniques have been designated mu (μ), delta (δ), kappa (κ) and sigma (σ) (see Chapter 15).

The various endogenous and exogenous opiates have differing affinities for these receptors and these are listed in Table 22.3.

Naloxone, the opiate (competitive) antagonist has the highest affinity for the μ receptor with much weaker effects on the δ and κ subclasses. It has also been suggested that the μ and δ receptors may be linked, possibly being differing conformational forms of a single receptor; although active, μ and δ receptors have not been located on the same neuron casting doubt on this concept.

The μ and δ mediated effects are similar with the central effects leading not only to analgesia to thermal, chemical and mechanical stimuli but to respiratory depression, dependence and constriction of the pupils. However, at least in animals, μ agonists reduce tidal volume whilst not

Table 22.3.

Receptor	Potency series of agonists
mu (μ)	β endorphin > morphine > enkephalins
delta (δ)	Enkephalins > β endorphin > morphine
kappa (κ)	Dynorphin Pentazocine

markedly changing respiratory rate whereas the converse occurs for δ agonists. The effects mediated from the κ receptor are markedly different since the κ and μ have quite selective analgesic actions, κ agonists being effective mainly only against chemical nociception. Also κ agonists, or indeed δ agonists, cannot substitute for μ agonists in preventing withdrawal from morphine and there may be less respiratory depression with pentazocine than morphine. The κ agonists do however produce psychomimetic effects unlike morphine-like compounds. There are also indications that κ agonists may be antagonists at the μ receptor, both in the peripheral nervous system and also at CNS sites.

Autoradiographic mapping of the location of the μ receptor has shown close parallels with the distribution of the enkephalins and in the spinal cord both are strategically placed to modulate incoming nociceptive information. The enkephalins are predominant in the substantia gelatinosa where high levels of opiate receptors are found. However, from studies using dorsal rhizotomy it is clear that about half of the opiate receptors in the cord are located in or on the terminals of the primary afferents since rhizotomy reduces their numbers.

Some ganglion cells have opiate receptors and axonal transport to the terminals has been observed in the sciatic nerve. A presynaptic site for the μ receptors is borne out by studies in which the systemic or iontophoretic application of morphine or opiate peptides has been shown to reduce the responses of nociceptive neurons to noxious but not innocuous stimuli, although there is evidence for a postsynaptic site of action as well. However, clinical reports and behavioural evidence suggests no impairment of tactile sensitivity by opiates. This direct or spinal action of morphine has led to the epidural or intrathecal application of opiates in order to prevent access to the brainstem and peripheral nervous system and so avoid some of the side-effects of these drugs. It is clear from a variety of electrophysiological and behavioural studies that both μ and δ agonists are active in the spinal cord in eliciting antinociception. The role of κ agonists is less compelling and motor deficits produced by these compounds may confound interpretation of antinociception using reflex tests such as the tail flick test. In fact, in many studies, morphine (μ agonist) and enkephalins (δ agonists) produce very similar effects despite the clear separation of receptors, although it would seem that δ mediated effects may be less effective than μ events in inhibiting noxious messages.

The seemingly predominant presynaptic effect of opiates indicated by behavioural and electrophysiological studies (Fig. 22.3) has not been borne out by anatomical approaches and no axo-axonic contacts between enkephalin containing and primary afferent terminals have been found. This may not be necessary, however, since LHRH (luteinizing hormone releasing factor) in some ganglia of the autonomic nervous system can influence neurons despite a lack of synaptic contact — presumably enough peptide is released in the vicinity of the sensory terminal to reach the receptors and this may occur also in the spinal cord.

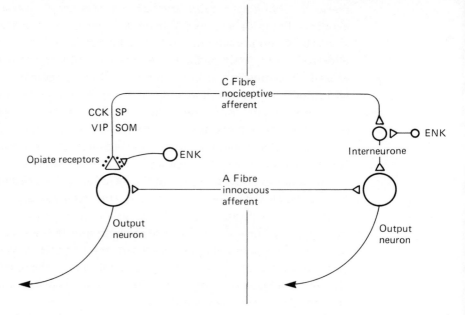

Fig. 22.3. Possible sites of action for the anti-nociceptive effect of opiates in the dorsal horn of the spinal cord. Opiate receptors are found on the terminals of nociceptive C fibres that might release substance P (SP), or some other peptide such as cholecystokinin (CCK) and somatostatin (SOM) or vasoactive intestinal peptide (VIP). The enkephalins released from local neurons (ENK) could then reduce nociceptive input by inhibiting the release of such peptides or by a direct depression of an interneuron on the afferent (nociceptive) pathway. It is assumed that the enkephalin neurons do not modify the inocuous (tactile) A fibre input.

One of the major actions of opiates in both the PNS and CNS, is to inhibit neurotransmitter release and this has been demonstrated for ACh, NA, DA and 5-HT. If opioids act presynaptically in the cord and nociceptive afferents release substance P, although as discussed previously the evidence is not entirely convincing for a role of substance P as the 'pain transmitter', then opiates should inhibit substance P release. *In vitro* studies have shown that the K^+ evoked release of substance P from slices of the trigeminal dorsal horn containing sensory terminals is inhibited by opiates in a naloxone reversible manner as is the release *in vivo* from the cord following high intensity stimulation of peripheral nerves. However, some electrophysiological studies have not been able to reduce substance P elicited excitations by local or systemic opiates.

The mechanisms by which opiates reduce transmitter release seem to be twofold; the relative contribution of each is as yet unknown. Firstly recordings from dorsal root ganglion cells in culture indicate that opiates reduce the calcium component of the action potential. This would result in a reduction in intracellular calcium and so reduced neurotransmitter release would be expected. However, in recordings from substantia gelatinosa neurons in a cord slice preparation and from the other central cells, a direct and rapid hyperpolarisation of the cells, by increasing potassium conductance, is observed following opiate application. It is possible that these cells are interneurons in the nociceptive pathway but yet presynaptic to the output or projection cells and indeed enkephalin terminals have been located on substantia gelatinosa cells. Whether a reduced release of neurotransmitter at the terminals or this direct inhibition of interneurons causes the behavioural analgesia is unknown: both may operate in a synergistic manner.

This spinal action of morphine and opiates is now relatively well elucidated and forms the basis of the epidural or intrathecal route of administration of opiates. However, its relevance to the effectiveness of systemic opiates is unclear since the ED_{50} for C fibre inhibition in the rat is high, much higher than that required to produce behavioural analgesia. Furthermore patients receiving morphine report that they are still aware and able to locate the noxious stimulus but it no longer bothers them. This subtle and selective action is unlikely to result from a block of C fibre transmission in the cord which would be expected to result in an abolition of noxious sensations. It is possible then that the spinal action is more relevant to the profound analgesia produced by very high doses of opiates (often in conjunction with neuroleptics) in anaesthesiology. However, there are supraspinal sites of actions of opiates which can indirectly influence the spinal cord via descending pathways. These will now be considered.

Neurotransmitter candidates for descending pathways

Early studies using restricted injections of opiates into the cerebral ventricles not only led to analgesic effects, but implicates supraspinal sites of action for the opiates in analgesia. Microinjection and other studies have now indicated that these sites are mostly found within the midbrain and brainstem (Fig. 22.4). In the midbrain, the ventral zone of the periaqueductal grey matter (PAG), overlying the nucleus raphe dorsalis and in the caudal brainstem the nucleus raphe magnus (NRM; see Fig. 9.1) and closely associated nucleus paragigantocellularis (NRPG) are all sites where opiates (morphine and enkephalins) can elicit analgesia following microinjection. Critical to a role in the effects of systemic morphine are the ability of naloxone microinjection or electrolytic lesions of NRM to reduce the analgesic effects of systemic opiates. The NRM contains most of the cells of origin of dorsal horn 5-HT and gives rise to bilateral projections to all levels of the cord which terminate onto dorsal horn neurons rather than the terminals of the sensory afferents. Supporting this post-synaptic influence are studies showing the ability of electrical stimulation of the NRM to inhibit all activities of convergent dorsal horn cells. It has been proposed that effects from the PAG are via the NRM but there may be direct independent projections from the PAG to the cord as well. This role of 5-HT in pain modulation is borne out by studies demonstrating analgesia by intrathecal 5-HT and the reduction in the

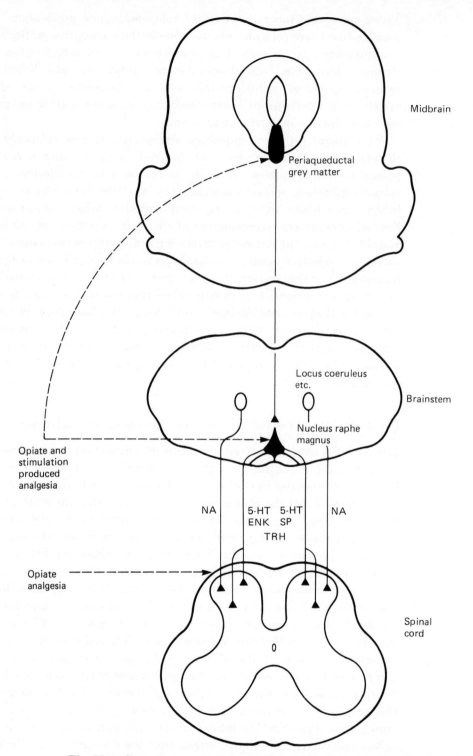

Fig. 22.4. Sites of action of opiates and descending influences on nociceptive input. Opiates may act in the spinal cord, on the raphe nuclei or in the periaqueductal grey matter. Part of their action is to modify descending influences on spinal cord activity either through the locus coeruleus and its descending NA axons or the nucleus raphe magnus and 5-HT neurons. Various peptides (enkephalin, substance P and thyrotrophin releasing hormone (TRH) may coexist with 5-HT in the appropriate descending fibre.

behavioural analgesia elicited by NRM stimulation by intrathecal 5-HT antagonists as well as those administered systemically. There is accumulating evidence that these descending inhibitions can be activated by a noxious stimulus and a release of both 5-HT and enkephalin into the lumbar CSF has been demonstrated. The supraspinal origin of these substances is indicated by the block and marked reduction, respectively, of their release following spinal section.

The precise interaction between opiates and these descending controls is controversial since the intuitive idea would be that these descending inhibitory influences would need to be enhanced by opiates — unfortunately there is evidence to the contrary. Electrophysiological and biochemical studies indicate that opiates reduce descending 5-HT mediated inhibitions although these have been interpreted on the basis that these pathways may have a role in nociceptive processing by a filtering action on spinal neurons. In brief it has been proposed that the transmission of nociceptive information by spinal neurons receiving both noxious and innocuous inputs occurs by the noxious inputs triggering serotoninergic inhibitions which then reduce the innocuous inputs so enhancing the noxious signals. The reduction in the descending inhibitions by morphine would dull the nociceptive messages.

In addition to the monoamines there are many peptide candidate neurotransmitters in the bulbospinal neuronal systems with enkephalins, substance P and thyrotrophin releasing hormone (TRH) found with 5-HT in the raphe nuclei. There are also hypothalamic oxytocin, vasopressin and angiotensin containing projections to the outer zones of the spinal cord. Functions of these systems remain unknown yet coexistence of substance P, 5-HT and TRH in the same neurons has been amply demonstrated by various techniques.

The implications for the co-existence of a peptide and another neurotransmitter are numerous. Some raphe-spinal neurons terminate on motoneurons and 5-HT, substance P and TRH can all increase excitability of cells without causing action potential generation. In the salivary gland VIP and ACh seem to act on different receptors to produce a synergistic response with an additional muscarinic presynaptic control of VIP release.

In addition to these 5-HT containing systems there are descending projections from the locus coeruleus and other brainstem noradrenergic systems. These monoamine pathways are independent of each other although there may be a noradrenergic innervation of raphe neurons. Noradrenaline, applied iontophoretically onto nociceptive neurons in the spinal cord is inhibitory and there are known to be α_2 adrenoceptor mediated presynaptic inhibitory effects on afferent C fibre transmission. Interference with noradrenergic mechanisms at the spinal level reduces the analgesic effects of systemic morphine and the available evidence indicates that 5-HT and NA act independently but synergistically to mediate some of the effects of opiates. In addition to spinal α_2 adrenoceptors there are α_2 autoreceptors on neurons in the locus coeruleus which reduce the release of NA. Clonidine (an α_2 agonist) not only produces analgesia but can block opiate withdrawal symptoms possibly because opiate receptors being located presynaptically in the locus coeruleus and spinal cord parallel the distribution and function of α_2 receptors in these areas.

It must not be forgotten that high levels of opioids and opiate receptors are found in forebrain and other areas some of which are not associated with pain transmission. High levels of opioids are found in the basal ganglia which are believed to play some role in motor and possibly emotional behaviour. The rigidity or catatonia seen after high doses of opiates may result from actions at this level. Furthermore, the rewarding or reinforcing effects of opiates leading to dependence, may be due to actions in the ventral tegmentum. Animals will self-administer opiates into this area following implantation of injection cannulae and there are behavioural experiments indicating that this area and the locus coeruleus, may be involved in mediating reward systems. A possible effect of opiates on sensory transmission may be manifest at cortical levels where there is a strict segregation of μ, δ, σ and κ receptors according to the lamina arrangement of the cortex.

Thus to summarise, opiates, particularly morphine and other μ agonists can act at the spinal level both directly and through descending brainstem-spinal projections.

The direct spinal action of opiates seems most likely to involve a block of transmission from $A\delta$ and C fibres, sparing large A fibre mediated innocuous messages. Whether this results from a reduction in release of the C fibre transmitter by an action on the terminals or an inhibition of interneurons between the C fibres and the output cells remains unclear. However, it is clear that both motor reflexes and the sensation of pain are reduced by opiates acting at this level and the clinical use of epidural or intrathecal administration of opiates has stemmed from these basic findings.

A supraspinal action on the brainstem which then influences the dorsal horn via descending controls is also clear and although the details of this action remain a subject of much study the final effect is a reduction in the intensity of nociception (Fig. 22.5).

Side-effects of opiates

The side-effects of opiates are problematic in that they limit the doses of opiates that can be used and hence their analgesic efficacy. These effects are due to high levels of opiate receptors in the medulla and peripheral nervous system.

1 Respiratory depression.
2 Cough suppression.
3 Vomiting.

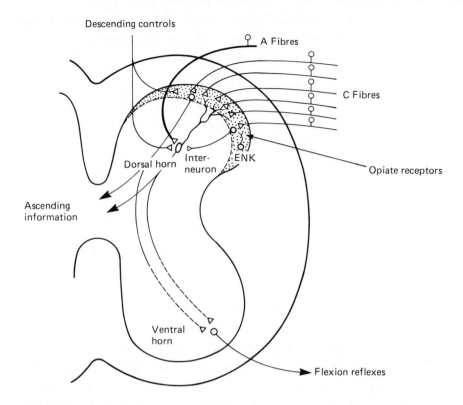

Descending controls

A Fibres

C Fibres

Opiate receptors

Dorsal horn

Inter-
neuron

ENK

Ascending
information

Ventral
horn

Flexion reflexes

Fig. 22.5. Summary diagram of control of nociceptive input and site of action of opiates in the spinal cord. Afferent transmission, relays in the dorsal horn and descending influences are all involved.

4 Constriction of pupils.
5 Constipation.
6 Contraction of sphincters.
7 Dependence.

1 *Respiratory depression.* This is due to action on opiate receptors in the medulla which leads to a decreased sensitivity of the respiratory centres to CO_2. It occurs at therapeutic doses and is the most common cause of death from overdose.

2 *Cough suppression.* This central antitussive action can be separated from the other actions of opiates, and codeine and dextromethorphan (which has no analgesic action) are used in cough suppression.

3 *Vomiting.* All opiates produce nausea or vomiting via an action on the chemoreceptor trigger zone of the medulla. This is then followed by a depression of vomiting. The morphine derivative, apomorphine (actually a dopamine agonist) is used as an emetic (vomiting agent).

PAIN TRANSMISSION AND ANALGESIA

4 *Constriction of the pupils.* Miosis or pin-point pupils results from pupillary constriction, and is an indicator of addiction as tolerance does not occur to this action of opiates.

5 *Constipation.* The general gastrointestinal effect of opiates is an increase in smooth muscle tone. The maintained contraction decreases motility and the decreased propulsion is the basis for the anti-diarrhoeal effects of opiates.

6 *Contraction of sphincters.* Opiates produce a constriction of sphincters throughout the gastrointestinal tract. Whereas opiate receptors and enkephalins are present in the gut some of the gastrointestinal effects of opiates may also have central components.

7 *Dependence.* Both physical and psychological dependence arise.

Nociceptive transmission and its implications for pain therapy

At first sight this daunting galaxy of neurotransmitters involved in the primary afferent transmission of painful messages, the local segmental controls and the descending controls acting on the spinal cord seems superfluous to the simple matter of getting a sensory signal from the receptor to areas of the CNS involved in conscious events.

Reflection on the complexities of pain makes this cornucopia of mediators seem less baffling. Examples abound; phantom limb pain where pain occurs in the absence of the leg or arm, causalgia where nerve damage leads to an excruciating burning sensation after tactile stimulation, troops on the battlefield who feel no pain after massive trauma and civilians in casualty departments where only 40% of accident victims report immediate pain after traumatic injury. Surgical sectioning of ascending spinal tracts has almost been abandoned since following an initial analgesic effect the pain soon returns with increased intensity. Many of these examples may be explained by the ability of the CNS to maintain function by homeostatic mechanisms.

The pharmacological basis for these complex controlling and modulating circuits are beginning to be understood in a rudimentary way. It is clear that peptide neurotransmission differs from classical transmission and many peptides are involved in the pain process. Since synthesis and breakdown are crucial to neurotransmitter function and as both the former and the axonal transport of peptides are slow, peptides may act over long time courses both in terms of latency and duration. There may be non-synaptic effects by release distant from the receptor and due to the slow production of peptides depletion may be common but replenishment will depend on the length of the axon. Even the synthesis of peptides in the cell body may by modulated by compounds which interfere with the propeptide synthesis, such as NA, 5-HT and ATP.

A good example of these problems is the attempt to assign a physiological role to the endogenous opiates, the enkephalins and endorphins. Many studies have used naloxone, the opiate antagonist, in an attempt to reverse effects produced by analgesia promoting manoeuvres or to alter the pain threshold. Whereas naloxone will clearly and reproducibly reverse morphine analgesia, experiments in animals and man have produced little evidence to support the idea that endogenous opiates modulate the pain threshold. Whereas this may be explained by true negative findings there may also be opioid systems aiding pain transmission especially as naloxone can produce analgesia when given alone under certain circumstances.

However, it is also quite likely that peptides in particular act over time courses much longer than those of classical or conventional neurotransmitters. From work on ganglion cells it is well demonstrated that the effects of some peptides are of long duration on ion channels (minutes) and in many systems they can modify neuronal excitability without initiating action potentials. If peptides do act to modulate other neurotransmitters or subtly change neuronal excitability then it would be naive to expect clear cut effects of naloxone on pain thresholds. Yet to further complicate matters enkephalins can hyperpolarise substantia gelatinosa cells via a prolongation of a potassium conductance and substance P can close K^+ channels, examples of relatively fast neurotransmission by any definition. Although it seems that peptides produce slow effects in many neuronal systems this example and indeed others, especially work on iontophoretic application of peptides to forebrain cells, illustrate that peptides can elicit firing or inhibitions of neurons over short time courses.

However, with evoked antinociception there is some evidence for an involvement of opioids. Low intensity and strictly segmental transcutaneous stimulation produces a local analgesic effect, which most research groups find is not naloxone sensitive. When high intensity or noxious stimuli are applied, however, a more widespread analgesia occurs which may be the basis for some forms of acupuncture, or indeed counterirritation. This form of antinociception seems to involve opiate release since high intensity stimulation results in increased CSF levels of enkephalin-like material and the resultant analgesia seems naloxone reversible. There is evidence for and against opioids being involved in placebo analgesia, analgesia produced by stimulation of the midbrain and the congenital insensitivity to pain found in a few people. Attempts to correlate CSF levels of endorphins with pain sensation have not been successful.

A recent major advance in this field has been the identification of the peptidases that degrade the enkephalins. As mentioned earlier the peptides seem to be removed from the synapse by enzymatic breakdown rather than reuptake. Three membrane bound peptidases have been identified which cleave between different amino acid links, enkephalinase, aminopeptidase M and a dipeptidylaminopeptidase. Inhibitors of the first two enzymes have been synthesised (thiorphan and bestatin, respectively) and a compound kelatorphan has been produced which inhibits all three enzymes. The relative ability of the three agents to protect both exogenous and endogenous enkephalins is kelatorphan > thiorphan + bestatin > thiorphan > bestatin which would indicate that enkephalinase is of more importance than aminopeptidases but that inhibition of all three enzymes is required for complete protection of these opioids. Interestingly this order parallels the ability of the agents to elicit analgesia in mice and inhibit nociceptive neurons in rat spinal cord. These studies might indicate a novel therapeutic approach. However, the multiple substrates for these peptidases may result in the enzyme inhibitors increasing the availability of other non-opioid peptides although it should be pointed out that the *in vivo* effects reported above were naloxone reversible. Of theoretical interest is the finding that the affinity of enkephalin for enkephalinase is in the micromolar range and the enkephalins have low affinities for the opioid receptors in *in vivo* binding studies, leading to the conclusion that for rapid repetitive enkephalinergic transmission (efficient receptor occupation and removal of enkephalin) high concentrations of the peptide are required in the synapse.

It is clear then that our knowledge of peptides involved in pain transmission and modulation is as yet insufficient to clearly assign a role to any of them in a defined facet of nociception. This may be due to the nature of peptide neurotransmission or to the complex synaptic relationship in nociceptive systems but also probably to the array of transmitters involved in this modality of sensation, both excitatory and inhibitory and also the number of CNS structures involved in pain transmission and modulation. The clinical relevance and basic interest in improving our knowledge of these systems lends impetus to the achievement of this end.

References and further reading

Akil H *et al.* (1984) Endogenous opioids: biology and function. *Ann. Rev. Neurosci.* **7**, 223–55.

Duggan AW (1985) Pharmacology of descending control systems. *Phil. Trans. R. Soc. Lond. B.* **308**, 375–91.

Duggan AW & North RA (1984) Electrophysiology of opioids. *Pharmac. Rev.* **35**, 219–81.

Kosterlitz HW (1985) Opioid peptides and their receptors. *Proc. R. Soc. Lond. B.* **225**, 27–40.

Martin TE & Hill R (1983) Neurotransmitter candidates of somatosensory primary afferent fibres. *Neuroscience* **10**, 1083–103.

Martin WR (1984) Pharmacology of opioids. *Pharmac. Rev.* **35**, 283–323.

North RA (1986) Opioid receptor types and membrane ion channels. *Trends Neurosci.* **9**, 114–17.

Schwartz JS, Costentin J & Lecombe J-M (1985) Pharmacology of enkephalinase inhibitors. *Trends Pharmacol. Sci,* 472–6.

Waksman G, Bouboutou R, Chaillet P, Devin J, Coulard A, Hamel E, Besselievre J, Costenesin J, Fournie-Zaluski MC & Roques BP (1985) Kelatorphan. A full inhibitor of enkephalin degrading enzymes. Biochemical and pharmacological properties, regional distribution of enkephalinase in rat brain by use of a tritated derivated. *Neuropeptides* **5**, 529–34.

Willis WD (1985) Nociceptive pathways: anatomy and physiology of nociceptive ascending pathways. *Phil. Trans. R. Soc. Lond. B* **308**, 253–68.

Yaksh TW & Noueihed (1985) The physiology and pharmacology of spinal opiates. *Ann. Rev. Pharmac. Toxicol.* **25**, 433–62.

Index

The abbreviations used in this index are those given on preliminary pages xii–xiv

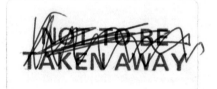
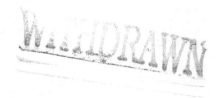